# THE FIVE OSTEOPATHIC MODELS

## Rationale, Application, Integration

From an evidence-based to a person-centered osteopathy

# THE FIVE OSTEOPATHIC MODELS

## Rationale, Application, Integration

From an evidence-based to a person-centered osteopathy

Raymond J Hruby (American Editor) Paolo Tozzi (European Editor)
Christian Lunghi and Giampiero Fusco

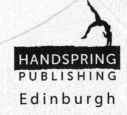

HANDSPRING
PUBLISHING
Edinburgh

HANDSPRING PUBLISHING LIMITED
The Old Manse, Fountainhall,
Pencaitland, East Lothian
EH34 5EY, United Kingdom
Tel: +44 1875 341 859
Website: www.handspringpublishing.com

Original Italian edition first published 2015 by EDRA SpA
English edition first published 2017 by Handspring Publishing

ISBN 978-1-909141-68-1
**British Library Cataloguing in Publication Data**
A catalogue record for this book is available from the British Library

**Library of Congress Cataloguing in Publication Data**
A catalog record for this book is available from the Library of Congress

**Commissioning Editor** Mary Law
**Project Manager** Morven Dean
**Copyeditor** Stephanie Pickering
**Cover and Design Direction** Bruce Hogarth, Kinesis Creative
**Typesetter** DSM Soft, India
**Printer** CPI Group (UK) Ltd, Croydon CR0 4YY

The
Publisher's
policy is to use
paper manufactured
from sustainable forests

# CONTENTS

## SECTION 1   Person-centered osteopathic medicine

# CONTENTS continued

# DEDICATIONS

I would like to dedicate my contribution to this work to:

My wife, Karen, who patiently and lovingly supports my passion for osteopathic medicine and helps me to not take on too many projects at once.

My parents, the late John J Hruby Jr and the late Helen Margaret Hruby – you raised me well, and I wish you were both still here.

My two cats, Serena and Gemma, who give the kind of unconditional support that only cats can give, and who are always glad to keep me company when I am writing, no matter what time of the day or night.

**Ray Hruby**

To Osteopathy, which taught me to listen as much as possible, to act when appropriate and to stop when necessary.

**Paolo Tozzi**

At times like these, in traditional native cultures, people meet with loved ones among the dancing and the beat of drums, food, good drink to celebrate all together... My celebration will be my gratitude to my fellow travelers with my love, my actions and next projects ... Thank you for having received the message hidden in this pathway ... Being compassionate.

COM PASSIONE VOLI (With passion you fly)

**Christian Lunghi**

To my daughters Greta and Sofia, thank you for the patience and the time granted to me for writing the book ... and for supporting me with your smiles.

**Giampiero Fusco**

**Raymond J Hruby**, DO, MS FAAO (Dist), graduated from the College of Osteopathic Medicine and Surgery in Des Moines, Iowa, in 1973. After a variety of clinical and academic posts, in 1999 he became Professor and Chair of the Department of Osteopathic Manipulative Medicine at the Western University of Health Sciences College of Osteopathic Medicine in Pomona, California. He recently "retired" from this position, but continues his work at Western University as a consultant to the Department of NMM/OMM. In this capacity he is involved with teaching, research, curriculum analysis and development, and mentoring of the new faculty and Predoctoral OMM Fellows. He is also involved with Western University's Interprofessional Education program, and he lectures part-time in the Graduate School of Basic Medical Sciences, among others.

**Paolo Tozzi** MSc Ost, DO, PT Is Principal of the First Italian School of Veterinary Osteopathy, Vice-Principal of the Italian Association of Posturologists, former Treasurer of the Osteopathic European Academic Network (OsEAN), and former Vice Principal of CROMON, the Centre for Holistic Research in Osteopathy and Natural Medicine, Rome. He lectures widely on osteopathy, biomechanics and manual therapy, and organized the first international congress on veterinary osteopathy (Rome 2012).

**Christian Lunghi,** DO, ND works as an osteopath and naturopath in Rome and Bracciano, Italy. He is a member of the Italian Advisory Board of the Centre for Osteopathic Medicine Collaboration foundation (COME), and a member of the Research Committee and of the National Examining Board of the Italian Register of Osteopaths (ROI). He lectures on osteopathic clinical reasoning and the rationale of osteopathic medicine. He is author and co-author of publications in several indexed journals. He is the co-author of a chapter in *Fascia in the Osteopathic Field*, edited by Liem, Tozzi and Chila, which is also published by Handspring Publishing.

**Giampiero Fusco,** DO, FT is an osteopath and physiotherapist. He teaches widely in Italy for both undergraduate and master programs of osteopathy. He is a member of the Research Committee of the Italian Register of Osteopaths, and has spoken at various national and international conferences. His work has been published in the *Journal of Bodywork and Movement Therapies*.

In 1986, The American Educational Council on Osteopathic Principles (ECOP) proposed a Core Curriculum for Osteopathic Education, for use in teaching osteopathic physicians to integrate osteopathic principles and philosophy throughout their training and into practice. The basis of this curriculum document is the Five Osteopathic Models – biomechanical, neurological, respiratory-circulatory, metabolic, and behavioral. These models provide a basis for the integration of basic and clinical sciences into an osteopathic thought process and a unique approach to the evaluation and treatment of patients.

The Italian language edition of this book is the first attempt, as far as is known and beyond the ECOP document, to thoroughly explain and explore these five models in depth and provide the most updated evidence base for their use. The success of the Italian language edition, and the increased teaching and usage of the five models in osteopathic education led to a demand for an English language version of the book, in order to make this important information more readily available to all those involved with the teaching and practice of osteopathic medicine, and the distinctive approach of osteopathic medicine to patient care. We are confident that readers of this book will find it most useful in furthering their understanding of osteopathic principles and philosophy through the five osteopathic models, and their application in daily practice and teaching.

Raymond J. Hruby, DO, MS, FAAO (Dist), US Editor
Pomona, California, USA.
Paolo Tozzi, MSc(Ost), DO, PT, European Editor
Rome, Italy
May, 2017

The World Health Organization has developed a 2014-2023 strategic plan that envisages the integration of biomedicine with complementary medicine. Complementary medicine is viewed as offering alternative approaches that are person-centered and therefore able to "take care" of the patient, in addition to "curing the disease".[1] Osteopathy, systematized on an anthropological basis of the "old doctor," makes a full entrance in this patient/person-centric process and, consequently, in this process of integration between the medicines. This approach provides a system of evaluation, diagnosis and manual treatment intended to promote health, or rather individual self-regulation, a postulation that *inter alia* allows you to search for health even in the presence of a wide range of clinical conditions.

Osteopathy is based on the principle that the structure and the functions of the body are tightly integrated, and that the well-being of the person requires adaptive capacity with respect to environmental questions.[2] In fact, when under stress, the body operates an allostatic accommodation (a vast variety of adaptive physiological changes, able to reach a new equilibrium), capable of guaranteeing better conditions to face the new environment context and the correlated challenges.[3] However, the allostatic accommodation has its cost, which is defined as allostatic load. Under conditions of chronic or repeated stress the physiological responses become less "elastic," no longer completely reversible; so that through adaptation they can in the short term, if persistent, become harmful and cause deleterious effects locally as well as throughout the entire body. This process will be the subject of development in Section 1 of this work. The adaptive response takes place through the work of the integrated systems of self-regulation, which the osteopath focuses on when applying specific models of investigation in the assessment of the patient and in activating corresponding forces in treatment (as will be detailed in Section 2 of this volume). These are the musculoskeletal, neurological, circulatory, metabolic and psychological systems:[2] a

dynamic group of functions that maintains health and is influenced by the interaction of body, mind and spirit; a cohesion of instances that when under stress, influences, determines and maintains a corresponding group of disorders often well known to practitioners of traditional medicine.[4] The complexity of these processes requires the integration of new knowledge from research areas such as psychoneuro-immunology and epigenetics. These sciences have transcended the separation between spiritual science and natural science, through observation of how cultural and biological dimensions communicate and influence in interdependent ways. Epigenetics, in particular, has facilitated the breach in the wall that overshadowed knowledge of the molecular processes underlying complex phenomena of human existence. Mental events, whether conscious or unconscious, epigenetically modulate the adaptive schemes of humans, from the hormonal axis to the neural processes,[5] affecting the mechanics of tissues: changes that the osteopath can perhaps perceive, or even influence. Not surprisingly, many experts have posed the question of how best to describe what happens when the hands of an operator are in action on the tissues.[6] Recent investigations into the mechanisms of the functioning of osteopathic treatment have reported how cultured cells subjected to tension and stress of various kinds can change their behavior, as well as after a manipulative treatment simulated in laboratory, revealing inflammatory reactions in the first case and inflammatory responses in the second.[7] Even if evidence such as this could actually support the theoretical efficacy of manipulative treatment, to proceed towards the observation of more complex phenomena basic researchers look for the "Rosetta Stone," or crucial key to understanding. In fact, watching the myriad of manipulative approaches described in the literature of the field, distinguished by the type of stimuli, such as compression, traction, slipping, twisting and untwisting, these researchers consider it appropriate to define and classify the "family of techniques." While on the one hand this would simplify the structure of research projects, on the other it ignores a crucial aspect: if different authors described similar technique modalities, through different viewpoints, they did so by applying the multiple nuances of common principles, the same nuances by which the complexity of a therapeutic relationship, such as that between patient and osteopath, is often benefitted by the application of an individualized treatment plan. So, for the purpose of research it is sometimes necessary to move osteopathy from its founding principles, to bring it together with other rehabilitative manipulation practices, as in "real" ambulatory life; however, this philosophy, as well as the art of practice, needs to preserve its peculiarities. The "Rosetta Stone" is a symbol of many things, from the culture of the past, at the crossroads of languages; it is in the vastness of meaning that the metaphor resides – everyone can choose the version they prefer, and we tend toward one that indicates the need to understand, as well as one that reminds us of the common reference, the basis by which we can understand and remember the "monolith" that gave us the base of common knowledge, shared by all humans. Tradition, scientific evidence and critical thinking provide a renewed approach, a rationale based on principles, far from being reduced to a mere protocol, but rooted in the flexible strength of an algorithm, a decisive process that shapes every operator–patient relationship, thanks to the art of osteopathy: the art of perceiving the other and accompanying him in movement; the movement is, and always will be, life.

Paolo Tozzi, Christian Lunghi and Giampiero Fusco
Rome, 2015

## References

1. World Health Organization (WHO), 2013. WHO Traditional Medicine Strategy: 2014-2023. WHO. Hong Kong.

2. Osteopathic International Alliance (OIA), 2013. Osteopathy and osteopathic medicine. A global view of practice, patients, education and the contribution to healthcare delivery. OIA. Chicago. Ch. 1.

3. McEwen, B.S., 2015. Biomarkers for assessing population and individual health and disease related to stress and adaptation. Metabolism. 64(3 Suppl 1):S2-S10.

4. Hardy, K., Pollard, H., 2006. The organization of the stress response, and its relevance to chiropractors: a commentary. Chiropr. Osteopat. 14:25.

5. Bottaccioli, F., 2014. Epigenetics and psycho-neuro-endocrine-immunology. The two faces of the ongoing revolution in the life sciences. EDRA, Milano. pp. 4.

6. Chaitow, L., 2014. Can we describe what we do? J. Bodyw. Mov. Ther. 18(3):315-6.

7. Standley, P.R., 2014. Towards a Rosetta Stone of manual therapeutic methodology. J Bodyw. Mov. Ther. 18(4):586-7.

# ABBREVIATIONS

**ACTH**: adrenocorticotropic hormone

**ANS**: autonomic nervous system

**ASIS**: anterior-superior iliac spine

**BLT**: balanced ligamentous tension

**BMT**: balanced membranous tension

**C1**: atlas

**C2**: axis

**C3, 4–7**: third, fourth to seventh cervical vertebrae

**cAMP**: cyclic adenosine monophosphate

**CGRP**: calcitonin gene-related peptide

**CNS**: central nervous system

**CO**: cranial osteopathy

**COMT**: catechol-*O*-methyltransferase

**CRF**: corticotropin-releasing factor

**CRH**: corticotropin-releasing hormone

**CRI**: cranial rhythmic impulse

**CRPS-I**: complex regional pain syndrome type I

**CS**: central sensitization

**CSF**: cerebrospinal fluid

**CV4**: compression of the fourth ventricle

**D1, 2–12**: first, second to twelfth dorsal vertebrae

**DDR**: dorsal root reflex

**DyFIR**: dynamics of fluids and involuntary rhythms

**EBV**: Epstein–Barr virus

**ECM**: extracellular matrix

**ERS**: extension, rotation, and sidebending

**ERSsn**: dysfunction in extension, rotation, and left sidebending

**EV4**: expansion of the fourth ventricle

**FCS**: fascial compensation scheme

**FPR**: facilitated positional release

**GABA**: gamma-aminobutyric acid

**GAG**: glycosaminoglycans

**GAS**: general adaptation syndrome

**GOT**: general osteopathic treatment

**HIV**: human immunodeficiency virus

**HPA**: hypothalamic–pituitary–adrenal axis

**HRMT**: human resting myofascial tone

**HSV**: herpes simplex virus

**HVLA**: high-velocity low-amplitude

**IgA/E**: A/E immunoglobulins

**IGF**: insulin-like growth factor

**IGFBPs**: insulin-like growth factor binding proteins

**IL-2/6**: 2/6 interleukins

**INE**: immune, neurological, endocrine system

**K1, 2–12**: first, second to twelfth ribs

**KAT**: kynurenine aminotransferase

**L**: left

**L1, 2, 3, 5**: first, second, third, fifth lumbar vertebrae

**LAS**: local adaptation syndrome or ligamenous articular strain

**LTP**: long-term potentiation

**LVHA**: low-velocity high-amplitude

**MET**: muscle energy technique

**MGF**: mechano growth factor

**MINE**: musculoskeletal, immune, neurological, and endrocrine system

**MSS**: musculoskeletal system

**MUS**: medically unexplained symptoms

**NK**: natural killer cells

**NMDA**: N-methyl-D-aspartate

**NSR**: natural sidebending rotation

**Oc**: occiput

**OCMM**: osteopathic cranial manipulative medicine

**OMT**: osteopathic manipulative treatment

**ORL**: otorhinolaryngology

**PAD**: primary afferent depolarization

**PAG**: periaqueductal gray

**PAN**: primary afferent nociceptors

**PINS**: progressive inhibition of neuromuscular structures

**PNS**: peripheral nervous system

**PRM**: primary respiratory mechanism

**PS**: peripheral sensitization

**PSIS**: posterior-superior iliac spine

**Rg**: right

**rNSR**: right neutral sidebending rotation

**ROM**: range of motion

**RSD**: reflex sympathetic dystrophy

**SAM**: sympathetic–adrenal–medullary system

**SAS**: sympathetic–adrenergic system

**SAT**: specific adjustment treatment/technique

**SD**: somatic dysfunction

**SNS**: sympathetic nervous system

**SOAP**: subjective + objective assessment and treatment plan

**SH**: somatotropin hormone

**TA**: transitional areas

**TART**: tissue texture abnormality, asymmetry, restriction of motion, tenderness/temperature

**TGF-β**: transforming growth factor β

**TMJ**: temporomandibular joint

**TRF**: thyrotropin-releasing factor

**THM**: Traube–Hering–Mayer waves

**WDR**: wide dynamic range

# 1
## SECTION

# Person-centered osteopathic medicine

## *From tradition to innovation through critical thinking supported by evidence*

*Christian Lunghi*

## INTRODUCTION

It has often been said that osteopathy is not a simple application of techniques, but a complete structured medicine, based on principles of application through a manual practice.[1] However, currently, worldwide, there seems to be a general disagreement within the osteopathic community on what the great osteopathic principles should be and how they should be applied clinically,[1,2] resulting in possible controversy when it comes to making a choice about, for example, which technique is best suited for a given patient.

This section aims to revisit the traditional osteopathic principles and their application in the light of a modern vision, supported by evidence and reinforced by critical thinking (see Chapter 1). These fundamentals are the essence of what makes osteopathy a unique profession that takes care of the person, centering treatment on health. The treatment is then focused on the adaptive capacities of the person treated, which are expressed through the functions of the hypothalamic–pituitary–adrenal (HPA) axis

of the sympathic-adrenergic system (SAS), and of the reflexes manifested on corporeal tissues from eventual overload of the regulatory systems. The osteopath observes the individual adaptive mode, trying to understand if this happens locally through somatic dysfunction (SD), or through functional alteration of the components of the somatic system in relation to each other as muscular-skeletal-fascial, vascular, lymphatic, and neural aspects (see Chapter 2); or if this is affected by factors that have a general effect on large parts of the body and are detectable in the fascial compensation schemes (FCS) and on the assessment of the dynamics of fluids and involuntary rhythms (DyFIR) (see Chapter 3).

Through knowledge of anatomy and physiology, the osteopath will try to interact with the tissue changes related to overloading of the self-regulating systems, with repercussions on neuropsychological, respiratory, circulatory, postural-biomechanical functions and the global economy of the body, so as to correct no longer sustainable dysfunctional patterns and changes of the individual chronobiology. The functions that can interact with the individual adaptive capacity represent five conceptual models of assessment of the relationship between structure and function, as well as activation forces which are based on biomechanical, neurological, circulatory-respiratory, metabolic-energetic, and biopsychosocial clinical approaches.[3] The osteopath, through the application of a decision-making process, selects the best mode of interaction with the person, proceeding sometimes with specific local approaches directed to the clinically relevant SD, sometimes with adaptogenic approaches aimed at balancing FCS and/or dynamics of fluids and involuntary rhythms (DyFRI). All this brings to light osteopathic manipulation as a medicine centered on the person, based on holistic principles and the global application of structure/function models, aimed at promoting health rather than curing disease (see Chapter 1).

## References

1.  Rogers FJ. Advancing a traditional view of osteopathic medicine through clinical practice. J Am Osteopath Assoc. 2005;105(5):255–9.

2.  Fryer G. Call for papers: an invitation to contribute to a special issue on osteopathic principles. Int J Osteopath Med. 2011;14(3):79–80.

3.  Educational Council on Osteopathic Principles (ECOP). Glossary of osteopathic terminology. Chevy Chase, MD: American Association of Colleges of Osteopathic Medicine (AACOM); 2009.

# Osteopathy: a practice based on tradition, research, critical thinking, and art

*Christian Lunghi*

## Synopsis

The "osteopathic principles" are crucial in defining the peculiar characteristics of osteopathy. However, the lack of sharing and embracing of these principles within the practice community has made these fundamentals vague and undeveloped; moreover, the lack of recognition of these principles in their application during practice has not helped to distinguish osteopathy from other health professions that likewise place anatomy, physiology, and holism at the base of their work. In this chapter, by observing the traditional principles and contemporary scientific evidence we have drawn a hypothesis of rational treatment based on these principles. There emerges an osteopathy based on salutogenesis: a traditional medicine, which, evolving on an anthropological basis, centers its work on the person. The text also attempts to answer questions related to the mechanism of action and clinical effectiveness of osteopathy in many areas of health: from pediatrics and gynecology to sports medicine and geriatrics, and so on. However, in order to outline the actual indications of osteopathic treatment, additional protocols are necessary to study the mechanisms of action of osteopathic manipulative treatment, its clinical efficacy, the reliability of palpatory procedures, the cost/benefit ratio, as well as the person's individual perception with respect to its discomfort, its adaptive capacity, and the osteopathic treatment received.

From reflections on the above principles there emerges a concept of adaptive health; consequently, the discomfort is considered a deficiency of the dynamic interaction within and between adaptive systems and is recognizable in the alterations of the relationship between structure and function, before the damage of the single system. The treatment has the objective of interacting with the adaptive biomechanical function, respiratory, circulatory, metabolic, and energetic, as well as psychological. Hence, the osteopath proceeds with either specific local approaches addressed to the clinically relevant somatic dysfunction, or with global adaptogenic approaches addressed to the balancing of the "fascial compensation schemes" and/or "dynamics of fluids and involuntary rhythms."

## Introduction: osteopathic principles and their applications

Osteopathy is based on the manual contact during the phase of evaluation and treatment of the patient with respect to the relationship between body, mind, and spirit in conditions of both health and disease.

The osteopath focuses his or her intervention on the structural and functional integrity of the organism and the inherent tendency of the body toward self-regulation. Osteopaths use a wide range of therapeutic manual techniques aimed at improving physiological functioning and/or supporting homeostasis that has been altered by somatic dysfunction (SD), indicated in the International Statistical

Classification of Diseases and Related Health Problems by the code M99,[1] namely a feature compromised or altered by somatic components in relation to each other.[2,3]

Osteopathic manipulative treatment (OMT) uses a series of manual techniques that can be combined with other treatments or modifications related to lifestyle. Osteopathy is a manipulative approach to patient care that has contributed to the body of knowledge of manual therapies and complementary and alternative traditional medicine. Osteopathic practice is distinct from other health care professions which use manual techniques, such as physical therapy or chiropractic care, although there are overlaps in terms of techniques and adopted interventions. Osteopathy is practiced in many countries around the world. In some of them, manual therapists use osteopathic techniques and claim to perform an osteopathic treatment, although they may not have received adequate training.[3] The lack of a shared definition of osteopathy has contributed to a lack of clarity surrounding the nature of the profession and its indications, which could add to the difficulties in identifying and promoting the features of the services provided by the profession in many countries. It has often been claimed that osteopathy is not a set of manual techniques, but rather the application of "osteopathic principles" crucial in defining the unique characteristics of osteopathy. In osteopathic practice, the latest scientific and medical knowledge is used to apply the principles of osteopathy to patient care. Scientific plausibility and evidence-based results have a high priority in the treatment of patients and the management of cases.

Osteopathy provides a wide range of approaches to health maintenance and disease management. It embraces the concept of unity of the structure (anatomy) and function (physiology) of the individual, in a patient-centered approach, rather than a disease-centered approach.

Osteopathy emphasizes the following principles:[4]

- The body possesses self-regulating mechanisms directed to self healing

- Structure and function are in an interdependent relationship on every level

- The human being is a functional dynamic unit, whose state of health is affected by the body and the mind

- Rational treatment is based on the above principles.

The principles described in Kirksville and reviewed here by Rogers,[4] however:

- do not seem to help in distinguishing osteopathy and the practice of osteopaths from other health professions

- do not appear to be shared in the different countries of the world. Many osteopaths in the UK and Australia seem to be familiar with "the principles of Kirksville," but there are other competing philosophical principles, for example those that are considered and taught in some European countries, such as the "three pillars" of osteopathy, namely structural, visceral and cranial influence.

These three pillars seem to distance the practice of the osteopath from the principles and their application, adding little to osteopathic practice, if not in stressing indirectly the importance of the biomechanical interdependence inside the body.[5] Probably this is related to the lack of shared principles within the community of practice, because they are vague, poorly developed, and do not clearly distinguish osteopathy from other health professions which place anatomy and physiology as the basis of their practice. Today osteopathy must clarify its professional identity;[6] in response, some put forward the view that it is a holistic approach to patient care that is the aspect that differentiates the approach of the osteopath from that exercised by the profession of allopathic medicine. The holistic approach can be practiced by various other professions, however, and so this argument is hardly convincing. In addition, the observation of the work of many osteopaths seems to be closely linked to the biomechanical model, which for many authors of scientific articles related to epistemological reflections would primarily not be supported by valid foundations, as well as being little based on holistic thinking.[7] The differences between osteopaths and other health professionals are perhaps sought in the application of osteopathic principles to the person in order to plan treatment by choosing special individualized manual techniques for the patient, from the practice of the pioneers to evidence-based practice, to ensure osteopathy is person-centered.

## The peculiar aspects of osteopathy

Although the above principles cannot be seen as exclusive to osteopathy, they are still part of its conceptual framework and a distinction might be found in the level of consideration and in the depths with which they are applied in practice. Although manual techniques are used by many professionals, such as chiropractors, physiotherapists, etc., the unique way in which the osteopathic manipulative techniques are integrated into the management of the patient, as well as the duration, frequency, and choice of technique, are all distinctive aspects of osteopathy.

This discipline is not limited to the techniques of vertebral "thrust" often associated with manual medicine. Different types of manual techniques are taught and used by osteopaths. These are techniques of thrust or impulse, as well as non-invasive techniques. Despite the fact that different forms of manual medicine each have their technical arsenal and their method of application, the continuous progress in interprofessional exchange has meant that, in the search for an effective manual therapeutic approach, only the techniques considered the most appropriate were chosen. Over time, this "technical evolution" has led to a significant transferring of techniques from one profession to another. They are only a part of the osteopathic practice. The way of thinking and the modalities of implementation of the technique are what distinguish osteopathic medicine from other forms of manual medicine,

far more than its procedures and the way they are carried out. Although the range of techniques, as indicated above, is not one of the characteristic features of osteopathy in comparison to the arsenal of other forms of manual medicine, continual reference is made within the profession to "perceptive palpation." This is a quite distinct concept from the execution of practical manual techniques, which results in an individualized osteopathic treatment for each situation. Other features, such as the holistic view of the patient and the salutogenic model, are not exclusive to osteopathy and can also be traced respectively to the principle of unity and the potential for self-regulation. Another important concept in the field of osteopathy is that of "function":[8] it is contextualized and related to the local function of a part of the body to the function of the whole person in his or her physical and social environment. Clinical decisions depend on the manner in which this context is generated and how it is understood. Osteopathy uses a specific approach regarding the contextual and relational nature of the function. On the one hand, evaluation and osteopathic diagnosis emphasize the importance of the whole to achieve a better understanding of the parts. On the other hand, the local dysfunctional systems are identified in a completely specific way. The above features are not only the prerogative of osteopathy, but the combination, and particularly their practical realization, certainly defines its identity.[9]

Osteopaths are active in primary health care, both for diagnosis and for treatment, acting as mediators in the maintenance and/or restoration of health, working closely with the patient, especially through "the touch." To this we add a manual technique which is aimed at restoring lost function at all levels of the body. Aspects of knowledge considered relevant for osteopathic practice include human dynamics, together with an understanding of how and why this is reflected in the anatomy of the individual and their interaction with the physical and social environments. Osteopathy is emerging through modern and relevant scientific sources, supported by a critical consideration of research evidence, which includes aspects of psychology, sociology, and other relevant disciplines. This knowledge allows the recognition and identification of disease and of the conditions that may lead to it. Osteopaths must constantly keep their knowledge up to date, to inform clinical reasoning and decision-making in order to provide an appropriate osteopathic treatment. This should be supported by research evidence whenever possible. The osteopath must have a detailed grasp of the concepts related to the structure and function of the human being. This should be enough to recognize, identify, and differentiate the normative and non-normative anatomical structures and processes in the living body. The operator considers that the reason for consulting a patient can hide underlying pathologies; thus he or she makes use of knowledge of human diseases sufficient for clinical judgment and for the recognition of diseases for which OMT may not be indicated. He or she also has a knowledge of human psychology and sociology sufficient to provide a context for clinical decision-making and patient management. The use of biophysical principles, along with the evaluation and implementation of the most relevant scientific evidence, enables him to understand the effects of the forces acting within living matter, especially in the application of OMT. This approach is not only aimed at the assessment and treatment of SD, understood as the area of discomfort, but also follows a decision-making process that allows the osteopath to assess the best access to promote salutogenesis, through the treatment of eventual decompensated areas if necessary, as, for example, through the stimulation or inhibition of self-regulatory functions and powers of activation, when it is preferable not to use specific approaches. The application of the following principles allows you to create a holistic, patient-centered practice, and not just state it in theory.

## Osteopathy: a traditional medicine centered on the person

According to the World Health Organization, in order to respond adequately to the new challenges of the twenty-first century, medicine has to focus on the health of the person rather than on the disease.

Some authors[10] have described historical evidence of the failure of biomedicine:

- in having pursued a practice based on the chemical and physical processes in the body, resulting in the depersonalization of the patient, so the doctor–patient relationship is suffocated by the practice of medicine centered on the disease

- in having renounced their origins and being unable to address the issue of global health, rejecting the contribution of thought and therefore of traditional medicines, and no longer being able to comprehend the vision of the human being, of every sentient being, that they encounter.

This resulted in patients starting to "turn back and within themselves" in a process of reappropriation of their dignity, integrity, and uniqueness as an individual, as a person, taking medicine not endorsed by the dominant medical model, and also returning to the need for health supporting and health promoting action in their lives. Practices such as mesmerism, phrenology, theosophy, and spiritualism took root and were practiced, as well as the art of the bonesetters, the eclectic and alternative medicines present in North America in the nineteenth century, and aspects of Shawnee traditional medicine;[11] it was within this context that the medicine of "the old doctor," osteopathy, was born and raised: a traditional medicine whose idea of good health was based on concepts that today are defined with the terms salutogenesis, resilience, proaction, sense of coherence, fairness, inside-out sustainability, awareness, responsibility, self-respect, individual value, participation – i.e., medicine centered on the person.

As is the case with anthropological medicine, defined as alternative, complementary, or traditional medicine (i.e., based on tradition), osteopathy has developed its own structure, which applies an analogical–observational model of the biological phenomena in the same way as Ayurveda or traditional Chinese medicine. Unlike the latter, however, osteopathic medicine does not use popular terms unknown to science in its nomenclature, but the language of anatomy and physiology to guide the manual approach intended to establish a helping relationship, an empathic salutogenic relationship. It is not the doctor that cures or the disease being cured, but the "taking care" that emerges from the relationship, accomplished by placing the person at the center of the therapeutic process employed to convey the salutogenesis. It is a common heritage, widely established both nationally and internationally, that traditional medicines have an established and stable role in innovation in the field of health. This is also demonstrated today by the enormous theoretical and practical interest that manifests itself increasingly in university, hospital, and community care areas in the private clinics of individual professionals. Traditional medicines share a commitment to education in, and dissemination and study of, salutogenesis, which is concerned with studying the sources of physical, mental, and spiritual health as an ethical and social responsibility, aware of the need for greater social empowerment, focusing on every single person.[12] Perhaps now is the time for biomedicine to develop a new scientific paradigm to research the real potential of approaches to health that engage with the person?

To produce evidence of the efficacy of traditional medicines we obviously need good-quality research. It is paradoxical for the academic and institutional establishment to ask traditional medical practices for evidence of their effectiveness when, except in rare cases, there are no state funds allocated for this purpose. The dominant biomedical system needs a new paradigm that allows the integration of knowledge gained from evidence-based medicine with that of traditional medicine. Biomedicine, the dominant medical system, as defined by the World Health Organization, should engage today, in a multidimensional, multifactorial, and multidisciplinary way, with the contribution to health of the anthropological health systems, such as traditional medicines, by virtue of their knowledge in observing nature and the sentient being and their interpretation in terms of the humanization of medicine. It should consider the totality of the human being, the intrinsic unity of

a person's being, on both the physical and the mental planes, for it is at these ceaselessly interacting levels that every human being is spiritually self-structured as a unique individual, and should be considered as such, so that they can be provided with the best possible approach to care.[13] We must also remember that the typical analogical observation of traditional medicines must be communicated using a common language that can be understood in the necessary overall observation of the person's health, avoiding any misinterpretation of the methods used for assessment. In this regard, the osteopath is confronted today with methodological studies of reliability[14] or of correlation of the results for his or her palpation with instruments for imaging diagnostics[15-17] that, on the one hand, tend to confirm the reliability of the approach, while on the other, requiring the operator to review the communication modes of his or her practice with the conventional medical world. In fact, the osteopath sometimes prefers to focus a technique on a specific anatomical structure, while the diagnostic tool cannot confirm the contact with such a landmark; on the other hand, however, it observes that the manual approach to the anatomical structure coincides with an improvement in the mobility and the local, segmental, and global functionality of the organ/system.[17] So the osteopath would perhaps be wise to remember that the teaching he or she receives is of a traditional medical nature, and in communicating his or her work he or she might use a suitable terminology so as not to be criticized by an outside party, such as a family doctor, for example.

Osteopaths must therefore:

- keep their knowledge up to date and in tune with the times and be able to guide their patients in choosing treatment, as well as being knowledgeable about health services as a whole[18,19]

- participate in the structuring of a research-assessment pattern of the functioning of the multiple physiological subsystems which contribute to determining the state of health by avoiding reliance on individual indicators

- be focused on a circular and non-pyramidal assessment for the study of health care globally, combining sociological, anthropological, and behavioral research, as well as cellular and molecular biology (observational studies, focus group studies, etc.).

## Osteopathy and health

It is necessary to outline the contribution that osteopathy can give to public health in order to understand how osteopaths observe the health-related process, its promotion and its maintenance. In the osteopathic field it is stated that the operator, in dealing with the person, is in the pursuit of health. This concept seems to alienate their practice from the disease, while in reality it outlines a unique approach focused on salutogenesis. Health is a tolerance to the variability of the environment; it is a biological luxury. Health is not being normal, but normative, i.e., being able to adapt physiological responses to environmental changes in order to allow the optimal execution of a function in the context in which it develops. Faced with change, we must not only be the possessors or bearers of values, but builders of new ones.

Value is what makes available skills, competencies, actions that increase tolerance to the variability of the environment and promote capacity for change. Health is therefore not only about the matching of the organism to an objective standard, but also about including the subjective dimension. It is a state of intrinsic adequacy and peace within oneself that cannot be surpassed by any other type of control.[20] By replacing perfection with adaptation, we approach a more compassionate, comforting, and creative program for medicine, one to which all health workers can contribute.[21] A biological pattern ready to describe this dynamic process of adaptation in finalizing health is represented by the theory of stress. This theory suggests that homeostasis and allostasis are endogenous systems responsible for maintaining the internal stability of the organism: homeostasis is a compound word deriving from the Greek words *omeos*, meaning "the same," and *stasis*, meaning "stable," i.e., "remain stable while remaining the same;" allostasis also has its roots in Greek, *allos* meaning "variable," thus "remain stable while being variable."[22] Homeostasis works to regulate daily bodily factors such as temperature or the rise in the cortisol level before awakening. The allostatic mechanism, however, responds to unexpected challenges, such as exposure to pathogens, or a mother's need to protect a child in difficult conditions. This allostatic response to stress is what we know as the "fight-or-flight" response, during which the body mobilizes energy: breathing accelerates, the heart rate increases, the superficial blood vessels constrict, the stored carbohydrates are released into the bloodstream, and the immune response is awakened. But what causes this response nowadays is not, for example, a tiger that is following us or the competition for food. Instead, it may be a demanding boss, children in difficulty, or a hectic agenda. Now we live in an artificial jungle, a concrete jungle. Our "tigers" look different, or they are manifested in a different way, but this does not make them harmless: quite the opposite. These stressors are different from those of survival because they can easily become more chronic, rather than short-term episodes. This type of stress does not involve the physical response of the normal fight-or-flight type, which requires extra glucose and lipids released into the bloodstream; rather it remains in a form of constant psychic energy tension. In addition, a substantial lack of blood circulation, coupled with non-escape and non-combat, produces deficiencies in the organs. Chronic stress of this nature can lead to depression, diabetes, and cardiovascular disease. The continued influence of the fight-or-flight mechanism creates an abnormal situation from which homeostasis is no longer able to protect us. Like homeostasis, allostasis helps the body to remain stable in confronting the changes. However, allostasis does this by varying the hormonal mediators and neurotransmitters of stress. The mechanism involved in the homeostasis resists changing, while allostasis responds to both change and the anticipating needs of the organism. The homeostasis regulation system does not have fixed parameters of adjustment in order to respond to unforeseen threats. This regulation system elicits behavioral physiological responses to anticipate and respond effectively to the challenges. Simply put, allostasis is a process used by the body to restore homeostasis when exposed to prolonged or extreme challenges. The goal of homeostasis and allostasis is to meet the energy and nutritional needs of the body, but each is designed to confront different types of change. The homeostasis theory attempts to explain the differences in individual responses to stress. For example, it investigates why some humans survive certain diseases and others do not. One explanation is that allostasis is vulnerable to severe and tough stressful events. It works well when needed and then turns off when it is no longer essential. However, chronic stimulation of the allostatic regulatory system creates tissue damage, and it is this damage that accelerates dysfunctional responses and leads to pathological conditions such as panic attack, heart disease, and memory loss (cf. Chapter 8). This deterioration is defined as "allostatic overload." It happens when the allostatic systems remain active, even though they are no longer needed. It is assumed that the origin of allostatic overload is due to the dysfunction of the neurotransmitters and hormones of the organs responsible for regulating allostasis. The concept of homeostasis demonstrates that the body's internal environment is maintained constant by negative feedback mechanisms, i.e., actions of self-correction of its constituent organs.

Allostasis demonstrates that the internal environment varies in order to meet the requirements of what is perceived and/or expected. This change is achieved by adaptive systems (biomechanical, neurological, respiratory-circulatory, metabolic-energetic, behavioral/biopsychosocial), which are mutually reinforcing in replacing the homeostatic mechanism. The allostatic model emphasizes the subordination of local feedback to control by the brain, providing a conceptual framework to explain the social and psychological modulation of the boundaries between physiology and pathology.[22] Internal stability responds to patterns of accommodation that can manifest in compensation or decompensation:

- with local adaptation in the tissue by altering the mobility, the location, the tissue texture, the sensibility of the components of the somatic system as skeletal, arthrodial, and myofascial structures, and the relative vascular, lymphatic, and neural elements; in other words, that which the osteopath refers to as SD[1-3,18]

- with general adaptation of the systems responsible for maintaining the internal stability of the body, leaving the memory of their energy consumption in postural organization with a particular fascial compensation scheme (FCS) and a relative dynamics of (biological) fluids and (biological) involuntary rhythms (DyFIR), detectable by the osteopath[23] (Fig. 1.1).

## Osteopathy and public health

Today, in many countries the professional osteopath is an independent practitioner, while in others the osteopath is one of those who practice primary care. Whenever possible, this professional will work alongside doctors, specialists, and/or other health disciplines, subject to the patient's consent. Osteopathy is independent in terms of actions (competence, diagnostics, safety, assistance, attitude, confidence, and awareness of responsibilities) and organization of work (efficiency, protection, right to bill for services). To which sector within primary health care does this traditional medicine belong? Osteopathy can be both complementary and alternative to standard medical treatments, with which it seeks an integrated approach (Fig. 1.2). In addition to its curative function, by virtue of its conceptual background, it can also be enlisted inside the area of preventive medicine. It is used to treat both

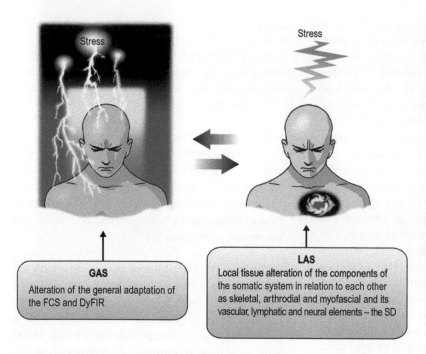

**Fig. 1.1**
Hypotheses of osteopathic assessment of health performance, the general and local adaptation syndromes (GAS and LAS), perceived through perceptive palpation and sometimes treated with local specific adjustments directed to the clinically relevant somatic dysfunction (SD), sometimes with general adaptive techniques addressing the normalization of compensating patterns or involuntary fluid movements. GAS and LAS are mutually dependent, so the evaluation and treatment must take into account the combination of all approaches.

**GAS**
Alteration of the general adaptation of the FCS and DyFIR

**LAS**
Local tissue alteration of the components of the somatic system in relation to each other as skeletal, arthrodial and myofascial and its vascular, lymphatic and neural elements – the SD

musculoskeletal and non-musculoskeletal conditions. As such, it has a clear role in the corpus of both curative and preventive medicine: health promotion. Osteopathy is concerned with health as the adaptive capacity of the person, or adaption difficulties that have affected health; therefore, the list of instructions that follow is not exhaustive and is suggested by European osteopathic institutions[18] as a general guide to the wide range of reasons for consultation that may lead patients to their osteopath, including:

- problems related to mechanical and nervous systems, such as pain, discomfort and dysfunction of muscles, joints, and their associated structures

- falls, injuries/lesions and stress, effects of poor posture, tension, emotional stress, and headache

- reduced functionality of the body systems such as digestive problems, circulatory disorders, respiratory diseases, ear, nose, or throat problems, especially in young people, stress-related

conditions or conditions related to infectious diseases and postoperative recovery

- problems related to sports at all levels, including elite athletes

- problems associated with pregnancy, pregnant women, infants and childhood

- when patients have no clear reason for consultation, but do not feel "balanced."

The above list[18] suggests that osteopathic treatment has an advantageous cost–benefit ratio and may reduce the patient's need for drug treatment, exposing the patient to less diagnostic testing and lowering the risk of complications. It is a much discussed contribution in the area of preventive health care.

The purpose of preventive medicine is to promote and maintain good health, prevent diseases, and combat their progression. The preventive function of osteopathy is determined by the osteopathic vision that sees illness and health as gradual phenomena

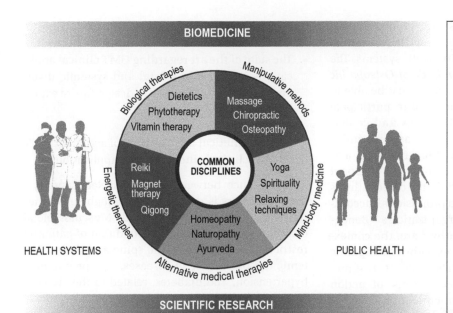

**Fig. 1.2**
Integration among the various types of medicine. Modified from: Exemplification of the five domains where the NCCAM classifies CAM. In: Roberti di Sarsina P, Morandi A, Alivia M et al., (2012) Conventional and non-conventional medicine in Italy. Considerations for a social choice to the person-centered medicine. Advanced Therapies. 1:3–29.

where it is believed that the patient's dysfunction is prodromal to the illness. The essence of this vision is that the organism holds within itself the potential for health, which can be vivified by the removal of SD and the allostatic load that it facilitates, in addition to being stimulated by global approaches. This vision leads to a form of prevention that is different from what today's society understands by prevention. The osteopath can also be employed in hospitals or in any other type of care facility, as he works within the entire spectrum of health and disease, together with other professionals, and is not limited to a certain area of health care. Osteopaths practice their profession in absolute independence. They work with diagnosis as well as with osteopathic treatment.

Osteopaths are professionals of first contact with a high degree of responsibility; a specialized training in the pathology of neurological and musculoskeletal systems, as well as in general semiotics, is aimed at building an adequate differential diagnosis, which allows the identification of those conditions in which it is appropriate (or not) to treat the person. They are aware of the possibilities, but also of the limits, of their profession and if during a consultation a medical intervention is determined to be of higher priority, they act accordingly, referring the person to the family doctor.[18]

## Research in osteopathy: demands, needs, and necessities

In the last decade, the international scientific community has witnessed the rapid assertion of evidence-based medicine, presented in 1992 as a methodology for applying the results of biomedical research to the individual patient.[24] In the drafting of this book the authors have questioned themselves on how far this paradigm has been accepted and how far the methodology of research has been applied in the osteopathic field. In everyday practice, should the osteopath have the knowledge, skills, tools, and methods of an evidence-based osteopathy? Should osteopathy adopt a methodology for the research of scientific information and its critical evaluation in the osteopathic field, integrating it into clinical care decisions for the osteopathic treatment that is to be applied to the patient? For many operators, professional registers, and schools, the answer is "yes."

According to the work of research groups at international level, such studies are needed in osteopathy to affirm the profession within health systems. The *European Framework for Standards of Osteopathic Practice*[19] states that the osteopath must be able to demonstrate awareness of the need to participate and contribute to structured courses and conferences in professional areas, as well as to organize and participate in group activities, research, and other educational activities to promote personal professional development and that of osteopathy as a profession. The key skills of a professional, according to the World Health Organization's "Benchmarks for training in osteopathy"[3] are: the contextualization of the basic sciences within osteopathic philosophy and the five models of structure–function; understanding the mechanisms of action underlying the manual therapeutic interventions, as well as the biochemical, cellular and anatomical response to the therapy; and the ability to critically assess the scientific and medical literature and to integrate the information into clinical practice. From the European Federation of Osteopath's document "Scope of osteopathic practice in Europe,"[18] it appears that the majority of osteopathic indications are within the sphere of locomotor apparatus functional pain. The purpose of osteopathic treatment is to bring the body back to normal function and, therefore, to limit the need for drugs or surgery. It is possible that other reasons for consulting an osteopath, linked to other functions such as the digestive and circulatory system, will eventually reach the same scientific level through further clinical and basic science research and therefore will be elevated to the rank of real and proper indications for osteopathic treatment.

Such research must be conducted in the university context and cooperation with medical specialties will be vital. A critical reading of the above-mentioned documents highlights the need for the community of osteopathic practice to continue the work already begun by some researchers in this area, by partaking actively as researchers, or as readers who contextualize the evidence in the ambulatory clinic.

The available literature provides the following:

- The state of the art regarding OMT clinical applications in musculoskeletal and systemic disorders, confirming the need to design future experimental studies

- The hypothetical mechanisms of action for OMT and the clinical outcomes of its application.

The difference between musculoskeletal and systemic disorders is quite simple, though sometimes the two are inextricably linked. Musculoskeletal disorders mainly refer to the condition of pain and restriction of mobility of the spine and limbs. Systemic disorders refer to diseases, e.g., pneumonia, hypertension, and diabetes, related to the visceral, vascular, endocrine, and immunological systems, usually with etiology in a specific organ. Related to systemic disorders is the interest associated with general physiological functions such as heart rate, digestion, and respiratory function.[25] There have been investigations, including a systematic review[26] and a meta-analysis,[27,28] that describe the benefit of manual therapy for low back pain. Most of the research projects on the impact of manual therapy on physiological functions and systemic disorders have not been sufficiently funded, and thus there are no clinical trials that would provide suitable material for a systematic review. Finally, there have not been sufficient qualitative studies aimed at studying "humanistic" approaches, to the perception and the satisfaction of both the operator and patient. You can often get valuable information through questionnaires and interviews. Studies of this type, although not experimental, are often the only way to detect tendencies in the population, distributions of certain professional practices, collections of experts' opinions, data about operators, and patients' perceptions.

Other tools that can provide valuable information include the following:

- *Historical analysis*: interviews with experts or the analysis of texts from authors of the past are useful for translating an archaic jargon into understandable terms. There are excellent examples of this historical analysis work carried out, as, for example, in the book by Jane Stark, written to help understand the ideas of Still on the "fluid of life" and on the fascia, in light of his knowledge and temporal context,[29] or a recent article describing how the model defined as "primary respiratory mechanism" (PRM) in osteopathic cranial manipulative medicine (OCMM), and described for the first time in the early twentieth century by William Garner Sutherland, repeats a certain number of theories previously enunciated by Emanuel Swedenborg. This has caused the opening of a critical dialogue aimed at the observation of how the OCMM model, and all manipulative osteopathic practices, are, as is all medicine, the evolution over time of the concepts of anatomy and of human physiology.[30]

- *Bio-behavioral research*: a complex web of relationships between genetic, physiological, environmental and behavioral factors influences the states of health and disease. The bio-behavioral mechanisms intervene in health and disease through physiological responses to stress that lead to the development of the disease. This can occur not only by means of behavioral choices that increase or reduce the risk of health impairment, but also by behavioral reactions to the disease that alter surveillance activities or the observance of recommendations and treatment regimens. The measurable variability of the individual response to the outcome of any disease is largely due to the behavior of the individual and his or her emotional response to stress that the disease involves.[31]

The behavior affects the physiological "landscape" and the physiological alterations produce important adaptations that cause repercussions on health and on the disease outcomes (see Chapter 8). The onset of a disease is a complex phenomenon, in which the pathologies of soft tissues and bones intervene (musculoskeletal abnormalities), as well as the psychosocial and behavioral responses to physical damage and environmental factors that maintain or strengthen disability even after the removal of its initial cause. From the point of view of osteopathic research, the studying of bio-behavioral interactions can promote the understanding of patients, improve treatment regimens and clarify, based on evidence, the principles of osteopathic medicine. The topics that will be the most subjected to measurements and bio-psychosocial studies will be the attitudes that lead to the development of an SD, attitudes derived from it, aspects related to quality of life, the effects of pain on the body's functions and the relationships between SD and the management, by the patient, of counterproductive behaviors.[32] The community of osteopaths must now establish and implement research that verifies the principles and beliefs on which it is based. These studies must be carried out within the osteopathic profession, not in other areas. They must answer the queries of the profession, verify its assumptions, and should only be interpreted by those who thoroughly know the theory and practice of osteopathic medicine. One cannot accept the risk of allowing others to conduct studies or to interpret the results from other points of view. Today, the future of the profession depends on this research effort as well as its commitment to teaching and clinical practice. Research that is coherent with the philosophy of osteopathy and that makes use of the knowledge derived from years of clinical experience will actively contribute to the most beneficial aspects of health care that osteopathy is essentially dedicated to, namely: the maintenance of health and optimal functionality of the whole person throughout life. One of the challenges is to actively defend the use of designs suitable for research on osteopathic manipulation and not be guided by preconceived ideas on how we should do research, or be forced to use unsuitable designs. Study protocols to investigate the basic science, to integrate the latter with clinical observation, for the construction of integrated models, epidemiological studies, clinical research, reviews and meta-analyses and qualitative studies are needed to investigate:

- OMT mechanisms of action

- clinical efficacy

- intra- and inter-operator reliability in palpatory procedures

- interactions between osteopath and patient

- cost—benefit ratio

- teaching methods of palpation and other osteopathic skills.

Osteopathic medicine and its principles have an important role in modern science. Society is waiting to see if and how the osteopathic profession chooses to respond to its dual responsibility to provide the best care possible based on current knowledge and make steady progress in knowledge. However, so far, the number and quality of research projects in basic science and the clinical area in this sector deserve examination, while the opportunity emerges to answer the questions of mechanisms of action and clinical efficacy in multiple areas of health.

## Applications of osteopathy in different clinical fields

### Specialization in the osteopathic field

Recently, there has been discussion about the use of a specialized approach in the osteopathic field.[33] The common view that is emerging today is that the osteopath should be able to apply the principles, models, and, finally, the techniques of osteopathy while individualizing them for every type of person. Everyone agrees to disagree with specializations such as "structuralist-biomechanic osteopaths" rather than "visceral osteopaths," as it is the "patient" and his or her relationship with the osteopath who chooses the approach, not the osteopath a priori. Nevertheless, the fact remains that certain clinical areas need proper training in order to allow the osteopath to know the peculiar aspects inherent to them (e.g., pediatrics, sports, geriatric, veterinarian, etc.).

### Osteopathy in gynecology and obstetrics

The ability to diagnose through palpation and treat an SD through viscerosomatic effects, vascular compromise, and the resulting pains ensures that the adjuvant osteopathic approach can represent a unique advantage to medical practice in the treatment of patients with gynecological and obstetric problems.[34] A significant number of patients with gynecological problems (endometriosis, adenomyosis, "ovulation pain," and several different types of pelvic infection) have pain in the pelvis and lumbar spine as a chief complaint. Underlying this algic/pain-dysfunctional symptomatology there can be observed viscerosomatic reflexes involving spinal segments that innervate the site of the disease.[35] Right from the earliest days of osteopathy,[34] practitioners have paid attention to the mechanical alterations of the musculoskeletal system the pregnant woman is subject to, especially changes in the spine and lumbar curvatures, presenting symptoms of functional dysmetria of the lower limbs, affecting the gait.[36] The load sustained during pregnancy makes back pain a major cause of complaints by pregnant women.[37] Although these conditions are inevitable, the effective treatment of SD relieves the discomfort without the need for drugs and makes pregnancy much more tolerable.[38] In particular, it has been hypothesized from the work of Hensel and colleagues that OMT can relieve pain in pregnant women, eliminating the SD and their viscerosomatic connections, balancing the autonomic and hemodynamic changes in the mother's body, reducing the duration of labor, and helping avoid complications.[39] The results of the observational study by King and colleagues confirmed that OMT reduces complications during pregnancy, labor, and delivery, such as pain during labor, its duration, the need for surgery, the presence of meconium in the amniotic fluid, and the use of forceps.[40] A study conducted in the Ruber International Hospital in Madrid, on urinary incontinence and other pelvic floor damage, focused on etiology and preventive strategies, studied the birth process and the way childbirth is currently managed in most Spanish hospitals.[41]

This study included, alongside other rehabilitation treatments, osteopathy in the postnatal period (puerperium), in order to:

- facilitate the proper return to normalcy of all soft tissues and pelvic joints involved in childbirth

- facilitate mobility or free up blocks in the pelvic joints.

A 2010 study conducted in the Department of Gynecology of the University of Campinas noted that application of high-velocity low-amplitude osteopathic techniques to the sacrum is associated with an increase in phasic contraction and perineal basal tone, measured by perineometer in women who did not have associated bone and joint diseases. This study, although preliminary, suggests future developments in the treatment of women with perineal hypotonia.[42] The results of a systematic review and a meta-analysis performed to evaluate the effects of OMT on symptoms involving the lower urinary tract are promising and encouraging, although the authors refer more definitive conclusions to future studies that should compare the osteopathic treatment with standard procedures, foreseeing studies with control groups.[43]

Based on the observation that carpal tunnel syndrome is extremely common during pregnancy, some studies have shown a reduction of the compression of the median nerve within the carpal tunnel.[44,45]

In 2010, Licciardone and colleagues observed that OMT slows down the deterioration and failure of the lumbar spine in women during the third trimester of pregnancy.[46] This study demonstrates the feasibility of offering OMT as a complement to conventional obstetric treatment during the third trimester of pregnancy, and is confirmed today by:

- a review of the literature[38] which concludes that the treatment of SD in pregnant women may improve homeostasis, and the comfort and quality

of life during the physiological and structural changes of pregnancy

- a further study of 2013 carried out according to the criteria of the Cochrane Collaboration, which also confirmed OMT effects in preventing the progressive dysfunction of the back during the third trimester of pregnancy, highlighting how they are potentially relevant to direct health costs and indirect costs of "disability/work" during pregnancy[47]

- a review published by the Cochrane Collaboration found that OMT, like other multimodal interventions, seems to relieve pelvic and back pain to a greater extent than the application of traditional therapy alone.[48]

## Osteopathy in pediatrics and prospects in neonatology

An area that has received attention from research and in clinical practice is OMT applied to children. Most of the techniques of OMT applied in pediatrics are non-invasive and directed to correcting SDs that may cause functional disturbances of the impulse streams of the cranial nerves. These are probably the cause of conditions such as infantile colic and compression of the cranial structures, which could alter the temporal bone position and disrupt the drainage of the Eustachian tube, resulting in recurrent otitis media.

Otitis media is a common condition in children and can have serious negative effects if not treated promptly. OMT applications in cases of otitis media were examined in two published reports.[49,50] It was found that children treated with OMT had a significant decrease of episodes of acute otitis media and an improvement in their tympanograms. These results span decades of clinical experience and research, and are still in progress.

Another common neonatal condition is colic. In its worst manifestation, it causes untreatable vomiting. Clinical success with this condition has been confirmed by research,[51] which showed a significant reduction in the symptoms of colic and an increase in the sleep duration of children undergoing treatment with OMT.

In slightly older children, sleep apnea symptoms were significantly reduced during 4 weeks of treatment with OMT. However, after the end of treatment there were no differences between those treated and the control patients. It is also evident that OMT improves cognitive function[52] and neurological development[53] in children. In studies by Lassovetskaia, children in a special education program reached higher scores in tests and behavioral assessment by the teachers whenever OMT was applied, and the effects appeared to be long lasting. Using Houle's Profile of Neurodevelopment, children who received OMT had a higher score than another group on a waiting list for treatment.[52] Data in a study by Philippi and colleagues in 2006 suggest that osteopathic treatment in the first months of life is useful for infants with idiopathic infantile postural asymmetry and that OMT methods can and should be evaluated in this age group.[54] However, to date, there have not been many studies on the application of OMT in pediatric disorders, although there have been decades of clinical positive observation. The mechanism of action that brings the benefits, as suggested above, is the return of altered neuromuscular structures to an anatomically normal configuration and function, which in turn can normalize visceral-somatic interactions. Although several studies document the effect of OMT in a population of pediatric patients, the medical literature lacks information on any potential benefits of OMT use in preterm infants. Some researchers considering the possible positive effects of OMT in reducing the risk of excessive length of hospital stay and gastrointestinal symptoms have recently published a multicenter randomized controlled study.[55] This study enrolled 695 preterm infants in three different neonatal intensive care units, and the result was a decrease of 4 days of hospitaliza-

tion for the group that received OMT, as well as a cost saving of around € 1,600 for each newborn, when compared to those who received only conventional treatments. From these studies emerge suggestions for future studies to assess, perhaps as a secondary outcome, the difference in daily weight increase, the number of episodes of vomiting and regurgitation, the use of enemas (clysters), and full enteral feeding time (breastfeeding and/or bottle).

## Osteopathy in geriatrics

The self-healing mechanism, a concept dear to osteopaths, varies from person to person and is, to a large extent, a manifestation of the individual's ability to compensate stress. This ability decreases with age, while the physiological sources of stress increase. A person may be old in years but young in their physiology, and vice versa. Osteopathy focuses on helping the patient to compensate for the inevitable failure caused by aging. So far, the evidence available confirms the improvement of pain and musculoskeletal function,[56] even in the presence of osteoporosis.[57]

Other studies have reported an increase in balance measured by clinical and stabilometry tests,[58] even in patients up to 75 years of age with persistent vertigo for at least 3 months.[59] In addition, after the experience derived from the pandemic influenza of 1918–19, the treatment of influenza and lung diseases was supplemented with lymphatic pump techniques, costal manipulations, and other OMT techniques. Therefore, today, many authors have described integrated complementary approaches with elective therapies[60] and investigated the effects of this approach on lung diseases, particularly pneumonia in the elderly,[61] including in the hospital setting.[62]

## Osteopathy in hospitals and for post-surgical patients

Osteopaths who operate on and take care of hospitalized patients have also contributed to the research literature on the effects of OMT. In the US, osteopaths hold a medical practice license. Many osteopathic physicians are surgeons and this has encouraged research on the application of OMT on hospitalized patients. The protocol used in these studies of OMT is directed to the areas of the axial skeleton, where the dysfunctions can have effects on the autonomic functions of the nervous system, as well as the peripheral areas that can affect the vascular flow. These areas are the atlanto-occipital joint and the sacrum, which possibly affect the functions related to the parasympathetic system (gastrointestinal tract, heart, lung, pelvic organs) and the spinal tract that goes from T1 to L3, associated with SD and functions related to the sympathetic system. A study of women who have had a hysterectomy noted that a preoperative treatment of OMT is able to significantly reduce the need for postoperative analgesics.[63] Unfortunately, due to insufficient availability of hospital records it was not possible to assess the subjective impression of faster recovery. In a study of the results in coronary bypass graft surgery, the researchers found that the preoperative application of OMT significantly improved drainage from the surgical site.[64] Oxygen saturation and postoperative cardiac efficiency were significantly improved in patients who had OMT compared to those who had not received it. The osteopathic protocol used included cervical and upper thoracic techniques to reduce tensions caused by the prolonged anesthesia and open air chest (thoracic) surgery. In a review study, patients who had had abdominal surgery with a diagnosis of postoperative ileus[65] were examined. The study showed that the participants who received OMT had a shorter hospital stay than the subjects to whom it was not administered. This study supports the clinical experience that postoperative OMT improves intestinal function. Another postoperative complication studied was atelectasis.[66] The results of the application of OMT have not reduced the onset of the disorder; however, this approach has been linked to a faster return to preoperative respiratory conditions.

Hospitalized patients with pancreatitis were also studied[67] and those who received treatment with OMT had a shorter hospital stay. In hospitalized and surgical patients OMT application can also be shown to save on related costs. Although the primary concern of research is the optimization of clinical results, the importance of cost savings through fewer medications and reduced hospital stay is certainly one more reason to consider the administration of OMT in hospitalized patients.

## Osteopathy in sports medicine

"Movement is life." In examining osteopathic principles, we can see a clear analogy with any kind of sport. Every athlete, amateur sportsperson, or practitioner of a sport sees the practical explanation of the axioms that shape and enrich an osteopath, day by day. The use of OMT in professional sports emerged at the turn of the nineteenth century, through the work of A. T. Still, who, through treatment provided to athletes in an osteopathic medical college, became one of the pioneers of sports medicine. One of the known figures of osteopathy in professional sports was Forrest "Phog" Allen, DO (1885–1974). Allen was the legendary basketball coach of the Kansas Jayhawks, known as the father of basketball coaches, with 24 championships won by his team at the University of Kansas. In addition to his work as head coach, he also covered the role of the team osteopath, a role that allowed him to introduce to the scientific community, and to athletes, coaches, and trainers, the impact that OMT has in the field of professional sport. Today, for the first time, osteopathy has been included in medical care services to the Olympic Games: 24 sports medicine osteopaths were selected to work with the London 2012 Olympic medical team. The athlete's problems are particularly suitable for osteopathic principles and concepts and their application;[68] the osteopath recognizes the existence of many factors that weaken both the ability and the natural tendency to recover. Among the most important factors are local disorders of the musculoskeletal system. The athletes who exercise in extreme temperatures and experience strong physical stress are often the victims of musculoskeletal injuries. These lesions represent the most recurrent problem in sports activities. However, in musculoskeletal problems of athletes for which no surgery is needed, the operator who has skills in osteopathic synthesis, who possesses a thorough knowledge of anatomy, physiology, and semeiotics of the human body and of manipulative treatment is well equipped for promoting the self-healing resources of the body. The supervision of athletes requires excellent collaboration between medical and paramedical professionals, including the osteopath,[69,70] after recognition of the skills of each operator in the sports medical team. The study of Larequi highlights how physiotherapy and osteopathy are complementary and inseparable activities in a framework aiming to provide real holistic care with evidence-based methods, safe both for traumatic or overload-induced pathologies and for functional disorders.[71] The sports osteopath is specially trained in biomechanics and sports-specific gestures, enabling him to make a structural assessment of the body to determine the SD. The use of OMT in athletes is biomechanically intuitive and physiological, since sport performance is mainly a function of the neuromusculoskeletal system. Several researchers are studying the effects of OMT in various kinematic parameters of spine, pelvis, and hip motion, suggesting that this approach could improve the range of motion, lessen pain, improve strength and spatial awareness, and lead to a better sports performance.[72]

### Osteopathic approach to the performance artist

Conventional medical treatments, including physical and occupational therapy, medication and surgery, can be beneficial in some cases of injuries to performing artists. These interventions, however, can sometimes be insufficient for a full return to health performance activity. This is probably related to the multidimensional nature of the performance movements that could benefit from a treatment plan of a holistic nature, focused on the patient.[73] The osteopathic approach of inclusion in a multidisciplinary rehabilitation plan also includes feedback of the tissue changes related to poor posture,

observing them as factors that may maintain or exacerbate a previous imbalance. It is necessary to structure approaches centered on the evaluation and treatment of the individual's allostatic load, its interoceptive capacity, its globality, and unique aspects of the art of manipulative osteopathy.[74] An approach structured in such a way helps optimize the rehabilitation of an artist, both in terms of posture and performative results.[75,76]

## Osteopathic practice

Recently, some authors have ventured into an interpretive representation of the factors that influence the decision-making process of osteopaths, through a qualitative study aiming at the analysis of this process.[77] The delicate interplay of instances aimed at establishing a relationship of mutual trust should be based on a balanced and shared relationship between operator and patient during the decision-making process. The osteopath must be simultaneously, and in equal measure, practitioner, communicator, and educator, claiming his or her ability to:

- listen to personal problems

- identify the coexistence of fear and catastrophic behaviors, as well as the person's sensitivity in respect to the real components of the disorder

- palpate and perform osteopathic technique

- communicate the therapeutic process to the person and to actively involve the patient, avoiding the risk of a passive approach to treatment.

## Osteopathic consultation

An osteopathic consultation is the taking charge of the patient by the osteopath, in the recording of present and remote anamnesis (see below) and conducting appropriate osteopathic tests. The osteopath formulates the diagnosis and prognosis, effectively communicates this to his or her patient and provides an OMT using methods consistent with clinical findings, and subsequently re-evaluates its results in terms of health promotion.[18]

## Anamnesis

The osteopath notes the details of the reason for consultation, the past and current medical history of the patient, including family history. This allows the patient to express himself and occasionally to elicit details about the symptomatic picture and beyond. It also asks a number of pertinent questions, including reports and conclusions of other specialists, useful for identifying any red flags[78,79] or yellow flags[80-82] (see Fig. 9.11) and for making a diagnosis of exclusion, a differential and a working one. Considerable attention is given to predisposing and maintenance factors that may have caused (or maintained) the problem, for example occupational factors, recreational factors, or stress. The osteopath maintains a comprehensive written record of the consultation and the consequent discussion with the patient. This information will be treated as strictly confidential and adequately protected and stored electronically and/or in paper format.

## Observation and clinical examination

Based on the history of the case, a range of possible diagnoses is generated and explored through a detailed osteopathic clinical examination, designed exclusively for the individual patient and his or her problem. When necessary, the osteopath will use the clinical examination procedures that are familiar and widely used by health professionals in order to examine all the systems of the body. In addition, the osteopath uses other specific evaluation techniques, such as observation and palpation, to assess the quality, status, mobility, and health of the mechanics of the joints, muscles, and other body tissues.

This will lead to an initial working diagnosis that the osteopath considers relevant in order to explain and solve the patient's problem. The operator then identifies the most important opportunities to deal with the discomfort of the person and communicates them to him. Diagnosis can be seen as the collection of a number of conclusions drawn from the history of the patient and from palpation, and

is used to identify the name of a condition, disease, or syndrome. This is useful in communicating predetermined signs and symptoms. The osteopath, however, strives to achieve an understanding and a complete and exhaustive explanation of the various factors involved, rather than just providing a label. In addition, the osteopathic interpretation of the patient's problem can evolve with the progress of the treatment and with a greater understanding of the conditions. At this point, the osteopath has sufficient results to identify the red and yellow flags and then proceed to treatment or referral to the family doctor or other health professional,[18] as appropriate (Fig. 1.3).

## Osteopathic evaluation of the person and perceptive palpation

Osteopaths summarize their assessments from the observations made in the palpatory examination to confirm or revise the working diagnosis, and therefore evaluate the overall health development of the person (allostatic load, posture, and energy level), correlate and prioritize the local area of adaptation (SD) across the patient's body systems, and design a treatment plan accordingly. At this point, they have a detailed discussion with the person about the diagnosis, treatment plan, and prognosis. From the beginning of their training, osteopaths continually develop their sense of touch, to be able to hear the information relevant to the patient's health. Diagnostic palpation plays a central role in practice: it is the highly qualified and practiced sense of touch, the mark of the osteopath. There is much known about the human sense of touch as the basis of perceptual osteopathic palpation. A study published by Skedung and colleagues in 2013, in the journal of the editors of *Nature, Scientific Reports*,[83] measured the sense of touch from a psychophysical point of view, analyzing which physical properties come into play in distinguishing a protuberance on a surface. The authors discovered 16 identical chemical planar surfaces on which invisible and very small wrinkles had formed, ranging from 7 to 4,500 nanometers. These "nano-wrinkles" (which

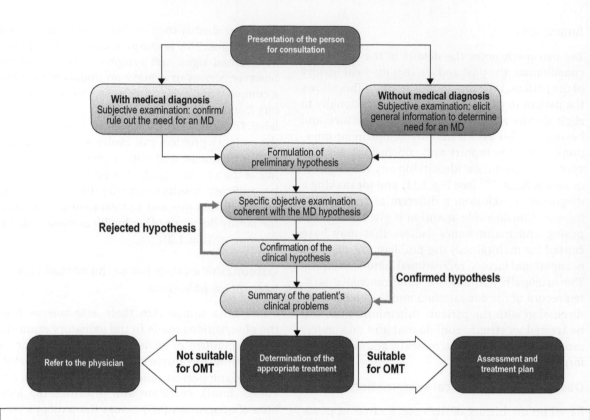

**Fig. 1.3**

Enrollment of a person in osteopathic manipulative treatment (OMT). In the evaluation phase, particularly during the first session, the operator proceeds with anamnesis and physical examination to assess any potential red flags or need for referral to other specialists without enrollment in OMT. Considerable attention is paid to the principle of *primum non nocere*, with particular reference to the medical history and the reason for the patient's consultation. The terms of confirmation or denial of medical diagnosis (MD) and differential diagnosis hypotheses do not have a connotation of abuse of the medical profession, rather a desire to understand whether the patient can be enrolled in OMT or whether it is more appropriate, rational, or simply more useful to refer the patient to the primary care physician or other specialist/therapist.

were quite far apart from each other – between 300 and 90,000 nanometers) create a surface reminiscent of the undulating surface of the sea. Afterwards, a group of volunteers was able to notice the (palpatory) difference between a flat surface and another which had lines of 13 nanometers with less than a micrometer distance between them. This study confirms that we can perceive, only by touching, objects of the size of a few nanometers. However, in the same year, Rosanna Sabini and colleagues brought our attention to how experi-

ence sometimes does not positively affect discriminative tactile ability, noting no difference between osteopathic professionals and students in the discriminative accuracy of objects suitably disguised for the experiment.[84] Experience, therefore, is not enough to elevate the human sense of touch to a reliable, sensitive, specific, and valid diagnostic tool. There are other qualities that have to grow with experience in order to be integrated into decision-making based on touch. Authors who are knowledgeable on the subject suggest that it is possible to achieve improvements in the development of palpatory perceptual skills ensuring that the teaching of palpation is not dissociated from the development of clinical reasoning skills.[85] Such a process should take into account knowledge about the quality of tissues both in normal structure and function integration conditions and in conditions where there is less interdependence of these instances of health.

This is due to the ability to integrate the palpatory information with all other sensitive information available to the professional. In fact, we know that we get information (including tactile information) about the world through all five of the senses: sight, hearing, touch, taste, and smell. It is known, furthermore, that we are able to train these senses, as we do the sense of sight when we learn to read; we know that a tea taster or wine taster trains the sense of taste, a perfumer trains the sense of smell, and a musician trains the ear. Similarly, from the beginning of their training, osteopaths develop their sense of touch to be able to sense the information that is not immediately evident (perceptible) to an untrained hand. These are all primary senses, which cannot be described simply by comparing them with each other or with other senses, but must be integrated with one another. The afferent information that comes to the osteopath from different senses is processed and interpreted at a central level, taking into account related anatomical, physiological, and pathological knowledge of osteopathic models of care and clinical experience. Considering the plastic nature of the human brain, it can be argued that the development of diagnostic palpatory skills is probably associated with adaptive behavioral, neuroanatomical, and neurophysiological changes. It is therefore likely that the osteopath's nervous system will undergo both functional and structural alterations, resulting from a long exposure to multi-sensory experience, continuous learning and decision-making processes. This process of integration among the senses, as well as the coherence between touch, scientific knowledge, and a good relational

capability, allows the osteopath to have an effective perception of:

- the areas where the lack of structure and function integration is expressed by alteration of mobility, sensitivity, and tissue viability

- the individual's totality, rather than focusing on an isolated single section.

Understanding the nature of competences in diagnostic palpation has implications for the quality of service offered by the osteopathic community. This is why students and professionals should be encouraged to use all available opportunities to experience normal and altered patterns of structure and function, thus reflecting on the validity and the reliability of their diagnostic judgments (Box 1.1).

## Osteopathic decision-making process

The osteopath tries to understand the person's health trends by assessing its adaptability, both in physiological systems of stress management (global tests) and in possible areas of "tissue memorization" (local tests). The practical application of the concepts and principles has been described by various perceptual models[33] that osteopaths use in the assessment of the area in which the patient experiences a loss of adaptive capacity, or alteration of the interdependence between structure and function. The five osteopathic models[2] describe the postural and biomechanical effects on the patient's ability to compensate for the stress factors or disease (biomechanical model), the influence of the nervous system in the field of physical-cognitive-emotional health (neurological model), the importance of the respiratory-circulatory system in the proper maintenance of cellular and tissue functionality (respiratory-circulatory model), the role of psychosocial factors in the prevention and treatment of diseases (behavioral/biopsychosocial model) and the factors affecting bioenergy needs such as oxygen and the consumption of nutrients (metabolic-energetic model). Thus, the osteopath tries to have a clear picture of the patient's condition through:

- communication aimed at creating a relationship of confidence between the osteopath and the patient (see Chapter 8)

- observation of the person through a "magnifying lens" that includes the instance or instances (well described by models) that are conditioning the patient's self-regulating systems, self-healing,

the ability to adapt to external and internal environmental stimuli – in other words, the person's entire health (see Chapter 9).

This allows the operator to perform an evaluation and select the appropriate model (see Chapter 9), approach, and techniques (Fig. 1.4), through assessment of general adaptation (global test) and local adaptation (regional, local, and specific tests), as well as a structure/function inhibition test.

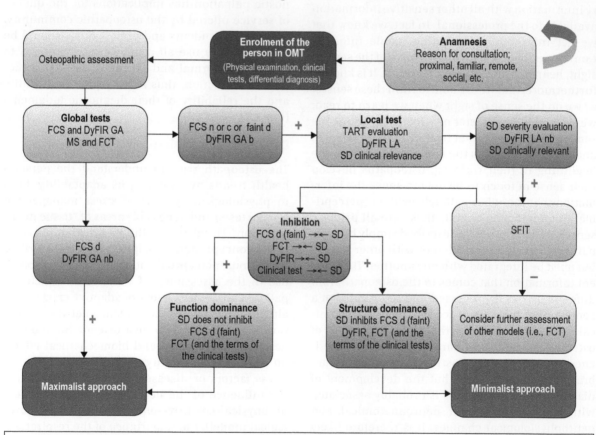

**Fig. 1.4**
Process of evaluation. The osteopath finalizes a clear representation of the patient's condition through evaluation and selection of the model, approach and techniques. FCS: fascial compensation scheme (n: neutral; c: compensated; d: decompensated); FCT: fascial compartments test; DyFIR: dynamics of fluids and biological involuntary rhythms (GA: global assessment; LA: local assessment; b: balanced; nb: not balanced); MS: model selection; SD: somatic dysfunction; TART: tissue texture abnormality, asymmetry, restriction of motion, tenderness; SFIT: structure/function inhibition test; +: positive test; –: negative test.

## Box 1.1

## Method for learning palpatory skills

Palpatory skills, the central component of osteopathic clinical practice, are essential to properly assess somatic dysfunction and select the most appropriate treatment techniques. In addition, they ensure the efficiency of the operator, determining the accuracy of clinical reasoning.[1] It takes a long time to achieve a level of competence in professional practice, whether in arts or in sports. The evidence relating to skills development shows that it takes about 10,000 hours of intensive deliberate practice to become expert in a particular field.[2] Understanding the way that osteopaths have to produce and interpret diagnostic information is important for the implementation of teaching strategies and effective learning. The imperceptible nature of the palpation process could be compared to the hidden part of clinical reasoning.[3] It has been shown that the results of clinical reasoning are in relation to the health care professional's ability to represent the clinical problem according to semantic qualifications.[4] As a result, it has been hypothesized that the value of palpation processes can be linked to the number of relevant qualifications that students choose among their points of reference in order to describe the palpatory results. Cognitive and motor learning theories, technical guidelines, considerations concerning the neural and behavioral correlates of the diagnostic skills of osteopathy, evidence relating to the field of cognitive neuroscience, experimental psychology, and medical knowledge have all inspired Aubin[3] in structuring a method of learning and monitoring perceptual palpation.

Palpation techniques can be divided into two distinct components:

1. A motor component, where the operator acts on the patient's tissues (information travels from the brain of the operator to the patient's tissues)

2. A perceptive component, where the operator checks the status of the tissues (information travels from patient's tissues to the operator's brain).

Self-control practices and external focusing (i.e., with focus on the effect of the movement) are the factors that have been shown to improve the learning of motor skills. In addition, motor automatism of the palpatory technique, where the action can be performed without conscious thought, allows enough cognitive space for perceptive exploration. However, it is critical that the method of palpation becomes a learning tool rather than a strict protocol to follow or additional data to learn. The purpose of a method like the one whose principles are being described would be greatly compromised if it were to increase the cognitive load in learning palpation techniques, rather than reducing it.[5]

The seven steps are as follows:

1. *Comfortable positioning of the operator*: discomfort related to postural constraints of the practitioner must be avoided in order to ensure the quality of palpation.

2. *Three-dimensional anatomical view*: during palpation there must be an external focus of attention (in the direction of the motion's effect) to maximize the learning of motor skills.[6] For less experienced operators, the mental representation may be limited to the fundamental characteristics of the structure or the joint, while for advanced operators it may be more complex, since it includes, for example, its relationship with adjacent structures and/or the axis of movement, or even the individual anatomical variations.

3. *Contact depth level*: to ensure the effectiveness of the technique, the palpation should be performed to the depth that allows perception of the movement.

4. *Target identification and maintenance of it for the entire duration of palpation*: the combination of the operator's positioning stages, its focus on the objective and the use of the principle of visualization decrees the success in learning complex movements in sports, in music and in surgery.[7–9] Moreover, visualization techniques are efficient enough to cause a cerebral reorganization that helps to improve the skill in palpation.[10]

5. *Integration of the evaluation of the parameters of an area with respect to the parameters of the surrounding areas*: the operator should use an initial point of contact to mobilize or normalize the structure to be tested and simultaneously monitor the effect of such movement on a corresponding reference point. This process promotes self-control, self-learning, and self-evaluation.

6. *Optimization of the five steps above and perceptive exploration*: integration of the quantitative components of motion (amplitude, asymmetry, etc.) with the qualitative components (tissue surface, sensitivity, response to touch, be it of defense or pleasure, changes in the structure of the tissue, density, elasticity, heat, vitality, etc.) for understanding the normal state of the explored tissues.

7. *Evaluate, standardize, and evaluate*: comparison of the state of tissues before and after normalization.

### References

1. Esteves JE, Spence C. Developing competence in diagnostic palpation: perspectives from neuroscience and education. Int J Osteopath Med. 2013;17.

2. Ericsson KA, Prietula MJ, Cokely ET. The making of an expert. Harv Bus Rev. 2007;85(7–8):114–21, 193.

3. Aubin A, Gagnon K, Morin C. The seven-step palpation method: a proposal to improve palpation skills. Int J Osteopath Med. 2014;17(1):66–72.

4. Bordage G. Prototypes and semantic qualifiers: from past to present. Med Educ. 2007;41(12):1117–21.

5. Lee TD, Swanson LR, Hall AL. What is repeated in a repetition? Effects of practice conditions on motor skill acquisition. Phys Ther. 1991;71(2):150–6, (1): 52–60.

6. Wulfs G, Shea C, Lewthwaite R. Motor skill learning and performance: a review of influential factors. Med Educ. 2010;44(1):75–84.

7. Hall JC. Imagery practice and the development of surgical skills. Am J Surg. 2002;184(5):465–70.

8. Driskell JE, Cooper C, Moran A. Does mental practice enhance performance? J Appl Psychol. 1994;79(4):481–92.

9. Sanders CW, Sadoski M, Bramson R et al. Comparing the effects of physical practice and mental imagery rehearsal on learning basic surgical skills by medical students. Am J Obstetrics Gynecol. 2004;191(5):1811–14.

10. Jackson PL, Lafleur MF, Malouin F et al. Functional cerebral reorganization following motor sequence learning through mental practice with motor imagery. Neuroimage. 2003;20(2):1171–80.

## Evaluation of general adaptation: global tests

Global tests are aimed at assessing the state of health of the person and their capacity for general adaptation to endogenous and exogenous environmental stresses. This includes performing procedures such as the Zink test on the fascial compensation scheme (CFS) or the evaluation test on the dynamics of fluids and involuntary rhythms (DyFIR) (see Chapters 3 and 6) as well as the fascial compartments test.

### "Fascial compensation scheme" (FCS) test or assessment of the dynamics of fluids and involuntary rhythms (DyFIR) (see Chapter 3)

Environmental stresses are stored within compensating fascial patterns, both in persons capable of adaptation and in those subjected to high allostatic load. It is believed that fascial compensation represents a useful answer, beneficial, functional (in the absence of obvious symptoms), by the musculoskeletal system, as a result of anomalies such as a shorter lower limb or excessive use. Decompensation describes the same phenomenon except that the changes of adaptation are dysfunctional, symptomatic, and highlight the failure of homeostatic mechanisms (adaptation and self-repair).

Through tissue preference tests (tension/laxity) in different transition areas, Zink and Lawson[23] argue that it is possible to classify patterns in a clinically useful way. For each region the test induces a slight rotation and/or alternating inclination to the left and to the right, as if it were applied on a cylinder, choosing which of the two directions is qualitatively preferred.

Thus, the following are detected:

• Neutral FCS: not affecting distant regions with tissue tensions (see Fig. 3.7)

• Compensated FCS: referring to a capacity to adapt to environmental stresses, in which the osteopath detects an allostatic process of the first type through the alternated tissue preference between one area and another (see Fig. 3.8)

- decompensated FCS: referring to an allostatic load of the second type, detectable through the non-alternating tissue preference between one area and the other. The osteopath interprets this condition as a probable loss of the ability of the person to adapt to stimuli (see Chapter 3).

The test can also be done intentionally, inducing an alternating of fluid dynamics. This latter modality can be used as a confirmation of the results obtained with the classic procedure described above.

Global and local evaluation of DyFIR can instead detect:

- harmony of the fluid rhythm on the longitudinal axis; or fragmentation of the rhythm on the vertical orientation of the person's body (often associated with decompensated/failed patterns), directing the osteopath toward the use of adaptogenic techniques with a global focus on balancing the DyFIR (the function dominates the structure). The test can be performed with bimanual catches along the poles of the midline, or testing the harmony or the fragmentation of the rhythm of the fluids of different cavities between the transitional areas (craniocervical, thoracic, abdominal, and pelvic)

- an area (e.g., between two transitional areas) with DyFIR more inert with respect to the other, driving the osteopath to proceed toward local tests that could confirm the presence of a dysfunctional area. In this case the osteopathic would perform a targeted treatment to regenerate the vitality of local or segmental self-regulating systems (the structure dominates the function).

The transitional areas also represent a functional unit that finalizes the corporeal alignment to the central line of gravity by modulating the energy expenditure in achieving stability. In addition to being connected to the articulating junctional areas of the spine and to transverse diaphragms, they are connected to the entire connective tissue system of the body, through organization in longitudinal tubular compartments, such as the visceral and meningeal fascia, through fascial junction areas that may experience fibrotic adhesions in case of high stressed metabolic load, such as emotional and neuroendocrine. A distortion of a transitional area implies a myofascial torsion of the entire longitudinal axis. Consequently, its function will be altered by corporeal vascular pumping, respiratory efficiency, and the corresponding fluidic dynamics, with consequent increase of mechanical stress on the longitudinal axis. For this reason, if the test of preferential rotation detects decompensated areas of transition, which consecutively rotate in the same direction, it is considered necessary to integrate the FCS evaluation with the test of the fascial compartments (FCT), i.e., the tubular longitudinal organization of the fascia in its axial, visceral. and meningeal components.[86]

## Test of fascial compartments

In this work we classify the fascial system of the body as pannicular, axial, meningeal, and visceral fascia, as described by Willard and colleagues[86] (Fig. 1.5).

The axial-appendicular fascia comes from the somatic mesenchyme and resides inside the pannicular fascia, where it covers the epimysium, the periosteum, and the peritendineum.

1. The axial component is organized into two tubular compartments, separated from the spine (notochord in the embryonic stage):

   - a front portion surrounding the hypaxial muscles (long neck, scalene, intercostals, and oblique and rectus abdominus) and inserting on the transverse processes

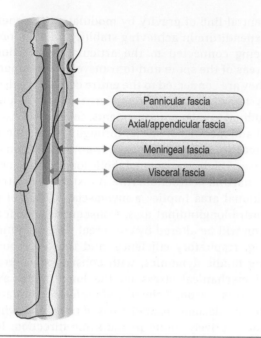

**Fig. 1.5**
Tubular fascial compartments. Pannicular, axial, visceral, and meningeal fascia. The figure refers to the classification of: Willard FH, Fossum C, Standley PR. The fascial system of the body. In: Chila A, editor. Foundations of osteopathic medicine. 3rd ed. Philadelphia: Lippincott Williams and Wilkins; 2010. ch. 7, fig. 7.13, p. 81.

– a rear portion surrounding the epaxial muscles, organizing themselves into two tubes that insert on the transverse processes and spinous process.

2. The appendicular component surrounds the nerve plexuses, such as the brachial and lumbar plexus, and organizes itself with a soft tissue skeleton that unfolds from the thoracolumbar fascia in the midline to the limbs through a tendinous junction system and multiplanar connective interconnections, defined with terms such as "ectoskeleton," "super-tendon," "dynament" (see Chapter 4). The osteopath applies the test over this fascial plan, focusing his or her attention on the effect of rigidity/tension on the tissue's resilience, which today is well described by parameters of tissue mechanics, such as viscoelasticity, thixotropy, and the ability

to resist a deformation that follows from the application of a compressive or tensional force. The test approaches the appendicular component through internal-external rotation, flexion, extension, compression, and tensioning, applied to the kinematic thoracic-lumbar-femoral and cervical-thoracic-brachial chains, to assess the degree of fluidity of the movement, of the gliding of the fascial planes on the underlying tissues, or an eventual restriction of it, be it general or in a particular region. This permits a further assessment with a second phase of the test, during which, through the pressure locally exerted on the previously identified region, it identifies the rigidity to pressure and release of a particular area compared to the surrounding areas. The test of the appendicular/ectoskeleton component is performed in different phases with the patient in the supine and/or prone position (Fig. 1.6). During scanning of this compartment the dysfunctional component of the axial portion is also tested, including any possible adhesion with the visceral fascial compartment, through a procedure that in the osteopathic tradition is defined as the central tendon test (see Chapter 6). This procedure involves scanning of the superior-posterior, superior-anterior and inferior portions (see Chapter 6) and rating the degree of tissue elasticity and the emergence of vectors of deviation and twisting in dysfunctional conditions.

3. The meningeal fascial band is the third layer and surrounds the nervous system. This layer includes the dura mater and the underlying leptomeninges, derived from the primitive meninges surrounding the embryonic nervous system. In particular, the spinal meninges are derived from the somatic mesoderm, while the meninges of the brainstem arise from the cephalic mesoderm and the telencephalic meninges from the neural crest[87] (Fig. 1.7). The meningeal fascia is continuous with the epineurium surrounding the peripheral nerve. The meningeal sac suspends the spinal cord in its continuity with the bulb at the level of the occipital foramen, with the nerves that pass into the conjugate foramen and denticulate ligaments, or pial expansions that

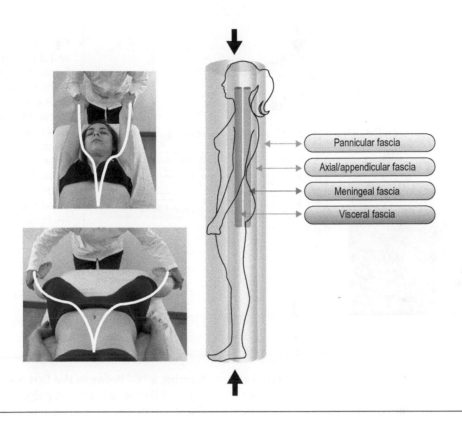

Pannicular fascia

Axial/appendicular fascia

Meningeal fascia

Visceral fascia

**Fig. 1.6**
Test of the axial-appendicular/ectoskeleton. With the patient in supine and then in prone position, the osteopath proceeds with the phase of passive mobility through internal-external rotation, flexion, extension, compression, and tension applied to the thoracic-lumbar-femoral (a) and cervical-thoracic-brachial (b) kinematic chains. The degree of fluidity of the movement is rated, and then further evaluation is done to determine any restricted areas of kinematics, thanks to the palpatory phase of the test. During the latter, by means of pressure exerted locally, the objective is to note the rigidity to pressure and release of an area compared to the surrounding areas. The objective of this phase is to assess the status of elasticity of the entire compartment, i.e., its property of returning to its original shape after a force is applied. Elasticity expresses the static (linear) and dynamic (viscoelastic) relationship between stress and tension of the tissue. The figure refers to the classification of: Willard FH, Fossum C, Standley PR. The fascial system of the body. In: Chila A, editor. Foundations of osteopathic medicine. 3rd ed. Philadelphia: Lippincott Williams and Wilkins; 2010. ch. 7, fig. 7.13, p. 81.

are carried toward the outside by the two lateral columns of the cord to the deep arachnoid fascia fixed to the dura mater, which are inserted by means of fibrous arch systems. These ligaments do not reach as far laterally as the arachnoid and in fact are so named because, while the medial ends are continuous and always adherent to the entire length of the spinal cord, the lateral edges are attached in some points and free in others. For this reason this structure has a festooned appearance when viewed from the side (laterally). The free margin is located at the levels where nerve roots emerge. In performing the test of the meningeal fascia (see Fig. 1.7), the osteopath asks the person to take a supine or lateral decubitus position, and listens with simultaneous palpation on the vertex and coccyx. The evaluation aims to perceive harmony of the longitudinal fluctuation

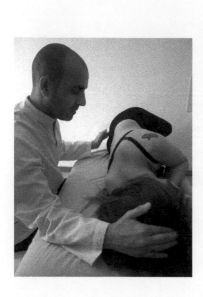

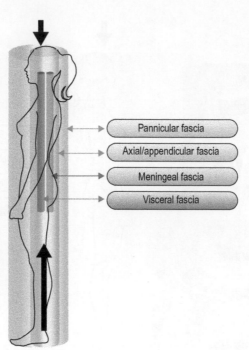

Pannicular fascia

Axial/appendicular fascia

Meningeal fascia

Visceral fascia

**Fig. 1.7**
Test of the meningeal fascia. The osteopath is positioned with hands resting on the vertex and coccyx. The evaluation aims to perceive any harmony or disharmony of the fluid dynamics of the posterior midline. The figure refers to the classification of: Willard FH, Fossum C, Standley PR. The fascial system of the body. In: Chila A, editor. Foundations of osteopathic medicine. 3rd ed. Philadelphia: Lippincott Williams and Wilkins; 2010. ch. 7, fig. 7.13, p. 81.

or any lateral fluctuations, twists, deviations, or interruptions of that median line between the selected contact points. The evaluation includes a second phase of deepening of the test, during which, through pressure locally exerted on the previously identified region, the objective is to evaluate the rigidity to pressure and release of an area compared to the surrounding area.

4. The visceral fascia is described as the fourth fascial plane, with embryological derivation from the splanchnic tissue. It is located on the anterior midline, extending from the base of the skull to the pelvic cavity, surrounding the pleural, pericardial, and peritoneal cavities. In performing the test of the visceral fascia (Fig. 1.8), the osteopath asks the person to take a supine position and stands at the side of the table. For a general evaluation, one hand palpates the anterior cervical region, forming a "C" between the first and second fingers, while the other hand palpates the anterior presacral area, again forming a "C" outlet between the first and second fingers. For an assessment of the cervicothoracic portion, one hand approaches the anterior cervical region,

forming a "C" between the first and second fingers, while the other hand palpates the body of the sternum. For an assessment of the thoracic-abdominal portion, one hand will be placed at the xiphoid process and sternal portion of the seventh and eighth ribs, while the other hand will be placed at the anterior presacral area. The osteopath induces an initial oscillation and then notes:

– under normal conditions, there is oscillatory uniformity along the anterior midline of the entire visceral fascial "tube;" fluid dynamics should be homogeneous along the anterior midline of the entire visceral fascial "tube"

– in the case of minor dysfunction, however, it feels like a fascial twist of the region, with a slight lateral deviation with greater amounts of dysfunction. In severe cases, one will experience a large lateral deviation. The assessment includes a second phase of the test's progression, during which, through pressure locally exerted on the previously identified region, one notes a rigidity in the cervicothoracic or abdominopelvic portion of the visceral fascia.

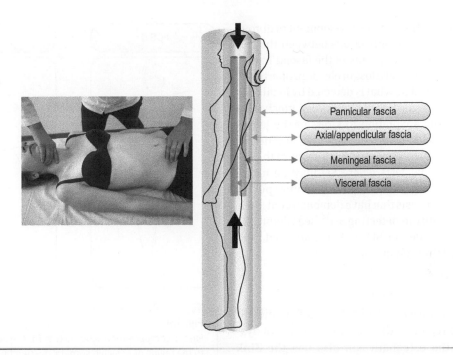

**Fig. 1.8**
Test of the visceral fascia. The osteopath induces an initial oscillation and then notes the oscillatory homogeneity or fascial twist/deviation along the anterior midline of the entire visceral fascial "tube." In this illustration, for a general evaluation, the right hand approaches the anterior cervical region, forming a "C" between the first and second finger, while the left hand, also forming a "C" between the first and second finger, approaches the anterior presacral area. For an assessment of the cervicothoracic portion, the right hand approaches the anterior cervical region of the neck, forming a "C" between the first and second finger, while the right hand is positioned on the sternal body. For an assessment of the thoracoabdominal portion, the right hand is placed on the xiphoid process and sternal portion of the seventh and eighth rib, while the left hand is placed on the anterior presacral area. The figure refers to the classification of: Willard FH, Fossum C, Standley PR. The fascial system of the body. In: Chila A, editor. Foundations of osteopathic medicine. 3rd ed. Philadelphia: Lippincott Williams and Wilkins; 2010. ch. 7, figs. 7.12–7.15, pp. 82–3.

## Evaluation of local adaptation: regional, local, and inhibition tests

Local tests are aimed at assessing the presence of SD or local adaptation of tissues to endogenous and exogenous environmental stress. Louisa Burns reported, in 1948, the ability to detect SD in the tissue, which under certain conditions becomes hyperemic, congested, and edematous. These conditions were defined as "petechial hemorrhages" that emerge as a result of coagulation processes and are organized through fibrosis and ischemia.[88] In essence, it could be the process that produces fibrotic adhesions over time as a result of chronic inflammatory processes.[89]

Activated immune cells release cytokines that stimulate fibrocytes to generate additional collagen during the repair process. The collagen manifests an irregular shape and, when these cells are excessive, can form adhesions that reach pathological proportions. Adhesions can occur in any region of the body, both visceral and somatic. Adhesions can wrap the tubular intestine and hamper the movement within its lumen or interfere with the functions of the reproductive organs, similar to the synovial sheaths, for example, in the carpal tunnel, interfering with the movement of the digital flexor tendons. A dysfunctional memory may be imprinted in the tissues, prior to the formation of true adhesions, through the development of fibrous infiltration with cross-connections between the collagen fibers in the nodal points of the fascial bands, together with a progressive loss of elastic properties.[90] This condition could be what is detected by local tests that assess the tissue and biotensegrity mechanics which govern the adaptation to stress of the joints, soft tissues, fascia, and visceral, vascular, and neural related structures. In this regard, the osteopath proceeds with regional tests where SD may be manifested. The following are descriptions of some specific tests selected from tests that have demonstrated inter-examiner reliability in detecting SD[14] (see Chapter 2). The severity of different SD is then evaluated, and finally verified through inhibition tests.

### Regional tests

- *Localization through the FCS*   As a first indication of the region with probable presence of dysfunction, the osteopath can also use the Zink test. In fact, the FCS may sometimes present as decompensations, for example, in only two of the four transition areas, pointing the osteopath to the likely presence of SD in the corresponding cavity between the two diaphragms (Fig. 1.9). The test is also used in osteopathic practice to identify the origin and nature of the dysfunctional component, although this was far from the objective for which the test was originally conceived. Some authors, for example, suggest the use of the FCS test even with the patient standing, comparing its results with those obtained in the supine position. This is to rule in or out any interference of the lower limbs on the test and then consider possible ascending dysfunctional patterns from the hips, knees, and ankles. In this case, decompensated patterns in standing should improve significantly in the supine position, while primary descendant dysfunctions would show decompensated patterns both in standing and in supine positions.[91]

- *The Gait test*   When applying the regional test, the osteopath is centered on the fascial network,

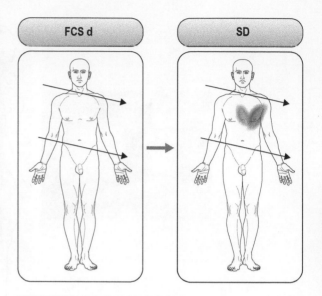

FCS d          SD

**Fig. 1.9**

Fascial compensation scheme test for the approach to the region of possible somatic dysfunction (SD). In cases where the Zink test shows a mild degree of decompensation, or between two transitional areas, the osteopath will proceed with other tests to assess the likely presence of SD in the cavity between the two diaphragms.

a system that extends and permeates from capsules to internal organs and could therefore be involved in both the origin and the resolution of somatic and visceral disorders. Recent work by Finando and Finando[92] suggests that the fascia is the medium involved in the effects of acupuncture on organ pathology. When the body is stressed or traumatized, the fascia responds by synthesizing new fibers to provide support to the injured area and "gluing" tissues, organs and muscles adjacent to each other.[93] Thickening and sticking of fascial layers can persist long after an injury has healed and leave behind clumps of non-resilient bands that can be perceived by palpation deep into the tissues.[94] These palpable densities may correspond to SD at the trigger points and at the stretched bands described by Travell and Simons[95] or at the inflammatory pockets described by Selye[96] as an expression of the local adaptation syndrome. Residual local tensions and fascial network adhesions can lead to compensatory tensions that extend throughout the musculoskeletal system. Such compensations can disrupt structures more distant from each other, leading to compromised movement patterns that leave the body vulnerable to further injury. The regional tests allow you to access any part of the living system from any location by palpating and applying light forces,[97] through the perception of adhesions in the fascial network of horizontal diaphragms, cables, and longitudinal tubes, which leads the operator to the regions where there are one or more SDs. For this evaluation, the authors propose the use of the gait test (Fig. 1.10), in which the osteopath asks the patient to walk, and observing weight-bearing on one leg, while the other shows a slight flexion of knee and hip. The osteopath maintains anterior–posterior contact with both hands and notices any restrictions of the harmonic movement observed in the patient's tissues during the execution of the movement. Any pivotal areas could probably be detected inside the cavity delineated by the two transitional areas that demonstrated decompensation (non-alternating) in the SCF test previously performed. The fascial tubular compartments may experience fibrotic adhesions that the osteopath can detect by testing the presence of alteration of the gliding, in the cavities between the transition areas, between the axial, the visceral and the meningeal fascia. The osteopath perceives a rotational movement/inclination alternating between the two hands in the absence of adhesions; conversely, in the presence of adhesions, the osteopath perceives a block or an alteration of the rotational movement/inclination, which suggests a possible presence of SD in the region, which can be investigated and eventually confirmed before the test of attraction/fascial listening and then by specific tests of the area.

- *Test of attraction/fascial listening* Following the same rationale,[97] one can perform another regional test, called the test of attraction/fascial listening test (Fig. 1.11). In this phase of the evaluation, the modus operandi is based on two essential material properties of the retention zone (SD): retraction and density/laxity. Resting on the area in dysfunction, the hand of the operator will identify the density during contact, and, if palpating at a distance, it will be attracted by the altered density. When the operator's hand is attracted, it analyzes two important things: (1) the direction of the traction in a region of the body; (2) the width of the traction that indicates whether the area "calling" is near or far, meaning that the longer the traction seems, the further away is the dysfunctional area. Such sensation results from the fact that, by approaching a restricted region, one can perceive the alteration of the tissue's texture. A period of comprehensive listening is then performed: the direction and magnitude indicate the dysfunctional area. The subject in orthostatic position keeps the legs slightly apart and a horizontal gaze. The osteopath, positioned behind the patient, gently places a flat hand on the subject's head, inducing a small compression such as to allow the hand to take the shape of the underlying structure, to follow any eventual movement of the body in an anterior, anterior–lateral or posterior direction, and to create a vector of tension between the head and the ground. Sometimes, the tissues included between the two points show a traction force that can provide an indication of the presence of SD in the region. A period of local listening is then performed: when the area is detected, we apply a slight compression between the hands. The force vector that emerges is perceived between the hands and indicates the dysfunctional area, where specific tests for the assessment of somatic dysfunction are performed.[14]

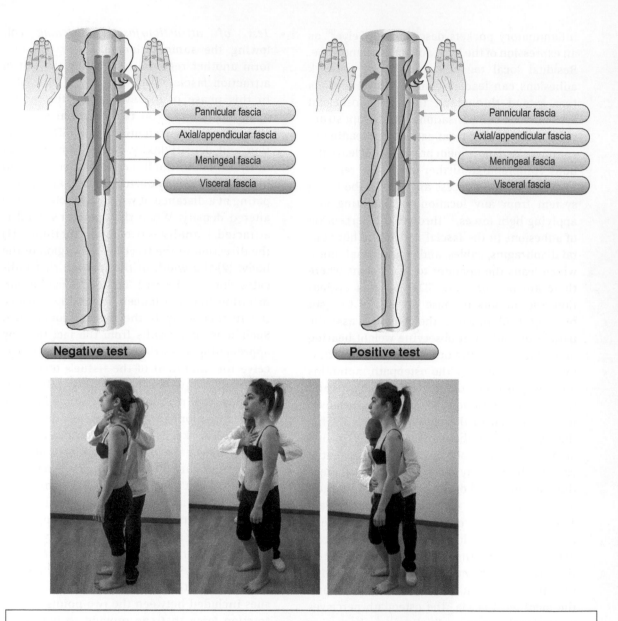

**Fig. 1.10**
Gait test for the approach to the region with possible presence of somatic dysfunction (SD). The osteopath asks the patient to make movements standing on the spot, shifting the weight from one inferior joint to the other, the latter flexed alternately. Using a two-handed anterior-posterior approach, the osteopath assesses tension areas that limit the kinetics of movement. *Note*: in the execution of the test phase, in which the operator approaches the cervical area with a two-hand palpation in anterior-posterior mode, one must take care not to compress the anterior and lateral aspects of the visceral region of the neck, so as to avoid any kind of discomfort to the patient.

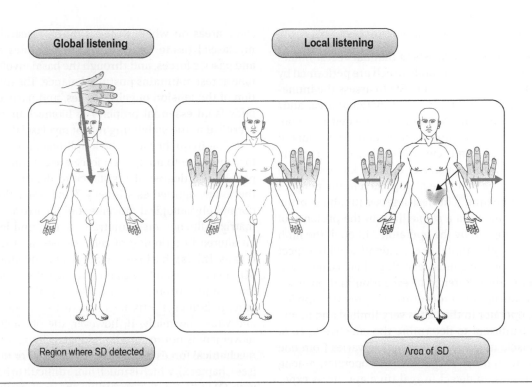

Global listening

Local listening

Region where SD detected

Area of SD

**Fig. 1.11**
Test of fascial attraction/global and local listening. Using a slight compression and release of tissues, the operator's hand is drawn to changes in tissue texture of dysfunctional areas, sensing the direction and magnitude of the traction that directs it toward a body region with the possible presence of somatic dysfunction (SD).

## Local tests

The specific tests used in the area are determined from theoretical considerations concerning the ways in which the presence of SD can affect the performance of the tissues, preventing the movement of fluids (causing edema or hardening and hindering the elimination of waste through the venous and lymphatic system), irritating the nerve endings (both chemically with the accumulation of toxins and mechanically with the accumulation of fluids). The resulting nociceptive impulses cause the activation of additional impulses from the central nervous system, which simultaneously affect the activity of visceral organs and the connective tissue throughout the sympathetic nervous system. Viscerosomatic and somatovisceral reflexes can lead to an irritation that originates from an organ and involves the connective tissue, and vice versa (see Chapter 2). The objectification of SD is the result of a palpatory investigation into whether there is at least one of the four criteria described by the acronym TART (tissue texture abnormality, asymmetry, restriction of motion, tenderness), i.e., alteration of tissue structure, asymmetry, restriction of mobility, and hyperesthesia or tenderness caused by palpation.[14] During the decision-making process, at the end of the local tests, the osteopath can detect different SDs in a person. One must also assess their severity, accessibility, and clinical relevance for the patient. This can be evaluated by the osteopath with reference to the severity of SD, i.e., by the detection of one or more parameters of the TART acronym in the dysfunctional area (see Chapter 2). In this regard, some professionals also practice the inhibition test.

## Dysfunctional hierarchy: inhibition test

The inhibition test consists of manual vector induction stimuli of a few seconds which are performed by the osteopath on an area of SD to assess the immediate response in another dysfunctional area, and/or a compensated area, and/or a related function. Many osteopaths, chiropractors and other manual therapists use the muscle provocation test, classically described in the context of applied kinesiology, to select the area and type of approach to the person's area of complaint.[98] The test assesses the ability of the person to maintain a stable limb in the presence of pressure applied by the operator. Although the limb position may be similar or even identical with respect to a corresponding muscle testing, there is, however, an important difference of execution and purpose. In fact, during the procedure, the pressure applied by the operator in the test is very limited and in any case insufficient to determine the effective force of the muscle involved. This response varies from one person to another and allows the operator, among other things, to detect in real time any stress experienced by the person, which can be physical, structural, biochemical, nutritional, emotional, mental, or even purely energetic. The change in response to muscle testing would occur due to changes of facilitation/excitation and inhibition of the motor neuron path, anterior horn and muscle; this does not seem to be the same as for kinesiology tests.[98] The inhibition test practiced by many osteopaths is also a challenge test. However, in the decision-making process, the operator is guided by agreement between the patient's history, clinical reasoning and the results of different tests, among which is a confirmatory test, such as the inhibition test. This test is performed by the osteopath in order to assess the most relevant and accessible SD, not necessarily to evaluate approaches to the disease. However, as with other tests, we need to rely on evidence obtained from methodological studies on diagnostic reliability and evaluation of inter-operator agreement, as well as studies relating to the mechanisms underlying the tissue responses that the operator uses to guide the treatment plan. In this regard, the current evidence relating to the physiology of mechanical tissue[99] allows us to hypothesize some areas on which to focus future research: the myofascial tissue network, which integrates active and passive forces, and through the basal myofascial tone at rest maintains postural balance. The integration of the tension of cells, tissues, and parts of the body is an essential property of biomechanics and is critical to the stabilizing role of myofascial tone at rest. The frequency and the amplitude of the vibratory response to an applied force are determined in part by the degree of resistance to deformation of the tissue, defined as stiffness.[99] The restrictions to normal physiological movement of the extracellular matrix influence mechanotransduction and lead to an altered functioning of cells, tissues, and related organs. This is what in osteopathy could coincide with SD. If you re-establish the physiological movement, for example, through the use of osteopathic manipulative treatment, the tissue returns to its previous state and works normally. If, however, the physiological movement is not restored, prolonged changes in the mechanical forces may lead to chronic SD or fibrosis (see Chapter 2), which is much more difficult to handle with OMT.[100] Studies regarding the contractile and sensory mechanical properties of the fascial network are extremely important for the understanding of disorder or somatic and visceral dysfunction. However, although on the one hand they help us in understanding the long-term responses that are obtained from the application of osteopathic and complementary techniques, such as acupuncture, on the other they do not explain the response of immediate improvement in tissue texture found by different studies.[101] McMakin and Oschman say that such quick reflexes might have an energy base in specific paths of the fascial network[101] and underlie the rationale of the inhibition test. Non-neurological communication occurs throughout the entire fascia. Because of their piezoelectric nature, the collagen fibers and ground substance create an instant communication outside of that provided by the nervous system. Thus, electric currents can be effectuated up to the intracellular level.[102] This occurs thanks to the effect of semiconductor bioelectric currents that differ from the ionic currents of nerves and neuromuscular junctions as they travel across the fascia and on the perineurium surrounding nerve fibers.[102] The movement of electricity along a conductor or semiconductor (nerves, fascia) produces bio-electromagnetic fields that can be detected with sensitive instruments or certain sensory receptors of the skin. These fields extend into and out of the body indefinitely and may be influenced by external electromagnetic fields.[103] Bioenergetics of the SD component can then be perceived during osteopathic palpation through the emergence of vectors of forces of attraction and amplitude greater than the inherent movements perceptible in a normal tissue.[104] The execution of the inhibition test (as the procedure used for the hierarchization of the SD; see Chapter 2) requires that the operator simulate vectors of forces for a few seconds, in an area of severe dysfunction, up to what could be equal to the

improvement of the stiffness of the matrix, a probable stabilization of the fascial tone at rest. Thus even related dysfunctional distant areas can temporarily improve their structure and functionality in terms of mobility, plasticity, viscosity, thixotropy, and vibratory resonant frequency.[99] The operator also decides if the stimulus on the SD area improves signs related to the clinical condition reported by the person, such as, for example, the amplitude of joint movement, muscle strength, or level of pain reported as a result of a semeiotic orthopedic test (Lasègue, Soto Hall, etc.). In this case, the operator defines the primary area as being that which, if stimulated, produces an improvement of structure and function in both the same and related areas of focus during treatment (Box 1.2).

---

**Box 1.2**

## Decision-making: the somatic dysfunction hierarchy and approach selection

Consider, for example, low back pain arising, in the absence of trauma, in a 40-year-old athletic male. No particular sign of stress is reported in the history except for a change of eating habits with increased consumption of red meat and milk products. Lab tests are normal, and diagnostic imaging tests in the lumbar area are negative for instability or space-occupying masses. Let us assume, for example, that the osteopath detects a positive result during the physical examination in the Lasègue test, with mild tenderness caused by 30° of passive flexion of the patient's right hip. In the global osteopathic evaluation there is a compensated FCS, a dysfunctional right hypochondriac region. The patient is also evaluated using regional tests, gait test and test of the lumbar-femoral (crural) kinematic chains, in which, with a contact on the feet of the patient, internal rotation of the limbs is performed to see if one of them is limited by tissue tension in a limb, abdomen, or other body part (Fig. 1.12). The execution of local tests permits the diagnosis of SD of the first lumbar vertebra (the parameter of dysfunction detected by palpation is the alteration of the structure of the tissue), SD of the right kidney (the dysfunctional parameters detected by palpation are alteration of the structure of the tissue

and restriction of mobility, causing sensitivity). The osteopath considers the renal dysfunction to be more severe, but proceeds by performing an inhibition test (Fig. 1.13) to confirm his or her deduction. At first, with the patient in supine position, with the palm of his or her right hand, the operator inserts vector parameters addressing them, e.g., on the kidney area, while the left hand perceives any changes in tissue tension in the area of the first lumbar. Any one change confirms the primary area of restriction to be the kidney. Next, the osteopath asks the patient (still in the supine position) to position the volar side of his or her right hand in the posterior area of the right hypochondrium and the palmar side of the left hand cupped with the palmar and digital side placed on the abdomen, in the border region between the right hypochondriac area and the hip. The patient is asked to perform a small anterior-posterior compression and to continue normal breathing. Meanwhile, the osteopath repeats the regional tests of the lumbar-femoral kinematic chain and evaluates whether there are changes in the previously perceived restriction. Finally, still with the patient in supine position, with the palm of his or her left hand, he or she inserts vector parameters addressing them on the renal area, while with his or her right hand he or she repeats the Lasègue test previously performed to evaluate any change in the result. If there is disappearance of the tenderness with 30° of passive flexion, or tenderness occurs with a higher degree of passive flexion, for example 60°, the osteopath observes that the SD of the renal area is able to interact with the other dysfunctional areas, and there may be possible involvement of the nerves (e.g., sciatic, tibial, sural, common peroneal). The operator concludes that the SD detected as a result of this integrative process between history, observation, and testing is clinically more relevant to the patient at that moment. Therefore the osteopath will give a treatment using a minimalist approach, probably also considering an approach to the symptomatic area, for example through techniques on soft tissues and articulations of the lumbar area, as well as the continuous management of the case with any specific exercises.

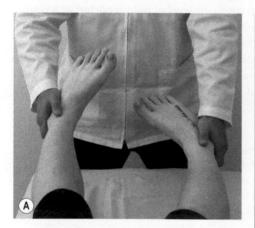

(A)

**Fig. 1.12**
Regional tests of the lumbar – femoral (A) and thoracic-cranial-cervical-brachial (B) kinematic chains. (A) The osteopath, positioned at the patient's feet and with the patient in the supine position, makes bilateral contact with the calcaneal/Achilles tendon areas and internally rotates the limbs to evaluate whether there is limited motion in one of them, due to tissue tension in a limb, in the abdomen or in another part of the body. (B) The osteopath, positioned at the patient's head and with the patient in supine, makes bilateral contact with the palms of hands and flexes and internally rotates the wrists, arms, and shoulders, to assess any limitations due to tissue tension in a limb, in the chest or in another body part. (C) The osteopath performs internal rotation of the limbs to evaluate if one of these is limited by tissue tension exerted on a limb, from a region of the body. (D) In this example, the osteopath detects a restriction of the kinematics of the left lower limb, probably linked to a restriction in the lumbar area/left hip; the operator will proceed with specific local tests of the area to assess the presence of any somatic dysfunction (SD).

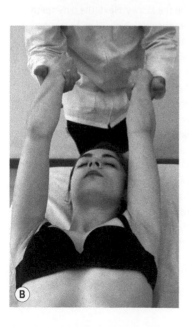

(B)

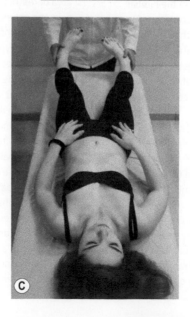

(C)

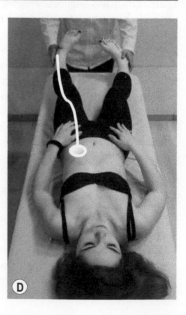

(D)

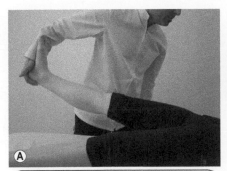

(A)

Lasègue test execution with mild tenderness outcome caused by the 30° passive flexion of the right hip of the patient.

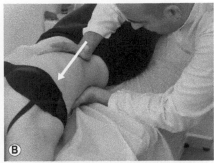

(B)

The insertion of vector parameters in the kidney area (right hand) evokes changes in tissue tension in the area of the first lumbar (left hand); we can deduce a primacy of the area.

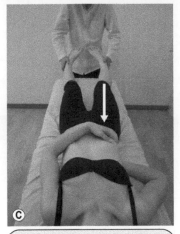

(C)

A small compression exercised by the patient on the kidney area previously highlighted normalizes the amplitude of the joint's movement.

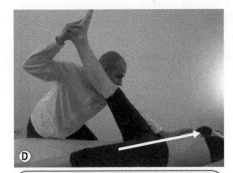

(D)

The insertion of vectorial parameters on the kidney area (left hand) previously highlighted coincides with a negative result of the clinical test (e.g. the test of Lasègue).

**Fig. 1.13**

Inhibition test: example of testing to confirm the dysfunctional hierarchy. (A) Lasègue test execution with mild tenderness provoked by 30° passive flexion of the patient's right hip. (B) The patient is in supine position, the osteopath is positioned at the right side of the table; the operator proceeds with an inhibition test that allows him to verify the hierarchy among the different dysfunctions previously hypothesized through the assessment of severity; in this example, the palm of his or her right hand inserts vector parameters addressing the kidney area, while his or her left hand perceives any changes in tissue tension in the area of the first lumbar. Any change confirms the kidney area as the primary area of somatic dysfunction (SD). (C) Next, the osteopath asks the supine patient to place the volar side of her right hand in the posterior area of the right hypochondrium and the palmar side of the left hand cupped with the palmar and digital side placed on the abdomen, in the border region between the right hypochondriac and hip. The patient is asked to perform a small anterior-posterior compression while breathing normally. Meanwhile, the osteopath repeats the regional tests of the lumbar-femoral kinematic chain and evaluates whether there are changes in the previously perceived restriction. Finally, with the patient in supine, with the palm of his or her left hand, the osteopath induces vector parameters, addressing them to the renal area, while with his or her right hand repeats the Lasègue test previously performed to evaluate any change in the result. If the tenderness disappears at flexion of 30°, or there is tenderness at a higher degree of passive flexion, for example 60°, the osteopath concludes that the SD of the renal area is the primary one.

## Interdependence between structure and function: inhibition test

Regarding the assessment of the interdependence between structure and function we shall proceed with a test to evaluate the dominance between decompensation noted in the FCS test and clinically relevant SD, which we will call the structure/function inhibition test (Fig. 1.14). In some cases, the operator proceeds with a structure/function inhibition test specific for each model that will be discussed in detail in Section 2. In structure/function inhibition tests specific for each model, the alteration of a function, or particular use of a model, for example postural control in the biomechanical model, is confronted with the clinically relevant SD. The operator evaluates whether or not the response of the function improves by applying direct and/or indirect vector parameters on tissue affected by SD. Improvement of the functional assessment (e.g., better postural control by retesting after inhibition of the SD) is interpreted by the operator as the dominance of the structure or of the SD over the function. This suggests a minimalist approach to the osteopath, with treatment of the SD through a specific technique. If inhibition of SD does not produce improved function, the operator will proceed with maximalist approaches. Inhibition tests of structure/function specific for each model therefore have the purpose of discriminating between the use of a maximal or a minimal approach in treatment.[33]

- *Maximalist approach*: this is used when function dominates one or more related structures, undermining salutogenesis. The choice will be to use techniques of stimulation of physiological functions capable of resolving the SD or correlated dysfunctions.

- *Minimalist approach*: this is used when one or more structures dominate a related function, undermining salutogenesis. The choice will be to use techniques that, by normalizing an area of SD that is dominant compared to other patterns, i.e., of high energy expenditure for the functions related to it and for the whole person, will modulate the activity of previously dormant self-regulating systems.

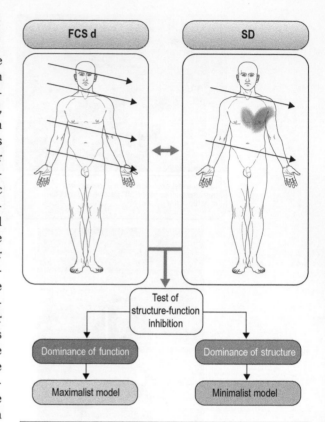

**Fig. 1.14**
Test of structure/function inhibition. This is applied through procedures that utilize the principles of inhibition. The osteopath assesses the interdependence between structure and function and is guided toward a maximalist or minimalist approach.

The techniques that derive from this algorithm can have global, regional/local, and segmental focus:

- *Global*: generally adaptogenic (this term is proposed in this text in place of the more commonly used term "homeostatic") techniques, not used to directly normalize an SD, but to stimulate the body's self-regulation systems, physiological functions of energy supply and elimination of waste products, and the optimal relationship between the individual and environmental chronobiology.

- *Regional/segmental*: approaches that focus on myofascial, joint, neural, and vascular units that connect and influence the areas affected by SD with other areas, including the symptomatic area, through metameric relationships.

- *Local*: approaches that focus on SD areas recognized as clinically relevant for the person's presenting complaint and for his or her overall health.

So, in conclusion, in treatment each model can be applied with:

- maximalist emphasis: using standard adaptogenic, global, regional, sometimes a set of global, regional, and local techniques not addressing the SD, but focused on the modulation of a function

- minimalist emphasis: using standard local techniques to directly focus on the SD.

However, the uniqueness of the osteopathic approach puts emphasis on the decisional algorithm, which allows the operator to contextualize the principles by individualizing each treatment; the reader should therefore consider the techniques described in Section 2 not as being exclusive to a model, but rather as an example of the application of the problem-solving process that can be different each time, as it represents the relationship between different patients and operators (see Chapter 9).

## Treatment and techniques

Osteopathic treatment is focused on the mobility of the patient's body tissue, correlated with the state of general health. Osteopathy offers a range of manual techniques that address the SD that can be classified as direct, indirect, and combined,[2,3,18] as well as adaptogenic techniques, focused on the dynamics of (biological) fluids and the involuntary rhythms (DyFIR) related to them, in order to improve the general adaptive response (Fig. 1.15):

- **Direct techniques**: employ active forces to correct SD, engaging the joint restriction barrier or tissue elasticity.[2] Push, impulse, muscular

contraction, fascial loading, or a vast range of passive motions can be used to get the response of the tissues.

- **Indirect techniques**: the restrictive joint barrier or the tissue elasticity is disengaged to correct SD, until the tissue tension is equal in one or all of the planes and directions.[2] The functional method is an indirect treatment approach that requires the discovery of the point of dynamic balance plus one of the following: apply an indirect force, maintain the position or add compression to exaggerate the position, wait for spontaneous correction. The osteopath guides the manipulative procedure while the dysfunctional area is palpated in order to obtain continuous feedback of the physiological response to the induced movement. The osteopath guides the part in dysfunction so as to create a sense of decreasing resistance of the tissues (increased compliance).

- **Combined techniques**: these are applied in sequence.[2] First, the facilitated dysfunctional vectors are exaggerated until they reach the physiological barrier. Then the latter is maintained, while the operator applies a compression/traction force in an orthogonal direction with the dysfunctional tissue plane. Such a contact point is used as a pivot around which to apply the maneuver, conducting the tissues toward the restrictive barrier.

- **Adaptogenic techniques**: the term "adaptogenic" is proposed by the authors to replace the one usually used ("homeostatic"). "Adaptogen" in medicine originally refers to natural substances which have been proven to be able to normalize body functions and strengthen systems compromised by stress. They are reported to have a protective effect on health against a wide variety of environmental stressors and different stress-generating emotional conditions. The term adaptogen was originally created by Lazarev in 1947.[105] The general pharmacodynamic characteristics of an adaptogenic substance were described by Brekhman and Dardymov in 1969[106] as follows:

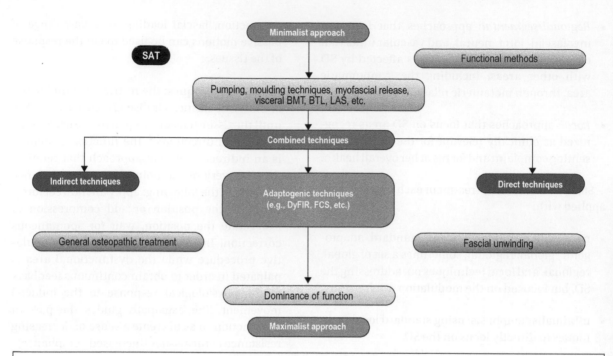

**Fig. 1.15**

Classification of techniques. Osteopathy offers a range of manual techniques that can be classified as: direct, indirect, or combined, to address somatic dysfunction (SD); also, adaptogenic techniques focused on the dynamics of fluids and involuntary rhythms (DyFIR) related to them and utilized to improve the general adaptive response. BLT: balanced ligamentous tension; BMT: balanced membranous tension; LAS: ligamentous articular strain. Modified from: Parsons J, Marcer N. Osteopathy: models for diagnosis, treatment and practice. Edinburgh: Elsevier Churchill Livingstone; 2006. p. 178.

– an adaptogen is non-toxic to the recipient

– an adaptogen tends to be nonspecific in its properties and acts by increasing the body's resistance through the modulation in a broad spectrum of different coordinating biological functions

– an adaptogen tends to be a regulator and normalizer of various systems of the receiving organism.

In osteopathy, homeostatic techniques are sometimes referred to as those approaches that do not focus on the SD, but on stimulating self-regulating systems. In the author's opinion, such techniques favor the adaptation by balancing the meta-system of homeostatic/allostatic regulation, and, for this

reason, in this text they will be defined as adaptogenic techniques. The techniques on the DyFIR focused on the balancing of autonomic and vascular functions related to tissue mechanics and aiming at the optimization of allostatic load serve as an example. The DyFIR can also be used by the osteopath as an activating force in combined mode together with direct and indirect approaches to the barriers identified in an SD, for example in some cranial techniques, where, in addition to the maintenance of a vector balancing point, one also uses tissue vitality defined as cranial rhythmic impulse (CRI). There are some techniques described in biodynamics that use an approach referred to as "potency" to release SD by harmonizing biological fluids.[107] These approaches, defined by the authors as DyFIR techniques, will be discussed from a contemporary point of view, including principles and applications, in the section dedicated to the osteopathic approach to fluids and involuntary rhythms in Chapter 3. Manipulative techniques are used to influence the patient's health in accordance with the structure/function models listed above. In the ongoing management of a case, maintenance of the osteopathic treatment also includes the utilization of therapeutic exercise. In osteopathy there are many types of techniques, some of which will be briefly described in the following section. Some of these techniques have been selected from those described in literature,[2,108,109] while others will be described in the section dedicated to osteopathic models.

### High velocity low amplitude technique (HVLA) – thrust[110]

These are direct techniques that use high velocity/ low amplitude forces, also referred to as thrust or mobilization with impulse techniques by the Educational Council on Osteopathic Principles. The osteopath performs a procedure to:

- identify the restricted joint movement in all possible planes of motion

- bring the articulation to the restrictive barrier in all planes

- apply the thrust along a plane, or a combination of restricted movement planes

- retest for improved mobility.

### Soft tissue techniques[111]

A system of diagnosis and treatment indicated for soft tissue as well as for skeletal or joint elements. The osteopath performs a procedure to:

1. identify soft tissue tension and/or edema

2. apply a force to the tensioned and/or edematous area by:

- longitudinal elongation (tension)

- kneading (lateral elongation)

- inhibition (prolonged pressure)

- effleurage (touch)

- petrissage (kneading)

3. retest for reduction or alleviation of the tension and/or edema.

### Muscle energy technique[112,113]

Muscle energy technique (MET) is a system of diagnosis and techniques developed by Fred Mitchell senior, DO, in which the patient voluntarily moves the body under specific direction from the operator. This direct action of the patient is performed from a precise and controlled position against a determined resistance by the osteopath. The osteopath performs a procedure in order to:

- identify the restricted joint movement

- apply a joint movement toward the restriction on all planes

- isometrically resist the patient's attempt to move away from the restriction, for 3–5 seconds

- reposition the patient at the next restriction barrier

- perform 3–5 repetitions of isometric contraction and relaxation

- retest for increased mobility.

### Percussion vibrator technique[114]

This is a manipulative technique developed by Robert Fulford, DO, which uses the application of a mechanical vibratory force to alleviate the SD. The osteopath:

- identifies tissue tension or restricted movement

- positions the percussion vibrator perpendicular to the body surface of the bone

- changes the speed, pressure, and angle of the instrument, until the vibrations are not felt firmly in the monitoring hand (located on the opposite side of the tension or restriction)

- maintains contact until the strength and rhythm of the vibrations produce release of the restricted tissues. Alternatively, the monitoring hand presses in the direction of the vibratory surface, resisting every other direction of pressure; the percussion is maintained in this position

- retests, after tissue release is perceived, for improved motion.

## Facilitated oscillatory release[115,116]

This is a manipulative technique developed by Zachary Comeaux, DO, which consists of the manual application of oscillatory forces to normalize neuromuscular function. The treatment goal is similar to that of ligamentous or myofascial techniques. The osteopath:

- identifies the tension and asymmetry related to the restriction of movement

- applies oscillatory movement to the restricted region, using a certain mass of tissue to produce a lasting (harmonic) wave

- monitors the quality of the motor response in tissue to locate any additional restriction

- continues the rhythmic oscillation or changes its strength, up to the point at which the tension has been reduced or the rhythmic mobility increased. Other activating forces may also be included

- retests for decreased tension and improved mobility.

## Techniques of functional osteopathy[74,117]

If the tissues are found to have increased tension, hardening, hypertonicity, shortening or contracture, the therapeutic intent typically consists of producing the release of these states, so as to encourage a regression of restriction barriers. The involved soft tissues can be stretched, massaged, mobilized, or manipulated using dozens of direct or indirect techniques. However, if the tissues present are painful, inflamed, in spasm, or have recently suffered trauma, and the use of direct manual methods is painful, it is more appropriate to use one of the methods categorized as positional release, which, by producing a minimal discomfort, allow a spontaneous resolution of the dysfunctional condition, passively inducing change in the tissues rather than forcing it. Osteopathy has contributed to three of the principal approaches of positional release defined as functional: strain/counterstrain, functional technique, and positional release.

## Strain/counterstrain or Counterstrain®[118,119]

This is a system of diagnosis and treatment developed by Lawrence Jones, DO, which considers dysfunction as a continuous and inappropriate reflection of strain (tension, stretching), which is inhibited by the application of a slight strain position in the direction exactly opposite to that of the reflex. This is achieved through the direct and specific positioning on the tender point to get the desired therapeutic effect. The osteopath performs a procedure as follows:

- Assessment of the presence of an area of sore/painful or hypersensitive (tender point) soft tissue and then classifying it according to the pain response of the patient (10/10 or 100%)

- Passive positioning of the body toward the tissue release until the tenderness at the tender point is reduced up to 2/10 (20%) or less

- Maintaining the position of relief for 90 seconds

- Passive return of the patient to a neutral position

- Retest for reduced pain and increased motion; repeat the treatment if not fully improved.

## Functional technique[74,117]

This was promoted by Harold Hoover and reworked by Charles Bowles to describe what was achieved when the tissues associated with dysfunction were placed in a position of "rest," which is defined by them as dynamic neutral. The functional osteopathic technique of "ignore the pain" does not monitor the tissue quality by palpating the tender point as a guide to the position of comfort, but rather relies on the reduction of the palpated tone of stressed tissues (hypertonic/with spasm), while the person being treated is placed in a position of ease relative to all potential directions of movement of the given region. The procedure consists of the following steps:

- While one hand "listens" and the other produces the movement, the tissues are brought into a position of maximal comfort with respect to all possible directions of movement – the dynamic neutral point, in which the various directional components are in the best possible position

- The "stacking" process (literally: "stack," "stacking"), which is reached by evaluating successively the position of ease relative to the various directions of motion, starting from the point of comfort obtained by the previous assessment

- After having maintained (for a suggested minimum of 90 seconds) the dynamic neutral position until achieving a feeling of warmth, pulsation, or greater vitality, the entire sequence is repeated at least once more, with variations of the comfort positions as determined by the first application of the sequence.

## Positional release[74,120]

This is an indirect myofascial release system developed by Stanley Schiowitz, DO. The body region is positioned in a neutral position, which decreases the tissue and articular/joint tensions in all the planes of motion, followed by the addition of an activating force. The procedure involves:

- identification of the regions of restricted mobility

- positioning of the joint or region in its neutral position

- palpation of maximal reduction of tissue tension in all planes

- addition of compression or torsion to facilitate the release of the tissue

- maintaining the release position for 3–5 seconds until all tension is released, followed by a slow return to the neutral position

- retesting for reduced tension and increased mobility.

## Osteopathic cranial manipulative medicine[121,122]

This is a system of treatment developed by William Sutherland, DO, using the primary respiratory mechanism (PRM) and the balancing of membranous tensions. The PRM is perceived through subtle palpation and has been described according to biokinetic and, later, biodynamic mechanics. The oscillatory rhythm of the tissues seems to be related to the Traube–Hering–Mayer wave, an expression of the chronobiological rhythms of tissues throughout the individual, influenced by factors such as age, health, lifestyle, and stress. When these factors are negatively reflected on health, changes can be detected in these oscillatory rhythms. The operator, by means of osteopathic cranial procedures which have been proposed to make use of the entrainment phenomenon, is able to reestablish the normal rhythm of the involved tissues. The restricted tissues/structures are taken toward the direction of greater ease of motion or against the barrier and held in this position, until they gradually and spontaneously return to a neutral position. Sometimes the mobility or the intrinsic motility of tissue restriction requires the application of pumping forces, molding, disengagement or direct forces. Subsequently the barrier resolves and the tissues are brought into a normal position. When necessary, the process is repeated.

### Still techniques[123,124]

These are described as indirect and articular long lever techniques. They are performed at low speed and at medium-high amplitude. They were developed by Andrew Taylor Still (minimalist model), and use a process in which a joint is mobilized within its entire range of motion, with the therapeutic intent of increasing the freedom of amplitude. The procedure includes the following steps:

- Identification of restricted joint movement in all possible planes of motion

- Slow movement of the joint toward its relaxed/released position in all planes

- Slow movement of the joint toward the restriction in all planes

- 3–5 repetitions as one harmonious movement until joint mobility is restored

- Retest of the involved joint for improved mobility.

### Articulatory techniques[125]

Articulatory techniques may be used individually or used in the maximalist approach, as suggested by Littlejohn and further developed by Wernham, who have described a specific routine, as for example GOT (general osteopathic treatment), aimed at the treatment of the whole patient (total body adjustment). In other words, the articulatory corrective forces are used to stimulate the whole body physiology (blood supply and neurological support, venous-lymphatic drainage of toxins).

Articulatory techniques can also be used with a minimalist focus to normalize movement restric-

tions, especially in patients who manifest circulatory and lymphatic congestion in the presence of articular and myofascial SD.

### Myofascial release[126,127]

This is a system of diagnosis and treatment that uses continuous palpatory feedback to achieve the release of myofascial tissues. This approach emphasizes the perception and recruitment of motility inherent in myofascial structures for the identification and treatment of proximal and distal mobility patterns, diaphragms, compartments, visceral/internal organs, structures, etc. The electric potential of the fascia produces palpable changes in its mobility. These changes relate to the homeostatic state of the internal environment and the biomechanical response to the external environment and can facilitate the diagnosis and treatment of visceral and musculoskeletal disorders. The procedure includes the following:

- Identification of the tissue restriction or limitation of joint movement among all possible planes of motion

- In the case of indirect technique a release point is found in all planes and any tissue release is followed until all tissue tension is released

- In the case of direct technique, it is necessary to slowly move the affected part of the body toward the restrictive barrier in all planes and apply a constant force until the release of the involved tissues is achieved

- Retest of the involved area for improved motion.

### Visceral techniques[128]

This is a system of diagnosis and treatment directed toward the internal organs to improve their physiological functioning. These techniques in particular, much like osteopathic manipulative treatment in general, pay a lot of attention to somatovisceral/viscerosomatic relations, i.e., to the effects of dysfunction of the autonomic nervous system. Generally, the viscera are brought to a fascial balancing point that can be detected by engaging vectors in the direction of the restriction of mobility or in the facilitated direction.

### Balanced ligamentous tension (BLT), ligamentous articular strain (LAS)[129,130]

This is the set of myofascial release techniques described by Howard and Rebecca Lippincott, Becker and Wales, which further developed work by Still and Sutherland. They can be considered distinct techniques as it seems that geographical distance and lack of contact between the two groups led to the development of the same technique under two distinct names. In the central United States (Texas), ligamentous articular strain (LAS) is the preferred term, while in the northeastern United States (New Jersey and New England), the name balanced ligamentous tension (BLT) is used. The term LAS seems to describe the dysfunction, while the term BLT/BMT (balanced membranous tension) identifies the process or the goal of the treatment. Tissue parameters are used in both cases to access what in this text is defined as DyFIR in order to normalize the SD. After the identification of the SD, in the form of both ligamentous and myofascial tension, it is necessary to:

- exert traction or pressure on the tensioned area in order to *disengage* the tissues

- slowly move the affected part of the body to its point of *balance* in all planes

- *hold* the balanced position until the tissue tension is released or until the DyFIR is palpated as homogeneous in itself and the surrounding tissues

- retest the region for decreased tension.

### Lymphatic techniques[131,132]

Initially these were considered to be visceral techniques, but later, with further understanding of the lymphatic system, they became a separate technique modality. Zink, for example, described the myofascial aspects of lymphatic congestion (of all the fluid systems, the lymphatic one, at low pressure, is more likely to get obstructed and to benefit from OMT). Dalrymple's pedal lymphatic pump and Miller's thoracic lymphatic pump are historically regarded as unique techniques for manipulative treatment of the immune system, and were extensively used in the influenza pandemic of 1918–19. The Galbreath mandibular drainage technique is historically regarded as a technique for the treatment of Bell's palsy. The lymphatic techniques can be applied:

- to remove obstacles to lymphatic flow, through the treatment of SD

- to promote lymphatic flow by promoting the flow with methods such as stimulation, percussion, vibration, effleurage, petrissage, thoracic and pedal pump, and drainage of myofascial components.

### Exercise techniques in the osteopathic field[133]

These are determined from the structural examination and the results of OMT and are presented here in the form of general concepts and guidelines, while some of their variants will be described in Section 2, which is dedicated to osteopathic models (see Chapter 7). The type of exercise recommended depends on the patient's assessment and the results of OMT. It will focus on SDs detected and/or on improvement of health in general. The techniques are distinguished by the following characteristics:

- *Positional release*: the hypertonic tissue is maintained in a shortened position for 2–5 minutes to obtain tissue release and reduction of pain. This is helpful for the myofascial tenderness associated with acute problems, as well as for the relief from pain caused by subacute or chronic problems. It is contraindicated in acute fractures.

- *Elongation*: a gentle force is exerted on the restriction for 10–20 seconds to reduce tension and restore mobility. It is useful for tension associated with subacute or chronic problems, and contraindicated in fractures or acute dislocations and in the presence of joint/articular instability.

- *Mobilization*: a small amplitude movement is performed, fast or slow and repetitive. It is useful in articular restrictions associated with subacute or chronic problems and contraindicated in fractures or acute dislocations, and in the presence of joint instability, inflammation, degeneration, or severe osteoporosis.

- *Postural strengthening*: this is performed by contracting postural muscles against gravity, until fatigued, and is repeated every day to restore muscle strength.

## Treatment plan

The above-mentioned techniques can be applied by the osteopath at different tissue or structural levels of the body: e.g., specific techniques on soft tissues, such as muscles and ligaments, to balance tissue tension; articulatory or positioning techniques to improve the range and quality of joint movement; quick controlled pressures to improve restricted movements of the joints (thrust); visceral techniques to restore the function of organs and glands, etc. The choice of treatment techniques or modalities is influenced by many factors, including the operator, the patient, and the context in which the therapeutic action occurs (see Chapter 9). At this point the treatment plan and the subsequent choice of techniques will be specific to the patient, who is made responsible, among other things, for maintaining health through education and counseling on general lifestyle. It is important that the patient is constantly updated and clearly informed about the diagnosis and treatment protocol, treatment strategies or alternative treatment methods. The patient is informed of the potential risks, side effects and timing of the treatment, and also required to give consent before starting any treatment.[18]

## Ongoing case management

At the beginning of each consultation, the patient is encouraged to report any progress or change related to the reason for consultation. The osteopath then performs a new examination and starts further treatment accordingly. The initial diagnosis is reviewed at the end of each treatment. The duration and frequency of the treatment plan depends on the patient's progress and on a number of other factors (see Chapter 9). The patient is kept informed throughout this process and will be notified of any need for referral.[17]

## Adequacy of treatment, objective examination, and osteopathic evaluation

The indication for osteopathic treatment is the presence of clinically significant SD. The clinical significance is determined by using the models of osteopathic practice. When employed by trained and competent personnel, the principles of osteopathy and osteopathic models of health care can be applied in particular clinical conditions. As providers of primary health care, osteopaths are responsible for referring the patient for a medical consultation or other therapeutic intervention, when the patient's condition requires it or when the case falls outside the field of the osteopath's training. These aspects are determined through physical examination. The osteopath needs to recognize when specific approaches and techniques may be contraindicated in certain conditions. It is important to understand that a contraindication to OMT in an area of the body does not preclude osteopathic treatment in a different area. Similarly, a contraindication for any specific technique does not preclude the use of a different type of technique in the same patient. Absolute and relative contraindications to osteopathic treatment are usually based on the technique used. It is the responsibility of the osteopath to discern what kinds of techniques are safe and appropriate in a clinical situation. Direct techniques, such as muscle energy, thrust, and articulatory maneuvers present different risks from indirect, fluid movement and reflex techniques. There are few published data on the conditions in which techniques should be avoided. Understanding of the pathophysiology of the patient's condition and the mechanism of action of the technique allows the osteopath to determine the biological plausibility for safety, and the absolute and relative contraindications,[18] which are listed in Box 1.3 (see also Chapter 9).

The methods most often used by osteopaths during the objective examination are:

- inspection

- range of motion (ROM)

- classic orthopedic tests

- classic neurological tests

- percussion and auscultation.

With respect to the general osteopathic evaluation, and in particular of SD (see Chapter 2), this is followed by:

- static and dynamic morphological inspection (with an assessment of quality and quantity of motion)

- palpation of position and movement/static and dynamic

- analysis of muscle function and tissue in general

- tender points (Jones techniques) and trigger points

- assessment of the intrinsic mobility of tissues and related involuntary movements

- assessment of joint mobility and soft tissues, their sensitivity, asymmetry, and movement

restriction throughout the body, including the head (neurocranium and viscerocranium)

- examination of neurolymphatic reflexes (Chapman's reflexes).

## Box 1.3

### Safety

The osteopathic profession has a reputation for safety since it involves less high-speed manipulation/handling when compared to other professions. The use of these techniques of high-speed manipulation/handling, addressed, for example, to the cervical spine has contributed to a much lower occurrence of adverse events compared to those associated with other manual therapy professions. These effects have not been reported with the application of OMT on patient populations such as pregnant women and hospitalized patients. Other studies show more cautious observations, indicating that there is a benefit in the use of spinal manipulation in patients with herniated disc, even if there are not enough quality tests that allow you to reach definitive conclusions.[1–18]

### Contraindications, risks, side effects

The patient's refusal or the absence of informed consent (verbal and/or written) is an absolute contraindication to inclusion in any research project, as well as to the application of any technique or osteopathic treatment. The document drawn up in 2010 by the World Health Organization describes absolute and relative contraindications to osteopathic techniques.[19] However, no absolute contraindications to OMT have been reported yet. The consultations which allowed the drafting of the document cited above consider the osteopath to be able to evaluate and choose the most appropriate technique for each case or, if necessary, refer the client to a medical specialist. It also highlighted, as shown by scientific publications, the safety of OMT applied to different types of populations, e.g., pediatric patients, emergency room patients, and women suffering from mood disorders related to menopause.[16,18,20]

## Direct techniques (19)

### Absolute contraindications to any direct technique (systemic conditions)

- Disorders of uncontrolled or suspected clotting/coagulation
- Prolonged bleeding time
- Treatment with anticoagulant pharmacotherapy without recent evaluation of therapeutic level
- Coagulation disorders
- Congenital or acquired diseases of the connective tissue, expressed in the integrity of the compromised tissues
- Compromised bone, tendons, ligaments or joint stability, as might occur in metabolic disorders, metastatic disease, and rheumatic diseases.

### Relative contraindications to direct techniques

- Osteoporosis
- Osteopenia
- Pediatric patients who have not reached puberty, elderly patients.

### Absolute contraindications to direct techniques, especially at local level

- Aortic aneurysm
- Acute hydrocephalus
- Undiagnosed hydrocephalus
- Acute intracerebral hemorrhage
- Acute and transient cerebral ischemia
- Suspected arteriovenous malformation
- Cerebral aneurysm
- Acute cholecystitis with suspected leakage or rupture
- Acute appendicitis with suspected leakage or rupture
- Acute or subacute closed head trauma
- Acute herniated disc with progressive neurological signs
- Evidence of vascular impairment (carotid, aortic, and ocular bruit)

- Suspected vertebral artery impairment (syncope, dizziness, known congenital malformation)
- Acute cauda equina syndrome
- Ocular lens implant (first postoperative period)
- Uncontrolled glaucoma
- Neoplasm
- Suspicion or risk of osseous impairment such as osteomyelitis, osseous/bone tuberculosis, etc.

### Absolute contraindications to direct techniques that primarily include HVLA/thrust and locally applied pulses

- Specific technique at a site with an internal fixation
- Bone or joint stability impairment, as might happen in cases of focal tumor, metastatic disease, suppurative arthritis, septic arthritis, rheumatoid diseases, osteomyelitis, bone tuberculosis, etc.
- Acute fractures
- Intramuscular hematoma.

### Relative contraindications to direct techniques (HVLA, thrust or pulses) locally applied

- Hernia of a vertebral disc without progressive neurological signs
- Injured ligaments
- Acute cervical injury/lesion by trauma from acceleration–deceleration (whiplash).

## Indirect techniques[19]

Contraindications relative to indirect techniques are usually related to the acuteness of the problem.

### Absolute contraindications to indirect techniques applied locally

- Undiagnosed acute hydrocephalus
- Acute cerebral hemorrhage
- Acute intracerebral vascular accident (or ischemic hypoxia)
- Suspected arteriovenous malformation
- Cerebral aneurysm
- Suspected acute peritonitis

- Acute appendicitis or other visceral diseases with suspected leakage or rupture

- Recent closed head injury with internal derangement suspected.

Relative contraindications to any indirect technique applied locally

- Metastatic disease

- Neoplasm

- Acute closed head trauma.

### References

1. Vogel S, Mars T, Keeping S et al. Clinical risk osteopathy and management scientific report: the CROaM study. National Council for Osteopathic Research (NCOR), London, February 2013. Available from: www.ncor.org.uk/wp-content/uploads/2013/05/croam_full_report_0313.pdf.

2. Carnes D, Mullinger B, Underwood M. Defining adverse events in manual therapies: a modified Delphi consensus study. Man Ther. 2009;15:2–6.

3. Carnes D, Mars TS, Mullinger B et al. Adverse events and manual therapy: a systematic review. Man Ther. 2010;15(4):355–63.

4. Cagnie B, Vinck E, Beernaert A et al. How common are side effects of spinal manipulation and can these side effects be predicted? Man Ther. 2004;9(3):151–6.

5. Rajendran D, Mullinger B, Fossum C et al. Monitoring self-reported adverse events: a prospective, pilot study in a UK osteopathic teaching clinic. Int J Osteopath Med. 2009;12(2):49–55.

6. Froud R, Rajendran D, Fossum C et al. How do patients feel post-treatment? Pilot study at a UK osteopathic teaching clinic of self-reported adverse events. Int J Osteopath Med. 2008;11(4):151–2.

7. Gibbons P, Tehan P. HVLA thrust techniques: what are the risks? Int J Osteopath Med. 2006;9(1):4–12.

8. Leach J. Risk and negligence: a minefield or an opportunity? Communicating risk in osteopathic practice. Int J Osteopath Med. 2006;9(1):1–3.

9. Oliphant D. Safety of spinal manipulation in the treatment of lumbar disk herniations: a systematic review and risk assessment. J Manipulative Physiol Ther. 2004;27:197–210.

10. Lisi AJ, Holmes EJ, Ammendolia C. High-velocity low-amplitude spinal manipulation for symptomatic lumbar disk disease: a systematic review of the literature. J Manipulative Physiol Ther. 2005;28(6):429–42.

11. Snelling NJ. Spinal manipulation in patients with disc herniation: a critical review of risk and benefit. Int J Osteopath Med. 2006;9(3):77–84.

12. Hensel KL, Pacchia CF, Smith ML. Acute improvement in hemodynamic control after osteopathic manipulative treatment in the third trimester of pregnancy. Complement Ther Med. 2013;21:618–26.

13. Sabino J, Grauer JN. Pregnancy and low back pain. Curr Rev Musculoskelet Med. 2008;1:137–41.

14. Sandler S The osteopathic approach to obstetrics. Man Ther. 1996;1(4):178–85.

15. Licciardone JC, Buchanan S, Hensel KL et al. Osteopathic manipulative treatment of back pain and related symptoms during pregnancy: a randomized controlled trial. Am J Obstet Gynecol. 2009;202(1):43.e1–8.

16. Roberge RJ, Roberge MR. Overcoming barriers to the use of osteopathic manipulation techniques in the emergency department. West J Emerg Med. 2009;(3):184–9.

17. Kronke K. A questionnaire to evaluate the professional field of osteopathy in Austria. Unpublished pilot study, 2006.

18. Hayes NM, Bezilla TA. Incidence of iatrogenesis associated with osteopathic manipulative treatment of pediatric patients. J Am Osteopath Assoc. 2006;106(10):605–8.

19. World Health Organization (WHO). Benchmarks for training in osteopathy. Geneva: WHO; 2010.

20. Plotkin BJ, Rodos JJ, Kappler R et al. Adjunctive osteopathic manipulative treatment in women with depression: a pilot study. J Am Osteopath Assoc. 2001;101(9):517–23.

## Communication and metaphor

The new generation of osteopaths cannot practice without considering communication as a powerful instrument to accompany the "hand" in order to establish a helping relationship. Appropriate communication is translated into a real re-socialization of the patient, as occurs after a discomfort, a trauma, a more or less severe psychophysical impediment/obstacle.[134] This theme will be discussed in detail in Chapter 8, dedicated to the biopsychosocial model; however, the authors believe some premises are necessary. Questions such as "What is health?" or "What is disease?" are challenging the philosophical, scientific, and professional concepts of osteopaths. Both osteopathic thinking and practice are influenced by the philosophical principles of Still, Sutherland, and Littlejohn and their students, who have often coined words or phrases in their teaching in order to pass their palpatory experiences on to others. In osteopathic literature, abstract and complex terms such as "health" are expressed mainly by metaphors. For example, when osteopaths commit themselves to improving the conditions of SD, they report that to finalize a technique they seek a feeling of swelling, softening, of the increase of space in a tissue level, loss of contact with the single unit that merges with everything, assonance with the central notochordal units. In this case, in the osteopathic language, in defining a balancing stimulus of the tensions of a dysfunctional area, which is implemented by a manipulative gesture that interacts with the tissue mechanics, reference is made to an embryonic structure, which by virtue of its function of induction is considered a balancing instance of tissue differentiation. Metaphorical concepts help to transfer osteopathic thinking, speaking, and acting regarding health into a simpler way of perceiving and understanding. In spite of the fact that osteopathic experience seems to be better articulated and discussed through the use of metaphors, this seems, for other reasons, to represent a major problem in the conceptualization of issues such as health and illness in the communication used by osteopaths in their profession. In a study by Risch in 2012 a metaphorical analysis was carried out, using one of the latest research methods in cognitive linguistics aimed at obtaining information about osteopathic health concepts. This was done by systematically analyzing the metaphorical concepts commonly used by osteopaths in their daily clinical practice.[135] The study by Risch concludes that metaphors, by highlighting some aspects and hiding others, create a partial knowledge of reality, but at the same time demonstrate a selective nature, allowing a differentiated point of view. The study notes how it is impossible not to use metaphors in conversations focused on the concept of health. Recent research studies of cognitive linguistics are taking into account metaphor as an important tool for the generation of a meaning and understanding of abstract contents. Risch reveals a high degree of the metaphorization of health in osteopathic language, with particular reference to concepts such as interoception, the sensory experience, the experience of the physical body oriented and associated with the sociological field. The most important metaphorical concepts used are: health as an experience, health as awareness, health as change, health as a process. The analysis of the most used metaphorical concepts by osteopaths suggests a paradigm shift that seems to move from a "biomechanical model" to a "salutogenic model." There emerges, however, difficulty with integration of the single subjective experiences of the practitioner and common professional osteopathic knowledge. This gives rise to a deficit in the intra- and interdisciplinary communication between different professionals and between osteopath and patient. In the absence of the awareness of common osteopathic language, the use of a metaphorical language can lead to conflict and confusion within osteopathy, slowing the process of development of a unified professional identity.[135]

## Osteopathy and the health adaptive model

The final considerations in this chapter are an introduction to the next, in trying to outline the philosophical and biological concept of health and a consequent salutogenic osteopathic rational approach based on the encounter between philosophy and scientific evidence. The practical application of the concepts and principles has been described by various models of structure-function relationships[33] that osteopaths use to influence the collection of diagnostic information and interpretation of the meaning of the neuromusculoskeletal results in the overall health of the patient.[2] What is the task of a health provider? This question was answered by the founder of osteopathy, Andrew Taylor Still, more than a century ago, reminding his students to leave the disease-centered approach to other professionals and to focus their attention on health. The latter is defined as a state of complete physical, mental, and social health and not merely the absence of disease. Philosophers have often ventured into the definition of health, without seeking a correlation with biological meanings: the concept of maintaining the stability of physiological systems by means of adaptation, i.e., self-regulation of the system with respect to questions asked of the organism by the environment in a natural selection scheme.[136,137] This homeostatic/allostatic adaptation is the principal element of the stress response. It is a biological mechanism that is used to restore balance and minimize internal effects of stress. The close relationship between the immune system and the nervous system has long been noted. Ancient Hippocratic medicine, as well as Indian and Chinese medicine, has always taken into account the close connection between body and brain. Western medicine, however, only began, to examine this relationship in the 1930s, with the studies of Hans Selye.[136] In the first decades of the 20th century, Cannon studied the alarm reaction concept and also described the concept of critical level of stress to indicate the maximum tolerable level of stimulation from the body's compensatory mechanisms. Selye defined stress as the body's nonspecific response to each request made of it. Stress is considered a normal reaction, with an adaptive function with respect to stressors from the environment. In the alarm phase, the bodily and mental defense mechanisms are mobilized in order to cope with stress through a "fight-or-flight" (neuroendocrine-type) response and an increase

in alertness and mental energy available. If stress is not resolved, it will pass into the phase of resistance, where the person tends to adapt to stressors by modifying homeostatic systems (heart rate, hormone levels, blood pressure, etc.) in order to repair the damage done to the body. If the person fails to recover, the body will enter the exhaustion phase, where the physiological responses are intensified, but the energy levels will deteriorate, with a reduction of the levels and adaptability of physiological regulation, which in time could lead to illness or even death. In some cases, therefore, stress can become pathological, when the environmental demands exceed the adaptive capacity of the individual.[137] Two different physiological systems manage stress: the hypothalamic–pituitary–adrenal (HPA) axis and the sympathetic–adrenal–medullary (SAM) system. These two systems are interfaced between the sympathetic nervous system (SNS) and the adrenal glands.[22] When the hypothalamus senses something as "stressful" it triggers a hormonal cascade that is defined as a "hormonal response to stress." The stress systems (HPA and SAM) produce different physiological changes in response to the influence of the stressor or stressors, which cause the body to adapt and to strive to restore physiological balance. Stress is perceived by the limbic system in the brain almost immediately after the stressful event has occurred.[22] The neurons activate the HPA and SAM axes, while the latter releases various hormones that are filtered by the HPA axis and travel through all the tissues and bloodstream. At the level of the hypothalamus, stressors stimulate the release of corticotropin-releasing hormone (CRH); CRH travels to the pituitary gland, where it stimulates the release of the ACTH (adrenocorticotropic hormone); in turn, the ACTH stimulates the production and release of glucocorticoid hormones (corticosteroids that include cortisol, cortisone, and corticosterone), principally cortisol from the adrenal cortex. The hypothalamus stimulates the adrenal glands, through the SNS, to release catecholamines, such as epinephrine (adrenalin) and norepinephrine (noradrenaline), into the bloodstream. To meet the challenges, the stress response increases the heart rate and breathing, the energy stores, and hormones such as glucocorticoids, while lower priority functions, such as gastrointestinal and reproductive functions, are decreased. The immune system is stimulated in the short term, but can be suppressed by prolonged and severe stress. The combination of the release of adrenaline and noradrenaline triggers the "fight-or-flight" response. Catecholamines and glucocorticoids induce a series of behavioral, biochemical, and physiological changes.[22] Selye denominated this reaction the local and general adaptation syndrome, describing an alarm stage, a stage of resistance and a stage of exhaustion.[136] The authors of this work observe that as OMT is carried out, one can assess, encourage, maintain, and restore the person's ability to adapt, sensing the trend of health, i.e., the adaptation syndrome (see Fig. 1.1). The adaptation syndromes are therefore of two types: local and general.

- *Local adaptation syndrome (LAS)*: the action of a specific stressor causes a localized effect only in some parts of the body, for example the painful shoulder of a swimmer subjected to functional overload. In the osteopathic field investigations have been pursued in this regard, studying the physiology of tissue adaptation to local stresses, namely the SD, understood as impaired or altered function of components of the somatic system in relation to each other as skeletal, arthrodial, and myofascial structures, and the related vascular, lymphatic, and neural elements.[1-3,18]

- *General adaptation syndrome (GAS)*: this is produced by agents that have a general effect on extensive parts of the body. The osteopath observes and assesses general global adaptation through the analysis of the FCS and the energy expenditure that follows,[138] considering its chronobiological agreement with the environment,[139] through the perceptive palpation of biological fluid dynamics and associated involuntary rhythms (DyFIR). Moreover, intervention is made with treatment aimed at stimulating

a less costly, more comfortable and painless adaptation, using procedures aimed at inherent movements, body fluids, and reduction of afferent stimuli. These are the specific objectives of adaptogenic osteopathic approaches such as the techniques used in the cranial, fascial, and visceral lymphatic fields.[3]

GAS and LAS are interdependent. A general stress can affect local reactions and, on the other hand, a local stress can (if strong enough) stimulate or aggravate a general reaction. The osteopath, through perceptive palpation, strengthened nowadays by scientific evidence, recognizes the best ways to interact with the person, proceeding as follows:

- Sometimes with local specific approaches directed to clinically relevant SD/s. The use of knowledge of anatomy and physiology allows the operator to recognize the functional alteration of a structure and to facilitate normalization

- Sometimes with global adaptogenic approaches aimed at balancing the FCS and/or DyFIR. Through knowledge of anatomy and physiology, the osteopath will attempt to interact with any abnormal functioning of the HPA axis, perhaps with circadian rhythm altered, increased levels of psychological activity, a reduced ability to relax, with repercussions on respiratory and circulatory function and on the global economy and posture of the body that will result in dysfunctional patterns and alterations of individual's chronobiology as a result of biologically unsustainable characteristics.

In both of these cases, which are often combined in a treatment, the osteopath seeks a state of attentiveness and compassion, a more relaxed and noninvasive state, which produces a neuroceptive and spontaneous relaxation of tension in the body, mind and spirit components of the entire spectrum of the person (Fig. 1.16).

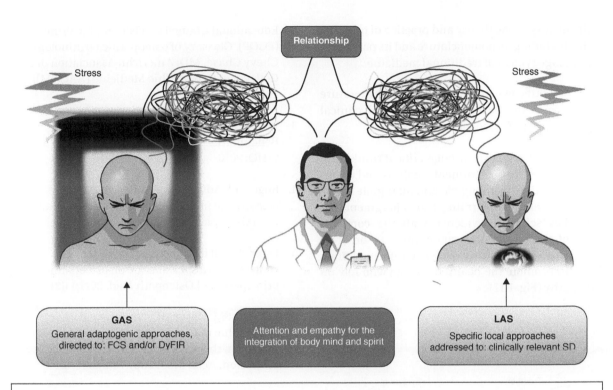

**Fig. 1.16**
Osteopathic approach to the general (GAS) and local (LAS) adaptation syndromes. The osteopath recognizes the best mode of interaction with the person and with his or her individual mode of adaptation, finalizing a treatment, sometimes with local specific approaches aimed at LAS, i.e., to the correlated structure with somatic dysfunction (SD); sometimes with general homeostatic approaches directed to GAS and to the anomalous HPA function, i.e., to the facial compensation scheme and related dynamics of fluids and involuntary rhythms. The osteopath combines the two approaches into a treatment seeking to establish an empathetic relationship that produces a state of balance of body, mind and spirit of the person as a whole.

## Conclusions

Disease arises from a lack of dynamic interaction within and among adaptive systems and is recognizable, before damage to a single system, by alterations in the relationship between structure and function. Topics covered in this book allow the observation of the process used by the professional to plan for rational OMT, based on the principle of interdependence between structure and function; a process that includes the use of perceptual models to recognize and to approach, with different osteopathic techniques, the multifactorial influences on health, including postural factors, nociceptive, circulatory-respiratory and metabolic requirements, as well as biopsychosocial and environmental influences. At the same time, the models reconfirm the importance of integration of structure and function in maintaining health. In order to propose a renewed osteopathic approach, but one consistent with osteopathy's nature as a person-centered traditional medicine,[140] the authors chose to observe the relationship between:

- the history of the theory and practice of osteopathy, including its nomenclature and its particular language typical of traditional medicine

- the scientific evidence available in the literature relative to the basic mechanisms and clinical applications of osteopathy.

We have tried to do this through critical thinking, a mental process of discernment, analysis and evaluation, reflection over tangible and intangible areas, with the intention of forming a solid judgment that reconciles scientific evidence with the common sense of the osteopathic community, in order to offer a fresh approach, an evidence-informed practice[141] to promote the health of people who rely on osteopathy (Fig. 1.17).

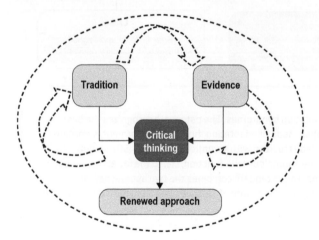

**Fig. 1.17**
From tradition to innovation. The authors propose a process of reflection on the historical and anthropological foundation of osteopathy, based on scientific evidence, and on their integration, mediated by critical thinking, in order to allow for a renewed approach.

## References

1.  World Health Organization (WHO). International statistical classification of diseases and related health problems. 10th revision. Geneva: WHO; 2011.

2.  Educational Council on Osteopathic Principles (ECOP). Glossary of osteopathic terminology. Chevy Chase, MD: American Association of Colleges of Osteopathic Medicine (AACOM); 2009.

3.  World Health Organization (WHO). Benchmarks for training in osteopathy. Geneva: WHO; 2010.

4.  Rogers FJ. Advancing a traditional view of osteopathic medicine through clinical practice. J Am Osteopath Assoc. 2005;105(5):255-9.

5.  Fryer G. Call for papers:an invitation to contribute to a special issue on osteopathic principles. Int J Osteopath Med. 2011;14(3):79-80.

6.  Johnson SM, Kurtz ME. Diminished use of osteopathic manipulative treatment and its impact on the uniqueness of the osteopathic profession. Acad Med. 2001;76(8):821-8.

7.  Chaitow L. Is postural-structural-biomechanical model within manual therapies, viable? A JBMT debate. J Bodyw Mov Ther. 2011;15(2):130-52.

8.  Tyreman SJ. The concept of function in osteopathy and conventional medicine:a comparative study [PhD thesis]. London: British School of Osteopathy; 2001.

9.  Wagner C. Exploring a European osteopathic identity:analysis of professional profiles of European osteopathic organizations [Masters thesis]. Vienna: WSO-DUK; 2009.

10. Roberti di Sarsina P, Morandi A, Alivia M et al. Traditional and non-conventional medicine in Italy. Considerations on a social choice for the person-centered medicine. Advanced Therapies 2012;1:3-29.

11. Gevitz N. The DOs: osteopathic medicine in America. 2nd ed. Baltimore, MD: Johns Hopkins University Press; 2004.

12. Antonovsky A. Health, stress and coping. San Francisco, CA: Jossey-Bass; 1979.

13. Roberti di Sarsina P, Alivia M, Guadagni P. Traditional, complementary and alternative medical systems and their contribution to personalization, prediction and prevention in person-centered medicine. European Association for Predictive, Preventive and Personalized Medicine (EPMA) Journal. 2012;3:15.

14. Degenhardt BF, Johnson JC, Snider KT et al. Maintenance and improvement of interobserver reliability of osteopathic palpatory tests over a 4-month period. J Am Osteopath Assoc. 2010;110(10):579–86.

15. Barnes L, Laboy F 3rd, Noto-Bell L et al. A comparative study of cervical hysteresis characteristics after various osteopathic manipulative treatment (OMT) modalities. J Bodyw Mov Ther. 2013;17(1):89–94.

16. Shaw KA, Dougherty JJ, Treffer KD et al. Establishing the content validity of palpatory examination for the assessment of the lumbar spine using ultrasonography:a pilot study. J Am Osteopath Assoc 2012;112(12):775–82.

17. Tozzi P, Bongiorno D, Vitturini C. Low back pain and kidney mobility: local osteopathic fascial manipulation decreases pain perception and improves renal mobility. J Bodyw Mov Ther. 2012;16(3):381–91.

18. European Federation of Osteopaths (EFO). Scope of osteopathic practice in Europe. Brussels: EFO; 2010.

19. Forum for Osteopathic Regulation in Europe (FORE). The European framework for standards of osteopathic practice. Brussels: FORE; 2010.

20. Canguilhem G. The normal and the pathological. New York: Zone Books; 1998.

21. Lancet [editorial]. What is health? The ability to adapt. Lancet 2009;373(9666):781.

22. Sterling P, Heyer J. Allostasis:a new paradigm to explain arousal pathology. In: Fisher S, Reason J, editors. Handbook of life stress, cognition and health. New York: J Wiley and Sons; 1988. pp. 629–49.

23. Zink JG. Applications of the osteopathic holistic approach to homeostasis. American Academy of Applied Osteopathy Yearbook, 1973. pp. 37–47.

24. Evidence-Based Medicine Working Group. Evidence-based medicine. A new approach to teaching the practice of medicine. JAMA. 1992;268(17):2420–5.

25. King HH, Janig W, Patterson MM, editors. The science and clinical application of manual therapy. Edinburgh: Churchill Livingstone/Elsevier; 2011.

26. Assendelft WJ, Morton SC, Yu EI et al. Spinal manipulative therapy for low back pain. Cochrane Database Syst Rev 2004;(1):CD000447.

27. Cherkin DC, Sherman KJ, Deyo RA et al. A review of the evidence for effectiveness, safety and the cost of acupuncture, massage therapy, and spinal manipulation for low back pain. Ann Intern Med. 2003;138:898–906.

28. Licciardone JC, Brimhall AK, King LK. Osteopathic manipulative treatment for low back pain: a systematic review and meta-analysis of randomized controlled trials. BMC Musculoskelet Disord. 2005;6:43.

29. Stark J. Still's fascia. Pahl, Germany: Jolandos; 2007.

30. Jordan T. Swedenborg's influence on Sutherland's "primary respiratory mechanism" model in cranial osteopathy. Int J Osteopath Med. 2009;12(3):100–5.

31. Spiegel D. Healing words:emotional expression and disease outcome. JAMA. 1999;281:1328–9.

32. Jerome JA, Foresman BH, D'Alonzo GE. Biobehavioral research. In: Chila A, editor. Foundations of osteopathic medicine. 3rd ed. Philadelphia: Wolters Kluwer/Lippincott, Williams and Wilkins; 2011. ch.73.

33. Parsons J, Marcer N. Osteopathy: models for diagnosis, treatment and practice. Edinburgh: Elsevier Churchill Livingstone; 2006.

34. Still AT. Philosophy of osteopathy [reprint]. Kirksville, MO: American Academy of Osteopathy; 1971 [first published 1899]. pp. 234–49.

35. Jarrell J. Demonstration of cutaneous allodynia in association with chronic pelvic pain. J Vis Exp. 2009;(28)ii:1232.

36. Tettambel M. Ostetrics. In: Ward RC, editor. Foundations of osteopathic medicine. 2nd ed. Philadelphia: Lippincott Williams and Wilkins; 2002. pp. 450–61.

37. Nelson KE. The management of low back pain: short leg syndrome/postural balance. J Am Osteopath Assoc. 1999;9(1):33–9.

38. Lavelle JM. Osteopathic manipulative treatment in pregnant women. J Am Osteopath Assoc. 2012;112(6):343–6.

39. Hensel KL, Pacchia CF, Smith ML. Acute improvement in hemodynamic control after osteopathic manipulative treatment in the third trimester of pregnancy. Complement Ther Med. 2013;21(6):618–26.

40. King HH, Tettambel MA, Lockwood MD et al. Osteopathic manipulative treatment in prenatal care: a retrospective case control design study. J Am Osteopath Assoc. 2003;103(12):577–82.

41. Amóstegui Azcúe JM, Ferri Morales A, Lillo De La Quintana C et al. Urinary incontinence and other pelvic floor damages: ethilogy and prevention strategies. Rev Med Univ Navarra. 2004;48(4):18–31.

42. de Almeida BS, Sabatino JH, Giraldo PC. Effects of high-velocity, low-amplitude spinal manipulation on strength and the basal tonus of female pelvic floor muscles. J Manipulative Physiol Ther. 2010;33(2):109–16.

43. Franke H, Hoesele K. Osteopathic manipulative treatment for lower urinary tract symptoms in women. J Bodyw Mov Ther. 2014;18(1):92.

44. Sucher BM. Palpatory diagnosis and manipulative management of carpal tunnel syndrome. J Am Osteopath Assoc. 1994;94(8):647–63.

45. Sucher BM, Hinrichs RN. Manipulative treatment of carpal tunnel syndrome: biomechanical and osteopathic intervention to increase the length of the transverse carpal ligament. J Am Osteopath Assoc. 1998;98(12):679–86.

46. Licciardone JC, Buchanan S, Hensel KL et al. Osteopathic manipulative treatment of back pain and related symptoms during pregnancy: a randomized controlled trial. Am J Obstet Gynecol. 2010;202(1):43.e1–8.

47. Licciardone JC, Aryal S. Prevention of progressive back-specific dysfunction during pregnancy: an assessment of osteopathic manual treatment based on Cochrane Back Review Group criteria. J Am Osteopath Assoc. 2013;113(10):728–36.

48. Pennick V, Liddle SD. Interventions for preventing and treating pelvic and back pain in pregnancy. Cochrane Database Syst Rev. 2013;8:CD001139.

49. Degenhardt BF, Kuchera ML. Update on osteopathic medical concepts and the lymphatic system. J Am Osteopath Assoc. 1996;96:97–100.

50. Mills MV, Henley CE, Barnes LLB et al. The use of osteopathic manipulative treatment as adjuvant therapy in children with recurrent acute otitis media. Arch Pediatr Adolesc Med. 2003;157:861–6.

51. Hayden C, Mullinger B. A preliminary assessment of the impact of cranial osteopathy for the relief of infantile colic. Complement Ther Clin Pract. 2006;12:83–90.

52. Lassovetskaia L. Applications of the osteopathic approach to school children with delayed psychic development of cerebro-organic origin. In: King HH, editor. Proceedings of International Research Conference: Osteopathy in pediatrics at the Osteopathic Center for Children in San Diego, CA, 2002. Indianapolis, IN: American Academy of Osteopathy; 2005. pp. 52–9.

53. FrymannVM, Carney RE, Springall P. Efficacy of osteopathic medical management on neurological development in children. J Am Osteopath Assoc. 1992;92:729–44.

54. PhiLippi H, Faldum A, Schleupen A et al. Infantile postural asymmetry and osteopathic treatment: a randomized therapeutic trial. Dev Med Child Neurol. 2006;48:5–9, discussion 4.

55. Cerritelli F, Pizzolorusso G, Renzetti C et al. A multicenter, randomized, controlled trial of osteopathic manipulative treatment on preterms. PLoS One. 2015;10(5):e0127370.

56. Knebl JA, Shores JH, Gamber RG et al. Improving functional ability in the elderly via the Spencer technique, an osteopathic manipulative treatment: a randomized, controlled trial. J Am Osteopath Assoc. 2002;102(7):387–96.

57. Papa L, Mandara A, Bottali M et al. A randomized control trial on the effectiveness of osteopathic manipulative treatment in reducing pain and improving the quality of life in elderly patients affected by osteoporosis. Clin Cases Miner Bone Metab. 2012;9(3):179–83.

58. Lopez D, King HH, Knebl JA et al. Effects of comprehensive osteopathic manipulative treatment on balance in elderly patients: a pilot study. J Am Osteopath Assoc. 2011;111(6):382–8.

59. Fraix M, Gordon A, Graham V et al. Use of the SMART Balance Master to quantify the effects of osteopathic manipulative treatment in patients with dizziness. J Am Osteopath Assoc. 2013;113(5):394–403.

60. Mueller DM. The 2012–2013 influenza epidemic and the role of osteopathic manipulative medicine. J Am Osteopath Assoc. 2013;113(9):703–7.

61. Hodge LM. Osteopathic lymphatic pump techniques to enhance immunity and treat pneumonia. Int J Osteopath Med. 2012;15(1):13–21.

62. Noll DR, Degenhardt BF, Morley TF et al. Efficacy of osteopathic manipulation as an adjunctive treatment for hospitalized patients with pneumonia: a randomized controlled trial. Osteopath Med Prim Care. 2010;4:2.

63. Goldstein FJ, Jeck S, Nicholas AS et al. Preoperative intravenous morphine sulfate with postoperative osteopathic manipulative treatment reduces patient analgesic use after total abdominal hysterectomy. J Am Osteopath Assoc. 2005;105(6):273–9.

64. Yurvati AH, Carnes MS, Clearfield MB et al. Hemodynamic effects of osteopathic manipulative treatment immediately after coronary artery bypass graft surgery. J Am Osteopath Assoc. 2005;105(10):475–81.

65. Crow WT, Gorodinsky L. Does osteopathic manipulative treatment (OMT) improve outcomes in patients who develop postoperative ileus: a retrospective chart review. Int J Osteopath Med. 2009;12(1):32-7.

66. Sleszynski SL, Kelso AF. Comparison of thoracic manipulation with incentive spirometry in preventing postoperative atelectasis. J Am Osteopath Assoc. 1993;93:834.

67. Radjieski JM, Lumley MA, Cantieri MS. Effect of osteopathic manipulative treatment of length of stay for pancreatitis: a randomized pilot study. J Am Osteopath Assoc. 1998;98(5):264-72.

68. Allen WA. Sports medicine. In: Ward RC, editor. Foundations of osteopathic medicine. 2nd ed. Philadelphia: Lippincott Williams and Wilkins; 2002. ch. 24.

69. Maffettone P. Complementary sportive medicine. Milan: Castello; 2002.

70. Zimaglia C. Sportive massage and complementary techniques. Milan: Edi-Ermes; 2011.

71. Larequi Y. Physiotherapy and osteopathy:a real holistic supervision of athletes. Rev Med Suisse. 2010;6(258):1504-7.

72. Brolinson GP, McGinley SM, Kerger S. Osteopathic manipulative and the athlete. Curr Sports Med Rep. 2008;7(1):49.

73. Fishbein M, Middlestadt SE, Ottati V et al. Medical problems among ICSOM musicians: overview of a national survey. Med Probl Perform Art. 1998;3:1.

74. Chaitow L. Manual therapy of soft tissue. Principles and techniques of the positional release. Milan: Elsevier; 2009.

75. Shoup D. Survey of performance related problems among high school and junior high school musicians. Med Probl Perform Art. 1995;10:3.

76. Shoup D. An osteopathic approach to performing arts medicine. Phys Med Rehabil Clin N Am. 2006;17(4):853-64, viii.

77. Thomson OP, Petty NJ, Moore AP. Clinical decision-making and therapeutic approaches in osteopathy. A qualitative grounded theory study. Man Ther. 2014;19:44-51.

78. Greenhalgh S. Red flags: a guide to identifying serious pathology of the spine. Philadelphia: Elsevier; 2006.

79. Sizer PS, Brismée JM, Cook C. Medical screening for red flags in the diagnosis and management of musculoskeletal spine pain. Pain Practice. 2007;7(1):53-71.

80. Kendall NAS, Linton SJ, Main C. Psychosocial yellow flags for acute low back pain: "yellow flags" as an analogue to "red flags". Eur J Pain. 1998;2:87-9.

81. Kendall NAS, Linton SJ, Main Newton-John TC et al. Early intervention in acute back pain: problems with flying the yellow flag. Physiotherapy. 2001;87(8):397-401.

82. Sowden M, Hatch A, Gray SE et al. Can four key psychosocial risk factors for chronic pain and disability (yellow flags) be modified by a pain management program? A pilot study. Physiotherapy. 2006;92:43-9.

83. Skedung L, Arvidsson M, Young Chung J et al. Feeling small: exploring the tactile perception limits. Scientific Report. 2013;3:2617.

84. Sabini RC, Leo CS, Moore AE. The relation of experience in osteopathic palpation and object identification. Chiropr Man Therap. 2013;21:38.

85. Esteves JE, Spence C. Developing competence in diagnostic palpation: perspectives from neuroscience and education. Int J Osteopath Med. 2013;17(1):52–60.

86. Willard FH, Fossum C, Standley PR. The fascial system of the body. In: Chila A, editor. Foundations of osteopathic medicine. 3rd ed. Baltimore: Lippincott Williams and Wilkins; 2010. ch. 7.

87. Catala M. Embryonic and fetal development of structures associated with the cerebrospinal fluid in man and other species. Part I: The ventricular system, meninges and choroid plexuses. Arch Anat Cytol Pathol. 1998;46(3):153–69.

88. Burns L.Pathogenesis of visceral disease following vertebral lesions. Chicago: American Osteopathic Association; 1948.

89. Wynn TA. Cellular and molecular mechanisms of fibrosis. J Pathol. 2008;214(2):199–210.

90. Tozzi P. Does fascia hold memories? J Bodyw Mov Ther. 2014;18(2):259–65.

91. Liem T, McPartland JM, Skinner E. Cranial osteopathy: principles and practice. Edinburgh: Elsevier, Churchill Livingstone; 2004. pp. 340–2.

92. Finando S, Finando D. Fascia and the mechanism of acupuncture. J Bodyw Mov Ther. 2011;15:168–76.

93. Wolff J. The law of bone remodeling [translation of the 1892 German edition]. Berlin: Springer; 1986.

94. Rolf IP. Rolfing. Reestablishing the natural alignment and structural integration of human body for vitality and well-being. Rochester, VT: Healing Arts Press; 1989. p. 129.

95. Simons DG, Travell JG. Travell and Simons' myofascial pain and dysfunction: the trigger point manual. 2nd ed. Baltimore: Williams and Wilkins; 1999. pp. 8–9.

96. Selye H. The stress of life. New York: McGraw-Hill; 1956. Plate 3, or revised edition.

97. O'Connell JA. Bioelectric fascial activation and release. Indianapolis: American Academy of Osteopathy; 2000. 22–25:59–78.

98. Rosner AL, Cuthbert SC. Applied kinesiology:distinctions in its definition and interpretation. J Bodyw Mov Ther. 2012;16(4):464–87.

99. Masi AT, Nair K, Evans T et al. Clinical, biomechanical, and physiological translational interpretations of human resting myofascial tone or tension. Int J Ther Massage Bodywork. 2010;16;3(4):16–28.

100. Swanson RL, 2nd. Biotensegrity: a unifying theory of biological architecture with applications to osteopathic practice, education, and research – a review and analysis. J Am Osteopath Assoc. 2013;113(1):34–52.

101. McMakin CR, Oschman JL. Visceral and somatic disorders: tissue softening with frequency-specific microcurrent. J Altern Complement Med. 2013;19(2):170–7.

102. Oschman JL. Energy medicine: the scientific basis. New York: Churchill Livingstone; 2000. pp. 1–40.

103. Oschman JL. Energy medicine in therapeutics and human performance. New York: Butterworth/Heinemann; 2003.

104. Hendryx JT, O'Brien RL. Dynamic strain-vector release: an energetic approach to OMT. Am Osteopath Assoc Journal. 2003;10(3):19–29.

105. Lazarev NV. 7th All Union Congress Physiol, Biochem, Pharmacol, Medgiz, Moscow; 1947. p. 579.

106. Brekhman II, Dardymov IV. New substances of plant origin which increase non specific resistance. Ann Rev Pharmacol. 1969;9:419–30.

107. McPartland JM, Skinner E. The biodynamic model of osteopathy in the cranial field. Explore (NY). 2005;1(1):21–32.

108. Nicholas AS, Nicholas EA. Atlas of osteopathic techniques. Philadelphia: Lippincot Williams and Wilkins; 2008.

109. De Stefano L. Greenman's principles of manual medicine. Baltimore: Lippincott Williams and Wilkins; 2010.

110. Nicholas AS, Nicholas EA. Atlas of osteopathic techniques. Philadelphia: Lippincot Williams and Wilkins; 2008. ch. 11.

111. Nicholas AS, Nicholas EA. Atlas of osteopathic techniques. Philadelphia: Lippincot Williams and Wilkins; 2008. ch. 7.

112. Nicholas AS, Nicholas EA. Atlas of osteopathic techniques. Philadelphia: Lippincot Williams and Wilkins; 2008. ch. 10.

113. De Stefano L. Greenman's principles of manual medicine. Baltimore: Lippincott Williams and Wilkins; 2010. ch. 8.

114. Yadava RL. Fulford percussion. In: Chila A, editor. Foundations of osteopathic medicine. 3rd ed. Philadelphia: Wolters Kluwer/ Lippincott, Williams and Wilkins; 2011. p. 866.

115. Nicholas AS, Nicholas EA. Atlas of osteopathic techniques. Philadelphia: Lippincot Williams and Wilkins; 2008. ch. 12.

116. Dowling DJ. Facilitated positional release. In: Chila A, editor. Foundations of osteopathic medicine. 3rd ed. Philadelphia: Wolters Kluwer/Lippincott, Williams and Wilkins; 2011. p. 813.

117. Johnston WL. Functional technique. In: Chila A, editor. Foundations of osteopathic medicine. 3rd ed. Philadelphia: Wolters Kluwer/ Lippincott, Williams and Wilkins; 2011. p. 831.

118. Nicholas AS, Nicholas EA. Atlas of osteopathic techniques. Philadelphia: Lippincot Williams and Wilkins; 2008. ch. 9.

119. Glover JC, Rennie PR. Strain and Counterstrain approach. In: Chila A, editor. Foundations of osteopathic medicine. 3rd ed. Philadelphia: Wolters Kluwer/Lippincott, Williams and Wilkins; 2011. p. 749.

120. Nicholas AS, Nicholas EA. Atlas of osteopathic techniques. Philadelphia: Lippincot Williams and Wilkins; 2008. ch. 12.

121. King HH. Osteopathy in the cranial field. In: Chila A, editor. Foundations of osteopathic medicine. 3rd ed. Philadelphia: Wolters Kluwer/Lippincott, Williams and Wilkins; 2011. p. 728.

122. Nicholas AS, Nicholas EA. Atlas of osteopathic techniques. Philadelphia: Lippincot Williams and Wilkins; 2008. ch. 18.

123. Nicholas AS, Nicholas EA. Atlas of osteopathic techniques. Philadelphia: Lippincot Williams and Wilkins; 2008. ch. 13.

124. Van Buskirk RL. 2011. Still technique. In: Chila A, editors. Foundations of osteopathic medicine. 3rd ed. Philadelphia: Wolters Kluwer/ Lippincott, Williams and Wilkins; 2011. p. 849.

125. Nicholas AS, Nicholas EA. Atlas of osteopathic techniques. Philadelphia: Lippincot Williams and Wilkins; 2008. ch. 17.

126. Nicholas AS, Nicholas EA. Atlas of osteopathic techniques. Philadelphia: Lippincot Williams and Wilkins; 2008. ch. 8.

127. O'Connel JA. Myofascial release approach. In: Chila A, editors. Foundations of osteopathic medicine. 3rd ed. Philadelphia: Wolters Kluwer/Lippincott, Williams and Wilkins; 2011. p. 698.

128. Nicholas AS, Nicholas EA. Atlas of osteopathic techniques. Philadelphia: Lippincot Williams and Wilkins; 2008. ch. 15.

129. Nicholas AS, Nicholas EA. Atlas of osteopathic techniques. Philadelphia: Lippincot Williams and Wilkins; 2008. ch. 14.

130. Crow WMT. Balanced ligamentous tension and ligamentous articular strain. In: Chila A, editor. Foundations of osteopathic medicine. 3rd ed. Philadelphia: Wolters Kluwer/Lippincott, Williams and Wilkins; 2011. p. 809.

131. Nicholas AS, Nicholas EA. Atlas of osteopathic techniques. Philadelphia: Lippincot Williams and Wilkins; 2008. ch. 16.

132. Kuchera ML. Lymphatics approach. In: Chila A, editor. Foundations of osteopathic medicine. 3rd ed. Philadelphia: Wolters Kluwer/Lippincott, Williams and Wilkins; 2011. p. 786.

133. Essig-Beatty DR, Steele KM, Comeaux Z et al. Pocket manual of OMT: osteopathic manipulative treatment for physicians. Philadelphia: Lippincott Williams and Wilkins; 2006. ch. 1.

134. De Santi A, Mendico S, Santilli V. CARE (Communication, Hospitality, Respect, Empathy) Rehabilitation, editors. Manual of evaluation of communication in rehabilitative field. Rome: Superior Institute of Health (Rapports ISTISAN 13/1); 2013.

135. Risch A. The metaphor analysis. A combination of quantitative and qualitative research. In: Hengel R, Tozzi P, editors. Teaching osteopathic research. Edinburgh: Handspring Publishing; 2010. p. 39.

136. Selye H. The stress of life. New York: McGraw-Hill; 1956.

137. Schulkin J. Rethinking homeostasis: allostatic regulation in physiology and pathophysiology. Cambridge: MIT Press; 2010.

138. Zink JG, Lawson WB. An osteopathic structural examination and functional interpretation of the soma. Osteopath Ann. 1979;7:12–9.

139. Glonek T, Sergueff N, Nelson KE. Physiological rhytms/oscillations. In: Chila A, editors. Foundations of osteopathic medicine. 3rd ed. Philadelphia: Wolters Kluwer/Lippincott, Williams and Wilkins; 2011. pp. 162–85.

140. World Health Organization. Traditional medicine strategy: 2014–2023. Geneva: WHO; 2013.

141. Fryer G. Teaching critical thinking in osteopathy – integrating craft knowledge and evidence-informed approaches. Int J Osteopath Med. 2008;11(2):56–61.

# Adaptive local response: somatic dysfunction

*Giampiero Fusco*

## Synopsis

Adaptation is the process that occurs when an individual has to respond to stress. Individuals are immersed daily in an environment where they may run into stressful stimuli. To preserve the state of health, the person uses strategies based on adaptive components of various types: physiological, psychosocial, cognitive, sociocultural, and spiritual. Selye described the local adaptation syndrome (LAS) as a chronic inflammation of the tissue in response to the action of stressful events represented by chemical, physical, biological, environmental, psychological, and emotional stimuli. These stimuli cause a locally irritative reaction that can lead to a reduction of blood flow and, consequently, to the retention of toxins. The basis for a vicious cycle that can lead to change in the tissue texture is thus created and change is produced by the interaction of tissues with daily superimposed stressor loads of various types.[1] The stressor load in itself represents a variable that, instant by instant, can lead the body to adaptation, or to constant activation of the intrinsic forces of self-healing. Therefore stress has repercussions on the human being, and is characterized on one hand by so-called polymorphisms (psychological, social, biochemical characteristics of the individual), and on the other hand by variable adaptive responses. Local adaptation is the tissue response to a stressor agent, which, in addition to bringing a readjustment of the functions *in situ,* can become an input intended to promote a general readjustment.[2] Adaptation allows us to understand the concept of health in biological, as well as philosophical terms. Moreover, it is one of the major theories that can describe the fundamentals of osteopathic medicine as handed down by Still.

## Somatic dysfunction viewed as key to local adaptation

The osteopathic lesion, now renamed somatic dysfunction (SD), was conceived as one of the primary factors that influence the economy of the body and as the root of many diseases. As described by Tasker,[3] the word "lesion" was used in osteopathy to identify "something more than an injury or a wound in any part of the body." Any structural change that negatively affects tissue functionality is called lesion. There may be structural changes noticeable on palpation, but which do not modify functionality and, consequently, are not lesions. Tasker illustrates how an anomaly of the vertebral development in itself does not correspond to an osteopathic lesion since it does not influence the functionality of the tissues, while a joint subluxation negatively affects the functionality of spinal mechanics and the neurophysiology of the annexed tissues and, in itself, corresponds to an osteopathic lesion. In the words of Tasker:[3]

The pressure of these structural lesions exerted on the media of communication and exchange, nerves and blood vessels, is believed to be the chief element active in producing and maintaining functional disorders. This is the central principle of osteopathic practice. Lesions may be present in any tissue, but their existence is most easily recognized in bone, ligament and muscle. Dislocations and subluxations of bones, thickened ligaments and contracted muscles constitute the usual varieties of lesions. A true lesion is usually palpable; the functional disturbance is related anatomically and physiologically; there is hyperaesthesia at the palpable area. These three conditions constitute the characteristics of the lesion as it is designated by the osteopath. Its palpability may vary between very wide limits; the anatomical and physiological association between the location of the structural change and functional derangement may be direct or indirect; the hyperaesthesia distinct or indistinct, still, the diagnostician is justified in centering attention upon the lesion if a reasonable amount of association can be detected.

By observing the SD according to the local adaptation syndrome (LAS), we could define it as a somatic mechanophysiological reaction intended to react, adapt and/or cause chronic exogenous and endogenous insults which affect the body. Tissue reactions would allow the individual's survival through the modification of four main parameters: (1) tissue texture change; (2) structural and functional asymmetry; (3) restriction of motion; and (4) tissue tenderness. From the beginning of the 20th century, clinical research, biological and pathophysiological analyses, as well as modeling the approach to SD, have been used to try to explain why these changes occur in the tissues and what might be the sequelae. We will analyze the studies and the descriptive models of SD, from the mechanical to the neurological and nociceptive, discussing the definitions shared by the practice community (Box 2.1) to describe contemporary models which focus attention on the fasciagenic origin of the dysfunction.

## Implications of reflexes in osteopathy

Since the very beginnings of osteopathic medicine, the nervous system has assumed a prominent role in attempts to explain the effects of both SD and osteopathic manipulative treatment (OMT). Both seem to be mediated by reflexes.[4] The four basic types of reflexes are at the base of complex reactions that occur in the body under physiological and pathological conditions. The concept of the reflex always includes an afferent branch, or coming from a sensory receptor, a spinal/central component and an output (efferent) branch which is normally a motor element of a somatic (musculoskeletal) or visceral structure that ends in synaptic connections which can both activate and inhibit the activity of the structure. Almost all reflex networks can be affected by a wide variety of other excitatory or inhibitory signals, including those from the highest and lowest levels of the central nervous system (CNS). The framework of a reflex as a simple signal that, rising from the neuromuscular spindle, causes contraction of the quadriceps muscle resulting in a patellar reflex of the kneecap is a stimulus/response interaction model. However, this reflex, defined as the myotatic reflex, represented by a tap on the patellar tendon and the subsequent knee jerk, is a simplified example of reflex.[5]

**Box 2.1**

Definition of somatic dysfunction and diagnostic criteria[1]

- *Somatic dysfunction (SD):* impaired or altered function of the components related to the somatic (body structure) system. Skeletal, myofascial, and arthrodial structures with their relative vascular, lymphatic, and neural elements may be involved. SD is treated by using osteopathic manipulative treatment. We can best describe the positional and dynamic aspects of an SD using at least one of three parameters: (1) the position of a part of the body determined by palpation and referred to a specific structure adjacent to it; (2) the directions in which the movement is more free; (3) the directions in which the movement is restricted.

- *Segmental dysfunction:* dysfunction in a mobile system located near precise segmental mobile units. The palpable characteristics of the segment in dysfunction are those associated with SD (see also STAR and TART, below). The answers to regional motor input at the level of the segment in dysfunction support the concepts of complete motor asymmetry and mirror-image motion asymmetries.

- *STAR*: acronym for the four diagnostic criteria of SD: sensitivity changes, tissue texture abnormality, asymmetry, and alteration of the quantity and quality of motion range.

- *TART*: acronym for the four diagnostic criteria of SD; tissue texture abnormality, asymmetry, motion restriction and tissue tenderness.

**Reference**

1. Educational Council on Osteopathic Principles (ECOP). Glossary of osteopathic terminology. Chevy Chase, MD: American Association of Colleges of Osteopathic Medicine; 2009. http://www.aacom.org/re-sources/bookstore/Pages/glossary.aspx.

The four basic types of reflexes include somato-somatic, somatovisceral, viscerosomatic and viscero-visceral reflexes:

- *Somato-somatic reflex*:[4] a stimulus (of any nature) applied to the outer surface of the body that elicits a response in the soma. The stimuli that can elicit such a reflex are of various origins, such as variations in temperature, chemical irritations, mechanical or environmental stresses. The basic criterion is that the stimulus must be sufficient to exceed the specific threshold (or resistance) of the reflex activity. The somato-somatic reflex was considered the most primitive reflex in humans.

- *Somatovisceral reflex*: the stimulus is applied to a receptor present in the soma while the effector is in the viscera. The efferent sympathetic cells of the intermediolateral column of the spinal cord represent the central synapses of the reflex. The hypothesis which is still under study[6] is that a stimulus applied to the soma would affect the visceral functions. In the presence of an appropriate stimulus the response is an autonomic activation, such as a vasomotor response; this is because the cells that are present in the intermediolateral column are the cells that initiate the sympathetic responses and are found in the border between the thoracic and lumbar spinal cord tract. Their endings arrive on the smooth musculature of the vascular system and, if activated, can lead to vasoconstriction.

- *Viscerosomatic reflex*:[4] the stimulus originates from a visceral structure and the response occurs in the soma. The stimulus activates an autonomic afferent response that, among its central connections, makes synapses with the anterior horn cells, which would cause the stimulation of a somatic efferent neuron. Among various connections, the autonomic pathway makes synapses with nociceptive afferent pathways, which may contribute to the onset of pain. It is unlikely that the reflex takes place in isolation, since the autonomic sensitive pathways of the viscera make synapses with the intermediolateral columns resulting in much more complex reflexes. The viscerosomatic reflexes may lead to tissue changes and are specifically considered as secondary effects that confirm the presence of SD in osteopathy. The effects taken into account in this regard were different, as extended (multisegmented) contracture of striated muscles, alteration of the tissue blood flow and activity of the sweat glands, which can be addressed, depending on the associated area of the dermatome, to the organ probably concerned. Although not enough to determine a differential diagnosis, in some cases these data were used in osteopathy to predict any complications or deteriorations in the visceral sphere.

- *Viscero-visceral reflex*:[4] is based primarily on an autonomic mechanism. This reflex is elicited by a stimulus coming from the viscera and the effect is associated with the same viscera through the autonomic nervous system. The visceral afferents reach the spinal cord/brainstem and through interneurons they cause efferent activity in the motor neurons of the sympathetic and/ or parasympathetic system. The spinal cord is the basis of integration of different reflexes. The gray matter of the spinal medulla is the convergence point of various stimuli of afferent and efferent nature, both somatic and visceral, and in some areas (areas of Rexed I and V) there appears to be considerable overlap of inputs coming from different nociceptors,[5] both somatic and visceral.

The stimuli, therefore, though creating different reflexes, travel in an integrated system, where afferent inputs from the skin, somatic and visceral tissues enter into direct or indirect communication with direct efferent pathways to the musculoskeletal system, autonomic effector cells (organs), neighboring or distant spinal segments, and supraspinal centers (brainstem, thalamus, and hypothalamus). In the spinal cord there is also integration of afferent/efferent pathways with descending pathways from supraspinal centers (brainstem and hypothalamus) that modulate the information processes from body tissues. The spinal cord thus becomes the programming and processing area of spinal reflex circuits[6] (Fig. 2.1).

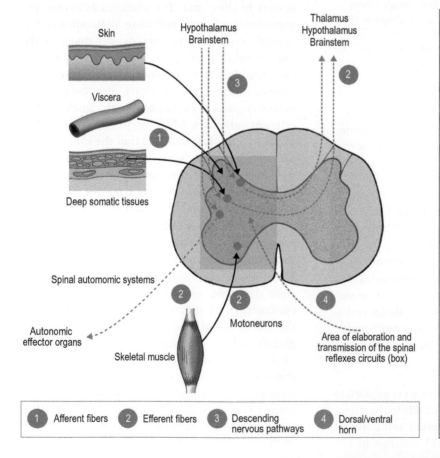

**Fig. 2.1**
Four types of reflexes and the spinal cord as a programming area. Modified by Jänig W. Vagal afferents and visceral pain. In: Undem B, Weinreich D, editors. Advances in vagal afferent neurobiology. Boca Raton, FL: CRC Press; 2005. pp. 465–93.

## Early research studies on somatic dysfunction

The first investigations related to the genesis of SD as a response to stress and possible somatic-visceral implication due to vertebral segments involved in dysfunction were conducted by Dr. Louisa Burns,[7] who dedicated her life to research in osteopathy. She defines the "bony lesion" (the name first given to SD, before it was renamed the osteopathic lesion) as an artificial lesion produced by holding one vertebra in an abnormal position compared to adjacent segments for a relatively short length of time. Early studies suggested that the duration of the "bony lesion" is important for understanding the spinal effects that may be present in the area of the involved segment, as well as for the reactions that may occur in the viscera affected by the respective autonomous innervation. Her research was conducted in laboratory using rabbits as test subjects; SD was experimentally "reproduced" in order to verify and quantify the effects of the tissues neurologically connected to the damaged segment in terms of cellular alteration. The changes included alterations in terms of organ functions neurologically related to the vertebral lesioned segment. The hypothesis was that these variations were mediated by the autonomic nervous system, because of its ability to interact with the organic blood support (vasoconstrictor action). Practically, what we now call somatic-visceral effects were verified and the results indicated congestion in the deep paraspinal muscles with adjacent physiological change (which Burns called "contraction"), muscle edema, and petechial hemorrhages in the areas of innervated organs. In the target tissues there was hyaline degeneration and hyperplasia of the connective tissue. Focusing on the changes in the muscles affected by the nerves coming from the area in the lesion, there was evidence of an increase in lactic acid content, and congestion of small blood vessels followed by chronic fibrosis. We reiterate that all lesions were assumed to be mediated by the autonomic nervous system. With regard to the viscerosomatic implications, osteopaths have shown special interest in the identification of SD associated with organic pathology.[8] These findings are similar for most autonomic innervation records. In a double-blind study conducted on 5,000 hospitalized patients who had been examined in order to find any SDs and their relation to the diagnosis, most visceral pathologies seemed to present more than one region with increased frequency in segmental relations. The oldest osteopathic research, consistent with facilitated segment(s)/viscerosomatic reflex findings, suggests a direct relationship between the OMT of T12–L2 dysfunctional segments and blood glucose levels.[9] Bandeen's research has been recently revised and reanalyzed[10] and it was suggested that if the pancreatic stimulation directed to ribs 2–5 is added to the stimulation of T12–L1, the blood glucose level is significantly affected.[11] Burns also conducted studies on visceral-somatic interactions,[12] implications in lung diseases,[13] and cardiac pathologies,[14] while Beal studied the prevalence of viscerosomatic dysfunctions in patients with heart disease, such as cardiac pathologies related to SD at T1–T3[15], coronary artery pathologies,[16] and lung diseases.[17] Additionally Hix[18,19] conducted research on specific musculoskeletal reactions to kidney and urinary tract stimulation in rats, in the laboratory of Denslow and Korr. In one of the studies[20] an osteopathic technique was applied to the T11 vertebral segment, intended to affect adrenal function, and the reduction of aldosterone levels in hypertensive patients showed a statistically significant result, but no reduction in blood pressure in the same patients. Johnston[21,22] studied the problem of how to identify visceral reflexes and then examine the spinal palpatory findings in patients with hypertension[23-25] and kidney disease.[26] Gwirtz and colleagues[27] have tested the hypothesis that myocardial ischemia induces an increase in paraspinal muscle tone located in the T2–T3 region and that this can be objectively measured with electromyography (EMG) and detected through palpation. Licciardone and colleagues[28] evaluated the palpatory results in 92 patients with type 2 diabetes mellitus, showing that the consistency of the tissues examined changed, including tissue tenderness on the right side at T12–L2. This was consistent with the viscerosomatic distribution of the kidney and diabetic renal pathophysiology.

## The neurophysiological basis of somatic dysfunction: the studies of Irvin M. Korr

According to osteopathic principles, the joints and soft tissues may be subject to functional and/or anatomical imbalances. Such imbalances may have local and/or distant effects. They are related directly or indirectly to pathological influences and can be detected by palpation and improved through OMT. The purpose of Dr. Korr's research[29] was to understand the neurophysiological basis that highlights the existence of SD. As stated in his studies, SD may have several aspects, among which are:

- tissue tenderness, especially muscular and spinal

- hyper-irritation as a reflex of an altered muscular activity and its state of contraction

- changes in the tissue texture of muscles, connective tissue, and skin

- changes in local circulation and exchange between blood and tissues

- alteration of visceral functions and other functions related to the autonomic nervous system.

In light of these statements that were established clinically and in previous studies, Korr wondered:

- How are these effects produced, and what are the key factors responsible for the manifestation of structural and postural abnormalities?

- What is the intrinsic nature of SD and the basis of the peripheral effects detectable by palpation?

- What are the real changes that take place as a result of effective manipulation?

Even today, many aspects have not been clarified, but it was Korr who encouraged and performed research in this area. He found in the nervous system most of the effects referring to the principles which underpin osteopathic treatment. After defining the nerve pathways that correlate the somatic and visceral afferents and efferents, and the connections between them on the segmental and axial planes, he declared that "the activity of skin, muscles, soft tissues, organs and cells is directly determined by motor nerve activity."[29] This activity is determined by the number of impulses conducted in each efferent fiber and the number of nerve fibers. The amount of contraction (tension produced or degree of shortening) at each moment is proportional to the number of motor neurons firing at that precise moment and to the average of number of impulses per second that each fiber is providing to the muscle. The principle that the "pulse" bombardment may lead to an increase in excitability is then extended to the autonomic system and various organs and systems. The common connection between muscles and organs is assigned to the sympathetic nervous system and, following in the footsteps of Burns' studies, Korr defines the spinothalamic tract as the pathway that can produce secondary effects because of pain, as well as psychological effects. The principles of reciprocity and convergence of the interneural networks also explain how one can have local and long-range effects, while an important role is assigned to both the proprioceptors and the afferent fibers coming from the viscera, such as receptors capable of generating increased impulses transmitted in the neural network. The final common pathway is represented by the motor system, which continually maintains a dynamic balance among all the excitatory and inhibitory influences from the many neurons that converge on it.[30] Proprioceptors and some superior centers, through their constant tonic control, act as modulators; the equilibrium, however, varies moment by moment, in accordance with the internal and external changes in the environment and in response to the will. Functional alteration results when the equilibrium is shifted too far in one direction or another (excitation or inhibition) for too long. The collective action of presynaptic fibers on the final common pathway is further reflected in the phenomena known as reinforcement and facilitation. Before any of the anterior horn cells can discharge impulses in the muscle fibers, they must simultaneously receive excitatory impulses from a number of presynaptic fibers. In other words: before a given stimulus (e.g., on the skin) can produce a muscle reflex response, the anterior horn cells must first be "warmed up" or "put on edge" (facilitated) by pulses coming from other excitatory fibers that make synapses with them. The efferent neuron must already be at a preliminary excitation threshold. To understand the role of SD in the genesis of nervous hyperactivity or hypoactivity and their consequences on the innervated organs, Korr recalls Denslow's studies[31,32] carried out at the College of Osteopathy and Surgery in Kirksville. Denslow starts from the clinical observation that the pressure applied to the spinous process of a dysfunctional vertebra produces greater contraction in the spinal extensor muscles. Additionally, the pressure required to elicit such a contraction is less than that applied to a non-dysfunctional vertebra. His studies were then designed to determine whether and to what extent a dysfunctional segment can be distinguished from a normal one in terms of reflex threshold. Muscular activity was determined electromyographically, i.e., by recording the electrical signs of muscular activity. Measured pressure stimuli were applied to the spinous processes by means of a calibrated pressure meter which simulated the action of thumb pressure. The pressure on the spinous process was applied to each segment gradually, until the appearance of muscular activity detected by the electromyogram: this accounted for the reflex threshold of the segment in question. The reflex arc thus comprised: the spinous process,

dorsal root, interneuron, anterior horn cells, and muscle fibers. This study showed that the reflex threshold of the segment in dysfunction was much lower than a normal segment and the greater the severity of the dysfunction was, the lower the activation threshold. It was also concluded, through further investigation, that the real center of dysfunctional convergence was given by the anterior horn cells of the dysfunctional segment, capable of being activated even if other normal segments were stimulated. Through additional experiments, a further hypothesis was developed, that a gamma-motor neuron circuit (or gamma-loop) maintained a low reflex threshold, and thus the played the predominant role of generating SD through a common final efferent pathway. Korr deduced, therefore, that other neurons could be facilitated, such as, for example, the sympathetic preganglionic fibers and the spinothalamic fibers that converge pain sensations onto the superior centers. The variation of the autonomic reflex threshold of the sympathetic nervous system was experimentally formed through the verification of the alterations in the activity of the sweat glands by measuring the skin electrical conductivity in dysfunctional and normal areas. Measurements were also designed to measure the change in the activity of the sympathetic fibers that control vasomotor activity. Other studies were performed to analyze the alterations of visceral functions due to changes in the activity of lateral horn cells, such as, for example, renal blood flow, glomerular filtration, and tubular secretion. Given the high number of sources that can cause and facilitate a segment in dysfunction, we can then understand that SD becomes a lens where physiological impulses, caused by irritation and conveyed to the related segment, converge and are channeled into the efferent flow. From a neurological standpoint, Korr then defined SD as "a facilitated segment of the spinal cord, maintained in that state by endogenous impulses entering the corresponding dorsal root; all the structures that receive efferent nerve fibers from such segments are, therefore, potentially exposed to excessive excitation or inhibition"[29] (Box 2.2).

## Box 2.2

Focal points described by Korr[1-4]

- SD is associated with a medullar spinal segment characterized by a low reflex motor threshold.

- The lowering of the reflex threshold is demonstrable by the hyperexcitability of motor neurons present in the anterior horn, which become hyperexcitable to different stimuli from all the neurons that make synapses with them, including, but not only, afferents from the involved vertebrae.

- SD, therefore, does not seem be the center of irritation but rather of focusing and convergence of stimuli both from the pertinent medullar segment and from distant stimuli.

- SD is associated with the concept of neurological spinal facilitation, i.e., with the spinal cord segment maintained in persistent excitation of endogenous origin by subliminal impulses, and whose structures, connected through efferent fibers, are potentially exposed to excessive excitation or inhibition.

### References

1. Korr IM. The neural basis of the osteopathic lesion. In: American Academy of Osteopathy Yearbook; 1953. pp. 76–85.

2. Sherrington CS. Correlation of reflexes and the principle of the common path. Brit Assoc Rep. 1904;74:728–41.

3. Denslow JS. An analysis of the variability of spinal reflex thresholds. J Neurophysiol .1944;7:207–15.

4. Denslow JS, Korr IM, Krems AD. Quantitative studies of chronic facilitation in human motoneuron pools. Am J Physiol. 1947;105:229–38.

Assuming the importance of proprioceptors in biomechanical imbalances, it is necessary to keep in mind the importance of afferents in establishing SD. In fact, any afferent related to or not through a segmental pathway may, through interneurons, exert an influence on the segment in dysfunction. To this we must add the influence of the superior centers and descending tracts on the inhibitory/excitatory equilibrium. Accordingly, SD should not be seen as the cause but one of the factors which in this context operate simultaneously; it is therefore an "adaptation" factor that "sets" the excessive informational, neurophysiological, and fluid load in the tissues in order to allow the individual to survive, to the detriment of health. According to the authors, therefore, we can find the complete concept of local adaptation in Korr's studies.

## The nociceptive model of somatic dysfunction

Subsequently, studies on Korr's research have gradually begun to bring attention to the nociceptive system as prime mover and maintenance factor of SD, since the free nerve endings are those that respond mostly to activation in the tissues by the sympathetic system. This makes it unlikely that the model for maintenance of SD is generated from the neuromuscular spindles, even though it does not exclude the simultaneous presence of the gamma loop. At this point, it was proposed that the etiology of SD is the unbalancing between the inputs of the various sensory receptors and the CNS. This immense variety of input and interactions between somatic and visceral systems makes it difficult to develop a standardized test for this. One possibility could be provoked pain, which almost always accompanies SD, and given the relationship between pain and the site of restriction, this would be a more appropriate way to investigate it, compared to the other epiphenomena. The model, proposed by Van Buskirk, has evolved from the neurological model of Korr, but emphasizes the nociceptors and reflexes as the sources of connective, gut, immune, and circulatory changes observed in the presence of SD.[33] The nociceptors (or PAN – primary afferent nociceptors) are primarily composed of C fibers and A-β fibers, with free nerve endings that terminate in all peripheral tissues and the stroma of all blood vessels, with the exception of the stroma of the brain, the nuclei of intervertebral discs, capillaries, and articular cartilage. They are well known for producing a muscular defense reaction and autonomic activation when a somatic or visceral tissue is stressed or damaged. In the case of trauma or damage to the peripheral tissues the following occur:

- There is release of pro-inflammatory components such as bradykinin, histamine, cytokines and prostaglandin that cause irritation of PAN, which in turn, if the stimulus is of minimum intensity, are able to inhibit the sensation of pain, while at high levels they are capable of generating, through spinal reflexes, increased sensitivity in the peripheral tissues.

- PAN, once stimulated, are able to release through an antidromic pathway (centrifugal action) sensitizing substances such as CGRP (calcitonin gene-related peptide), substance P, and somatostatin, which contribute not only to the sensitization of nociceptive peripheral branches, but also to the facilitation of the local inflammatory response.

- With increased peripheral activity of the C fibers there follows an increase of glutamate release in the dorsal horn that "facilitates" the system at a later episode of stimulation; metaphorically, it is as if a spring system was loaded for a higher intensity future action. This "spring" position is called wind-up and this hyperexcitability sensitizes the nociceptive signal transport system to the higher centers (centripetal action).

- Neurogenic inflammation is also mediated by interneurons in the dorsal root by GABA (γ-aminobutyric acid), which, when released in the central terminations of PAN, causes primary afferent depolarization (PAD), a phenomenon that at low amplitude reduces the feeling of pain through presynaptic inhibition, but at high amplitude is able to determine an antidromic action potential that also causes the release of pro-inflammatory substances in the peripheral endings. This phenomenon is also known as the dorsal root reflex (DRR).[34]

- The result of these phenomena will be increased sensitivity in the affected peripheral tissues or tissue tenderness, which we note as tissue tenderness.

- The inflammatory phenomenon causes abnormal defensive positions of muscles and variations of the motor range. The neuromuscular spindles will be influenced by the local humoral inflammatory response and by the autonomic reflex pathway, as well as the defensive muscle contraction caused by the α motor neurons, and in this context it may involve the aforementioned gamma loop described by Korr that can in turn lead to reflex muscle hyper-reactivity. This reaction will cause visible asymmetry and variation in the quality and quantity of motion detected during the osteopathic test.

- Finally, the maintenance of muscles, joint, and associated tissues in an abnormal defensive position causes a modification of the connective tissue or alteration of tissue texture. The most significant indicator of this change is variation in connective tissue by means of remodeling by fibroblasts. The altered tissue will have a random orientation and thus will be less able to maintain normal lines of force.

In the model proposed by Van Buskirk, the nociceptor is therefore able to "fabricate" SD. If the

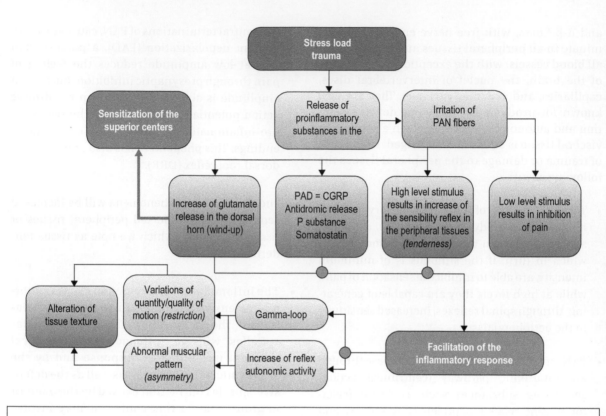

**Fig. 2.2**
Possible neurophysiological and tissue changes that can occur when the body is exposed to a stress load/trauma. Note the correlation between the release of pro-inflammatory substances, the neural, anatomical, and physiological changes and the quantitative/qualitative tissue variations.

abnormal position is maintained for a long time (hours to days) the dysfunction changes from acute to chronic. Now the dysfunction will be maintained by the nocifensive reflex and the connective variations and since the joint involved will no longer be balanced (at a functional, gravitational, and postural level), everything will facilitate nociceptive activation and pain perception[34] (Fig. 2.2).

## Central sensitization and neuroendocrine response

We learned that protracted inflammation of the peripheral tissues induces sensitization

of the nociceptors. This causes a lowering of the discharge threshold and the occurrence of spontaneous activities, as well as the recruitment of silent unmyelinated mechanosensitive fibers. This phenomenon further leads to the sensitization of second order neurons (interneurons) of the dorsal horn, amplification of the transmission of nociceptive impulses, and plastic/functional neuronal variations. This phenomenon is known as central sensitization (CS) and its clinical implications will be explored in Chapter 5, which examines the neurological model. As described by Jänig,[6] CS involves an increase in receptor capacity and the development of responses to new stimuli in peripheral tissues. Neural and glial cell changes can take place at different times, from hours to days, and many of these changes have been described by several authors.[35,36] Functional plastic changes in the dorsal horn can be followed by (or occur in parallel to) plastic changes in supraspinal centers such as the brainstem, hypothalamus, thalamus, and telencephalon, which will affect the control capabilities of the descending pathways. Whatever the specific mechanisms of chronic sensitization of the neurons of the dorsal horn, in pathophysiological conditions and the subsequent changes in supraspinal centers, it is not far-fetched to assume that these changes occur in all second order neurons that make synapses with the nociceptive afferent system and that transmit and process information directed to the neurons of the ascending tract, motor neurons or preganglionic neurons. So, in the presence of an organ or deep somatic structure dysfunction, the persistence of the activity of afferent nociceptive neurons may cause pain, discomfort, modification of the ongoing activities, and will be reflected in the autonomic spinal and somatic motor pathways.

These variations are seen in the projection areas of the efferent neurons: dermatomes, miotomes, sclerotomes, and viscerotomes. The sympathetic nervous system (SNS) also contributes to tissue changes present in SD and is a component of the fast and slow body defense systems present in the hypothalamus-midbrain system; in this regard, the regulation of pain is an integral part of these systems.[37] In fact, in the presence of a stress/harmful stimulus, both systems are activated for adjusting the perception of pain, whose higher centers used for such control are located in the periaqueductal gray matter (PAG) present in the midbrain. During the rapid defensive response, the system can choose a combat strategy (fight) or avoidance (flight), and both are characterized by the mobilization of energy sources, by activation of the sympathetic adrenal system (SAM), the hypothalamic–pituitary-adrenal (HPA) axis, and nonopioid hypoalgesia generated by the suppression of nociceptive impulses from the PAN. Such a response is also regulated by nociceptive peripheral sensitivity and is accompanied by an increase in vigilance, heart rate, blood pressure, and vasodilation in striated muscles. If the threat is inevitable, the rapid system can choose a passive coping strategy, where we see a decrease in the above-mentioned parameters. In the slow response, the organism is in a state of recovery and healing in which the physiological responses are similar to the passive coping strategy. Another important component is represented by the immune system, which through bidirectional communication promotes recovery and tissue repair. The brain is constantly influenced by immune cytochemical signals and modulates immune reactivity through the sympathetic neural pathway and the SAM and HPA systems; it is, therefore, fully involved in the recovery phase and in promoting self-healing mechanisms. The spinal reflexes, elicited by the sympathetic system in the presence of cutaneous, tissue, and visceral noxious stimuli, also fall within this protection system. The efferent sympathetic pathways regulate different parameters,[6] including: capillary blood flow, sweating, cutaneous tissue texture, consistence/edema of the subcutaneous tissue, tone, irritability, viscoelastic and fluidic properties of striated muscle tissue, variations in tissue texture of the deep fascial layers and joint capsules, and secretion and motility of the visceral organs. In practice, all the parameters taken into account during the osteopathic clinical diagnosis are considered. We can therefore imagine SD as an imbalance between the spinal systems and the supraspinal controls, which "leads" to functional disorders in somatic and visceral tissues, and that "induces" a defensive neuroendocrine response through the SNS, which, among other actions, modulates tissue inflammation (Fig. 2.3).

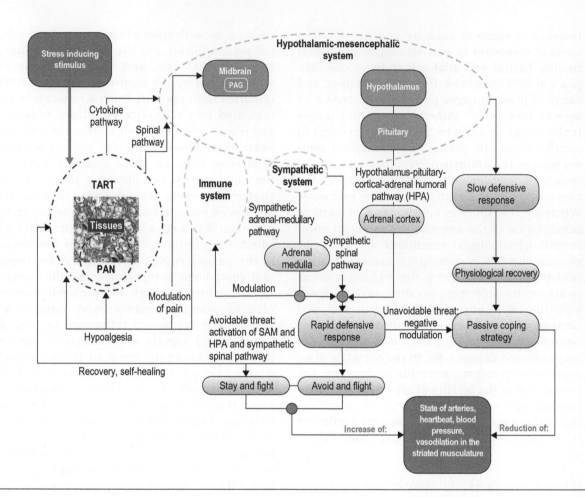

**Fig. 2.3**
Neuroendocrine-immunological systemic response that occurs in the presence of a stress-inducing stimulus and the correlation with tissue changes. Starting from the left: the tissues are presented together with the integrated primary efferent nociceptor (PAN) fibers in them; the arrows in the upper left represent the humoral and spinal communication between the tissues and the hypothalamus-midbrain system. The next ellipse shows the immune system in its role as "modulator" of tissue pain and "connector" between tissues and higher centers. In sequence we find the sympathetic adrenal medullary (SAM) systems, spinal sympathetic and HPA, which play a key role in the rapid and slow defensive responses and in the modulation of the passive coping strategy. Depending on the specific response, the systems modulate hypoalgesic functions, physiological recovery, and self-healing in tissues, and the modification of the systemic parameters described in the lower right pane. Please refer to the text for further details.

## The neurofasciagenic model of somatic dysfunction

Ever since the founding of osteopathy, the evaluation and the role of connective tissue has been considered fundamental in the treatment of a wide variety of conditions and essential to achieve desired clinical results. As founder Andrew Taylor Still said: "Fascia is the place to look for the cause of disease and the place to consult and begin the action of remedies in all diseases."[38] In addition to being valued as a source of self-healing properties of the body, such as the matrix of life, the fascia was also recognized as the ground for the spread of various harmful processes to the body.[39] The fascial concepts enunciated by Still continued to be developed by the early osteopaths who have created the basis for much of our clinical understanding of this tissue, which is widely recognized as the structural element of unification of the body, the key to understanding the mutual interrelationship between structure and function, and the innate ability of the body to self-regulate.[40,41] These principles have led to the development of manual approaches that go beyond the model of joint structural treatment. Unlike the aspects described in the previous paragraphs, where osteopathic research has been focused on the interrelations in neurology, there need to be investigations on the fascial aspects as mechanisms that underlie the establishment of SD. Tozzi proposes a neurofasciagenic model of SD[42] as a unifying model of the neurogenic aspects, long explored, and the mechanisms related to the fascia which underlie the establishment of SD. The following are the key points described.

## Fascial architecture

In the model of fascial architecture, it is noted that the fibroblasts have the ability to remodel their cytoskeleton and, in particular, when subjected to stress/tensional variations of a mechanical nature, a redistribution of actin and contraction of actomyosin can occur within a few minutes.[43] This would also lead to architectural change of the surrounding tissue, causing an increase in the number of stress fibers (contractile bundles of actin detectable in non-muscle cells)[44] with connections to focal adhesions. Any deregulation of the mechanisms by which cells sense mechanical signals and convert them into chemical response may then lead to the deregulation of the cellular metabolic processes and the degradation of connective tissue components.[45] This may cause an increase or a decrease of deposition of extracellular matrix (ECM), altered tissue architecture, dysfunction and, in some cases, significant morbidity.[46] In the neurofasciagenic model further

studies have been published which show that collagen deposition is modulated by physical activity, while degradation is modulated by immobility. It was also noticed that, in chronic musculoskeletal conditions, a variation of the relative thickness of the deep fascial layer is related to an increase in the amount of loose connective tissue located between the layers of dense collagen fibers, but without any increase of the collagen itself.[47] This process of fascial thickening and increase in density could explain the reduction in the sliding potential between the fascial layers involved and adjacent structures, as observed in patients with nonspecific cervical and lumbar pain.[48] The sliding reduction may be associated with, or induce, an asymmetric muscular activity, becoming a potential source of SD. These adhesions can lead to chronic fibrosis, manifesting some features of SD as changes in tissue texture and asymmetry: changes that become evident to the osteopath during palpation are therefore the result of changes involving the cytoarchitecture up to the extracellular matrix, causing repercussions in the entire body fascial network and requiring tissue adaptation to local stress, through a global connective reorganization.

## Fascial contractility

It has been suggested that the fascia may have contractile capabilities similar to smooth muscle regardless of the skeletal muscles' activity.[49] This is possibly related to the presence of smooth muscle cells in the fascial tissue.[50] The behavior and myofibroblastic contractility are highly sensitive to oxygen levels, vasoactive peptides, autonomic activities, pro-inflammatory cytokines and tension of the surrounding tissues.[51] It has been suggested that the force generated by the fascial contraction may extend to the intramuscular connective tissue in order to adapt muscular rigidity/stiffness to the changes of stress load.[52] This in turn can affect the muscle tone at rest and musculoskeletal dynamics through local redistribution of mechanical forces and the neurological influence on somatic motor neurons. The dysfunction of this apparatus could then lead to an altered myofascial tone, decreased neuromuscular coordination, with possible sequelae such as postural disorders, pain syndromes and pathologies of the musculoskeletal system, with subsequent readjustment of myofascial and tissue contractility that underlie the motion restriction characteristic of SD.

## Fascial viscoelasticity

Depending on the increase, the speed and duration of the load, the fascia shows elastic-plastic deformation capacity in a nonlinear fashion.[53,54] This viscoelastic property is based on the interdependence between the architecture and composition of the connective tissue and the water content.[55] Recently, researchers have discovered an inherent and independent viscoelastic property of the myofascia, regardless of the activity of the nervous system: it is defined as HRMT[56] (human resting myofascial tone or tension) and is determined by the molecular interactions of actomyosin filaments in myofibroblasts and the sarcomeric units. HRMT can make a substantial contribution to maintaining biomechanical postural stability (see below and Chapter 4). A persistent static load could lead to a variation of the viscoelastic sliding of the connective tissue, resulting in a transient alteration of the neuromuscular activity (spasm and muscle hyperexcitability),[57] as well as to a variation in terms of colloidal consistency of the fundamental substance which tends toward a solid state, thus changing the intrinsic biological activity of the connective tissue, as well as the tissue consistency, which predisposes to additional risk of damage.

## Dynamics and fascial fluid contents

The fascia also plays an important role in the balancing and physiology of fluids. The water contained in the fascial layer depends on the pressure changes of interstitial fluid resulting from the dynamic interaction between the osmotic attraction exerted by negative charges, due to the glycosaminoglycans being generally under-hydrated and abundant in the fascia, and the mechanical tension/stiffness of the collagen fibers, which resist the extrusion of water, resulting in tissue swelling.[58] It seems that any reduction of the tension of collagen leads to a reduction of the interstitial hydrostatic pressure and determines that fluids are reabsorbed by the ECM components. The role of the fibroblasts is also crucial in determining the collagen tension across the contacts between the matrix and the cells, by acting as modulators of the dynamics of the fluids through the adjustment of their dimension and tension of the matrix in response to changes in osmotic pressure,[59] as well as modifying the physical properties of the connective tissue and the transcapillary exchange during inflammation. Thus, there is a mutual influence between mechanical strength/force, response of the cells, and dynamics of interstitial fluids. A sustained static stretch applied to the fascia can produce an extrusion of water from the tissue followed by a compensatory increase in hydration of the matrix,[60] similar to a sponge effect, which can be significant for fascial function.[61] It has been shown that under normal physiological conditions, a lubricating hyaluronic acid layer is located between the deep fascia and muscles, as well as in the loose connective tissue, dividing several fibrous sublayers of the deep fascia. These hyaluronated layers promote normal fascial function and sliding movements. If compromised as a result of injury or chronic inflammation, alteration of tissue sliding and fluid dynamics occurs, leading to alterations of chemistry and tissue structure, contributing to the development of myofascial dysfunctions.

## Fascial pH and the factors that influence its level

Several free nerve endings in the fascia inform the insular cortex of the forebrain about the physiological conditions of the tissue, such as pH changes and warmth.[62] Variations in the pH, ionic content, and temperature may represent the main metabolic and environmental factors that influence fascial viscosity.[63] The changes of breathing patterns and temperature, and presumably of physical activity[64] and nutrition,[65] are able to modulate tissue pH levels through environmental and metabolic changes, and oscillations of these can strongly influence fascial function.

## Somatic neurofascial interaction

The presence of mechanoreceptors and PAN in the fascia[66] suggests a role in the dynamics of proprioception, force transmission, and motor control. However, abnormal mechanical stimulation can cause a pathological change of the fascial innervation, generating an increase in nociceptive fibers[67] within the fascia that would support fascial inflammation.[68] Therefore, the irritation of PAN, as described in the previous paragraphs, is able to initiate the release of neuropeptides and finally the creation of a neurogenic inflammation predisposing to peripheral and central sensitization, altering the texture of the surrounding connective tissue by the interaction of fibroblasts and immune cells.[69] The repercussions of this phenomenon through the neuroendocrine response were discussed in the relevant section and will be recalled in Chapter 5, dedicated to the neurological model, where we will analyze its clinical implications.

## Autonomic neurofascial interactions

Fascial tension can be adjusted by the activity of the autonomic nervous system, independent of skeletal muscle tone. This can occur through the interaction between the autonomic fibers and smooth muscle cells located in the fascia that can contract as a smooth muscle tissue.[49] It has been suggested that sympathetic activation may induce myofibroblastic contraction in the fascial tissue through the release of TGF-β1, just as other cytokines can modulate fascial stiffness.[60] Therefore, activity of the autonomic nervous system may be involved in the genesis and maintenance of pain and SD in the connective tissue.

## Metabolic influences

Different cells of the connective tissue respond to mechanical stress by inducing the expression of collagen and remodeling of the matrix under the influence of hormones and growth factors.[70] Such mechanically induced expressions of pro-collagen and collagen synthesis appear to be mediated in the myofascial tissue by an early upregulation of specific growth factors such as insulin-like growth factors (IGF), mechano growth factors (MGF), and IGF binding proteins (IGFBP).[71] In summary, several studies[72-79] show that various hormonal and metabolic factors may influence myofascial consist-

ency and stiffness, assuming a possible role in the genesis and maintenance of characteristic fascial and associated dysfunctions.

## Piezoelectricity

Thanks to piezoelectric properties (the capacity by which a mechanical force is converted into an electrical stimulus), collagen can exchange physical information at both macroscopic and cellular levels, directly or through biochemical processes.[80] It seems that the physical-chemical properties of collagen depend strongly on its hierarchical structure, and the piezoelectric response appears to be directly proportional to the level at which collagen fibril molecules are assembled.[81] In fact, the piezoelectric current generated by the mechanical strain on the collagen fibers during wound formation have been proposed as the driving forces in the early stages of tissue reparation, acting in concert with the TGF-β to determine the deposition and orientation of the collagen fibers.[82] It is plausible that the alterations of collagen architecture following injury, surgery, or chronic inflammation can lead to changes in the piezoelectric response of the affected area, with consequent repercussions on structure and fascial functionality.

## Epigenetics

Epigenetics is defined as "the collective heritable changes in phenotype caused by processes that arise regardless of primary DNA sequence."[83] These changes in the accessibility of genes and their expression are linked to the independent alteration of the germline of the chromatin architecture, which occur mostly through DNA methylation, modification of histones, and microRNA processes. The result is the remodeling of the organization of chromatin, which is preserved during cell division, then becomes inheritable. Although the mechanical signals are known to be a key regulator of behavior and of the cellular differentiation of connective tissue, the influences on gene regulation at the epigenetic level have been demonstrated only recently.[84] Epigenetic changes, including DNA and histonic methylation, may cause a permanent activation of fibroblasts capable of altering the immune function, thereby producing inflammatory responses until the development of chronic disorders of the connective tissue.[85] Altered epigenetic schemes may also be responsible for myofibroblastic differentiation and accumulation of extracellular matrix in chronic inflammatory conditions[86] and fibrotic disorders.[87]

## Hypothesis: water

Each collagen fiber in the body is embedded in layers of water molecules which, when they are associated with proteins, behave in an orderly and schematic, or crystalline manner.[88] As demonstrated by several studies, this system, based on the interaction of water and protein, can provide a dynamic framework for understanding various biological mechanisms, such as transcription and DNA replication, which are the basis of the various biophysical processes.[89] It is therefore hypothesized that fascial dysfunction could be generated by self-reinforcing dysfunctional circuits of proton-electron-hydrogen transfers following the structural alteration of the collagen network linked to water, such as may occur in injury, inflammation and scar tissue.

## Hypothesis: bioenergetics

The structural continuum of the collagen matrix with the intracellular skeleton can function as a semiconductor system by displaying coherent vibrations throughout the body, with a potentially regulatory role.[90] This communication system can affect the metabolism and the function of the cells,[91] viewing the metabolic activities as a result of interactions of electromagnetic and electromechanical forces.[92] With regards to fascia, fibroblasts in cell culture showed different patterns of proliferation under the influence of bone growth factors that may be correlated with an ultra-weak emission of photons following irradiation with a moderate dose of ultraviolet A rays.[93] This feature can be deregulated or altered in the event of illness,

in conjunction with many underlying pathogenic processes to various conditions, including those that affect connective tissue, related to a general high oxidative state of the organism.[94,95]

## Neurofasciagenic model: conclusions

In conclusion, all the fasciagenic factors described above can play a role in the genesis and maintenance of SD and its features that are certainly related, but not limited exclusively, to neural influences. These processes may also cause and maintain types of SD that have not yet been classified in terms of reduction of the quantity and quality of movement.[96] These processes can be organized into a unifying model of structural and functional changes of the fascia, under various influences and interactions, leading to palpable features of SD. This can be the result of a series of dysfunctional processes caused by interaction of various forces and of the subsequent responses to different dysfunctional events (Fig. 2.4).

## Local adaptive response: identification of somatic dysfunction

The osteopathic examination includes a screening intended to identify the region of the body in which an SD is present. The diagnosis of SD has a code (M99.00) in the International Classification of Disease (ICD-10).[97] The classification is based on the anatomical area in which the dysfunction is diagnosed (Box 2.3). During screening, a detailed visual investigation (scanning) is performed, in order to identify the specific location, followed by a local palpatory inquiry (perceptual palpation), to exactly define the type of dysfunction, by verifying the presence of at least one of following parameters:

- Alteration of tissue texture, identified with the letter T which in English indicates Tissue texture change

- Structural and/or functional asymmetry, identified with the letter A for Asymmetry

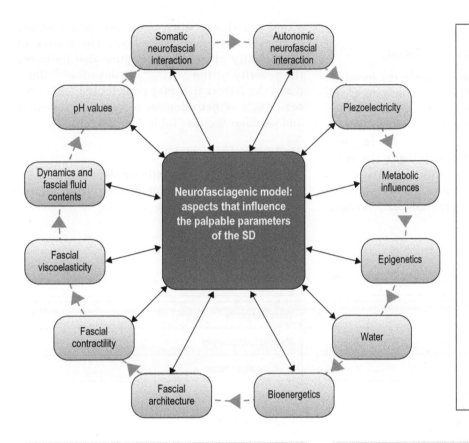

**Fig. 2.4**
Fasciagenic factors that may play a role in the genesis, maintenance, and determination of the palpable characteristic parameters of somatic dysfunction (SD).

**Box 2.3**

Somatic dysfunction classification according to ICD-10[1]

- M99.00 SD of the head region
- M99.01 SD of the cervical region
- M99.02 SD of the thoracic region
- M99.03 SD lumbar region
- M99.04 SD of the sacral region
- M99.05 SD of the pelvic sacral region
- M99.06 SD of the lower limbs
- M99.07 SD of the upper limbs
- M99.09 SD of the abdomen and other regions

Reference

1. ICD-10 CM. International Classification of Disease, 10th revision. Geneva: World Health Organization; 2010.

- Motion range restriction, identified with the letter R for Restriction

- Hyperesthesia or tissue tenderness, identified with the letter T for Tenderness (or Temperature in some cases).

The initials of the four parameters create the acronym TART, whose diagnostic significance is further described below.

## TART

### Alteration of tissue texture (T = Tissue)

The first information that we use in the formulation of the diagnosis of SD is the changing of the tissue texture. The tissues surrounding the joint(s), affected by SD manifest palpable tissue texture changes. These occur in the skin, fascia, muscles and vessels and vary according to the acute or chronic nature of the dysfunction. Increased heat, moisture, and hypertonia, etc., is typical in the acute phase, while decreased heat, dryness, atrophy, and stiffening of tissues are indicators of chronic dysfunctional stages. The degree of abnormality of the tissue texture also indicates the severity of the SD.[98-99] DiGiovanna[100] illustrates the factors that may contribute to this process, such as neurological (direct and referred) and vascular factors (Table 2.1).

### Asymmetry (A = Asymmetry)

On palpation, an articulation presenting with SD will be positioned asymmetrically with respect to contiguous joints. For example, a transverse

**Table 2.1**
Factors that may contribute to the genesis of the alteration of the tissue texture

| Neurological factors | Vascular factors |
|---|---|
| *Somatic manifestations* | *Macroscopic changes* |
| • Muscular hypertonia | • Temperature change |
| • Hyperactivity of neuromuscular spindles | • Erythema or blanching |
| • Alteration of sudomotor activity | • Edema (swelling) |
| • Alteration of neurologically induced vasomotor activity | • Variation of the pulse and heart rate |
| • Soreness or hypersensitivity of soft tissues | |
| *Referred manifestations* | *Microscopic changes* |
| • Referred pain | • Hyperaemia of soft tissues |
| • Stiffness of the tissues in the involved sites | • Congestion and dilatation |
| • Variations in arterial pulse | • Edema (swelling) |
| • Variations in skin temperature | • Minute hemorrhages |
| | • Fibrosis |
| | • Local ischemia |
| | • Atrophy |

Modified by: DiGiovanna EL. Somatic dysfunction. In: DiGiovanna EL, Schiowitz S, Dowling DJ, editors. An osteopathic approach to diagnosis and treatment, 3rd ed. Philadelphia, PA: Lippincott Williams and Wilkins; 2005. ch. 4.

process of a vertebra could be more posterior than those of the vertebrae immediately above or below it, or the interspinous space may be more restricted with respect to the immediately contiguous vertebral segments. Not all asymmetries can be considered indicators of SD, since many actually represent postural compensation or congenital anatomical variations (e.g., the different sizes of the spinous processes in the thoracic spine), and should always be assessed and considered in the global context of the individual. Finally, over time we have not only positional but also functional asymmetry.

## Restriction (R = Restriction)

A tissue or an articulation involved in SD has a reduction in range of motion, called the restrictive barrier. Normally in a joint there are two barriers: the physiological and the anatomical one:

- *The physiological barrier* is the highest point of joint movement that can actively be achieved by the patient. It is a functional limitation within the anatomical motion range. A further passive motion can be introduced over the barrier toward the anatomical barrier (elastic barrier).

- *The anatomical barrier* is the highest point that can be reached beyond the physiological barrier. This point can be reduced by the action of the ligaments, tendons, and bones. Movement beyond the anatomical barrier results in rupture of the attached tissues.

In this context, the osteopathic restrictive barrier occurs within the physiological motion range and prevents the joint from moving through the entire physiological motion range. The restriction may affect more planes of movement, but the movement in the opposite direction appears normal and relatively free. From a qualitative point of view, starting from a point farthest from the restrictive barrier, we could find a point that is called a "balancing point" or "dysfunctional neu-

tral" that corresponds to a tensional compromise between the dysfunctional vector parameters and the corrective forces of the surrounding tissues; usually this is the point to seek and maintain during the application of indirect techniques (see Chapter 1). Do not forget that even pain can be a restrictive barrier, so if a movement is painful, the body will try to compensate and provide relief by reducing the movement, restricting and "shortening" the myofascial tissues.

The restrictive barriers display different palpatory characteristics than normal physiological, elastic, and anatomical barriers and can give very different end-feel sensations. For example, congestion or edema lead to a widespread feeling of "sponginess"; chronic fibrosis will lead to a more solid and rigid end-feel while a barrier caused by a muscular physiological alteration, be it a spasm, hypertonicity, or contracture, will result in a tenser end-feel that evokes a marked rebound on palpation. We can find a restrictive barrier in the skin, fascia, muscles, and ligaments, in joint capsules and in articular surfaces.[101] The goal of osteopathic treatment in this context is to normalize the existing restriction in the direction in which the movement is limited.

Other key concepts to consider in joint movement are those of freedom and tension in the soft tissues. The ability to perceive these phenomena is at the basis of assessment and manipulative treatment: the more one moves in the direction of the neutral point of a motor range, be it normal or pathological, the more the homogeneous the tissue is, and the freer it is from tension. This concept is at the basis of the "functional" methods of treatment based on the variation of the neuromotor, rather than articular, response (Fig. 2.5).

We must also consider that, despite the presence of a restrictive barrier, the individual is able to overcome it by actively moving against this restriction (which differentiates it from a pathological barrier), but with greater energy expenditure and

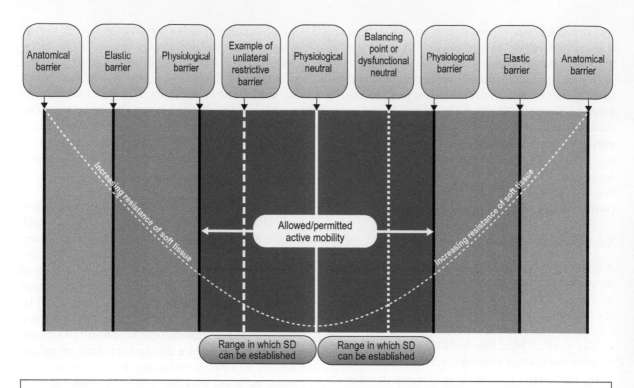

**Fig. 2.5**
Various types of barrier, the area where there may be a restrictive barrier characteristic of somatic dysfunction (SD) and illustration of increasing tone/resistance of soft tissues in relation to approaching/departing from the neutral point.
Modified from: Greenman P. Principles of manual medicine. Baltimore, MD: Williams and Wilkins; 1989. ch. 3.

by recruiting accessory movements (sidebending, rotation, translation, etc.). Finally, the restriction could in some cases be evident in all three planes of vertebral movement, and more evident in the minor movements of the joint. We may also find hypermobility or increased movement between the adjacent vertebrae as the result of compensation or persistent regional restrictions.[100]

## Tissue tenderness (T = Tenderness)

The tissue tenderness parameter may appear due to the applied pressure during palpation, or indicated by the patient in order to inform the operator of his or her pain. The perceived pain can manifest itself in the detected SD, or in a different area, for example by palpating the tissues in an SD of T1 the patient perceives

the pain in the T4 area. Tissue tenderness should not be confused with pain. Pain is the subjective awareness given by the activity of nociceptors and the relative psychoemotional state connected with it. Hypersensitivity is the pain provoked on palpation. As such, hypersensitivity is an objective physical phenomenon and it is often elicited as an involuntary response to pain, such as a muscle contraction or a facial grimacing on diagnostic palpation, which can be then used to confirm the diagnosis of SD after observation of tissue texture changes. It is believed that hypersensitivity is the less relevant criterion among those cited previously, and in osteopathic practice is used in a limited way to monitor the severity of the dysfunction and its performance during, and response after, treatment, especially in counterstrain techniques. The motion restriction of SD puts compensatory stress on adjacent structures, resulting in the perception of pain in them. However, due to mutual autonomic innervation, pain may be distant from the area of SD, a phenomenon that occurs when palpating a trigger point reproduces pain distally. As with tissue texture changes, hypersensitivity is an indicator of the severity of SD.

## A particular combination of the TART parameters: the somatic dysfunction of reflected origin

Tissue texture changes and tissue tenderness in the absence of asymmetry and motion restrictions are indicative of SD of reflex origin that is generated or supported by viscerosomatic or somato-somatic reflexes.[98,99] Osteopathic theory and practice defines the visceral reflexes that affect the soma as important causes of SD and of great diagnostic importance. There are differences between acute and chronic viscero somatic dysfunctions, but generally speaking, we say that the tissue response in a dysfunction where there is an acute viscero somatic reflex is indistinguishable from any SD,[100] while in a dysfunction where there is a chronic viscero somatic reflex we will have the following findings:

- The skin will tend to be more atrophic in the involved area.

- The tissues will be more "firm/still," dry, with an opposite feel to the one present in an acute dysfunction.

- The tissue texture will be very firm.

- Joint movement will be very small and will appear firmer when compared to a typical dysfunction.

- On motion testing, the joint will produce a slower and more rigid movement, and the end-feel will be "rubbery."

- The SD present may recur even after correction, until the reflex that tends to support/create it is normalized.

Beal[8] recommends focusing attention at the costotransverse area in the thoracic spine and suggests that viscerosomatic reflexes can be differentiated by the involvement of two or more adjacent vertebral segments; the restrictive barrier is not dictated so much by biomechanical phenomena as by deep muscle reflexes, an indicator of neuronal adaptation. The initial response to a viscerosomatic reflex may be limited to two adjacent segments, but with increasing duration and severity of underlying medical conditions, the findings will be spread to several adjacent segments through interneural connections. Changes of the tissue texture in the skin and in the subcutaneous area also give indications of the acuteness or chronicity of the visceral underlying pathology. An acute viscerosomatic reflex will lead for example to a temperature increase, vasodilatation and redness, while a chronic viscerosomatic reflex will lead to a decrease in temperature, reduced sudomotor reflex, fibrosis sensation detected by palpation, and hypersensitivity to deep palpation.[102] We will address in Chapter 5 the specific tests that allow us to identify the presence of such somatic influence. Stone[103] advances hypotheses regarding the correlation of the visceral pathological state with tissue changes, which can be summarized as follows: if the results indicate an acute viscerosomatic reflex, the viscera should be treated first; in contrast, in chronic conditions, the correlated vertebral SD should be the first to be treated, but one must still be aware of the imbalance of both viscerosomatic and somatovisceral reflex activities.

## Somatic dysfunction and vertebral mechanics

Among the research studies carried out by Fryette in osteopathy, the best known is that regarding the physiological movements of the spine.[104] Starting with the studies of Lovett[105] based on the entire spinal column, he described in detail the movements and biomechanical behavior of individual vertebrae. The conclusions are well-known and still used, known as the laws of spinal motion, or Fryette's principles, or Fryette's Laws. Below we briefly describe the laws and the vertebral mechanisms; for further details, the reader is referred to the text by Fryette.[106] Please note that the observations were based solely on palpation and without using objective measurements,[107] and further research is needed. Many osteopaths use the following principles as an aid in the diagnosis of SD of the spine and the application of treatment technique:

- *First principle*: when the spine, thoracic or lumbar, is in the neutral position (functional), the movements of sidebending and rotation for a group of vertebrae are such that the sidebending and rotation occur in opposite directions (the rotation goes toward the convexity).

- *Second principle*: when the spine, thoracic or lumbar, is in sufficient forward flexion or extension (not functional), the movements of sidebending and rotation in a single vertebral unit occur in the same direction (the rotation goes toward the concavity).

- *Third principle*: initial movement of a segment in one plane of motion will modify the motion of that segment in all other planes.

While the first and the third law seem to be generally accepted, there is considerable debate on the second law. In the words of Gibbons and Tehan:[108]

> There is evidence to support the laws of Fryette in relation to the coupled movements of sidebending and rotation in the cervical spine, such as rotation and sidebending to the same side,[109] but the evidence in relation to the lumbar spine is inconsistent.[110-113] As a result, these laws may be useful in predicting the biomechanical behavior of the cervical spine, but should be used with caution in regard to the movements of the thoracic and lumbar spine.

The conclusions of a systematic review by Harrison[114] indicate that "the investigations of the three-dimensional movement of vertebral patterns show that the vertebra rotates and moves in all three axes of movement and, therefore, the previous motion theories based on two-dimensional studies are inaccurate and invalid." Despite the fact that the laws that derive from Fryette's observations were challenged by many manual therapists, he is certainly credited with having organized an explanatory teaching model of vertebral dysfunctional features, useful for giving students an idea of the three-dimensional structures they palpate.

## Nomenclature

The nomenclature of SD uses abbreviations which describe dysfunctional movements. According to the principles of Fryette, they concern the lumbar and thoracic vertebrae, and the movement in these regions is determined by the patterns of forces generated by the discs, ligaments, and associated muscles. These principles describe the types of SD that can be derived, and these SDs are named according to the principles that describe their movement. The first principle describes a type I SD and the second a type II SD.[107]

## Local adaptive response: the somatic dysfunction

### Type I somatic dysfunction

Type I SDs tend to occur in groups, in the case of scoliosis, or in a single vertebra. Usually at the apex of the type I SD there is a type II SD. For the SD to be evaluated the spinal column must be in functional position, and when sidebending and rotation are introduced, the sidebending and the rotation will have opposite directions. For example, in neutral position, an SD at T9 will be present in relation to T10 with a right rotation and a left sidebend. We will say that T9 is NRrSl, or if it is the T2–T5 group that is affected by this SD we say that T2–T5 is NRrSl.

### Type II somatic dysfunction

Type II SDs tend to be present in single vertebral segments, although two similar adjacent SDs can occur simultaneously. It is important to note that the characteristics are not so much dictated by biomechanical phenomena as by deep muscle reflexes and by neuronal adaptation in the presence of viscerosomatic reflexes. For such an SD to occur, the thoracic or lumbar spine must be sufficiently out of the neutral position, or in flexion or extension, and in this position an SD can occur in which sidebending and rotation are in the same direction. If, for example, a type II dysfunction is present at T2, with dysfunctional movement in flexion coupled with right rotation and right sidebending, we say that T5 is FRrSr (Table 2.2).

## The cervical spine

Motion in the cervical spine is determined mainly by the shape of the joint facets. Motion of the occiput (Oc) on C1, for example, follows the first principle (rotation and sidebending will always be in opposite directions), while at C1 to C2 only rotation is considered; from C2 to C6 motion always follows the second principle (rotation and sidebending will always be in the same directions). Motion at C7 (with respect to T1) will tend to follow the classic thoracic and lumbar laws.

## Complex dysfunctions

There can also be restriction of a single plane of movement or compression (as, e.g., occiput and C1 compressed), and in the presence of trauma to the disc/ligament instability this can generate movements that go beyond the principles laid down by Fryette, generating complex dysfunctions[115] that need to be treated in a specific way depending on the clinical presentation and palpation findings (Table 2.3).

**Table 2.2**
Abbreviations and annotations that define vertebral somatic dysfunction

| Abbreviations (positions) | Annotations |
|---|---|
| N = Neutral | Type I SD (example): |
| F = Flexion | • T9 in neutral position, rotated to the left, sidebent to the right |
| E = Extension | |
| Lx = Left | • *Or* T9 iNRISr |
| Rx = Right | Type II SD (example): |
| R = Rotation | • T9 in flexion, rotated to the left, sidebent to the left *Or* T9 FRISl |
| S = Sidebending | |

Modified by: Ehrenfeuchter WC. Segmental motion testing. In: Chila A, editor. Foundations of osteopathic medicine. 3rd ed. Philadelphia, PA: Lippincott Williams and Wilkins; 2010. ch. 35.

## Somatic dysfunction hierarchy

In describing the complexity of dysfunctions and problems that can be found in the patient, it is often useful to create a hierarchy of SD, indicating the "generating" SDs as primary SDs and the compensation areas, which may present additional SDs, as secondary SDs. In fact, a primary SD (also called key

**Table 2.3**
Various types of vertebral somatic dysfunction, movements and units involved

| | Type I | Type II | Complex |
|---|---|---|---|
| Position of the spine | Neutral | Flexion/extension | Any |
| Coupled movements | Rotation opposite to sidebending | Rotation same as sidebending | Variable + compression |
| Vertebral regions | Thoracic, lumbar, Oc–C1, C2 (predominantly rotation) | Thoracic, lumbar, C3–C7 | Any |
| Vertebral units involved | Usually in groups, but it could be present as single | Usually single but in some cases two single units superimposed | Singular / single |

SD)[116] is the SD that maintains a global dysfunctional scheme and that according to Mitchell[117] causes a change of adaptation or compensation in the body, or directly causes dysfunctions or trophic changes in other parts of the body. In the *Glossary of Osteopathic Terminology*[116] we find the following definitions:

- Primary SD: (1) SD that maintains a global dysfunctional pattern (see also key injury, below). (2) The initial SD or that which appears first.

- Secondary SD: SD resulting from a mechanical or neurophysiologic response subsequent to, or as a consequence of, other etiologies.

- Key injury: SD that maintains a global dysfunctional pattern including secondary dysfunctions.

The concept of primary dysfunction underlies the SAT (specific adjustment technique), in which Tom Dummer[118] describes a treatment model that is based on three units: (1) the pelvis and lower limbs; (2) head, neck, chest down to the level of T4, upper limbs; and (3) chest and abdomen. After detecting the injury in each unit, the most severe of these is evaluated, namely the primary SD, on which a specific treatment is focused; the latter is usually associated with the accumulation of a traumatic force which causes a modification of the vertebral position beyond the physiological barrier, and in this approach is considered more important than the motion restriction. In different observations of osteopaths, different quantitative and qualitative evaluation methods of SD have been followed, sometimes giving emphasis to its positional parameters, as in the SAT, and at other times to the motion restriction, as in functional methods. This should not disconcert the osteopath who is faced with two different conceptual models; rather it should help him understand which of the models helps in understanding the nature of local adaptation in the presenting patient. According to Parsons and Marcer,[119] the logical consequence of this concept is the premise that, if the primary SD is treated, the compensations should move toward resolution. They add that such a resolution could actually occur in individuals with dysfunctional patterns of short duration and where the tissue changes did not become chronic. In case of long-term alterations, the fibrous tissue may create patterns that do not allow spontaneous healing after the removal of the generating SD. Therefore they reaffirm that the concept of "removal" of the primary SD as decisive is relative and should be analyzed according to the complexity of the dysfunctional model of the subject, where, in the presence of chronic disorders or long-term disruption, a secondary SD can become generating and supportive of the physiological imbalances, assuming the typical characteristics of a primary SD. From a diagnostic point of view, we may also consider a primary SD if it retains its dysfunctional parameters in every position assumed by the patient during the evaluation.

## Local adaptive response: perceptive palpation of somatic dysfunction

In order to manipulate soft tissue or articular structures, the osteopath should be able to perceive, assess, and evaluate quickly and accurately the range of parametric differences that differentiate physiological and pathological conditions. The osteopath must therefore acquire such information and then interpret it, in order to choose the appropriate manipulative technique. According to Greenman,[120] osteopathic diagnosis and palpation require serious consideration and practice in order to develop high-level diagnostic capacity, since palpation skills affect the ability to:

- perceive tissue texture changes

- detect asymmetry of position, by both visual and tactile methods

- demonstrate differences in the global motion range, in quality of motion, and in end-feel

- sense the position in space of both patient and examiner

- detect changes (both improvement and deterioration) over time.

Chapter 1 described the key that the osteopath will use in order to interpret the significance of local SDs in the evolution of the subject's health. Various specific tests will be described from time to time in the five models in accordance with the specific diagnostic picture for the "structure/function" relation that the lens of the model attempts to observe. The therapeutic approach will have the same criteria and examples of treatment will be described for each model. In this chapter, we report three examples of palpatory tests: articular, fascial, and visceral.

## Palpation of an articular/joint somatic dysfunction

For detecting an articular SD, we will use as an example the procedure adopted by Degenhardt and colleagues in their study of reliability[121] through the use of four tests designed to detect the presence of TART parameters in the lumbar L1–L4 region.

Tissue texture (T) is evaluated by palpating with the thumb directly on the inferior articular facets from L1 to L4. The presence of localized edema or fibrotic changes is considered a positive sign for the detection of tissue texture changes (Fig. 2.6A).

The detection of segmental static positional asymmetries of the transverse processes on the horizontal plane (A) is based on the position of the posterior portion of the transverse processes of each vertebra from L1 to L4 with the spinal column in the neutral position and the subject in the prone position. One notes whether the right or left transverse process is more posterior or prominent compared with that of the other side or if the processes are symmetrically positioned using the dominant eye (Fig. 2.6b).

Joint motion restriction (R) is detected by testing resistance to anterior springing of the spinous

processes. Basically, the palm of the hand (the area between the thenar and hypothenar eminences) is positioned on the midline of each spinous process from L1 to L4. The examiner induces an anterior springing motion. The motion is described as free movement (no restrictions) or restricted movement (Fig. 2.6C).

The provocation of pain to assess tissue tenderness on the spinous processes (T) was evaluated by applying a constant pressure with the thumb in an anterior direction on the spinous processes from L1 to L4. The subjects participating in the study notified the examiner as soon as they felt pain. Prior to the test, the amount of pressure necessary to palpate bone was determined to be 1.5 kg/cm$^2$,[122] and up to 4 kg/cm$^2$ was needed to detect tissue tenderness.[123] These measurements were used as a calibrated scale for purposes of determining intra-examiner reliability (Fig. 2.6D).

## Fascial palpation

Perceptual palpation is a tool that allows the osteopath to "listen" actively and passively to the tissue layers. Anatomical knowledge of the structure you want to palpate is of fundamental importance, in order to visualize the layers from superficial to deep, depending on the pressure that the examiner uses to assess the tissue change, both actively and passively. As suggested and described by Greenman,[120] it may be educationally useful to undergo consensus training in order to ensure correct assessment and identification of the different palpated anatomical structures. As Chaitow reminds us,[124] we should be able to perceive:

- motion range

- the type of restrictive barrier

- the relative weakness or tension in the muscles

- the amount of hypertonicity, edema, or fibrosis in the soft tissues

- the density and mobility of fascial structures

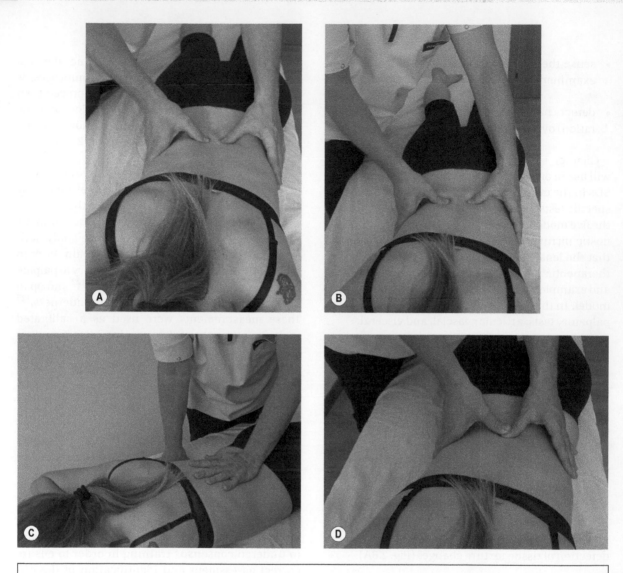

**Fig. 2.6**
The four stages of procedure for identification of joint SD. (A) T = detecting tissue texture changes; (B) A = detection of positional asymmetries; (C) R = test for joint motion restriction; (D) T = provocation of pain.

- regions in which reflex neurological activities are present and manifested

- the qualitative differences perceived in terms of vitality

- the changes in characteristics of each body region.

Fascial palpation allows the osteopath to capture sensory information that the brain interprets as the temperature, texture, surface moisture, elasticity, turgor, tissue tension, thickness, shape, irritability that has resulted in these changes in the tissues. To do this, it is necessary that the hands must be able to feel, think, see, and know; therefore we reiterate that it is necessary to have a visual image based on anatomical knowledge. Placing the hand on the affected area, we connect with the superficial fascial layer; by gradually increasing the pressure we contact the deeper fascial layers. For each layer, we may use the TART criteria adapting it to the global fascial system:

- evaluate the density of the tissue, testing its vitality (T)

- evaluate the presence of possible asymmetry (A), which in this case will be of a functional type and will show us a preferential direction of expansion/contraction

- listen to the intrinsic preferential movement that the tissue shows us, that "attraction" or indication of a specific motion vector, while the remaining perceived movements will be globally reduced (R)

- note whether during perceptual palpation the patient reports the onset of spontaneous tissue tenderness (T) or sense of irritation (in the tested area or elsewhere) (Fig. 2.7).

## Visceral palpation

Visceral evaluation involves four elements:

- Palpation, which gives information about the tone of the visceral cavity walls

- Percussion, which gives information about the location and size of the organ in question

- Auscultation, which gives information about other factors such as air flow, blood flow, and secretions (such as the bile secretion)[125]

- Pressure, which indicates possible venous congestion of the organ that is manifested as variation in the degree of viscoelasticity.

Barral and Mercier[126] underline the importance of visceral influence on muscle structure and vice versa. Two characteristics of an organ should be tested:

- *Mobility*, which represents the potential movement of an organ with respect to another muscle interface, a wall of another organ, or within the same organ (e.g., between the lobes of a lung). This mobility is directed by external muscle contraction forces or movements due to pressure differences. Knowing the position of the organ and its relative permitted movements, we will have information on characteristics such as elasticity, viscoelasticity, laxity/ptosis, spasm or trauma of the support structures (Fig. 2.8)

- *Motility*, which represents the inherent motion present in a specific tissue. To test motility, the hand rests on the specific organ, with a pressure of 20–100 g, depending on the depth of the organ. In some cases, the hand can fit the shape of the organ. The hand is totally passive, but there is an extension of the sense of touch used during this examination. The hand must listen passively, until a slow rhythmic motion (7–8 per minute in health) of low amplitude is perceived. To sharpen the perception, as soon as the movement is perceived you can stop and start again.

## Evaluation of the dysfunctional hierarchy

The severity of SD in a region refers sometimes to the detection of one or more characteristics of the TART acronym in the dysfunctional area. The ambulatory osteopathic module of documenting the subjective and objective data, and the assessment and treatment plan (SOAP), developed by the Louisa Burns Research Committee of the American Academy of Osteopathy as part of a grant from the American Osteopathic Association, was found to be valid and easy to use for research and training in the osteopathic profession.[127] The osteopathic SOAP note form suggests the following scale to describe a level of severity within the dysfunctional areas examined:

- 0/no SD: no detected parameter; equivalent to no SD present

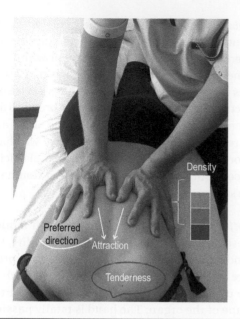

**Fig. 2.7**
Fascial palpation approach, noting the density of the
tissue, the direction of the preferential movement of
expansion/contraction/attraction, and the onset of pain.

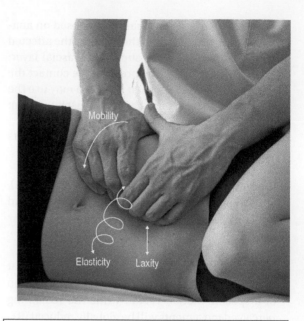

**Fig. 2.8**
Visceral palpation approach, noting the mobility
characteristics of an organ.

- 1/mild SD: minor elements of TART; equivalent
  to mild and asymptomatic dysfunction

- 2/moderate SD: obvious elements of TART, in particular restricted motion (R) and/or tissue texture
  changes (T); equivalent to moderate dysfunction

- 3/severe SD: significant elements of R and/or T
  present, identifiable with minimal palpation, as
  well as hypersensitivity to provocation; equivalent to severe dysfunction.

The osteopath tries to discriminate the SD keeping
in mind that the frequency and the amplitude of the
vibratory response to an applied force are partially
determined by the degree of resistance to deformation
of the tissue. If the osteopath detects different SDs in
a patient, there follows an assessment of the different
degrees of severity, its accessibility, as well as the clinical relevance to the patient's disorder. To optimize

this goal many osteopaths use the inhibition test (see
Chapter 1). The operator induces vector forces in an
area of severe dysfunction, until there is an improvement in the stiffness (the resistance of a material to
deformation provoked by the application of a compressive or tensile force) of the matrix, to stabilize the
fascial tone at rest, so the related dysfunctional distant
areas can improve their structure and functionality in
terms of mobility, plasticity, viscosity, thixotropy, and
resonant vibratory frequency. In such a case the operator will define as primary the area that, if stimulated,
produces an improvement of the structure and function both in the primary area and in any related areas,
and will focus his or her treatment on this.

### Test of inhibition

This test allows the osteopath to establish a possible
hierarchical relationship among identified dysfunctions, discriminating the compensatory/adaptive

from the primary/priority/causative. Put simply, the test is performed by contacting the two most relevant dysfunctions and applying and maintaining a slight pressure on one of them (inhibiting it), while the other is tested, by listening to any changes in involuntary rhythms or evaluating possible changes in tissue density via a pressure test. The test is then applied on the second dysfunction, evaluating the tissue responses of the first. The principle of the test is that, during the application of pressure (inhibition) on a dysfunction, it will eliminate or reduce temporarily the disturbing influences on the other (perhaps also thanks to the gate mechanism). During this time, it will reveal an improvement, worsening, or maintenance of its SD parameters. From this, the osteopath can gather the following information:

- Non-relationship ratio: in this case, when inhibiting one dysfunction the other dysfunction does not show changes in its SD properties. The test therefore suggests that there is no hierarchical dysfunctional relationship of any kind between the two zones, indicating a probable

separation of chronology, etiology, severity, and depth.

- Dominance ratio: if by inhibiting a dysfunction the second one gets better, but by inhibiting the second the first does not change, the first is probably dominant. Indeed, by inhibiting the disturbing influences, the second one improves its SD parameters. However, the opposite may occur.

- Co-dominance ratio: this type of relationship emerges when, by inhibiting alternately each of the two dysfunctions, the other improves its characteristics (Fig. 2.9).

In Section II, dedicated to the models, the inhibition test will be used in the context of the relevant model and including aspects such as the somatovisceral and viscerosomatic relationships, where osteopaths have tried to identify SDs correlated to visceral disorders through the interaction of nervous, fascial, and vascular systems.

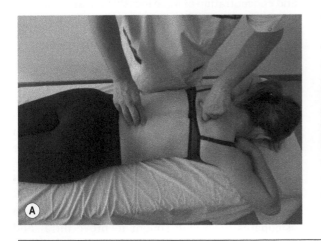 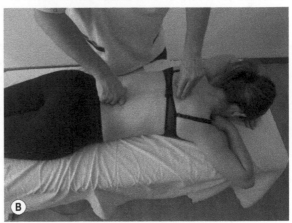

**Fig. 2.9**
Inhibition test, allowing the osteopath to compare the disorders considered clinically relevant. In (A) a slight inhibitory pressure is applied with the left hand on T4, while the right hand simultaneously detects whether there are tissue texture changes occurring at L1. In (B), applying the same procedure, a pressure on L1 is applied while monitoring T4.

## Palpation as an instrument: conclusions

It is possible to evaluate an SD from two main perspectives.[128] The first is represented by quantitative parameters, namely an objective approach that allows using, for example, a device such as the goniometer to record the effective differences in the symmetry of movement, even if a quantitative parameter, such as asymmetry, is often evaluated visually. The second perspective is represented by qualitative parameters, a subjective perspective which assesses the quality of the movement, or if the movement is free to flow, or if there is a disturbance in the quality of movement. If there is disorder, it is important to assess whether it is present throughout the motion range, or if it occurs at a specific point. The nature of the dysfunction may also involve fine or coarse mobility, or whether the barrier is found to be hard or soft, as well as the nature of the related soft tissue: elastic, hypertonic, swollen, hot, cold, etc. For example, the term "boggy," which in common language refers to soft and wet ground and is normally used in relation to a literal swamp or marsh, is used in osteopathy to define "an area that during palpation is identified as spongy," in order to create a vivid image of the abnormal sensation that has been perceived due to congestion caused by increased fluid.[100] During perceptual palpation, imagination and sense of touch are always used in unison. Osteopathic medicine has therefore developed its own language, in order to describe metaphorically the qualitative differences between an acute and a chronic SD. The tissue texture of a chronic SD is described as cold, dry, tense, or as a tissue that we imagine to be "stringy/filamentous" (ropiness). This language allows the operator and the patient to imagine how a tissue has been distorted over time and to correlate it to the pain experienced.

Moreover, when these palpatory responses are described, the palpatory diagnosis becomes more accessible to the patient's understanding because the osteopath uses a common language and promotes the establishment of a better osteopath–patient relationship. Osteopathic palpation therefore seeks to describe a wide range of conditions and different thermal and mechanical characteristics, trying to correlate them at first hypothetically (and subsequently after treatment) to the anamnesis made. Fig. 2.10 illustrates the unique and differential tissue characteristics present in acute and chronic SD.[129]

In modern terms, we could describe these modifications as conditions of alteration of tissue resilience, described by parameters of tissue mechanics, which include stiffness, or resistance of a material to deformation provoked by the application of a compressive or tensile force, elasticity, plasticity, thixotropy, and other features that encapsulate the ability of the muscular tissue to have an inherent passive tone (not generated by electric potentials) due to its molecular viscoelastic properties. In fact, as described in the work of Masi,[130] there exists an intrinsic viscoelastic property of the myofascial tissues, regardless of nervous system activity, which in humans gives rise to a resting muscle tone (HRMT). This parameter could be the basis for tension transmission through fascial containment elements; through tensegrity responses to stress, the HRMT mediates the maintenance of an efficient postural balance in the body, in the same way as a loss in conditions of excessive transmission and concentration of force localized in an area.

This would justify biomechanical adaptations, such as responses to environmental stimuli, clinically encountered in osteopathy (see Chapter 4). To verify the effective mechano-tissue changes, Barnes and colleagues[131] confirm that the use of the durometer can objectively measure the response of tissue texture to mechanical deformation, in order to provide numeric data representing tissue changes obtained through manipulation itself. The durometer could therefore be a useful tool for the evaluation of tissue hysteresis detectable by palpation in correspondence with SD; however, although osteopaths have long sought to prove intra- and inter-examiner reliability in the evaluation of SD, decades of research have not reached the level of reproducibility required to meet evidence-based criteria, until recently.[132]

Degenhardt and colleagues[121] observed an inter-operator concordance in the palpatory detection

**Chronic DS**

The past medical history shows symptoms of long duration, more than 6 months, sometimes years; the pain appears dull, aching, burning, itching; often the earlier pain occurs acutely/sharp (like acute- SD). The skin shows trophic changes (peeling, dryness, pigmentation changes, etc.); it is pale and cold due to the vascular changes which are due to the regional neural hyperactivity of the sympathetic system. The tissues are pasty, fibrotic, thickened, with chronic congestion and increased stiffness; mobility is qualitatively poor or normal and quantitatively reduced: the musculature has reduced tone and/or contractures. Somato-visceral and viscero-somatic effects may be present.

**Acute DS**

The next anamnesis shows a recent beginning, often of traumatic origin, with acute and sharp pain. The skin does not show trophic changes but is moist, reddened, inflamed and hot due to vascular alterations caused by the release of endogenous peptides and increased activity of the sympathetic nervous system with local effect dominated by bradykinin-s. The tissues are edematous and congested and mobility is qualitatively poor, while quantitatively can often be normal: the musculature shows increased tone and/or spasm with probable variation of fusal activity. The somato-visceral and viscero-somatic effects may be minimal, silent or absent.

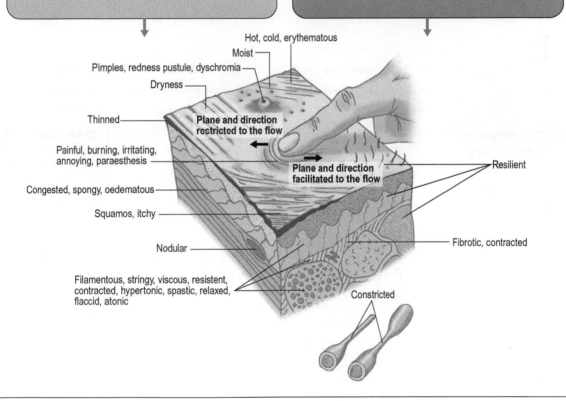

**Fig. 2.10**

Unique features present in acute and chronic somatic dysfunction (SD) detectable on palpation. Modified from: Kuchera ML, Kuchera WA. Osteopathic principles in practice. Columbus, OH: Greyden Press; 1994. pp. 20–5.

of SD in the lumbar area as a result of a consensus training of the examiners, while Tozzi and colleagues[96] were able to observe the relationships between reduced visceral mobility and musculo- skeletal pain, also suggesting that OMT can improve mobility and related pain. Diagnostic imaging could also be used to study the characteristics of the tissues where SD has been detected. A study by Shaw and colleagues[133] concluded that ultrasound is a reliable tool for evaluating SD of the lumbar spine. The data also confirm the validity of SD palpation performed by the osteopaths enrolled in the study. In addition, this study provides the first objective evidence of the effect of OMT focused on SD of the lumbar vertebrae.

## Hypothesis: somatic dysfunction as local adaptation

In summary, we look forward to "visualizing" SD as possible LAS. Imagine a clinical case concerning an athlete suffering from hyper-load in the right knee. We know that this will lead to a reduction in the efficiency of the quadriceps and, over time, to an imbalance of kinetic chains, which would affect the postural biomechanical efficiency of the entire individual. So we will have the following (Fig. 2.11):

- An acute phase (alarm phase) where the joint can be subjected to a high stress-producing load involving both the osteoligamentous profile and the recall of muscle patterns intended to "react" to the load imposed, with increased muscle tone, reduction of fluid drainage, possible

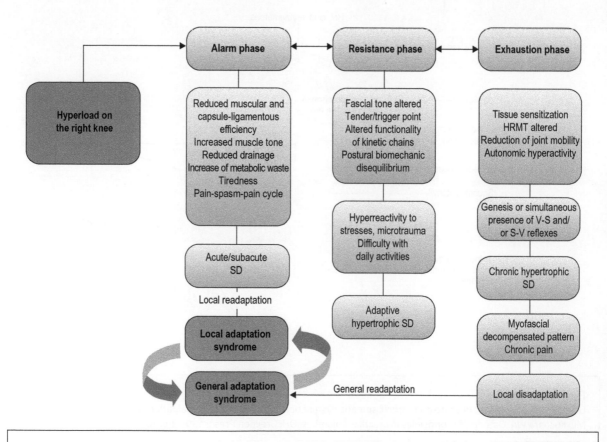

**Fig. 2.11**
Somatic dysfunction (SD) described according to local adaptation syndrome (LAS). Note the different alarm and resistance stages, adaptation, and specific neuroanatomical and physiological changes that underlie the implementation of acute, adaptive and chronic SD.

tissue ischemia and retention of metabolic wastes with fatigue. This will lead to irritation with possible inflammation that can result in the "pain–spasm–pain" cycle, with nociceptive hyper-reactivity and the possible beginning of an alteration of the minimum threshold of pain perception. The alarm phase can be made "silent" by adapting and fixing the imbalance, in the form of SD, in order to continue daily activities. Initially, therefore, the body adapts, appropriates, stores and limits locally the perceived stress (LAS). The SD can range from acute (0–72 hours) to subacute (3–14 days), with spontaneous tissue tenderness or reproducibility by palpation.

- Daily activities and training may be perceived as perpetual traumatic micro-stresses: the mechanosensory activation will lead to a collagen reinforcement intended to cushion the functional continuous demand and patterns of myofascial compensation (resistance stage) having an abnormal basal fascial tone will be established, which can promote the appearance of tendon, tendon-periosteal, and muscular trigger and tender points, as well as impact muscular synergistic–antagonistic activities. From the point of view of the tissue, SD in the resistance phase will be hypertrophic/adaptive (from 2 weeks to 3 months) with signs of tissue hypertrophy and subsequent adaptive tissue changes (3–6 months).

- If the tissues cannot compensate, chronic pain syndromes will manifest, in which the previous modification of the painful threshold may favor the genesis of peripheral and central sensitization through hyper-activation (centrifugal and centripetal) of PAN fibers in the extracellular matrix from the increase in sensitizing substances (inflammatory) present and the variation of HRMT, viscoelastic parameters, plastic and fascial thixotropy, decreased joint mobility and capacity to use the joint concerned (exhaustion phase). If a visceral disorder is present, this could further affect the spinal traffic through the autonomic (visceral-somatic) pathway and slow down the processes of adaptation by involvement of the descendant inhibitory pathways; or, whenever the systems of equilibrium of the autonomic circuits (e.g., control of the cardiac activity, pressure, etc.) become hyperactive, it could be further stimulated (somatovisceral) through the nociceptive ascending impulses from the area in SD and/or the spinal sensitization. In the exhaustion phase the SD will be chronic (from 6 months to 2 years) with signs of fibrosis, until the frank pathological response arises with manifested tissue atrophy (over 2 years).

- The adaptation to chronic pain, over time, can lead to the genesis of unbalanced postural patterns or to the overuse of the contralateral limb, creating imbalances that will affect the entire individual, representing a further body adaptive energy demand in the form of general adaptation syndrome (GAS).

## References

1. Selye H. The stress of life. New York: McGraw-Hill; 1978.

2. Chaitow L. Local adaptation syndromes holistic solutions depend on contextual thinking. massagetoday.com. 2006;1(2).

3. Tasker D. Principles of osteopathy. 2nd ed. Los Angeles: Baumgardt Publishing; 1905. pp. 144–5.

4. Cole WV. A reflex basis for osteopathic medicine. In: American Academy of Osteopathy Yearbook 1984: The Cole Book. pp. 15–9.

5. Patterson MM, Wurster RD. Somatic dysfunction, spinal facilitation, and viscerosomatic integration. In: Chila A, editor. Foundations of osteopathic medicine. 3rd ed. Philadelphia, PA: Lippincott, Williams and Wilkins; 2011. pp. 120–2.

6.  King HH, Jänig W, Patterson MM. The science and clinical application of manual therapy. Edinburgh: Churchill Livingstone, Elsevier; 2011. ch. 16.

7.  Cole WV. Louisa Burns Memorial Lecture. In: Beal MC, editor. American Academy of Osteopathy Yearbook 1994. pp. 2-10.

8.  Beal MC. Viscerosomatic reflexes: a review. J Am Osteopath Assoc. 1985;85(12):786-801.

9.  Bandeen SG. Pancreatic stimulation and blood chemical changes. Indianapolis: American Academy Of Osteopathy Yearbook. 1948;48:78-99.

10. Licciardone JC. Rediscovering the classic osteopathic literature to advance contemporary patient-oriented research: a new look at diabetes mellitus. Osteopath Med Prim Care. 2008;2:9.

11. Bandeen SG. Diabetes:report covering twenty-five years research on stimulation of pancreas, blood chemical changes. Osteopath Prof. 1949;17:11-15, 38, 40, 42, 44, 46-47.

12. Burns L. Qualities distinguishing muscles affected by primary vertebral lesions from those affected by viscerosomatic nerve reflexes. J Am Osteopath Assoc. 1928;27:542-5.

13. Burns L. Osteopathic case reports of pulmonary disease: a review. J Am Osteopath Assoc. 1933;33:1-5.

14. Burns L. Principles governing the treatment of cardiac conditions. J Am Osteopath Assoc. 1944;43:231-4.

15. Beal MC. Palpatory testing for somatic dysfunction in patients with cardiovascular disease. J Am Osteopath Assoc. 1982;82:822-31.

16. Beal MC, Kleiber GE. Somatic dysfunction as a predictor of coronary artery disease. J Am Osteopath Assoc. 1945;85:302-7.

17. Beal MC, Morlock JW. Somatic dysfunction associated with pulmonary disease. J. Am Osteopath Assoc. 1984;84:179-83.

18. Hix EL. A visceral influence on the cutaneous-renal receptive field. J Am Osteopath. Assoc. 1972;72:72-158.

19. Hix EL. Reflex viscerosomatic reference phenomena. Osteopathic Annals. 1976; 4:496-503.

20. Mannino JR. The application of neurologic reflexes to the treatment of hypertension. J Am Osteopath Assoc. 1979;79:225-31.

21. Johnston WL. Segmental definition: part III. Definitive basis for distinguishing somatic findings of visceral reflex origin. Am Osteopath Assoc. 1988;88(3):347-53.

22. Johnston WL. Osteopathic clinical aspects of somato-visceral interaction. In: Patterson MM, Howell JN, editors. The central connection: somato-visceral/ viscerosomatic interaction. Indianapolis, IN: American Academy of Osteopathy; 1992. pp. 30-46.

23. Johnston WL, Hill JL, Sealey JW et al. Palpatory finding in the cervicothoracic region: variations in normotensive and hypertensive subjects. A preliminary report. J Am Osteopath Assoc. 1980;79(5):55-63.

24. Johnston WL, Hill JL, Elkiss ML et al. Identification of stable somatic findings in hypertensive subjects by trained examiners using palpatory examination. J Am Osteopath Assoc. 1982;81(2):59-66.

25. Johnston WL, Kelso AF. Changes in presence of a segmental dysfunction pattern associated with hypertension: part A long-term longitudinal study. J Am Osteopath Assoc. 1995;95(5):315-8.

26. Johnston WL, Kelso AF, Hollandsworth DL et al. Somatic manifestations in renal disease: a clinical research study. Am Osteopath Assoc. 1987;87(1):61–74.

27. Gwirtz PA, Dickely J, Vick D et al. Viscerosomatic interaction induced by myocardial ischemia in conscious dogs. App. Physiol. 2007;103:511–7.

28. Licciardone JC, Fulda KG, Stoll ST et al. A case-control study of osteopathic palpatory findings in type 2 diabetes mellitus. Osteopath Med Prim Care 2007;1:6.

29. Korr IM. The neural basis of the osteopathic lesion. In: American Academy of Osteopathy Yearbook 1953. pp. 76–85.

30. Sherrington CS. Correlation of reflexes and the principle of the common path. Brit Assoc Rep. 1904;74:728–41.

31. Denslow JS. An analysis of the variability of spinal reflex thresholds. J Neurophysiol. 1944;7:207–15.

32. Denslow JS, Korr IM, Krems AD. Quantitative studies of chronic facilitation in human motoneuron pools. Am Physiol. 1947;105:229–38.

33. Van Buskirk RL. Nociceptive reflexes and the somatic dysfunction:a model. J Am Osteopath Assoc. 1990;90(9):792–4, 797–809.

34. Howell JN, Willard F. Nociception: new understandings and their possible relation to somatic dysfunction and its treatment. Ohio Res Clin Rev. 2005; vol.15.

35. Sandkühler J. Models and mechanisms of hyperalgesia and allodynia. Physiol Rev 2009;89(2):707–58.

36. Wolf CJ, Salter MW. Plasticity and pain. In: McMahon SB, Koltzenburg M, editors. Wall and Melzack's Textbook of Pain. 5th ed. Edinburgh: Elsevier Churchill Livingstone; 2006. pp. 91–105.

37. King HH, Jänig W, Patterson MM. The science and clinical application of manual therapy. Edinburgh: Churchill Livingstone, Elsevier; 2011. ch.2.

38. Still AT. Philosophy of osteopathy. Kirksville, MO: A.T. Still; 1899. p. 86.

39. Still AT. Philosophy of osteopathy. Kirksville, MO: A.T. Still; 1899. p. 164.

40. Page LE. The role of the fasciae in the maintenance of structural integrity. Indianapolis: American Academy of Osteopathy Yearbook 1952; 70.

41. Snyder GE. Fasciae – applied anatomy and physiology. Indianapolis: American Academy of Osteopathy Yearbook 1956; 65.

42. Tozzi P. A unifyng neuro-fasciagenic model of somatic dysfynction. Underlying mechanisms and treatment – Part I. J Bodyw Mov Ther. 2015;19(2):310–26.

43. Langevin HM, Storch KN, Cipolla MJ et al. Fibroblast spreading induced by connective tissue stretch involves intracellular redistribution of alpha- and beta-actin. Histochem Cell Biol. 2006;125(5):487–95.

44. Kreis TE, Birchmeier W. Stress fiber sarcomeres of fibroblasts are contractile. Cell. 1980;22(2):555–61.

45. Ingber DE. Mechanobiology and diseases of mechano-transduction. Ann Med. 2003;35(8):564–77.

46. McAnulty RJ. Fibroblasts and myofibroblasts: their source, function and role in disease. Int J Biochem Cell Biol. 2007;39(4),666–71.

47. Stecco A, Meneghini A, Stern R et al. Ultrasonography in myofascial neck pain: randomized clinical trial for diagnosis and follow-up. Surg Radiol Anat. 2014;36(3): 243–53.

48. Tozzi P, Bongiorno D, Vitturini C. Fascial release effects on patients with non-specific cervical or lumbar pain. J Bodyw Mov Ther. 2011;15(4):405–16.

49. Schleip R, Klingler W, Lehmann-Horn F. Active fascial contractility: fascia may be able to contract in a smooth muscle-like manner and thereby influence musculoskeletal dynamics. Med Hypotheses. 2005;65(2):273–7.

50. Staubesand J, Baumbach KU, Li Y. La structure fine de l'aponèvrose jambière Phlébologie. 1997;50(1):105–13.

51. Porter KE, Turner NA. Cardiac fibroblasts: at the heart of myocardial remodelling. Pharmacol Ther. 2009;123(2):255–78.

52. Schleip R, Naylor IL, Ursu D et al. Passive muscle stiffness may be influenced by active contractility of intramuscular connective tissue. Med Hypotheses. 2006;66(1):66–71.

53. Yahia LH, Pigeon P, DesRosiers EA. Viscoelastic properties of the human lumbodorsal fascia. J Biomed Eng. 1993;15(5):425–9.

54. Kirilova M. Time-dependent properties of human umbilical fascia. Connect Tissue Res. 2012;53(1):21–8.

55. Woo S, Livesay GA, Runco TJ et al. Structure and function of tendons and ligaments. In: Mow VC, Hayes WC, editors. Basic orthopaedic biomechanics. Philadelphia, PA: Lippincott-Raven; 1997. pp. 209–52.

56. Masi AT, Hannon JC. Human resting muscle tone (HRMT): narrative introduction and modern concepts. J Bodyw Mov Ther. 2008;12(4):320–32.

57. Sbriccoli P, Solomonow M, Zhou BH et al. Static load magnitude is a risk factor in the development of cumulative low back disorder. Muscle Nerve. 2004;29(2):300–8.

58. Mow VC, Ratcliffe A. Structure and function of articular and meniscus. In: Mow VC, Hayes WC, editors. Basic orthopaedic biomechanics. Philadelphia, PA: Lippincott-Raven; 1997. pp. 113–77.

59. Langevin HM, Nedergaard M, Howe AK. Cellular control of connective tissue matrix tension. J Cell Biochem. 2013;114(8):1714–19.

60. Schleip R, Duerselen L, Vleeming A et al. Strain hardening of fascia: static stretching of dense fibrous connective tissues can induce a temporary stiffness increase accompanied by enhanced matrix hydration. J Bodyw Mov Ther. 2012;16(1):94–100.

61. Stecco C, Stern R, Porzionato A et al. Hyaluronan within fascia in the etiology of myofascial pain. Surg Radiol Anat. 2011;33(10):891–6.

62. Craig AD. How do you feel? Interoception: the sense of the physiological condition of the body. Nat Rev Neurosci. 2002;3(8):655–66.

63. Thomas J, Klingler W. The influence of pH and other metabolic actors on fascial properties. In: Schleip R, Findley TW, Chaitow L, Huijing PA, editors. Fascia: the tensional network of the human body. Edinburgh: Churchill Livingstone Elsevier; 2012. pp. 171–6.

64. Shen CL, Chyu MC, Yeh JK et al. Effect of green tea and tai chi on bone health in postmenopausal osteopenic women: a 6-month randomized placebo-controlled trial. Osteoporos Int. 2012;23(5):1541–52.

65. Arent SM, Senso M, Golem DL et al. The effects of the aflavin-enriched black tea extract on muscle soreness, oxidative stress, inflammation, and endocrine responses to acute anaerobic interval training:a randomized, double-blind, crossover study. J Int Soc Sports Nutr. 2010;7(1):11.

66. Benjamin M. The fascia of the limbs and back: a review. Anat. 2009;214(1):1–18.

67. Sanchis-Alfonso V, Roselló-Sastre E. Immunohistochemical analysis for neural markers of the lateral retinaculum in patients with isolated symptomatic patellofemoral malalignment. A neuroanatomic basis for anterior knee pain in the active young patient. Am J Sports Med. 2000;28(5):725–31.

68. Herbert MK, Holzer P. Neurogenic inflammation II: pathophysiology and clinical implications. Anasthesiol Intensivmed Notfallmed Schmerzther. 2002;37(7):386–94.

69. Mense S. Pathophysiology of low back pain and the transition to the chronic state – experimental data and new concepts. Schmerz. 2001;15(6):413–7.

70. Kjaer M, Langberg H, Heinemeier K et al. From mechanical loading to collagen synthesis, structural changes and function in human tendon. Scand J Med Sci Sports. 2009;19(4):500–10.

71. Olesen JL, Heinemeier KM, Haddad F et al. Expression of insulin-like growth factor I, insulin-like growth factor binding proteins, and collagen mRNA in mechanically loaded plantaris tendon. J Appl Physiol (1985). 2006;101(1):183–8.

72. Doessing S, Heinemeier KM, Holm L et al. Growth hormone stimulates the collagen synthesis in human tendon and skeletal muscle without affecting myofibrillar protein synthesis. Physiol. 2010;588(2):341–51.

73. Skutek M, Van Griensven M, Zeichen J et al. Cyclic mechanical stretching modulates secretion pattern of growth factors in human fibroblasts. Eur J Appl Physiol. 2001;86(1):48–52.

74. Robbins JR, Evanko SP, Vogel KG. Mechanical loading and TGF-b regulate proteoglycan synthesis in tendon. Arch Biochem Biophys. 1997;342(2):203–11.

75. Leask A, Holmes A, Abraham DJ. Connective tissue growth factor: a new and important player in the pathogenesis of fibrosis. Curr Rheumatol Rep. 2002;4(2):136–42.

76. Van Snick J. Interleukin-6: an overview. Annu Rev Immunol. 1990;8253–78.

77. Duncan MR, Berman B. Stimulation of collagen and glycosaminoglycan production in cultured human adult dermal fibroblast by recombinant human interleukin 6. J Invest Dermatol. 1991;97(4):686–92.

78. Unemori E, Ehsani N, Wang M et al. Interleukin-1 and transforming growth factor beta: synergistic stimulation of metalloproteinases, PGE2 and proliferation in human fibroblasts. Exp Cell Res. 1994;210(2):166–71.

79. Yu WD, Panossian V, Hatch JD et al. Combined effects of estrogen and progesterone on the anterior cruciate ligament. Clin Orthop Relat Res. 2001;383:268–81.

80. Stroe MC, Crolet JM, Racila M. Mechanotransduction in cortical bone and the role of piezoelectricity: a numerical approach. Comput Methods Biomech Biomed Eng. 2013;16(2):119–29.

81. Denning D, Paukshto MV, Habelitz S et al. Piezo-electric properties of aligned collagen membranes. J Biomed Mater Res B Appl Biomater. 2014;102(2):284–92.

82. Farahani RM, Kloth LC. The hypothesis of biophysical matrix contraction: wound contraction revisited. Int Wound J. 2008;5(3):477–82.

83. Tollefsbol T, editor. Handbook of epigenetics: the new molecular and medical genetics. London: Academic Press; 2011. p. 1.

84. Arnsdorf EJ, Tummala P, Castillo AB et al. The epigenetic mechanism of mechanically induced osteogenic differentiation. J Biomech. 2010;43(15):2881–6.

85. Ospelt C, Gay S. Epigenetics in inflammatory systemic diseases [Article in German] Internist (Berl). 2014;55(2):124–7.

86. Cho JS, Moon YM, Park IH et al. Epigenetic regulation of myofibroblast differentiation and extracellular matrix production in nasal polyp-derived fibroblasts. Clin Exp Allergy. 2010;42(6):872–82.

87. Hinz B, Phan SH, Thannickal VJ et al. Recent developments in myofibroblast biology: paradigms for connective tissue remodeling. Am J Pathol. 2012;180(4):1340–55.

88. Pollack GH, Cameron IL, Wheatley DN. Water and the cell. Dordrecht: Springer; 2006.

89. Pang, XF. Properties of proton transfer in hydrogen-bonded systems and its experimental evidences and applications in biology. Prog Biophys Mol Biol. 2013; 112(1–2):1–32.

90. Pienta KJ, Coffey DS. Cellular harmonic information transfer through a tissue tensegrity-matrix system. Med Hypotheses. 1991;34(1):88–95.

91. Pienta KJ, Hoover CN. Coupling of cell structure to cell metabolism and function. J Cell Biochem. 1994;55(1):16–21.

92. Fröhlich H. Biological effects of microwaves and the question of coherence. Prog Clin Biol Res. 1982;107:189–95.

93. Niggli HJ, Scaletta C, Yu Y et al. Ultraweak photon emission in assessing bone growth factor efficiency using fibroblastic differentiation. J Photochem Photobiol B. 2001;64(1):62–8.

94. Van Wijk R, Van Wijk EP, Wiegant FA et al. Free radicals and low-level photon emission in human pathogenesis:state of the art. Indian J Exp Biol. 2008;46(5):273–309.

95. Popp. FA. Cancer growth and its inhibition in terms of coherence. Electromagn Biol Med. 2009;28(1):53–60.

96. Tozzi P, Bongiorno D, Vitturini C. Low back pain and kidney mobility: local osteopathic fascial manipulation decreases pain perception and improves renal mobility. J Bodyw Mov Ther. 2012;16(3): 381–91.

97. ICD-10 CM. International Classification of Disease, 10th revision. Geneva: World Health Organization; 2010.

98. Nelson KE, Glonek T. Somatic dysfunction in osteopathic family medicine. Baltimore, MD: Lippincott Wiliams and Wilkins; 2007. ch. 5.

99. Nicholas AS, Nicholas EA. Atlas of osteopathic techniques. Baltimore, MD: Lippincot Williams and Wilkins; 2008. ch 1.

100. DiGiovanna EL. Somatic dysfunction. In: DiGiovanna EL, Schiowitz S, Dowling DJ, editors. An osteopathic approach to diagnosis and treatment. 3rd ed. Philadelphia, PA: Lippincott Williams and Wilkins; 2005. ch. 4.

101. Greenman P. Principles of manual medicine. Baltimore, MD: Williams and Wilkins; 1989. ch. 3.

102. Beal MC. Incidence of spinal palpatory findings: a review. In: The principles of palpatory diagnosis and manipulative techniques. American Academy of Osteopathy Yearbook 1992. pp. 139–44.

103. Stone C. Visceral and obstetric osteopathy. Edinburgh: Elsevier Churchill Livinsgstone; 2007. p. 46.

104. Fryette HH. Physiological movements of the spine. In: American Academy of Osteopathy Yearbook 1950. pp. 91–2.

105. Lovett RA. Lateral curvatures of the spine and round shoulders. 4th ed. Philadelphia, PA: P Blakiston; 1907.

106. Fryette HH. Principles of osteopathic technique. Carmel, CA: American Academy of Osteopathy; 1954.

107. Ehrenfeuchter WC. Segmental motion testing. In: Chila A, editor. Foundations of osteopathic medicine. 3rd ed. Philadelphia, PA: Lippincott Williams and Wilkins; 2010. ch. 35.

108. Gibbons P, Tehan P. Spinal manipulation: indications, risks and benefits. J Bodyw Mov Ther. 2001;5(2):110–9.

109. Mimura M, Moriya H, Watanabe T et al. Three dimensional motion analysis of cervical spine with special reference to axial rotation. Spine. 1989;14:1135–9.

110. Pearcy M, Tibrewal S. Axial rotation and lumbar side-bending in the normal lumbar spine measured by three-dimensional radiography. Spine. 1984;9:582–7.

111. Plamondon A, Gagnon M, Maurais G. Application of a stereoradiographic method for the study of interverterbral motion. Spine. 1988;13:1027–32.

112. Panjabi M, Yamamoto I, Oxland T et al. How does posture affect coupling in the lumbar spine? Spine. 1989;14:1002–11.

113. Vicenzino G, Twomey L. Sideflexion and induced lumbar spine conjunct rotation and its influencing factors. Australian Physiotherapy. 1993;39:299–306.

114. Harrison DE, Harrison DD, Troyanovich SJ. Three-dimensional spinal coupling mechanics: Part I. A review of the literature. J Manipulative Physiol Ther. 1998;21:101–13.

115. Hoover HV. Complicated lesions. In: Barnes MW, editor. Michigan: Yearbook of the Academy of Applied Osteopathy 1950. pp. 67–9.

116. Educational Council on Osteopathic Principles (ECOP). Glossary of osteopathic terminology. American Association of Colleges of Osteopathic Medicine; 2009. http://wwwaacomorg/re-sources/bookstore/Pages/glossaryaspx.

117. Mitchell FL. Towards a definition of somatic dysfunction. Osteopathic Annals. 1979;7(1): 12–25.

118. Parsons J, Marcer N. Osteopathy: models for diagnosis, treatment and practice. Edinburgh: Elsevier Churchill Livingstone; 2006. ch. 11.

119. Parsons J, Marcer N. Osteopathy: models for diagnosis, treatment and practice. Edinburgh: Elsevier Churchill Livingstone; 2006. ch. 9.

120. Greenman P. Principles of manual medicine. 4th ed. Baltimore, MD: Williams and Wilkins; 2011. pp. 14–16.

121. Degenhardt BF, Johnson JC, Snider KT et al. Maintenance and improvement of inter-observer reliability of osteopathic palpatory tests over a 4-month period. J Am Osteopath Assoc. 2010;110(10):579–86.

122. Ehrenfeuchter WC, Kappler RE. Palpatory esamination. In: Chila A, editor. Foundations of osteopathic medicine. 3rd ed. Philadelphia, PA: Lippincott Williams and Wilkins; 2010. ch. 33.

123. Degenhardt BF, Snider KT, Snider EJ et al. Interobserver reliability of osteopathic palpatory diagnostic tests of the lumbar spine: improvements from consensus training. JAOA. 2005;105:465–73.

124. Chaitow L, Coughlin P, Findley TW et al. Fascial palpation. In: Schleip R, Findley T, Chaitow L, Huijing P, editors. Fascia: the tensional network of the human body. Edinburgh: Churchill Livingstone, Elsevier; 2012. p. 271.

125. Chaitow L. Palpation and assessment skills: assessment through touch. 3rd ed. Edinburgh: Churchill Livingstone; 2010. ch. 10.

126. Barral JP, Mercier P. Visceral manipulation. Seattle: Eastland Press; 1988.

127. Chamberlain NR, Yates HA. Use of a computer-assisted clinical case (CACC) SOAP note exercise to assess students' application of osteopathic principles and practice. J Am Osteopath Assoc. 2000;100(7):437–40.

128. Parsons J, Marcer N. Osteopathy: models for diagnosis, treatment and practice. Edinburgh: Elsevier Churchill Livingstone; 2006. ch. 2.

129. Kuchera ML, Kuchera WA. Osteopathic principles in practice. Columbus, OH: Greyden Press; 1994. pp. 20–5.

130. Masi AT, Nair K, Evans T et al. Clinical, biomechanical, and physiological translational interpretations of human resting myofascial tone or tension. Inter J Ther Massage Bodyw. 2010;16;3(4):16–28.

131. Barnes L, Laboy F, Noto-Bell L et al. A comparative study of cervical hysteresis characteristics after various osteopathic manipulative treatment (OMT) modalities. J Bodyw Mov Ther. 2013;17(1):89–94.

132. Lucas N, Bogduk N. Diagnostic reliability in osteopathic medicine. Int J Osteopath Med. 2011;14(2):43–7.

133. Shaw KA, Dougherty JJ, Treffer KD et al. Establishing the content validity of palpatory examination for the assessment of the lumbar spine usingultrasonography: a pilot study. J Am Osteopath Assoc. 2012;112(12):775–82.

# General adaptation syndrome: biological fluids, involuntary rhythms, and fascial compensation schemes 3

*Christian Lunghi*

## Synopsis

Osteopathy in its most traditional form was originally conceived to approach the patient by directly searching for the expression of health and not of disease. In this regard, osteopaths have described the possibility of evaluating the general adaptation capacity of the body through the organization of connective tissues in patterns related to the dynamics of body fluids. It is possible to palpate the degree of stress in fascial patterns as the amount of permitted macro-movement and also as the inherent motion within the tissues, i.e., the tissue's intrinsic involuntary rhythm. This field, unique to osteopathic practice, is in this text referred to as "dynamics of fluids and involuntary rhythms" (DyFIR).

## Introduction

More than a century ago, the old doctor replied to very current questions related to the osteopath's task, stating forcefully, with a stick in his or her hand, that the osteopath's goal was to find health. The goal of this approach is to maintain the stability of the adaptative systems.[1,2] The homeostatic-allostatic oscillation is the response to stress aimed at restoring equilibrium and minimizing dysfunction via two basic modes of adaptation:

1. Local adaptation, or reorganization of the tissue physiology mechanics of an area affected by SD (see Chapter 2)

2. General adaptation, when stress requires a generalized response of the physiological systems of the body. The osteopath also observes and assesses the general adaptation syndrome (GAS) through observation and palpation of fascial compensation schemes (FCS),[7] and of the dynamics of (biological) fluids and involuntary rhythms (DyFIR).

The intervention, in both cases, is a treatment intended to:

- encourage FCS toward neutral conditions

- stimulate a less expensive, more comfortable, and painless adaptation using procedures aimed at balancing the DyFIR and reducing dysfunctional afferent stimuli.

The available evidence[8] provides useful information for understanding the chronobiological rhythms of the whole body. Nevertheless, the approach to body rhythm in osteopathy refers almost exclusively to the model defined as the primary respiratory mechanism (PRM), which describes the craniosacral axis cyclical rhythm. Cyclic supply and drainage of fluids are also specific objectives of osteopathic techniques in fascial and visceral lymphatic areas.[6] The operator would therefore have the option of using the principles of health, such as the general (GAS) and local (LAS) adaptation syndromes, to evaluate the patient. In fact, before disease appears, there could be an alteration of the structure/function relationship, and this alteration would be recognizable even in the "tissue rhythmic behavior," which can be coordinated or fragmented. Following this principle, the operator uses an individual's global perspective. It is not difficult for an osteopath to make reference to his or her daily practice, where, in order to take care of health, he or she searches for and promotes movement using mainly manual approaches. With skilled and experienced hands, osteopaths try to recognize health in the individual's tissues, through the perceptive palpation of normal tissue, proceeding slowly, in contrast to some other therapeutic techniques.[9]

The old doctor always used to say that movement is that which expresses life itself. So, if life itself is expressed through the dynamics and kinetics of a living body (tensed to adaptation), we know that it is possible to perceive this dynamic through palpation. It is necessary to evaluate the integration of and between different areas, as well as how much their degree of compensation can affect the mechanical tissue and movement of biological fluids.[7] The osteopath can in this way come into contact with the vital forces of the individual, but must understand in how many ways the vital movement can be expressed. Starting from their experience with palpation, osteopaths have described the existence of body schemes or connective adaptations related to the dynamics of body fluids, consistent in stressed, ill, and healthy subjects/patients.

It is possible to palpate the degree of stress perceived in the fascial compensation patterns as permitted, or macro movement, of a tissue as well as the intrinsic involuntary rhythm of a tissue.[10] This vital motility, which osteopaths refer to as inherent therapeutic potency,[11] is explained by philosophical approaches, sometimes with reference to embryology in the case of the biodynamic osteopathic approach to the whole body,[12] sometimes with attempts at biomechanical modeling of the PRM, which concerns the craniosacral system.[13] This field, unique to osteopathy, is in this text referred to as DyFIR. After the work of Still, Sutherland[13] and Becker[11] have focused their attention and their palpatory experiences on these aspects.

These pioneers have focused on the concept of stillness over that of movement: the presence of movement implies, according to Becker, a point of stillness, the so-called still point from which the motion can start again.[11] The focusing of the therapist on the intrinsic "homeodynamic" processes and the health of the patient are essential foundations in therapy performed through palpation. If this happens in a state of attention and empathy, in a more relaxed and non-invasive state, and through synchronization of the therapist with the forces and intrinsic homeodynamic rhythms, there is great opportunity for the spontaneous introduction of stress relaxation in the body. Osteopaths inform the patient with the perceptive palpation of a moment/point of local or systemic rest.[11-13] Osteopathy in its most traditional form was originally conceived to approach the patient with the goal of seeking the expression of health and not disease.

There are many technical approaches designed to allow the user to directly access the "health system." If these are used appropriately, it is possible to witness a spontaneous therapeutic process through which health is restored. As reported by osteopaths, the most efficient access lies without doubt in the point of stillness, a well-known concept to those engaging traditional osteopathy. In order to access this point, one needs to be disciplined, transparent, and not simply focus attention on "lesions," i.e., the local adaptation areas to stress, well described in osteopathy as somatic dysfunction (SD). The operator learns to listen to the individual's vitality, with which he or she enters into a relationship, i.e., the relationship between its allostatic load and its homeostasis, in other words its capacity to adapt. To do so, the osteopath must be an observer, a witness of the therapeutic process, and patiently wait for the salutogenesis in this state of perception. Through palpatory experience it is therefore possible to perceive the existent movement and the point of stillness, but it is necessary to revise the way that is used to make this approach. We must learn to reflect on the act of observing, recognizing this condition as the experience of a true creative act: the genesis of a helping relationship based on listening to biological rhythms.

Through the observation of these phenomena it is possible to perceive the patient's vital dynamics creating the conditions that will re-establish his or her health and, as a consequence, will prepare him for the healing process. In the training courses for osteopaths, both curricular and extracurricular, there are basically two ways of describing the mechanisms that underlie osteopathic manipulative treatment (OMT), with particular reference to the biomechanical and biodynamic models used to describe osteopathic cranial manipulative medicine (OCMM) and the resulting relationship that is established with the patient. The first modality is "scientific," because it utilizes knowledge of science in order to advance the osteopath's professional knowledge and ambulatory clinical practice, "by stimulating the left hemisphere." The second modality is "historical-philosophical," because, according to the principles of Still, Sutherland, and others, it uses a metaphorical language in order to advance the osteopath's professional knowledge and ambulatory clinical practice, "by stimulating the left hemisphere." However, the scientific mode and the historical-philosophical mode, in the same way as the two cerebral hemispheres usually provide information independently, work in a complementary manner. The two hemispheres are specialized, but share and integrate information by communicating through a large bundle of nerve fibers known as the corpus callosum. This text aims to stimulate the "corpus callosum" of the osteopath in order to integrate history, philosophy, and science, systems that always evolve together, even if sometimes this is not accepted and integrated into practice.

The philosophy of science, or rather the philosophy of knowledge,[14,15] tries to explain the nature of concepts and scientific statements, i.e., the modality in which they are produced; how science explains nature, how it predicts and uses nature for its own purposes; the means for determining the validity of the information; the formulation and use of the scientific method; the types of reasoning that are used to arrive at certain conclusions; and the integration of scientific models with real models existing in human society.[16] One of the peculiar aspects of osteopathic practice is certainly represented by osteopathy in the cranial, fascial, visceral, and lymphatic areas.

As they evolved over time, these approaches embodied the dichotomy between science and philosophy. Osteopathic cranial manipulative medicine is practiced by the osteopath through a biomechanical (efferent) model and a traditional (afferent) biodynamic model that are both intended to promote health through the force of inherent activation, defined cranial rhythmic impulse (CRI), PRM, etc. While the biomechanical approach has seen a succession of theories in the attempt to be supported by scientific evidence, the traditional biodynamic approach, in which one is taught how to detect polyrhythms by increasing the "afferent" activity and decreasing the "efferent" activity (Fig. 3.1), has continued to be handed down in study groups and extracurricular courses. These are areas where the approach and the mechanisms that underlie the proposed treatment are explained with a metaphorical philosophical language. Compared to the basics of the biodynamic approach, McPartland[12] suggests paying attention to the embryo and generating external forces of its spatial orientation, that through fluid forces (hydrogen/water electromagnetic bonds) supplies a matrix which governs the embryo's development.

The embryo is therefore considered a biodynamic archetype, used as a template for the body's ability to heal itself, in terms of how formative and regenerative fluid forces that organize the embryological development are present throughout life.[12] Cranial biomechanical approaches observe the relationships between structures and functions in a totally different way, with particular emphasis on the structural relationships of the craniosacral region and their functional influences, venous and lymphatic drainage, glial rhythmic pulsations, any malfunctions involving suture joints, as well as muscular, dural, and fascial components that maintain the relationships between the skull, spine, and sacrum.[13] In this chapter, the author also proposes to reconsider the PRM model in order to open a critical dialogue aimed at the observation of how OCMM and OMT in general are an evolution in time of the concepts of human anatomy and physiology, like all the rest of medicine.

History is now considered a stimulus to the evolution of critical thinking and not to self-referenced thinking.[17] One of the objectives of this chapter is to overcome the concept that the birth of osteopathy is due to the "exclusive" ideas of some great men. The critical readings of some historical documents confirm that the model defined as the PRM in OCMM, described for the first time in the early years of the twentieth century by William Garner Sutherland, repeats a number of theories previously enunciated by Emanuel Swedenborg.[18] These facts hint that osteopathy is part of the historical path of medicine, which, starting from Hippocrates and passing through Still and Sutherland, arrives at the present day.[19] However, nowadays, the concept of PRM has caused many difficulties.

It is hard to explain this concept to both students (future professionals) and osteopaths and similarly to other health professionals. In addition, the scientific, historical, and philosophical findings seem to converge into a unifying model. The efficiency of a session in the context of DyFIR depends not only

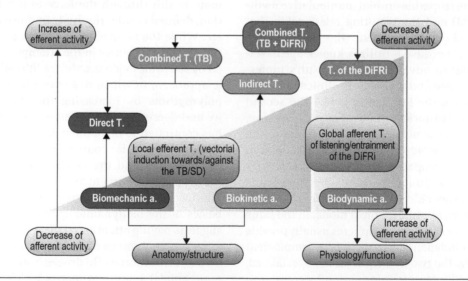

**Fig. 3.1**
Global afferent approaches, local efferent approaches, and their combinations. Description of the evolution from the technical approach based on a biomechanical, biokinetic, and biodynamic rationale, to the approach based on efferent/afferent focus and application of the direct, indirect, and combined techniques. TB: tissue barrier; DyFIR: dynamics of fluids and involuntary rhythms; SD: somatic dysfunction. Modified from: Parsons J, Marcer N. Osteopathy: models for diagnosis, treatment and practice. Edinburgh: Elsevier Churchill Livingstone; 2006. p. 178.

on the degree of the operator's specific biomechanical knowledge, but especially on the ability to conduct interpersonal processes (philosophy), i.e., the capacity to understand and observe changes in the autonomic nervous system (ANS) and in vasomotion.[20] So, the microvascular dynamics of spontaneous, autonomous, and indigenous oscillations of arterioles, nutritional capillaries and venules of the extracellular matrix (science) are equally important.

## Osteopathic approach to the "dynamics of fluids and involuntary rhythms"

### Historical background

The development of manipulative medicine flourished in the United States in the early 20th century. Within the osteopathic and chiropractic professions, many therapists began to apply manipulative techniques on the cranial structures. Charlotte Weaver, DO,[21] and Nephi Cottam, DC,[22] developed the first models for diagnosis and treatment in the cranial field. At the same time, William Garner Sutherland, DO, created a model called the "primary respiratory mechanism" (PRM). Through the efforts made by academies[23] and foundations[24] that came into being

around the 1950s, the classical model of osteopathic cranial manipulative medicine spread into most of the osteopathic training institutions. The conclusions of a historical review in 2009[18] suggest that Sutherland was inspired by the physiology explained in the anatomical studies of Emanuel Swedenborg (Fig. 3.2). Although Sutherland has never openly stated the use of any source for his ideas, careful examination reveals striking similarities between his writings and those of Swedenborg. This connection helps in explaining some of the most unique and vague aspects of the origins of the PRM model. This is an invitation to stimulate critical thinking,[25] intended to review, update, and revise the PRM model and OCMM through understanding of human anatomy and physiology, especially in light of the history of a community of practice and the evolution of its thinking.[26] Jordan,[18] in his historical review, mentions the important people who have established the connection between Swedenborg and Sutherland:

- Rudolf Tafel, who in 1882 translated *The Brain*, by Swedenborg

- Ida Rolf, who claimed that Sutherland made use of Tafel's translation to formulate his PRM model

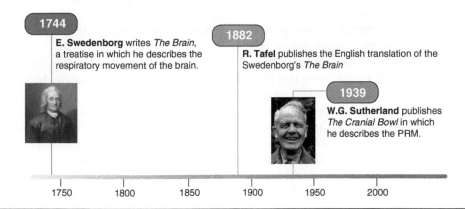

**1744**
E. Swedenborg writes *The Brain*, a treatise in which he describes the respiratory movement of the brain.

**1882**
R. Tafel publishes the English translation of the Swedenborg's *The Brain*

**1939**
W.G. Sutherland publishes *The Cranial Bowl* in which he describes the PRM.

1750  1800  1850  1900  1950  2000

**Fig. 3.2**
Chronological connections between the writings of Swedenborg and Sutherland. This connection helps in explaining some of the unique and more vague aspects of the genesis of the primary respiratory mechanism (PRM) model described by Sutherland. Modified from: Jordan T. Swedenborg's influence on Sutherland's "primary respiratory mechanism" model in cranial osteopathy. Int J Osteopath Med. 2009;12 (3):100–5.

- The reverend Alfred Acton, noted for his knowledge, teaching, and translations of the works of Swedenborg, who had contact with several osteopaths, including Isabelle Bibble and Howard and Rebecca Lippincott, who were students of Sutherland.

Also cited are the similarities and differences between the writings of Swedenborg and the PRM model described by Sutherland,[13] divided into five basic components:

1. Inherent motility of the brain and spinal cord

2. Fluctuation of cerebrospinal fluid

3. Mobility of the intracranial and intraspinal membranes

4. Joint mobility of the cranial bones

5. Involuntary movement of the sacrum between the hip bones.

The first four components of Sutherland's cranial concept are similar and consistent with the descriptions by Swedenborg written two centuries earlier. Swedenborg described the brain and spinal movement and the fluctuation of the cerebrospinal fluid as did Sutherland, who reported a synchronous pulsation of the cerebrospinal fluid containing a higher principle; a principle which gave it more meaning and abilities than a simple liquid. Swedenborg and Sutherland's descriptions of the reciprocal tension of dural membranes were essentially the same. Both authors described the movement of cranial bones in response to the movement of the brain, although Sutherland's descriptions were more detailed and sophisticated than those of Swedenborg. Swedenborg described the "circle of life" as the circulation of the cephalorachidian fluid, which, after being produced in the cerebral cortex, spread and vitalized the cerebrospinal fluid and finally ended up in the bloodstream. The circle ended, according to his observations, in the cortex of the brain, where it could be extracted and put back into circulation.

Sutherland observed a special principle or power of the cerebrospinal fluid as it fluctuated from the brain to the periphery of the nervous system and body, although he did not emphasize any kind of return circulation, but did underline that the fluctuation occurred in a semi-closed system. The contemporary literature on the subject[27] reports evidence for a hydrodynamic model of production, circulation, and absorption of the cerebrospinal fluid (CSF) and interstitial fluid in the brain parenchyma: these would also be produced by hydrostatic and oncotic exchanges, through the endothelial walls of the arterial capillaries in the central nervous system (CNS).

Secretion would be from the choroid plexuses and capillary brain circuit, while absorption would occur in the arachnoid membrane/villi and lymphatic and venous capillary endothelium. These findings could be of interest to osteopathic practice that addresses the fluids and involuntary movements in the cranial region, reassessing even the insights provided by Swedenborg and Sutherland in light of this "renewed" model of CSF secretion and reabsorption described by contemporary scholars.[27] Sutherland described a sacral involuntary movement that corresponds to the movement of the sphenobasilar joint of the PRM, a concept not found in the writings of Swedenborg.

The latter worked diligently over the years to better understand the human body, and how its structure and function were connected and interdependent, although he did not develop any specific therapeutic application of his work. Sutherland also devoted himself to the understanding of human structure and function and also applied this understanding in the context of the osteopathic tradition and philosophy of Andrew Taylor Still, developing a sophisticated and effective system of diagnosis and manipulative treatment, based on the perception of involuntary movements of the skull and of the entire body. The influence of Swedenborg on Sutherland was significant. Four of the five basic components of Sutherland's skull concept are found in the writings of Swedenborg, published nearly 200 years earlier.

Swedenborg was one of the brightest students of the human form and function. He described the rhythmic animation of the brain as a mechanism for the interaction of soul and body, connecting it with all the other movements of life. He studied the brain's movements, the motion of the reciprocal dural membranes and cranial bones, as well as the cerebrospinal fluid qualities, described as "pulsating liquid animation," which in turn animates the entire body. This brilliant anatomical work was the springboard from which Swedenborg tried to move beyond anatomical science to explore an organic theology that is still influential and significant today. Sutherland had his initial intuition on the cranial mechanism in 1898 and then integrated and deepened it later with further studies. The quotations show that he knew and appreciated the anatomical writings of Swedenborg. He found the latter's ideas in line with his own point of view and perception of osteopathic structure/function. It can be said that Sutherland developed his cranial concept by blending the brain paradigm of Swedenborg with an osteopathic treatment approach, a sophisticated system of diagnosis and treatment that has continued to benefit many patients up to the present day.

This knowledge provides different cues and explains some vague aspects of the PRM model, such as, for example, the relationship between the "breathing" of the skull and that of the lung, the insistence of Sutherland on the fact that the "breathing" of the brain precedes that of the lungs and the origin of the concept of the "breath of life." A greater knowledge of the ideas of Swedenborg allows us to improve our understanding with respect to some aspects of OCMM. Many osteopaths consider the contribution of William Sutherland related to the PRM model as one of the most important contributions to osteopathic thinking, unlike any other model of the skull, as it went beyond simple anatomy and mechanics. By attributing the driving force of this cranial mechanism to the intrinsic movement of the central nervous system he introduced a powerful and elusive mechanism, which generated a philosophical treatise and scientific discussion. The PRM model, as originally described by Sutherland, is most likely the applied restatement of a physiological hypothesis of the mid-18th century.[18]

The purpose of this dialogue is to advance the science of osteopathy by also reconsidering the philosophical aspects of this science. It is a science that deals with the "spirit" and its physiological manifestations, the "breath of life" that contemporary osteopaths call "present movement," the possibility that a rhythm, the expression of the sum of involuntary movements, is palpable by expert hands, as now advanced by experimental studies.[28] The philosophy of 18th-century science has stimulated the evolution of the concepts of osteopathy, which today are found in the research on biological rhythms. Those who practice manual therapy are aware of the importance of oscillatory rhythms in different aspects of osteopathic theory and practice. This of course reminds us of the low-frequency oscillations of the CRI.[29] Contemporary experimental studies suggest that the professional osteopath must take sufficient time when performing an examination of the tissues and take into account the presence of the relationship of these tissues with the circadian rhythms.[8,30]

Contemporary medicine considers the individual's allostatic load and defines disease as energy expenditure as a consequence thereof. As such, therapies are commonly directed to lower or raise the abnormal physiological processes. We recall that even John Martin Littlejohn pointed out how the body responded optimally when the procedures were applied rhythmically and at an appropriate frequency. He proposed the use of physiological frequencies to influence these oscillations as a therapeutic effect, so that the osteopathic treatment could be synced to a higher harmonic resonance and avoid dissonance.[31,32] This historical review aims to reconsider the PRM model and open a critical dialogue aimed at the observation of how the cranial osteopathic model, and all of manipulative osteopathic practice, is an evolution over time of the concepts of anatomy and human physiology.

## Evolution of biomechanics: tissue mechanics from the skull to the rest of the body

Existing research in the field of tissue mechanics represents a potentially interesting source for understanding the working mechanisms of all of osteopathic treatment, not only cranial. For example, the extent to which an object is stretched or compressed is expressed as a percentage of the initial size of the object in terms of the strain measurement unit: a measurement unit extremely sensitive to stress. To get an idea, we can report that a reasonable value for the elastic modulus of a rigid living tissue, such as cortical bone, in humans is 15,000 pascal.[33,34] This principle has been widely applied to understand the role and development of the cranial sutures and the distribution of stress and strain on the skull. The key points of the well-known applications[35] of tissue mechanics on the cranial area are as follows:

- The skull bones are deformed according to their viscoelastic properties[36-38] during normal functioning and most obviously during trauma.[35]

- The sutures can affect the way in which the skull is distorted in shape, but the head may still be distorted if they are fused.[35] The bony movements hypothesized in OCMM assume a certain degree of patency of the sutures, but this condition is not always true in the course of the whole life. The closing of a suture is a complex and gradual process; moreover, osseous trabeculae (cancellous bone) appear before their complete fusion.[39-42]

- Contractile fibers, such as those of the cranial muscles, are the main cause of the loading[38,43,44] and the deformation of the skull, with the exception of what happens in traumatic events.[45-49]

However, these considerations are also found in other body areas. For example, although it is among the hardest materials in the body, bone, including the cranial bone, if subjected to stress and tension, distorts and may alter its structure. All of this can also lead to deductive thinking so as to reconsider whether it is necessary today to have a specific model of cranial diagnosis and treatment, or if a model applicable to the whole body would make more sense: "Why do we consider the head differently from the rest of the body?"[35]

### Unifying model

Osteopathic cranial manipulative medicine (OCMM) was born in the 1930s through the work of Sutherland, who, under the tutelage of Still, while studying human skull models, came to describe in 1939, in his first work, *The Cranial Bowl*,[50] a biomechanical model of this particular approach of osteopathy still practiced today. However, there are still controversial issues with the PRM original model. Even if we logically hypothesize the mobility of cranial bones in relation to the shape of the sutures, as has been shown in animals, through the action of the chewing muscles,[51-53] the assumptions about bone deviations due to an intrinsic motility of the CNS are not consistent with current knowledge of the cranial bones.[54,55] It is true that there is some research to support the PRM model.[56] These contributions of science to OCMM did not come from researchers within the community of osteopathic practice, but from other fields of scientific research, in particular:

- discoveries in biochemistry and a further understanding of the physiology of the extracellular matrix (ECM).[57] The understanding of the CRI, which is perhaps not only cranial,[35] continues to grow with continuous scientific advances

- discoveries in the field of biomechanics, which is not the mere application of kinematics to the human body, but also includes the study of the continuous plastic and elastic changes of living tissues, in response to internal and external environmental stresses. With tissue mechanics we can describe the way in which the tibia is deformed during running or jumping,[58] the mechanisms by which stress fractures,[59,60] disc degeneration,[61,62] damage to, and remodeling of, bone occurs.[63,64] Tissue mechanics aims to describe the way in which living tissues are modified under different types of load,[65,66] and in particular to understand the role and development of cranial sutures and the distribution of stress and strain on the skulls of primates[67,68]

- evidence[27,35,57,69] from physiology is now emerging and could be used to explain the concepts of the fluid balancing point, balanced exchange of fluids, and point of "peace," which the osteopath refers to as the still point.

This chapter, along with the work of Lee,[57] Gabutti,[35] Hamm,[69] Chikly Quaghebeur,[27] and other authors, proposes and adopts a line of deductive reasoning, starting from the collection and analysis of the evidence relating to the physiological, chemical, and mechanical properties of tissues, in order to update the concept of OCMM. Our goal is to promote further research, providing information that is broadly shared and accepted by the scientific community, with the hope of developing future models for the practice in DyFIR areas in terms of palpation, evaluation criteria, and treatment techniques. In reference to the limited research resources that we have in osteopathy, many authors suggest giving priority to research about the clinical efficacy of these approaches before exploring the possible mechanisms.[70] However, in this work we discuss the biochemical, mechanical and physiological findings, in an attempt to verify whether there is any evidence for the methods of DyFIR, and for the "internal forces" and "inherent powers" of which Sutherland, Becker, and other authors speak,[13,71] with the aim of stimulating the community of practice to encourage research on related clinical aspects.

## Extracellular matrix

Within the extracellular matrix (ECM) structures we find cells, fibers, and ground substance. The fundamental cell of the matrix is the fibroblast, which produces essential elements: its fibers (e.g., colla-

gen) and the ground substance. There are also other cells that move in and out of the matrix, such as the white blood cells that are found in the bloodstream, macrophages, and mast cells. These "resident" cells, the (wandering) lymphocytes and polymorphonuclear leukocytes fulfill the usual functions of detoxification and immunity in the matrix.[72,73] The most common fibrous product of fibroblast is collagen, a structural protein, not very stretchable, which repels water in its dense form as its most notable characteristic.

This offers stability by providing a scaffold around which the more malleable part of the ECM and the parenchymal cells are organized. In addition, collagen provides the essential piezoelectric properties for the matrix. Along with elastin and other structural proteins such as fibronectin, collagen demonstrates polarity within its molecular structure. A part of the molecule has a positive charge with respect to another, relatively negative, part. Collagen molecules are aligned so that the positive charges lie in the direction of the organism's growth, development, and healing forces.[74,75] Piezoelectricity is a form of electrical power produced by the deformation of certain solid materials: a biomechanical structure with a shape possesses a certain charge; if the shape changes, there is change in the charge, and vice versa; if the position changes, there are changes in shape.

Tissue piezoelectric properties have been observed showing that when a tissue is deformed, there is a separation of electric charges in the mucopolysaccharide chains.[76] The piezoelectric effect caused by the deformation produces an electric charge, which, in a closed system such as the fascial system, tends to dispersion, for which the energy is released quickly. However, an applied stress produces a voltage across the tissue. The impulse obtained after a deformation would be brief and polar: the concave side of the compressed tissue would have a negative charge, while the convex side, where the tissue is stretched, would have a positive charge.[77]

This explains clinical and experimental observations, where compression and tension forces applied to the bone would result in the reconstruction of tissue on the concave side and reabsorption on the convex side.[77-79] Another product of the fibroblast is the "ground substance," consisting mainly of proteoglycans that are associated with long chains of hyaluronic acid by means of special proteins, called the link protein. Proteoglycans have the ability to "trap" substantial amounts of water, forming a gel that has the functions of mechanical support, resistance to compression, and acting as a filter that regulates the diffusion rate of liquids through the connective tissue. Proteoglycans present in the ECM are associated in non-covalent mode, and in large numbers, in a single molecule of hyaluronic acid. Interspersed between the hyaluronic and proteoglicanic aggregates are fibrous proteins such as collagen, fibronectin, and elastin, which form a complex network able to confer mechanical resistance.

Hyaluronic acid, which is located in the ground substance, is one of the main elements of connective tissues in humans and other mammals. It confers resistance and shape retention properties, being the only glycosaminoglycan to be present in the ECM which is not linked to a protein nucleus to necessarily form a proteoglycan. In the amorphous matrix of a connective tissue, hyaluronic acid is responsible for maintaining the degree of hydration, firmness/turgidity, plasticity, and viscosity, for it is organized as an aggregate conformation in space, thus attracting a considerable number of water molecules.[80] "It fills the space between cells" and is also capable of acting as a cementing substance, a shockproof molecule and also as an efficient lubricant (e.g., in the synovial fluid), preventing damage to the tissue cells caused by physical stress.[57] The extreme length of the molecule, together with its high degree of hydration, allows many hyaluronic acid polymers to organize themselves to form a reticular type of structure that has two main functions:

1. To create a molecular scaffold to keep the shape and tone of the tissue

2. To function as a filter against the free diffusion into the tissue of particular substances, such as bacteria and infectious agents.

Together with proteoglycans, they form aggregates of a size comparable to that of a bacterium, with a weight of tens of millions of Da for different μm in length. These proteoglycanic complexes, by virtue of their structure, viscosity, and permeability, are excellent molecular filters that can spread some of the low molecular weight substances, and trap other substances that are more voluminous, including viruses and bacteria. It should be noted that many bacteria have hyaluronidase, an enzyme that can break down hyaluronic acid, which allows them to invade the cells. Hyaluronate has a high polarity and solubility, allowing it to join with many molecules of water, reaching a high degree of hydration. Hyaluronate consists of macromolecules of a mass greater than 1,000 kDa that give rise to clear high viscosity solutions.

This polymer aggregates itself in proteoglycans by tying them to its protein dorsal structure, by means of "bristles" of structures in the form of a "brush," composed of glycosaminoglycans (GAGs): heparin, keratin, chondroitin, and dermatan. Since GAGs are sulphated, the matrix becomes negatively charged and thus able to attract water.[80] We can more easily conceptualize some of the key features of the ECM in the cartilage. The latter is very smooth and gelatinous and acts as a sponge, absorbing large volumes of water, thus allowing the introduction of oxygen and nutrients, which influence, in a beneficial way, the tissue viability. The ECM and the connective tissue in general create the form of the organism[81] by means of structural interactions,[82] from the generic physical level to subcellular mechanisms.[83,84]

The structures were created as the "architecture" of the function at all levels of organization, from the motor functions of general activity to the enzymatic functions of cells. Although initially function precedes structure, sometimes it is controlled by the process of growth and evolution, thus becoming dependent on the structure.[81] The ECM creates the structure-form pattern, creating proteins such as collagen. It is also closely allied to function on the cellular and subcellular level. These influences include morphogenetic activities and metabolism.[85] Furthermore, the matrix is piezoelectric: by applying an electrical stimulus on it, it causes a mechanical movement (vibration) and by applying a physical force (stretching, compression, or torsion) electricity is generated.[81] It is a semiconductor and the electrons are equally shared by all of the structural proteins and other loaded elements in this complex network. The energy fluctuations diffuse through the matrix by means of the changes in liquid crystalline water.

The energy transmissions are used by the cells as information.[80] Since the ECM is open to influences and is unstable, it is also subject to oscillations. The macromolecules are capable of oscillation that is favored by their spiral structure and influenced by cyclical variations of the pH and concentrations of ions, and the degrees of polymerization.[86–88] The ECM is also viscoelastic. The changes of viscosity appear in the changes of swelling of the hyaluronic acid and other glycosaminoglycans.[89] From this we can deduce that the changes in viscosity occur in terms of variations of the polymerization of macromolecules and in terms of the redox potential fluctuation.[90]

Since these enormous polymers swell or are depolymerized, the "pore sizes" of the ECM allow larger molecules to pass through the extracellular fluid.[91] The most obvious example of gelation occurs when there is maximum polymerization, a process that has been observed in the state of rigor mortis, which occurs after the vital functions leave the body. During life, the matrix is revitalized and liquefied by factors that allow the movement of nutrients and waste products from and into the parenchymal cells. The polymers contain sulfated parts that carry a strong negative charge when they are polymerized into gel. This attracts relatively large volumes of water that bind to the macromolecules of the matrix and help the formation of gel.

The concentration of calcium ions is inversely proportional, and is linked, to the size of the polymers of hyaluronic acid and the increase of the water that is carried by the polymers.[92] When the calcium ion concentration decreases, the water binds more tightly to the macromolecules of the matrix; conversely, when the concentration of calcium ions increases, the bound water is free to flow. When the intensity of the negative charge of the ECM decreases along with its depolymerization, the calcium ions and water flow toward the presence of the negatively charged elements in the region of the next cell membrane.

The water that "flows" supplies nutrients to the parenchymal cells.[80] This delivery mechanism is more efficient than a simple diffusion. When water "flows," the concentration of calcium ions by dilution decreases; this will play a depolymerizing function. Therefore, macromolecules will repolymerize once again, increasing the viscosity of the matrix and "attracting" relatively large volumes of water. Thus, we can observe how in the ECM there is a palpable movement cycle that is shown in the state transition between gelation and solidification[57] (Fig. 3.3).

The influence of the matrix on the neighboring cells is demonstrated in part by the extracellular cyclic adenosine monophosphate (cAMP), in part by calcium ions that stimulate intracellular functions through the cell membranes associated with the glycosaminoglycans and through the surface receptor cells. Integrins are a group of surface receptor cells, localized inside the bilaminar cell membrane, which transmit the signal from the ECM to the intracellular structure. The extracellular calcium ions should interact with integrin molecules to initiate a process called mechanotransduction.

The latter integrates mechanics and biochemistry at the molecular level;[83] it is piezoelectricity in action. Close to the integrins are found the focal adhesion complexes: these are groups of special proteins that act as "spot welds" in strategic places, such as on the outskirts of the adjacent cell and

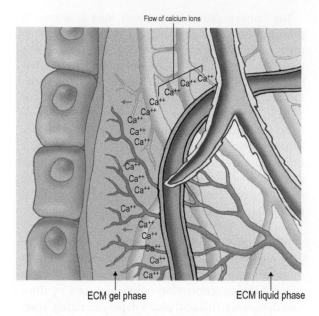

Flow of calcium ions

ECM gel phase                    ECM liquid phase

**Fig. 3.3**
Gelation and solidification in the extracellular matrix (ECM). Schematic representation of the theoretical model of a normal phase transition that occurs in the ECM. On the left, parenchymal cells require a liquid phase of the matrix in order to receive nutrients from the capillary (red structure on the right) and to discharge the waste to the terminal lymphatic vessel (green structure to the right). A gel phase of the basic substance is depicted in the extracellular matrix adjacent to the parenchymal cells and a liquid phase adjacent to the capillary. In the middle is shown a flow of calcium ions, from right to left, that is causing a change of the basic substance phase. Modified by: Lee PR. The living matrix: a model for the primary respiratory mechanism. Explore. 2008;4(6):374–8.

within the cell membrane. In conjunction with the microtubules, intermediate filaments, and microfilaments, the complex of focal adhesion ensures the shape of the cells. Microtubules, intermediate filaments, and microfilaments act as tensegritive elements within the cell. They determine the size and shape of the cells through tension and compression. Microfilaments, being composed of actin, have contractile properties. Microtubules act as support in compression against the preset tension of actin filaments. Actin filaments adhere to these welding points, as well as to integrins that functionally connect the inside of the cell with the outside.

Through mediation of the focal adhesion complexes, actin filaments contract in response to influences coming from integrins, "tuning" the cell to a preset vibration. This setting determines the response of cells to mechanical and electrical stimuli. The extracellular fluctuations in pH, ion concentration, etc., induce a flow of intracellular calcium ions, influencing many intracellular functions, even in the nucleus and its genetic material.[57] Moreover, each subsequent influence on the integrin molecule will distort the cytoskeleton by means of a contrac-

tion of the actin filaments, with the mediation of the focal adhesion complex. Like dew drops on a spider web, the enzymes that perform the primary functions are carefully arranged on actin filaments and microtubules within the cell.

During the movement of the cytoskeleton, the actin filaments, microtubules, and intermediate filaments reorganize a chain of enzymes from one filament to the adjacent one, so as to create important sequences of chemical reactions. When "the chain" meshes are separated from each other, other series of enzymes could be activated. In this way, mechanics stimulate and regulate the metabolic functions. The "swelling" of a cell and its "retraction" have been associated with the concentration of calcium ions in the intracellular level.[84] Streams of intracellular calcium waves are responsible for many metabolic functions in the cell. Many other secondary messengers induce metabolic functions, also stimulated by the cell membrane, through cAMP. In this way the calcium waves are auto-stimulated. In this model, the calcium-activated contraction of actin filaments in the cytoskeleton is associated with cell volume changes.[82]

Calcium wave cycles in the cell were recorded at frequencies of 0.1 to 12 cycles per minute.[88] Cycles of electrical potentials, having periods of four cycles per minute, were recorded in anesthetized dogs through microelectrodes in tissues of various organs, particularly the serous membranes of stomach, liver and kidneys.[90] Even the terminal lymphatic channel is controlled by the matrix, both in terms of growth (lymphangiogenesis) and of function.[57] Waves of calcium cause contraction of actin filaments that suspend the endothelial cells of the terminal lymphatic channel, thus opening the fenestrations between cells. Water that has been ejected from parenchymal cells adjacent to the contraction of intracellular actin filaments flows through the fenestrations into the lymphatic vessels. As soon as the calcium wave dissipates, it closes the fenestrations and traps the loading–unloading water inside the lymphatic vessel. With the subsequent calcium wave, more water flows in the terminal lymphatic channel, forcing and pushing the previous bolus of lymph along the channel. In this way, we have a pulsatile movement in the lymphatic vessels. (See chapter Appendix.)

## Hydrodynamics of the cerebrospinal fluid and relationships with bodily fluids

The traditional hydrodynamic model of the CSF assumes that CSF is mainly produced by the choroid plexus; it flows from the ventricles of the subarachnoid spaces, and is mainly absorbed in the arachnoid villi. The transcoroidal secretion of fluid, ions, and macromolecules guide the liquid along the "ventriculo cisternal" axis.[93] Recent scientific findings challenge this model, stating that it is apparently based on faulty research and misinterpretation of the data.[27] Some experiments of the 1980s found that the choroid plexus is responsible for 60–85% of the total production of CSF.[94] Studies have shown that around 15–30% of CSF has an extrachoroidal origin.[95] Other researchers have suggested that it can be formed and reabsorbed anywhere within the central nervous system.[96] Different experimental models have concluded that the capillary endothelium of the CNS can be an important source

of production.[97] Other research has shown that the increase of hydrostatic intracranial pressure considerably reduces production, and vice versa.[98] It was also noted that the osmolarity elevation of this fluid greatly increases its production.[99] Oreskovic and colleagues used a cannula with tap that allowed the transit of the CSF in cats, but occluded the flow in the Sylvian aqueduct.[100] They were monitoring the flow in the aqueduct of Silvio but could not recover the CSF via the inserted cannula. They observed that flow did not occur within the CSF spaces, but was absorbed very quickly in the neighboring brain capillaries. These data, in addition to their distrust of the classic model, made them skeptical about the circulation of the CSF.[100] Subsequent studies found that, if insulin was injected into the subarachnoid space, it was very slowly eliminated in the bloodstream and redistributed in a multidirectional mode because of its long elimination time from the subarachnoid space.[101]

Conversely, the injection of water at any part of the CSF system may result in the distribution of the CSF in a multidirectional way, including a "retrograde" path into the lateral ventricles.[102] These results were confirmed by Iliff and colleagues,[103] who found and described a network of special cells, similar to the lymphatic cells, capable of pumping action in order to remove fluid and waste material from the brain. This glymphatic system is similar to the lymphatic system, but is managed by brain cells known as glial cells. Astrocytes use projections, or "end-feet," consisting of aquaporins, to form a network of pipelines around the outer perimeter of the arteries and veins that are located in the brain. Thanks to this system, the CSF is pumped from the brain along the channels surrounding the arteries.

This fluid gently bathes the brain tissue before being gathered in the canals around the veins and thence being downloaded outside of the brain. In the first half of the 20th century, Weed showed how the arachnoid villi and granulations are not the main source of absorption.[104] Although this hypothesis is established, most researchers still consider the reabsorption as a passive process mostly located in the arachnoid villi and granulations.[105] The idea that the arachnoid villi and granulations are among the main sources of absorption of CSF is still in dispute: they do not seem to exist before birth, either in ovine animals or in humans; their development, in fact, begins with birth and they increase in number with age.[106,107]

Recently, lymphatic vessels were found in the dura mater, pia mater, pituitary capsule, orbit, nasal mucosa, and middle ear and a large collection of studies, conducted both on animals and on humans, prove that absorption also occurs in the lymphatic vessels and that this path may become more impor-

tant in conditions of high intraventricular pressure.[106,107] A recent review of the literature[27] presents extensive evidence about a new hypothesis of the physiology of this biological fluid: it is produced and reabsorbed from the entire functional unit consisting of CSF and interstitial fluid. The latter are largely formed and reabsorbed through hydrostatic and oncotic exchanges in all the endothelial walls of the blood capillaries in the central nervous system (Fig. 3.4).

Thus, the choroid plexus, arachnoid villi and lymphatic vessels become smaller sites for the hydrodynamics of the CSF. Lymph vessels can play a larger role in its absorption when the CSF-interstitial fluid

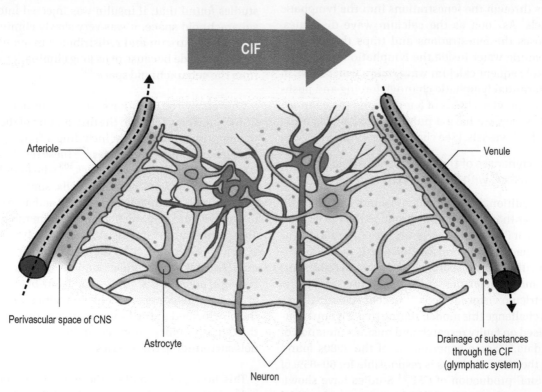

**Fig. 3.4**
Gliovascular system of compensation: drainage of cerebral interstitial fluid (CIF) from arterioles to venules. Modified from: Chikly B, Quaghe-Beurs J. Reassessing cerebrospinal fluid (CSF) hydrodynamics: a literature review presenting a novel hypothesis for CSF physiology. J Bodyw Mov Ther. 2013;17(3):344–54:1360–8592.

pressure increases. We believe that future studies will allow us to understand the exact percentage of:

- the CSF secretion by the choroid plexus from arterial-lymphatic and venous cerebral capillaries

- the CSF reabsorption at the capillary endothelium.

But it seems that these results favor the cerebral capillary endothelium.[27] Fluid flowing from the spinal and cranial subarachnoid space drains through a meta-system that uses both the classically described system and the glymphatic system:[103] a pump system, through which the liquids are absorbed from the brain tissue and are actively pumped up through special channels into the blood system, through the mediation of fascial collagen tubules. Erlingheuser observed the presence of the CSF in the connective tissue fibrils of glial cells.[108] Collagen, surrounded by extracellular matrix, provides a means through which substances are exchanged between the blood and the cells.[109,110]

## Biological autonomic rhythms and baroreflex oscillations

Some studies show that the variability of autonomic rhythms, such as the heart rate, can be modulated at several levels:[111,112] by the circadian rhythm,[113] hepatic and renal peripheral clocks,[114] blood pressure, and by the synthesis of nitric oxide.[115] Some studies suggest changes following a cranial osteopathic treatment.[116] Many of the conclusions derived from different authors argue for a correlation between the hemodynamic autonomic rhythms and their variation over time.[117-119] Osteopathy considers the consistency of autonomic rhythmic oscillatory signals as a control mechanism which, if disrupted, stimulates the components of the entire network to create an adaptive-corrective response.[8] There is strong evidence of the presence of a central oscillatory biological synchronizer which generates an oscillation of about 0.1 Hz. Other studies support a resonance phenomenon[120,121] in the baroreceptor reflex. During the observation of this model, it must

also be considered that the entire mechanism so far described is controlled by the autonomic nervous system, present everywhere in the matrix through nerve endings.

Traube–Hering–Mayer waves (THM) (first described in the mid-19th century by Siegmund Mayer, Ewald Hering, and Ludwig Traube) are expressed as oscillations of the autonomic nervous system. THM are cyclical changes or arterial pressure waves caused by oscillations in the control systems of the chemo-baroreceptor reflex;[122,123] they are visible both in the ECG and in the Doppler laser as continuous waves of blood pressure and have a frequency of about 0.1 Hz (10 waves/sec). They can be defined as oscillations of the arterial pressure with slower respiratory rate frequencies; they show significant coherence with efferent autonomic nervous activity. In humans, oscillations in arterial pressure which satisfy these properties have a characteristic frequency of about 0.1 Hz, and in rabbits and rats 0.3–0.4 Hz.[123] THM are oscillations in blood pressure during respirations.

There are two peaks, one at 15/min and another at 6/min. The first is the Traube–Hering, wave associated with breathing and vagal tone, while the second, low-frequency wave is due to the sympathetic system and is connected to the baro-chemoceptors of the carotid sinus and the sympathetic control of arterioles. The hemodynamic basis of Mayer waves is in the oscillation of the autonomic vasomotor tone of arterial blood vessels: some studies have observed that these are strongly attenuated by the pharmacological blockade of α-adrenergic receptors.[123] Within a given biological species, their frequency is quite stable. In humans it has been shown that this frequency does not depend on sex, age or posture. It has been suggested, in fact, that in the moment in which cyclic force changes on the vascular endothelium are manifested, Mayer waves trigger the release of endothelium-derived nitric oxide. This may be useful in order to ensure good functioning of the perfused organs. Mayer waves are correlated with heart rate variability.[123]

Fluctuations of the blood pressure in the arteries seem to oscillate in search of a medium pressure. Slow fluctuations of the pulse pressure in arteries appear to be controlled by oscillations in autonomic tone, as reported by Guyton and Harris.[120] It has been shown that THM are consistent with tissue oscillatory rhythmic phenomena that osteopaths perceive when practicing cranial osteopathy.[124] The PRM has the CRI as manifestation, which seems to have a remarkable resemblance to the THM oscillations. For this reason, in light of current knowledge of physiology, the CRI and PRM are considered part of the same context of the THM and associated biochemical phenomena oscillations. Today we tend to consider that baroreflex oscillations most likely represent the wave perceived by Sutherland,[13] called the "fast tide" of the CRI, while Mayer waves and oscillator thermal reflexes can be considered the "slow tide" of CRI as described by Becker.[11]

The central nervous system is expressed through the sympathetic and parasympathetic branches of the autonomic nervous system, and the cardiovascular system. We can observe how the phenomenon defined by osteopaths as the PRM can be explained in the context of the THM and how from the palpation of vasomotion in tissues[8] there emerges a model that transcends the classical biomechanical aspects of osteopathy, and brings it closer to its holistic-systemic nature. Vasomotion is defined as the rhythmic oscillation of vascular tone caused by local changes in the constriction and dilation of smooth muscles, which can occur 5–10 times per minute.[125,126] Some researchers have found that vasomotion is calcium-mediated: it can be interrupted due to the interruption of the flow of $Ca^{2+}$,[127,128] for example in the basilar artery.[112] We also know that it can be affected by electromagnetic fields at low intensity of the autonomic nerve fibers.[129]

Oscillations result from changes of neural discharges and are synchronous in large parts of the body, but vasomotion can also be a local phenomenon. Sympathetic tone is a prerequisite for vasomotion, as it provides a basic tone and a direct stimulus

necessary for the oscillation.[130,131] Its activity is in tune with the decreased activity of smooth muscles;[132] however, not all the tone variations are caused by nerves and external signals to the vessels, in addition they can be generated by local factors.[133] So, in the palpation of a zone, it becomes difficult for the practitioner to distinguish a systemic vascular oscillation from a local one.[134] This may explain why inter- and intra-examiner correlation studies in palpatory procedures, with two practitioners that palpate a model in two different physical locations, show poor results.[135]

One or both operators can palpate a response of the locally produced vasomotion, rather than the real autonomic oscillation of the basic THM, which is expressed synchronously throughout the body. Also the amount of pressure that the OCMM practitioner applies with his or her hands to palpate the expression of the intrinsic motion of the tissues makes it difficult to discriminate related tissue responses from the rhythm of the heart, and vasomotion.[136,137] In order to assess the individual's health status through the expression of vasomotion responses, the osteopath tries to understand the basic autonomic status and the relationship with local autonomic responses. Expert operators' advice during "tissue listening," using a metaphorical language, consists of having a "peripheral vision," or "divided attention," not focusing only on the dysfunction, but "listening to health" during perceptual palpation, i.e., the synchronous expression of the THM. The eventual perception of spasms in some areas, which also express attraction vectors (see Chapter 1, the fascial attraction/listening test), is viewed by the operator as an expression of the local alteration of vasomotion. Thus, genesis of the baroreflex waves seems dependent upon the synchronized action of a multitude of singular regulators and cellular oscillators.

The concept of calcium release and the absorption of calcium reserves of smooth muscle, synchronized by ion channels of the sarcolemma, and sometimes influenced by endothelial factors, may provide a better understanding of this phenomenon;[138–140] it is generated within the vascular wall and is not a consequence of the heartbeat, respiration, or neural input.[141] It is the basic, intermittent, oscillator of the sarcoplasmic reticulum that releases calcium through the cell. In the presence of cyclic GMP (guanosine monophosphate), this calcium is able to activate chloride channels in the plasma membrane. If this current is activated simultaneously in a sufficient number of cells, the cells will be depolarized. Even the cells which at that moment are not contracted depolarize, because they are electrically paired. All this requires the coordination of the activities of vascular smooth muscular cells of the vessel wall through an electrical connection.[141]

This phenomenon may help explain the dominant entrainment phenomenon, favored by centering procedures such as osteopathy.[32] Coordination between the electrically connected cells, asynchronously oscillating, may lead to entrainment through these interconnections. Chaytor and colleagues found that this interconnection could be interrupted by the introduction of blocks in the gap-junctions.[142] Vasomotion is usually more diffuse in reduced perfusion conditions, absent at rest, and accelerated during metabolic stress conditions,[143-145] and is considered palpable by expert osteopaths.[146]

## Autonomic nervous system, social involvement, and general adaptation syndrome

The previous paragraphs presented an involuntary rhythms model that does not focus exclusively on the craniosacral axis. The proposed model collects different observations on the physiology of the extracellular matrix, on the links between different biological fluids, the relationship between tissue, fluid flow, and the autonomic nervous system (ANS) observable in the THM baroreflex waves. In describing the polyvagal model, Porges[147] considers the autonomic nervous system as the phylogenetic substrate of a social system involvement. This section considers his proposal as a rational basis for the evaluation of the individual's adaptive capacity, considering the

interactions between behavior and physiology of the ANS. According to the classical neurophysiological view, the ANS is divided into a sympathetic and a parasympathetic system. In this model, the two systems have opposite and balancing functions, similar to the two plates of a balance.

The sympathetic system has activating and catabolic functions (energy use), increases arousal (bodily activation system), activates the responses to danger (attention and consciousness focus), preparing the body to initiate "avoidance" reactions, such as those of fight-or-flight mediated by adrenaline (epinephrine) and noradrenaline (norepinephrine). This involves all the concomitant physiological reactions to adrenergic stimulation, starting with an increase in heart rate. On an emotional (limbic) level, this activation is linked to fear, terror (escape), or anger (attack). The presence of sympathetic hyperactivity, called hyperarousal, can reach the so-called hypertonic freeze, with complete blockage and muscular rigidity, like the "deer caught in the headlights," which stands paralyzed in the sudden light of the main beam, in the middle of the road, unable to move.

The parasympathetic system, by contrast, has saving and recovery energy (anabolic) functions, decreases arousal, slows the heart rate, and facilitates rest and digestion. It acts via the vagus nerve, in cholinergic transmission and facilitates the attachment, socialization, and submission action systems, inhibiting the defensive reactions of sympathetic mediation. The presence of parasympathetic hyperactivity, called hypo-arousal, activates the reactions of "passive avoidance," with a sense of detachment, lowering the level of consciousness, along with emotional and sensory hearing loss. Hypo-arousal can reach clear dissociative states with severe alteration or loss of bodily sensations, depersonalization, unreality, and loss of consciousness. Another reaction from intense hypo-arousal is the so-called tonic immobility, or "fake death" triggered by situations of extreme danger, with no possibility of escape, during which the animal seems lifeless. Since it is a defensive reaction often used by the opossum, it is also called "playing possum."

This reaction is also present in humans and is at the basis of total vulnerability situations, with inability to react to an attack, or a threat experienced as absolutely overwhelming and insurmountable. This reaction is automatic; it is in no way associated to a conscious choice and should not be mistaken for a willing attitude of acceptance of the attack that one is experiencing. On an emotional level, parasympathetic activation is correlated with feelings of guilt and shame. We can define as "binary" this classic pattern of the autonomic nervous system, while Stephen Porges, a neuroscientist and psychophysiologist from Chicago, proposed a tripartite model, the so called polyvagal model, using laboratory data and following arguments on anatomical, phylogenetic, and neurophysiological bases. The polyvagal theory presupposes a separation into two parts of the vagal system. The first part is phylogenetically older; it is called the dorsovagal tract and arises from the dorsal motor nucleus of the vagus in the medulla oblongata. It corresponds, in terms of distribution and functions, to the vagal system as described by "classic" neurophysiology. The second system, the so called ventrovagal, is present only in mammals and is therefore much more recent in the evolutionary sense.

Unlike the dorsovagal system, it is composed mainly of myelinated fibers, functionally more effective; it originates from the nucleus ambiguus and innervates the face, larynx, and heart. It has a key role in modulating affective states and social behavior, being involved in mimicry and voice control, linking them to the neurovegetative state, especially to heart rate variability and certain functions of the hypothalamic–pituitary axis. It decreases the reactivity of the sympathetic system and action systems related to defense, attack, and escape. We can therefore say that, through contact with the other systems (sight/voice/hearing), the ventral vagal system adjusts, by calming, the sympathetic system. For these reasons, Porges talks about the

different parts of the autonomic nervous system as phylogenetic substrates of a social nervous system and, in particular, defines the ventral vagal innervation as a social involvement system.

This system is already present at birth and is evidently important in the adjustment of the dyadic interaction between mother and infant, mediating part of the mode of attachment. Since the ventral vagal system needs maturity (myelination), i.e., a favorable environment, it is conceivable that the quality of early care by a parent affects the quality of the individual's future functioning, including the level of autonomic nervous system regulation. In fact, in abused or neglected children, even years later, we can detect serious alterations at the level of visceral functions coordinated by the protoreptilian brain (failure of arousal, and pulse and respiratory rate modulation, altered perception and processing of stimuli, in particular hunger, sleep, thirst, pain, and proprioception). From the point of view of behavior interpretation, the polyvagal system proposes the presence of three activation levels:

1. A secure environment: there is a prevalence of the ventrovagal system over the sympathetic system and dorsovagal system. As for avoidance reactions, neither active nor passive types are necessary. Social interaction is the fundamental mediator of autonomic modulation. The action systems of attachment, socialization, games, and exploration are facilitated, which allow maturation and growth of the nervous system through cerebral neuroplasticity, also present in adulthood.

2. An insecure environment: perceived danger activates the sympathetic system, facilitating the reactions of active avoidance, at that time adaptive, as they give the opportunity to attack or to escape more effectively. The ventrovagal system is inhibited because the reactions it mediates are not adaptive in this situation. In case of excessive activation, the sympathetic system can lead to maladaptive responses in the form of

hyperarousal (uncontrollable fear, panic, block/hypertonic freezing).

3. A life-threatening situation: in such situations, the reactions of fight-or-flight are not an option because the threat is overwhelming and insurmountable. It is facilitated by the ancient vagal pathway (dorsovagal system) with reactions of passive avoidance (submission, emotional and sensorial hearing loss, dissociation, and tonic immobility), which can sometimes be adaptive, since predators tend not to take action against or be aggressive toward still or dead prey, sometimes even not noticing them. From this description, it is evident how the polyvagal model provides a very interesting description, based on the neurophysiological and neuroanatomical aspects, even when applied to the traumatic dysregulation of arousal.

Through the tripartite division of Porges it is possible to describe the reactions that occur during many traumatic situations that are repeated in the body after any reactivation of traumatic memories (including treatment sessions). The polyvagal model also provides a way of comprehension and development of the therapeutic potential related to the possibility of "hooking" the patient in the state of arousal that the patient is experiencing, by understanding, at least in part, the manifestations and dynamics. Therefore, body-centered care modalities with a neurophysiological basis can be proposed. This is the case with osteopathy with particular reference to the model focused on DyFIR.

## Hypotheses correlated to treatment

It is not the author's intention to describe the performance of osteopathic techniques that are already detailed in classic treatises.[11,13,50] However, they will be cited and revisited within the chapters of Section II, on models and their clinical application. In this section we proceed with the use of a deductive model to review the tradition inherent to treatment in the field of DyFIR, in light of contemporary developments in science. Lee says that what osteopaths listen to in tissues and call "tide" is linked to the waves of calcium ions in solution, and is associated with changes in viscosity and matrix charge.[146] Other authors suggest that the application of subtle compression or the disengagement of the osteopath's hands on specific tissues, for example during specific techniques such as OCMM, causes ionic movement through the fluids and the fibers of the ECM.[69] A net negative charge in the collagen matrix may cause a change of state from gel to sol. This is attributable to the thixotropic properties of collagen and to the changes in polarity resulting from the reorganization of collagen molecules, generated by compression exerted manually.

"Structure governs function"[13] is a basic osteopathic principle. When tissues are subjected to direct or indirect trauma, the physiology, normal mechanical function, and normal organization of a tissue are impaired.[148] Palpatory contacts on the skin can cause a change in the distribution of cations through mechano-chemical transduction processes, which may lead to changes in the ionic distribution, in the permeability of the plasma membrane, generating an increase of potential and change in vasomotion. The skin is a charged membrane that generates a fluctuation potential when it is deformed.[149]

A light contact pressure, less than that necessary to compress collagen, can produce an electric charge, and the resulting ionic movement can generate changes in the cellular plasma membrane, as well as a vasomotion response;[150] a response that might be entrained.[69] Internal and external tensions in the epidermis and dermis also give rise to active mechanical interactions between the extracellular matrix and cells and between cells themselves, as well as mechano-chemical transduction processes that can be an important part of the homeostatic processes of the connective tissue.[149] With the introduction of contact pressure on the skin, the OCMM practitioner introduces a pre-stress, increasing the fixed charge density, the pressure, and the electric potential in the tissues.[150-152] This may begin to explain how light contact can evoke a feeling of expansion from the increased pressure of the fluid.[69]

The response of local vasomotion harmonization with the dynamic fluid flow is due to both the increased fluid pressure within the ECM and the higher fixed charge density, and would be perceived by the osteopath as tissue expansion and tuning with the CRI. So, we have a basic oscillation through the THM oscillations, perhaps palpable by some operators as movements of "flexion, external rotation and extension, internal rotation," but it should also be noted that as soon as the osteopath applies light pressure, the compression through tissues also induces a response in vasomotion.[69]

Moreover, changes in the cellular membrane and in the plasma, leading to a continuous oscillation between the adjacent cells, effectively alter the pH, the volume, or the temperature, through linear thermodynamic effects, which in turn activate a response of vasomotion.[125] It is hypothesized that this is perceived as a change in the quality of DyFIR, of PRM/CRI, perhaps as the "phase tuning" of OCMM treatment, where flexion and extension are more easily palpable.[69] A gradient of ion concentration would be the result of the net effect of ions moving against a concentration gradient. When the latter approximates equilibrium, there follows a gradual decrease in the movement amplitude of the tissue perceptible as flexion/extension, resulting in a tensional equilibrium point defined by osteopaths as the still point, or quiet/stillness. By keeping this point of tensional balance, the free movement of all ions across membranes against their usual gradients would be facilitated, resulting in the achievement of a point known to OCMM operators as balanced fluid interchange.

When this is achieved, the redox and electrical potentials are cleared everywhere, simultaneously, and free electrons recharge the fluids, raising the pH and recalling minerals. Hypothetically, if the compression between the hands of the practitioner is still present, "calcium ion pumps" can actively bring calcium to optimal saturation levels. With the free active ionic movement, through all of the plasma cell membranes at the point of fluid balance, all other ionic levels could return to optimal levels. In this case, the basal THM oscillations go back to normal and the osteopath registers a change in DyFIR. With ionic concentrations at their optimum levels within the intracellular and extracellular environment and the lymphatic fluids, it could result in the optimization of the ionic concentrations in the cerebrospinal fluid and interstitial fluid,[108] as well as the action potentials through collagen fibers.[57] There would be a production of optimal ionic compositions in the ECM, with an optimal tissue perfusion, which most likely means that vasomotion would cease. As stated earlier, vasomotion is not common in normal physiological conditions, and a basic level would be observable in the THM oscillations.

This, we assume, would be palpated by the osteopath as a better quality in the PRM/CRI, most likely perceived as a slow wave. Charman suggests that dysfunctional information stored inside of the liquid crystals may be canceled with the increase in temperature, of piezoelectric events, and transferred again to a homogeneous fluid.[153] The process should ideally depolarize the interstitial tissue and reset the control system to be more efficient in the transmission of information and eliminate any false signals produced by a dehydrated crystalline matrix. The ion flow and the fluctuations of fluids appear to be closely related to electromagnetic fields, which in turn are responsive to mechanical-elastic tension activated through calcium channels. The liquid-crystalline continuity of the ECM can generate vibrations and currents, as well as work as a means of a quantum hologram, recording local activities that interact with a globally coherent field. During an osteopathic treatment there occurs a vibrational interaction of bioelectric and biomagnetic fields between therapist and client. This would allow an exchange of information with the present state of the living matrix, which is codified in the cellular and tissue structure and is holographically accessible if the appropriate frequencies are recognized (see Chapter 7). Arguably, the OCMM practitioner, which we could now redefine as osteopathy in the DyFIR field, might be in a privileged position from which to achieve these changes in the body physiology.

Injuries, malfunctions, insults, and stress can directly or indirectly affect the bone, fascial, or fluid structures and alter joint mobility, vascular circulation, arterial supply, venous and lymphatic drainage, and influence the trophism of the nerves inside the motor and sensory nerves of the central nervous system and the autonomic nervous system.[148] An overload of the central and autonomic nervous systems will lead to musculoskeletal problems and disrupt the normal tone of vasomotion in vascular structures and the ECM, which in turn may immunologically compromise and disturb cell physiology through the plasmatic membranes.[154,155]

## Example of the evaluation process and technique selection

The purpose of OMT is to normalize structure in order to improve function, and improve function to normalize structure. The perception of physiological phenomena, tissue and DyFIR mechanics guides the osteopath in the decision-making process (Fig. 3.5). During the evaluation process, the osteopath can examine the integrated function between different dysfunctional structures, considering that the one with more inert DyFIR could be the key, if treated, to regenerate the vitality of the local self-regulation systems (structure dominates function). These dysfunctional areas could sometimes benefit from a stimulus to the overall vasomotion with adaptogenic techniques, not addressed to SD, but with a global focus toward balancing the DyFIR (function dominates structure).

During perceptual palpation, the osteopath performs a global assessment/evaluation of the DyFIR. The test can be performed with bimanual contact along the poles of the midline, or by testing the harmony or the fragmentation of the fluid rhythm of the different cavities between the transitional areas (craniocervical, thoracic, abdominal, and pelvic). The operator can perceive a fragmentation of the rhythm on the vertical orientation of the patient's body, through the presence of latero-lateral fluctuations, for example of the different cavities between the transition areas, perceived in some areas as spasms, while in others as DyFIR inertia. In the presence of fascial compensation scheme overload, one perceives the loss of resilience of multiple regions, through the lack of expression of primary respiration by tissues and fluids. Inertia or rhythm spasms are perceived through distortions organized around fulcrums in a unified field of motion. These areas are interpreted as autonomic rhythm and vasomotion disharmonies, related to allostatic overloads. The osteopath defines this detection as a imbalanced global DyFIR, therefore proceeding with a comprehensive approach directed to the homeostatic processes rather than dysfunction. For this purpose we use techniques to expand longitudinal fluctuation (e.g., midline techniques) that tend, through afferent approaches by the operator, to overcome the perception of "latero-lateral fluctuation" with a global harmonic oscillation, a " longitudinal fluctuation" from which a state defined as "neutral" would emerge. The latter is the condition which, through a meditative, calm, and present attitude and maintaining rhythmic oscillatory contact with the patient, leads to the point of fluid balancing. The approaches in the field of DyFIR tend to achieve this state, to finalize the "therapeutic process:" an autonomic balancing, vasomotion response and normal tissue mechanics, probably achieved by the entrainment phenomenon.[32] During the evaluation process, the osteopath can perform an "attraction test/fascial listening" (see Chapter 1) and recognize connective tensions in a single region (e.g., a cavity between two transition areas). Then the osteopath performs a DyFIR local evaluation, where he or she estimates the amount of rhythm fragmentation with spasm or inertia in a region, a condition traditional osteopaths refer to as "latero-lateral fluctuation."

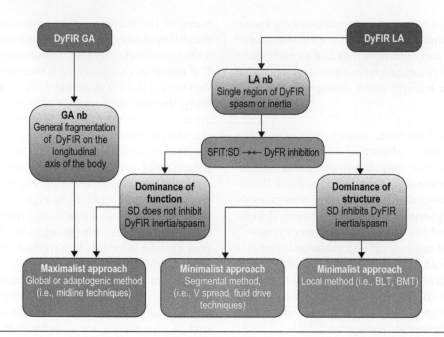

**Fig. 3.5**
Process of evaluation and selection of techniques for dynamics of fluids and involuntary rhythms (DyFIR). The perception of physiological phenomena and tissue mechanics and DyFIR guide the osteopath in decision-making. The osteopath examines the integration between structure and function. The global (GA) and local (LA) assessment of fluid dynamics and involuntary rhythms may detect: (1) an area with dysfunctional fluid dynamics and more inert involuntary rhythms than another; this guides the osteopath to a targeted treatment to regenerate the vitality of local or segmental self-regulating systems (structure dominates function); (2) a rhythm fragmentation on the vertical orientation of the patient's body; this guides the osteopath to homeostatic techniques, with a global focus toward balancing DyFIR (function dominates structure). TIS/F: structure/function inhibition test (inhibition of the vector parameters of SD/DyFIR).

When the longitudinal fluctuation of a fluid encounters the resistance of an inertia or spasm fulcrum, different movement patterns are generated with respect to the surrounding tissues, with attraction vectors perceptible to the operator's hands. With both hands positioned at the poles of the region (craniocervical, thoracic, abdominal, and pelvic), the operator induces a slight oscillatory impulse in accordance with the fluctuation direction. The way in which the fluids react to the stimulus allows the osteopath to locate a possible fulcrum which, if present, produces a palpatory feeling of attraction. This fulcrum, detected through a local not balanced DyFIR, may indicate a region of possible presence of one or more SDs. The operator proceeds by linking multiple areas affected by SD, sensing which of these manifests greater inertia of vasomotion and which presents greater rhythm spasm, therefore discriminating, for example, the one with the most inert inherent motility, less vital (in respect to tissue global rhythm and other dysfunctions), as the dominant among these. In other cases, the osteopath may detect as dominant an SD that manifests more excitability, heat, rhythm spasm, compared to the general tissue rhythm of the individual being examined, and with respect to the other dysfunctional areas. The point is not to evaluate as dominant the most inert, or the most excited, but the one that has lost the ability to adapt and affects the tissues and functions related to it, with its altered vasomotion, its fluid-electric vitality, and whether it is exhausted or overexcited.

The operator then evaluates the integration between structure and function through an inhibition test, i.e., if the inclusion of direct, indirect, or combined vector parameters on the dysfunctional area is detected as dominant, does or does not evoke an improvement of inertia or spasm balancing, by harmonizing the quality of the local rhythm with the general rhythm. Based on the result, one chooses the most appropriate approach for access to the therapeutic process:

- If the insertion of vector parameters evokes an improvement of inertia or local DyFIR balancing by harmonizing the quality of the rhythm with the global one, the operator is directed toward a local approach (e.g., membranous or ligamentous tension balancing), using compressions and/or disengagement (efferent approach) and allowing the DyFIR to express itself within the barriers to reorganize until there occurs a homogeneous motion between and within tissues (afferent approach).

- If the insertion of vector parameters does not result in a harmonization of the local/general rhythm, we proceed with a homeostatic global approach.

- Sometimes, the inhibition test result is not clear, so the osteopath is directed toward the application of segmental techniques, by exercising compression or disengagement with one hand in the SD area (efferent approach), while the other hand leaves the tissues of the symptomatic area or the related regional tissues (afferent approach) free to expand, sensing a DyFIR flow between the two hands (e.g., Fluid Drive, V spread).

## Example of local techniques in DyFIR: general principles of performance and possible mechanisms of operation

After contact with the dysfunctional tissue, if it is fascial[69] it will produce effects on different planes, among which is a piezoelectric change within the collagen matrix: compression or disengagement of fascia creates mechanochemical effects which are integrated into the whole system through the ECM. The altered cationic distribution modifies the permeability of the cell membrane and produces a vasomotion response through adjacent cells. The osteopath can further engage this response using the thixotropic properties of collagen. Manual contact is made with the tissue through gentle movements of compression, torsion, lateral bending, and cutting movements, to gently encourage the collagen fibers toward the "maximum scroll potential" or, in OCMM terms, toward a point of ease: the "point of balanced membranous tension," where the amplitude is reduced until the flexion/extension perceived by the osteopath and the tissue autonomic hyperactivity cease.

The still point is probably perceived when the ions return to an equilibrium point of the concentration gradient. Thermodynamic changes occur within the ECM through the pH, volume, heat, and ionic exchange across cellular plasmatic membranes. The fluid viscosity of the collagen matrix is optimized for the maximum cutting potentials obtained at the equilibrium point. The viscosity of the fluid can be verified for a few seconds to several minutes. It has been suggested that this is a feeling of liberation within the tissues. As the still point is reached, the balanced exchange of fluids is now noted; this is associated with the ionic movement of the free solute across the plasmatic membranes.

Some osteopaths suggest that when a still point is reached, the redox potential is set to zero everywhere simultaneously; electrical potentials are normalized, free electrons recharge fluids by raising the pH; the calcium pumps facilitate a return to a supersaturated concentration in the ECM;[146] vasomotion slows as a result of regular tissue perfusion and normal calcium oscillations are perceived as THM return oscillations; the ion balance is optimal at the cellular plasmatic membrane and in the cerebrospinal fluid. The piezoelectric effects and temperature changes associated with thermodynamic events and the return of the ECM to a more homogeneous fluidic state cancel the dysfunctional information stored in the liquid crystal matrix. The process of balanced liquid exchange has depolarized the interstitial tissue and reset the control system, to be more efficient in the transmission of information, eliminating any disturbance signals produced by the crystalline matrix.

### Example of segmental and global techniques in the DyFIR context: general principles of performance and possible mechanisms of operation

In the context of DyFIR, OCMM describes tissue compression techniques/suppression-diminution of rhythm (e.g., compression of the fourth ventricle – CV4) and of expansion/disengagement/increase in speed (e.g., expansion the of fourth ventricle – EV4). However, clinicians are well aware that during the execution of the procedures both passages are frequently exercised; the osteopath, with one hand in a specific area, in agreement with the tissue dynamics, can compress or disengage a "fulcrum" and wait for the emergence of the intrinsic movement. As already mentioned, there are procedures where the phases are alternated, or even segmental techniques where an operator's one hand compresses, while the other releases (Fluid Drive, V spread).

As reported by some authors, negative and positive ions are concentrated in the compressed or stretched collagen tissue.[69] The piezoelectric influences affect the overall network of fibers; the viscosity of the fluid within the collagen matrix is optimized; the osteopath perceives a longitudinal fluctuation, a homogeneous harmonic rhythm within an anatomical segment. The operator can

sometimes proceed from the fragmented vasomotion rhythm, without focusing on the area of SD. The osteopath removes his or her hands from the dysfunctional area, places them along the midline of the body, and, during the emergence of the intrinsic motion, simply listens, leaving space for expansion, and waits for the perception of an integrated homogenous flexion–extension rhythm: this is the balancing point of fluids, the still point.

What has been described is not a technique in itself, but rather an approach in which the operator lowers the degree of efferent activity in order to increase the afferent listening mode, through contact with longitudinal anatomical structures, such as the fascial compartments. There are several approaches:

1. At the posterior midline, the meningeal fascia, with contact on the vertex and coccyx (see Fig. 1.7)

2. At the anterior midline, i.e., the visceral fascia, with the osteopath positioned with bimanual contact forming a "C" between the first and second fingers of one hand, contacting the anterior cervical region, and the other hand on the anterior presacral area (see Fig. 1.8).

In both compartments, the osteopath tries to perceive in different stages:

1. The eventual emergence of tensional and inertial fulcrums of the intrinsic movement that is also detectable by testing the harmony of the fluctuation with small inductions at the poles, which could give rise to lateral rhythm fluctuations and sheer vector forces

2. The removal of attention from the dysfunctional fulcrums, with increased attention to the rhythm between the operator's hands (called "division of attention") (see Fig. 3.1). In the context of DyFIR, the therapist must have a light and ample feel, a neutral intention and a wide perceptive vision. The operator tries to maintain a vigilant attention to the rhythmic expression of the tissue vitality,

noting whether it is harmonic throughout the entire body or disharmonious in an area that expresses tissue tension, spasm or rhythm inertia. The operator tries to perceive this by focusing his or her attention, whether it is global or local. This awareness is a process in which the focus moves along a continuum that goes from the particular to the general: selective attention with circumscribed focusing to observe an area and panoramic attention with enlarged focusing to observe the whole individual and the individual's relationship with the operator (Fig. 3.6). The attention required during palpation is therefore such that it floats freely between local and global, and may take different degrees of focus. The opening of the field of attention is a condition that promotes a state of relaxation and deep breathing in the patient, with a power influx perceived between the two poles in the space between the hands (called "prolonged inhalation")

3. The emergence of a "homogeneous tissue density", i.e., a "neutral" state, characterized by the absence of tensions in the space around the meningeal visceral or posterior anterior midline

4. A phase of adjustment, of dynamic equilibrium of the DyFIR tissue tensions, with a slowdown of the lateral fluctuations and tensional vectors previously perceived around an inertial fulcrum (still point)

5. A reorganization of the intrinsic tissue motion starting from the state of rest, with the perception of free longitudinal fluctuation of the vasomotor rhythm along the midline, perceived with cyclical movements of expansion and contraction, flexion and extension of the tissue between the operator's hands. We know today that homeostatic techniques not addressed to SD, but focused on the balance of fluids and involuntary rhythms, may be effectively applied to relieve excessive intracranial pressure, reducing fluid flow or cerebral blood volume.[156]

In fact, during afferent global approaches addressed to DyFIR in the form of methods using meditative movements, the operator and the patient reach a relaxed state, where the interceptive/proprioceptive sensations become progressively more intense.[157,158] In this regard, in osteopathic practice

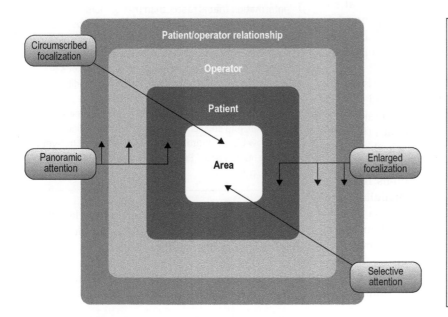

**Fig. 3.6**
Local and global attention on palpation. The necessary attention the operator must have during palpation should fluctuate between local and global observation: the operator can assume different states of selective attention. Attention with a circumscribed/limited focus on a dysfunctional area, and panoramic selective attention with enlarged focus to observe the entire individual and the individual's relationship with the operator.

techniques of fascial unwinding are used,[159] during which spontaneous movement reactions in response to the therapist's touch are activated in the patient; these are ideomotor reflexes mediated by the autonomic nervous system which address the myofascial tone at rest to achieve a more comfortable posture of the entire body.

The osteopath who performs a fascial unwinding technique proceeds with:

- the assessment of tissue tensions and vector forces emerging from dysfunctional areas and reflected on the entire connective structure

- induction of slow and alternating movements of compression and distraction, exceeding the reactive postural tone, evoking tissue relaxation which is then amplified by movements of tension "unwinding" up to a harmonization of the kinematics and a general state of relaxation of the individual.

The necessary attention the operator must have during palpation should be fluctuating between local and global observation. The operator can assume different states of selective attention: attention to a circumscribed/limited area, or panoramic selective attention to observe the entire individual and the individual's relationship with the operator.[160]

We recall that interoceptive stimulation is detected from free nerve endings (demyelinated C fibers with low mechanical threshold), the majority of which are localized in the fascial tissues throughout the entire human body.[160] Researchers have observed in primates a path of interoceptive information faster than that of other mammals: from free nerve endings and lamina 1 of the medulla, information arrives at the thalamus and insula with no need to be processed in the parabrachial nucleus of the brainstem (Fig. 3.7). Fascial disorders may thus affect proprioceptive and interoceptive sensory functions.[161] As a result of stimulation of the interoceptive endings, changes of the autonomic output

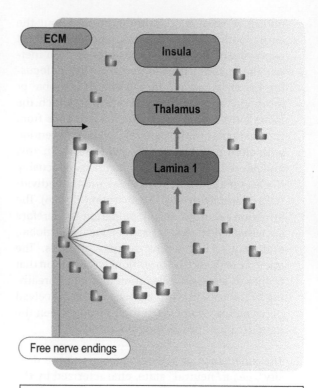

**Fig. 3.7**
From the fascia to body sensations. In primates there has recently been observed a path of interoceptive information that is faster than that of mammals. Via free nerve endings located in the fascial tissue, information passes from lamina 1 of the medulla to the thalamus, to finally arrive at the insula, with no need to be processed in the parabrachial nucleus of the brainstem. ECM: extracellular matrix. Modified from: Schleip R, Jager H. Interception. A new correlate for intricate connections between fascial receptors, emotion, and self recognition. In: Schleip R, Findley W, Chaitow L et al., editors. Fascia: the tensional network of the human body. Edinburgh: Elsevier; 2012. fig. 2.3.2., p. 91.

occur, with an increase in extravascular plasma, i.e., plasma extrusion from the small blood vessels in the extracellular matrix.[161]

The operator, during the execution of the technique, must therefore pay attention to the individual's autonomic and limbic-emotional (or insular) responses by monitoring the direction, speed, and touch so as to achieve a level of uniform hydration in the fascial tissue, as well as other systemic autonomic effects.[161] During a treatment that is set up in this way, attention should also be paid to facial expressions, expansion/contraction of the pupils, spontaneous micromovements of the limbs, changes in breathing, as well as the individual's verbal responses, such as feelings of warmth, lightness/heaviness, density/fluidity, nausea, throbbing, spontaneous emotions, or a general sense of well-being, considering that these interoceptive perceptions can be activated by meditative movements, from fluid approaches or visceral and gentle manipulations of the myofascial tissues, and may be related to physiological and psychoemotional effects.[161]

In addition, cranial osteopathic treatments were seen as more relevant than just specific exercises aimed at producing relaxation and decreasing the frequency of tension headache attacks.[162] This relaxation response to osteopathic treatment was observed with EEG readings that reported changes in sleep latency and autonomic activity.[163] Thus there emerges a similarity of the effects of this treatment to meditative practices. These practices induce a "state of mind" that is distinct from both the vigil state and the sleep state, in relation not only to the specificity of the EEG pattern, but also to the prevalence of hemispheric activities, which "move" from left to right, resulting in enhancement of the somatovisceral, psychological, and cognitive functions that fall within the influence of the right side of the brain.[164]

The hemispheric shift is accompanied by important changes in the reactivity of the autonomic nervous system and major changes in the reactivity of the hypothalamic–pituitary–adrenal (HPA) axis, which, in turn, lead to changes in the quality or quantity of many different physiologic processes, including immune, respiratory, and cardiovascular.[165]

The reactivity of the sympathetic nervous system and endocrine structures involved in the stress reaction – pituitary and adrenal gland, initially – are subject to complex regulation by the diencephalic (such as the hypothalamus, the limbic system, the amygdala) and neocortical (frontal lobes and association areas) areas, which process and modulate the body's response to stimuli within wide limits, so that the same response can be amplified or even cancelled. The character of the reaction to stress depends on the perception one has of the stimulus in question, and it is well known how equal stimuli elicit different responses, of eustress and distress, consisting of a reaction that potentially protects or threatens homeostasis and the integrity of the organism itself. A reaction from prolonged stress, supported by the parallel hyperactivation of the HPA axis, contributes to the etiopathogenesis of the major degenerative diseases that plague modern man, from mental to cardiovascular and neoplastic disorders.[166]

Numerous studies demonstrate how the practice of meditation is accompanied by a significant attenuation in the activity of the HPA axis, even in the presence of a potentially stressful stimulation.[167] In all studies, cortisol, the main hormone involved in stress reaction, is significantly and drastically reduced compared to that observed in the control groups.[168] The reduced secretion of cortisol is accompanied by other changes in important neurotransmitters, involved not only in the regulation of stress response, but also involved in the maintenance of mood and in the modulation of cardiovascular and immune system components,[165] such as ACTH, serotonin, prolactin, aldosterone and β-endorphin.[169,170] Most of the studies related to meditative practices show that the reduced reactivity of the HPA is accompanied by a significant attenuation of sympathetic tone, with a greater focus on autonomic activity rather than the parasympathetic system.[171] Some studies have also observed how osteopathic treatment is related to a reduction in stress levels measured 5 days after the treatment, by documenting alterations in pain biomarkers such as β-endorphin,[172] and better autonomic balance.[173]

However, despite the immediate effects of meditation on physiological functions,[174] it seems that a few years of operation are required in order for the HPA axis responsiveness to be "remodeled" on significantly lower levels than normal.[175] These reflections lead us to consider that non-experts, or people not used to performing meditative practices, can achieve the same results in terms of allostatic load reduction[176] through osteopathic approaches to DyFIR. As shown in the descriptive examples of technical approaches in the DyFIR field, classification of local or global techniques in this domain refers to the operator's focus rather than the rationale of the therapeutic process, which is always designed to improve the individual's adaptive capacity through the harmonization of the dynamics of biological fluids and individual chronobiological involuntary rhythms.

## Osteopathic approach to fascial compensation schemes

It was often stated by the old doctor[177] that the human body does not work in separate units, but as a harmonious whole, and that osteopathy observes it in its entirety. In the previous paragraphs we have observed how one of the areas developed within the evolution of osteopathic medicine, from its pioneers,[19] is the ability to evaluate health and treatment, which from the local may be reflected on the general and vice versa. We proceed in this chapter with a description of another approach born with the intention to answer questions relating to the application of osteopathic principles:

- How does the osteopath observe the body in its unity?

- How does the osteopath treat it as a whole?

- Which are the global tests (those which assess the integration between structure and function of the parts into one)?

- How do you know if and when a subject or an articulation has reached the limit?

We know that, if stressors on an organism are constant and increasing, all the adaptation potentials reach a stage of exhaustion, as happens with a length of elastic that breaks when it is stretched too much. The fascial compensation schemes (FCS) proposed by Gordon Zink[178–180] are one of the tools that can be used to provide information on the degree of advancement of decompensation. Zink, osteopath and lecturer at the Department of Osteopathic Manipulative Medicine at Des Moines University in Iowa, was the first to provide a written explanation that was understandable and clinically useful, relating to the fascial rotational trends, forming a method of evaluation and treatment of the body's fascial pattern in relation to the degree of stress.[181] Fascial tension of any origin can determine the local alteration of the tissue, and tissue memory,[153,182] perceptible to palpation,[146,183] which inevitably ends up affecting other tissues at a distance. Zink noted four transition areas of the body where fascial restriction could be verified. The fascial restriction takes place in regions in which we find anatomical or functional transverse diaphragms, playing a prominent role as active pumps in the circulation of fluids (see Chapter 6). Transition areas also include the articular junction areas, in which a lordosis is converted into a kyphosis or vice versa. There are areas of inversion in scoliotic curvatures as well.

Moreover, as we know, the diaphragms are related also to the whole axial visceral and meningeal corporeal fascial longitudinal organization. It is the fascial junction areas that may experience fibrotic adhesions.[184] Zink's research had focused on posture, on fascial tensions and their effects, particularly on the movement of biological fluids. SD or tissue stiffness, for example, of the transitional areas may affect vasomotion.[150–153] A restriction of abnormal twisting of the passing paths of veins, arteries, and lymph vessels may hamper the flow of biological fluids. Trauma, chemical modifications of the fluid, immunological changes and other stressors or pathogens alter the fascial organization and modify the intersections of fascial bands, maintaining fascial tension, which in turn alters the interstitial fluid, blood circulation, and efficient function of organs.

These requirements have led to the recognition of one of the unique principles of the osteopathic approach, the law of artery supremacy[177] in one of the perceptual models of which Zink was definitely a pioneer; the respiratory-circulatory model.[180] For this reason, in the chapter devoted to this model (see Chapter 6) the basic concepts described here, as well as the practical implementation of the FCS test, will be explained in more detail. The following paragraphs outline some osteopathic considerations on FCS and their basis, which should be integrated with knowledge of the circulatory-respiratory pattern to be expertly applied in clinical practice.

## Osteopathic considerations on the composition of the fascial compensation scheme

As previously mentioned, tissue stress interferes with the circulation of any body fluid and can affect tissue health. It is believed that fascial compensation represents a useful, beneficial, and functional response (i.e., in the absence of obvious symptoms) by the musculoskeletal system, for example as a result of abnormalities, such as an anatomically short lower limb or excessive use of a structure. The failure of these processes describes the same phenomenon, the difference being that the adaptive responses are dysfunctional and symptomatic and represent the failure of homeostatic mechanisms (i.e., adaptation and self-repair). In fact, Zink was also questioned about the physiological changes following treatment based on the FCS, as shown in the study by Ortley in 1980, in which Zink himself took part. This study showed positive physiological changes in "healthy" subjects, such as a decrease in respiratory and cardiac frequency, an increase in tidal volume, and decreased skin resistance.[185]

This approach may also be useful in planning preventive treatment for a general population not suffering from manifested disease or musculoskeletal disorders, as in the study by McPartland in which this mode was applied, resulting in

cannabimimetic, anxiolytic, sedative and analgesic effects. This study suggests that OMT may be associated with changes in the endorphin system and, in particular, may actually be mediated by the endocannabinoid system.[186] Through the application of tissue preference tests of the tension/laxity ratio, performed in the transition areas, it is possible to assess the health trend by observing the FCS in a clinically useful way (Fig. 3.8). The test is also carried out to assess the alternating cycle of fluid dynamics in the transition areas and the evaluation of the harmony–disharmony of the fluid rhythm on the longitudinal axis, i.e., between the different cavities that are created between the transition areas (craniocervical, thoracic, abdominal, and pelvic).

The osteopath can detect:

• neutral fascial compensation schemes (Fig. 3.9)

• compensated fascial compensation schemes (Fig. 3.10)

• decompensated fascial compensation schemes (Fig. 3.11).

In order to evaluate the ability of individual adaptation, through postural tissue responses (see Chapter 1), the osteopath observes the individual, considering the possible correlations between:

• neutral FCS and maintenance of homeostatic/allostatic process alternation. The response to environmental stressors occurs through the occurrence of altered homeostatic activity by allostatic mediators, which integrate physiology and associated behaviors. This activity maintains the fitness of physiological systems in response to the changes in the environment. Once this activation has achieved a new level of adaptation, the body exits from the allostatic state to return to homeostasis

• FCS and allostatic load. This is the cumulative result of an allostatic state. It has a functional

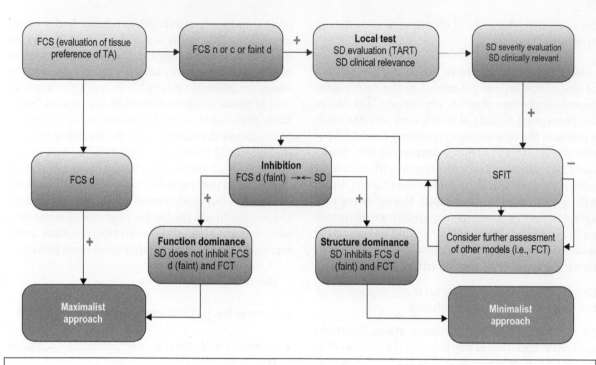

**Fig. 3.8**
Evaluation process of the integrated fascial compensation scheme (FCS). The osteopath finalizes a clear picture of the patient's condition, through the application of an evaluation process that, through the FCS assessment integrated with other osteopathic tests, provides a guide to the selection of the model, approach and techniques.
FCS: fascial compensation scheme; TA: transitional area; n: neutral; c: compensated; d: decompensated; SD: somatic dysfunction; TART: tissue texture abnormality, asymmetry, restriction of motion, tenderness; FCT: fascial compartments test; SFIT: structure/function inhibition test; +: positive test; -: negative test.

significance in response to environmental changes. It integrates the unpredictable events in the normal life cycle, through what is called the alarm stage in the Selye's theory of the general adaptation syndrome: a body must be able to vary all parameters of its internal milieu and match them appropriately with environmental requirements

- decompensated FCS and allostatic overload. This is a condition that exceeds the individual's ability to cope with adversity, and corresponds to the phase of resistance or exhaustion in the Selye's theory of the general adaptation syndrome. It occurs when there is exceptional or unexpected

noise overlapping with allostatic load, resulting in a harmful overload.

In the case of neutral FCS, there is an absence of tissue preference in the transition areas, which is interpreted as a condition of minimum adaptation loads transferred to the other regions. Probably the reason for the individual's consultation will be correlated to an area of local adaptation, for which SD, if present, is rated as clinically significant, even if it is not severe enough to globally destabilize general function, and thus will be dealt with by the osteopath with a minimalist approach. The compensated FCS present a preference of alternated rotation-lateral inclination of the transition areas. This result is

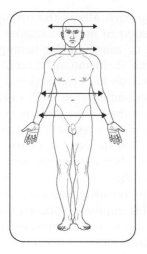

**Fig. 3.9**
Neutral fascial compensation scheme.

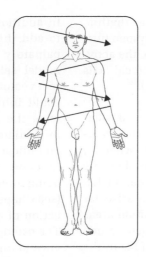

**Fig. 3.10**
Compensated fascial compensation scheme.

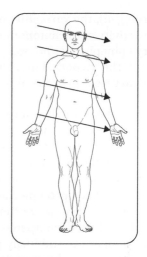

**Fig. 3.11**
Decompensated fascial compensation scheme.

evaluated as a tissue indicator that the individual is subject to an allostatic load to which it responds with adaptability.

The osteopath proceeds with local adaptation area evaluation, searching for clinically significant SD which may be treated with a minimalist approach. The decompensated FCS manifest a lack of alternation of the transition areas that will present with a non-alternating rotational-lateral inclination preference. In these cases, the connection of the operator with the rhythm of the fluids often detects a fragmentation of the fluctuation along the midline, with regions of spasm and/or inertia in the cavities between the transition areas.

This could be the result of a stimulus/sudden trauma or microstimulus/repeated microtrauma. Obviously the sole detection of a decompensated FCS does not, by itself, help to deduce a high degree of stress: focusing of the osteopathic treatment requires the evaluation of cognitive and emotional processes of the individual being treated. The strong individual difference that is found in the subjective component of stress forces us to look at other factors, such as personality, cognitive styles, and anxiety, which can affect the process. This extreme variety of stress components is reflected significantly in the kinds of stress reactions, which include, but are not limited to, psychological ones. In turn, the way in which stress is measured today reflects, on one hand, the theoretical framework in which stress is defined (scales and questionnaires on perceived stress, on life events, interviews, autonomic physiological parameters, endocrine, immunological) and, on the other hand, the specific effect on the individual's complexity (see Chapter 8).

Then, through an interdisciplinary approach, during the evaluation of the individual's adaptive potential, we may also consider certain physiological parameters, considered today as biomarkers of allostatic load, such as blood pressure, or metabolic parameters (glucose, insulin, lipid profile, waist–hip circumference), as well as parameters of inflammation (interleukin-6, C-reactive protein, fibrinogen), the variability of the cardiac rhythm, the activity of the autonomic nervous system (urinary epinephrine and norepinephrine), the activity of the hypothalamic–pituitary–adrenal axis (salivary free cortisol, epinephrine, etc.).[187]

The osteopath therefore collates the information derived from the medical history, the evaluation of the decompensated fascial schemes, and unbalanced DyFIR and detects an allostatic overload that guides him toward a maximalist approach. The decompensated FCS may arise, for example, in only two of the four transition areas (mild failure/decompensation), which guide the osteopath to the likely presence of SD in the cavity between the two diaphragms (Fig. 3.12).

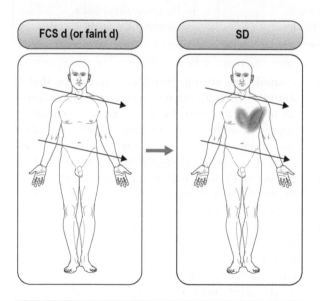

**FCS d (or faint d)**        **SD**

**Fig. 3.12**
Testing the fascial compensation scheme (FCS) and approaching the somatic dysfunction (SD) region. The FCS test could detect a non-alternating mode in two of the four transition areas, which guides the osteopath to the likely presence of SD in the cavity delineated by the two diaphragms. FCS: fascial compensation scheme; d: decompensated; SD: somatic dysfunction.

In addition, this approach allows the osteopath to add this information to medical history and palpatory data and to use them for perceptual model selection. The inclusion of direct/indirect vector parameters on the dysfunctional area could inhibit the decompensated FCS, normalizing the response to the tissue preference test immediately after being re-executed, thus giving an indication of the dominance of structure over function. This result, when perceptible and after being integrated with the remaining assessments (see Chapter 9), guides the osteopath to the application of a minimalist approach focused on SD. The osteopath determines, for example, the presence of an uncompensated FCS with cervicothoracic and thoracoabdominal non-alternating transition areas; this could be related to the respiratory-circulatory function, tending to confirm medical history data. Through the structure/function inhibition test (Fig. 3.13), sometimes specific to each model (Fig. 3.14), the operator can relate the uncompensated FCS, high load index of the stress function (in this case respiratory-circulatory), to any identified SD.

The inclusion of direct/indirect vector parameters on the dysfunctional area may not inhibit the decompensated FCS, leaving unchanged the response to the tissue preference test immediately after being re-executed, thus giving an indication of the dominance of function over structure. The osteopath then proceeds with a maximalist approach, characterized by adaptogenic techniques which will be described in the sections regarding the models.

For example, a metabolic function overload could be confirmed by a non-alternating pattern between the two thoracoabdominal and abdominopelvic transition areas. The FCS test provides further information during the clinical evaluation, if we consider that the diaphragms are related to the entire body's axial fascial organization and its visceral and meningeal components. The fascial tubular compartmentalization may have fibrotic

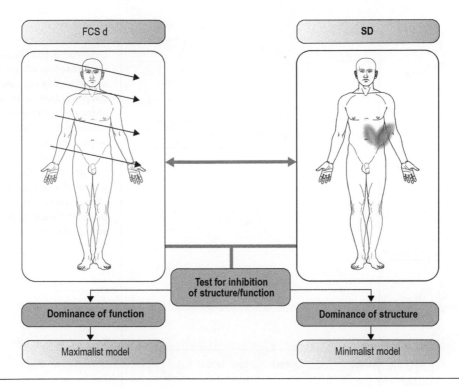

**Fig. 3.13**

Test of structure/function inhibition (SD/FCS). Testing the interdependence between structure/function by evaluating the dominance of failure/decompensation noted during the fascial compensation scheme (FCS) tests and the clinically relevant somatic dysfunction (SD). The test is aimed at discriminating the approach to be used: minimalist or maximalist. FCS: fascial compensation scheme; d: decompensated; SD: somatic dysfunction.

adhesions,[184] which the osteopath can detect by testing, in addition to the transition areas in the complex, and the fascial junction areas (see Chapter 1), i.e., the component related to the visceral fascia and its reflections from the head to the sacrum (see Fig. 1.5) and the meningeal fascia (see Fig. 1.6).

By crediting Zink with the description of the circulatory-respiratory model, the choice was made to describe in the chapter dedicated to it (Chapter 6) the testing of the tissue preference on the transition areas (tested globally or its components such as the diaphragm and fascial junction areas) and its utilization in different evaluation areas of osteopathy, as well as in its evolution during clinical application by the authors. The chapter devoted to the biomechanical model refers to how the Zink test is used to understand the level in which the rotation/preferential inclination pattern is manifested most clearly: in this case the test is used to determine whether the dorsal or ventral muscles maintain the tissue preference of two transition areas, or to assess if myofascial chains of cranial flexion or extension maintain an entire decompensated scheme (see Chapter 4).

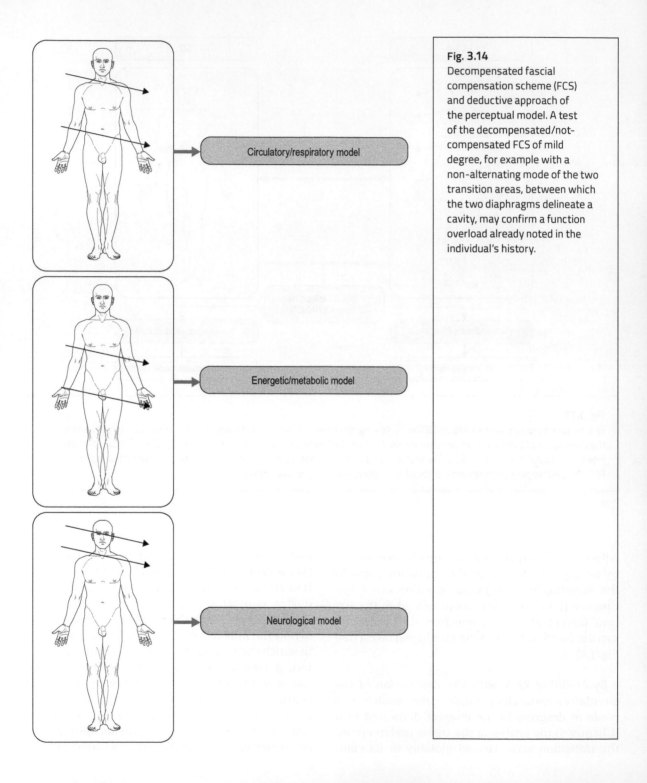

Circulatory/respiratory model

Energetic/metabolic model

Neurological model

**Fig. 3.14**
Decompensated fascial compensation scheme (FCS) and deductive approach of the perceptual model. A test of the decompensated/not-compensated FCS of mild degree, for example with a non-alternating mode of the two transition areas, between which the two diaphragms delineate a cavity, may confirm a function overload already noted in the individual's history.

## Origin of fascial compensation schemes

The causal component of the inability of the organism to adapt to micro- or macro-solicitations or trauma described by Zink[181] was attributable to instances such as vestibular lateralization, cerebral lateralization, and fetal growth and birth:

- *Vestibular lateralization*: early signs of vestibular control would be observed in the labyrinthine reflex of the newborn. It is known that the reflection reflex depends on stimuli from both vestibular organs, to finalize the automatic extension of the head and hold it in an orthostatic posture. This exerts specific control over the extensor postural antigravity musculature and it is known that there is a dominance of the vestibular laterality in the world's population, as opposed to a motor laterality correlated with the flexor muscles. This factor would be related to the cephalic positioning of the fetus during pregnancy, with one side – thus an ear, a labyrinth, a vestibular apparatus – sensing the acceleration during the mother's labor and thus being stimulated more than the contralateral side.[188] Therefore, in the daily work of the mature individual there will be a leg mainly used for postural control (vestibular dominance), the other for voluntary activities (motor dominance). This condition could facilitate the FCS with alternation of the transition areas.

- *Cerebral lateralization*: there is a hemispheric lateralization predominant in the human brain, which corresponds to a dominant laterality and thus to an increased use of hands and feet.[189] This condition could keep and maintain FCS with alternation of the transition areas.

- *Fetal growth and birth*: fetal growth can be divided into three phases, hypertrophy, hyperplasia, and a third phase where both instances are present, with a dominant hypertrophic growth starting at the 32nd week, in which the fetus takes on postural characteristics, defined attitudes or habitus, relative to growth and accommodation into the uterine cavity. The latter, with each passing day, accommodates the increasing size of the fetus with a corresponding decrease in amniotic fluid. Therefore, the fetus, often positioned caudally, adheres more to the uterine cavity.[181] In most cases, the fetal presentation at delivery is either occipital-left anterior iliac (60%) or occipital-right posterior iliac (30%).[190]

The habitus of the baby would imprint a tissue memory in its helical posture with a FCS showing an alternating pattern between the transition areas. It would also appear that, during childhood and development, as the child reaches the ability to crawl, stand, and walk, the child adopts the rotational pattern which is more adaptable than the alternating FCS.[181] In the literature,[191] several authors describe mechanical adjustments with reference to rotational models. For example, the gravitational force due to body weight compression is not transmitted through the femur in a vertical line; rather, it is transmitted as a curved force that extends from the hip to the knee. As a tensegrity structure, the medial aspect of the femur resists compression, while the lateral aspect is under pressure. In addition, in the proximal and distal end of the femur (and of all long bones), the bone widens and the compact bone is replaced by a spongy bone. It is important to note that cancellous bone is not casually present but is organized around a geometric triangulation, with some structures under tension and some that are resistant to compression.

This triangulation provides maximum stability of bone and helps to receive and distribute the force through a joint. Therefore, the femur is a tensegrity structure composed of a combination of pre-compressed and triangular components that fits by arranging itself as a spiral.[191] This tensegritive system is maintained from the macroscopic to the microscopic level: the cellular rigid substrate exerts opposing tensile forces to points of resistance in the ECM, creating a mutual mechanical isometric tension.[192] This dynamic system, with its phases of mechanotransduction, alters the cellular microenvironment, thereby promoting the remodeling of the ECM in conditions of both homeostasis and tissue disorders.[192] It creates a geodesic tensegritive structure of triangles and spheres, inherently self-stabilized, thanks to the level of pre-compression between the cell and ECM.

This autostabilization, in turn, allows the tensegrity systems to transfer the forces applied through the spiral torsion responses of their structures, allowing flexibility, while minimizing damage to the structure. Furthermore, due to the pre-compressed nature of the system, the tensegrity structure immediately regains its previous shape when a force that has been applied ceases. Finally, the continuous tension with intermittent compression allows tensegrity structures to be extremely efficient, normal, and heavy.[191] Biotensegrity is viewed as a natural extension of the concepts expressed by Selye;[193] this model provides a conceptual understanding of the human body's hierarchical organization and of how much of its ability to adapt to change is maintained or lost.

## Fascial memory

Assumptions about the genesis and maintenance of the FCS help to formulate the idea, described by different authors, that the tissues could possess a kind of memory.[182] Fascia can encode memory traces through its contractile capacity related to spinal reflex activity and central control. After the discovery of myofibroblasts in connective tissue,[194] the presence of α-actin of smooth musculature in the myofibroblast cytoskeleton has also been demonstrated,[195] together with its reactivity to mechanical stress. This supports a fascial contractile capacity similar to that of smooth musculature, and its potential influence on musculoskeletal dynamics,[196] i.e., on the resting muscular tone.[197] In addition, the finding of smooth muscle cells and intrafascial nerves supports the hypothesis that a fascial pre-tension can be adjusted via autonomic activity, regardless of muscle tone.[198]

So, as the fascia seems to be organized in myofascial tension bands, which are organized in a single structure,[199] the repercussions of an intrafascial restriction could be global in the body and potentially create stress on any structure involved or attached to a fascia. A dysfunctional memory could then be imprinted by the development of fibrous infiltration and cross-links between collagen fibers at the nodal points of facial bands, together with a progressive loss of elastic properties. Therefore, these changes in myofascial tissue can alter the activity of the higher centers correlated with both sensory integration[200] and motor control.[201] The result is the origination of a FCS related to tissue tensions resulting from fetal growth, from the birth process, and vestibular and cerebral lateralization, and then maintained by a fascial memory.

The latter deductive jump allows us to advance the hypothesis, already known to clinical osteopaths, which states that a therapeutic touch may produce a stimulation of the mechanoreceptors sensitive to pressure in fascial tissue, followed by a response of the parasympathetic system.[202] Under autonomic influence, a change in local vasodilation and tissue viscosity can occur, together with decreased tone of intrafascial smooth muscle cells. Finally, in response to proprioceptive input, the central nervous system can change the muscular tone, allowing the therapist to follow myofascial paths of minor resistance, up to the point where the dysfunctional correction of the cross-linked matrix is reached.[203,182]

## Example of fascial scheme decompensation treatment

If the individual's state of high allostatic overload, noted during the medical history, is confirmed during osteopathic assessment through the detection of a decompensated scheme, the operator can opt for a maximalist approach. The decompensated FCS can be normalized with facilitated positional release technique,[204] in which the operator encourages each of the four transition areas toward the vector of tissue preference involving the fascial diaphragmatic transverse structures and related spinal segments (Fig. 3.15). The operator proceeds with the following steps:

- Positioning, finding the tensional balance of each transition area and maintaining each neutral point via a comfortable placement, or even through the aid of a pillow or other support placed below the lifted side that allows for the preferential rotation

- Treatment, seeking a point of balanced tension. Once the release is obtained, the operator continues with another transition area, until a neutral tissue preference of all areas is obtained. To facilitate the full release and the simultaneous use of all four areas of transition, the operator requires deep breaths and suggests holding the breath in inspiration or expiration, if one of these respiratory states contributes to the tissue tension release.

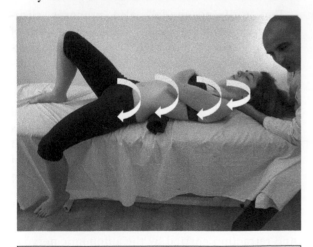

**Fig. 3.15**
Positional facilitated release treatment of the uncompensated fascial scheme. The osteopath approaches the patient via long lever positioning and through the use of pillows, approaching each of the four transition areas toward the tissue preference carrier that involves cross-diaphragmatic fascial structures and related spinal segments. He or she then proceeds with the treatment of each individual station with indirect inductions, aimed at obtaining global tensional balance.

## Conclusions

In this discussion we addressed the osteopath's approach to globalization. Trying to "dig" with the scientific evidence "spade" in the fertile soil of tradition, we tried to understand the approach to the FCS. This allows the osteopath to approach the individual in his or her entirety, before diving in in search of peripheral disturbances which on many occasions determine the normalization of the debilitated self-regulating systems potential (as when conditioned by the presence of SD). This approach is aimed at assessing the degree of adaptation, stress load, the autonomic balance, and the individual's response to micro- or macrotrauma, impressed upon, and thus detectable and treatable in the fascial organization, tissues and their related physiological rhythms. In the domain of physiological rhythms there emerges a particular concept of osteopathy: the PRM, commonly viewed by osteopaths as a motion mechanically governed by pressure changes in the cerebrospinal fluid system and which manifests itself in synchronization throughout the body.[205]

More recent studies have revealed a strong correlation between the "respiratory pulse palpated in the skull" (and the rest of the body) and rhythmic variations in the circulatory system. Vasomotion, through the oscillations of THM, can be measured in the whole body, and seems to represent the mechanism that controls what is perceived as a pulse in the tissue, including the skull. In other words, the biological rhythm, described in OCMM using the PRM model, is now seen as a side effect of rhythmic changes in the blood vessels, both in the brain and in other parts of the body.[8,27–29]

Another manifestation of the same phenomenon is the variability in heart rate, which proved to be a valid index of good health (in fact, a patient who presents zero or very little variability has an 18 times greater chance of dying within a year). In the cardiovascular system there seems to coexist two separate oscillations:[8] while one usually tends to be slower than respiration and appears to be associated with blood pressure variations, the other, the vascular one, seems closely related to respiratory sinus arrhythmia, namely the variability of heart rate as a response to respiratory cycles. The rhythm of vasomotion is slower and is also coordinated by the autonomic nervous system. Stephen Porges has studied respiratory sinus arrhythmia for decades, demonstrating that these rhythmic changes express the state of regulation of the autonomic nervous system. His "polyvagal theory" states that these fluctuations in blood flow are an expression of the "ventral vagus complex."[147]

Contrary to the "dorsal vagus" (which is not myelinated and is of anterior phylogenetic origin), the complex of the ventral vagus constitutes a more recent development for mammals, and is characterized by a myelinated vagus that is able to quickly adjust the cardiac output to favor both interaction with the environment and insulation.[147] It is neuroanatomically related to the nucleus ambiguus and the cranial nerves that govern social relations through facial expression, head turning and voice, and also the regulation of neuropeptides such as oxytocin and vasopressin, which influence social bonding. Post-traumatic stress disorders are usually characterized by significant changes in the autonomic nervous system that occur with the passage from ventral vagus regulation to the older vagal-dorsal system (that is relevant to immobilization), and can be measured by the reduction of both "vagal tone" (respiratory sinus arrhythmia), and the slower THM waves.[206]

This correlation of tissue pulsation with the autonomic nervous system, the extracellular matrix, the tissue mechanics and the studies on tissue viscoelastic and thixotropic responses in response to stress, and the allostatic load memorization in individual fascial organizing, open up some interesting perspectives in the clinical field:

• Instead of just focusing on local alteration research, which sometimes may not be accessible, the global assessment guides the osteopath

in choosing, if necessary, approaches aimed at vitalizing or stabilizing the individual with adaptogenic techniques.

• Rather than focusing solely on the biomechanical model, as determining the palpable rhythm in cranial motion, and instead of explaining human physiology exclusively with metaphysical and vitalistic concepts of life force, energy flow, potency,[207] perhaps one should consider that the current discoveries provide a more comprehensive and organic basis for further clinical research for new applications, which integrate neurobiology and philosophy into a unifying model within the DyFIR. This new model includes the powerful effects of manual therapy at the level of the fascial system, the autonomic nervous system, and related systems, including emotions.

The "unifying model" also proposes clinical applications to assess the effectiveness of disorders related to a high allostatic load, post-traumatic stress disorders, and similar conditions.[208] For example, the measurement of autonomic balance by way of heart rate variability is noninvasive and can be done very easily and inexpensively.[209-211] Another interesting aspect is that the effectiveness of an osteopathic treatment session depends not only on the operator's level of specific biomechanical knowledge, but also the ability to conduct interpersonal processes, palpate tissue changes and observe tissue viability,[186] and recognize the oscillation of tissue expansion and retraction carried by the autonomic nervous system and tissue physiological mechanisms of vasomotion.[27-29]

From this point of view, one should expect major changes in curricular priorities in future training courses in osteopathy.[211-213] Although few studies have yet been completed of those intended to correlate visceral motility with vasomotion, it seems very likely that the visceral organs' rhythmic movements (which according to the assertion would be independent of breathing, heartbeat, or peristalsis) are also governed by biological forces.[203] Since visceral functioning, as much and perhaps even more than cranial functioning, is linked to the autonomous system, it is very likely that visceral motility is in a strong interdependent relationship with vasomotor oscillations controlled by the autonomic nervous system.[155,214] The "unifying model" of "DyFIR osteopathy" explained in this chapter offers the operator a way of understanding the development of therapeutic possibilities that allow the osteopath to "engage the patient and his rhythms."

The osteopath can assess the integration of mind, body, and spirit of the patient, and propose a person-centered and neurophysiologically founded treatment mode:

- perceiving the state of arousal that the individual is expressing

- assessing his or her general state of adaptation to stress

- "listening to" the degree of the patient's adaptation to the environment

- comprehending, at least in part, manifestations and physiological dynamics.

This is the case of osteopathy with particular reference to cranial, fascial, visceral, and lymphatic spheres, from which there seems to emerge a treatment model that includes fluid dynamics, involuntary rhythms, and fascial compensation schemes.

## References

1. Selye H. The stress of life. New York: McGraw-Hill; 1956.

2. Schulkin J. Rethinking homeostasis: allostatic regulation in physiology and pathophysiology. Cambridge, MA: MIT Press; 2003.

3. World Health Organization. International statistical classification of diseases and related health problems. 10th revision. Geneva: WHO; 2011.

4. Educational Council on Osteopathic Principles (ECOP). Glossary of osteopathic terminology usage guide. Chevy Chase, MD: American Association of Colleges of Osteopathic Medicine (AACOM); 2011.

5. European Federation of Osteopaths (EFO). Scope of osteopathic practice in Europe. Brussels: EFO; 2010.

6. World Health Organization. Benchmarks for training in osteopathy. Geneva: WHO; 2010.

7. Zink JG, Lawson WB. An osteopathic structural examination and functional interpretation of the soma. Osteopath Ann. 1979;7:12–9.

8. Glonek T, Sergueff N, Nelson KE. Physiological rhythms/oscillations complementary, alternative, and integrative considerations of biorhythms. In: Chila A, editor. Foundations of osteopathic medicine. 3rd ed. Philadelphia, PA: Wolters Kluwer/Lippincott, Williams and Wilkins; 2011. pp. 162–90.

9. Gadamer HG. Dove si nasconde la salute. Milan: Cortina Editore; 1994.

10. Cozzolino V. Hands on health. Pre-congress courses. Oral presentation at the First International Congress on Biological Mechanisms of Osteopathy – BIOMECH'O 2014.

11. Brooks RE. Life in motion. The osteopathic vision of Rollin E. Becker DO. Portland, OR: Rudra Press; 2010. pp. 181–2.

12. McPartland JM, Skinner E. The biodynamic model of osteopathy in the cranial field. Explore. 2005;1(1):21–32.

13. Sutherland WG. In: Wales A, editor. Teaching in the science of osteopathy. 1st ed. Fort Worth, TX: Sutherland Cranial Teaching Foundation; 1990. pp. 166–89.

14. Geymonat L. Lineamenti di filosofia della scienza. Milan: Mondadori; 1985.

15. Lentini L. Il paradigma del sapere. Conoscenza e teoria della conoscenza nell'epistemologia contemporanea. Milan: Franco Angeli; 1990.

16. Ludovico A. Dalla fisica alla filosofia. Rome: Editore Nuova Cultura; 2011.

17. Kang S. Tao of medicine? Cultural assumptions in medical theory and practice. In: Evans M, Louhiala P, Puustinen R, editors. Philosophy of medicine: applications in a clinical context. Oxford: Radcliffe Medical Press; 2004. pp. 67.

18. Jordan T. Swedenborg's influence on Sutherland's "primary respiratory mechanism" model in cranial osteopathy. Int J Osteopathic Med. 2009;12(3):100–5.

19. Gevitz N. The DOs: osteopathic medicine in America. Baltimore, MD: Johns Hopkins University Press; 2004.

20. Nilsson H, Aalkjaer C. Vasomotion: mechanisms and physiological importance. Mol Interv. 2003;3(2):79–89, 51.

21. Weaver C. Cranial vertebrae. J Am Osteopath Assoc. 1936;35:328–36.

22. Cottam C, Smith EM. The roots of cranial manipulation: Nephi Cottam and "craniopathy". Chiropr Hist. 1981:31–5.

23. http://wwwcranialacademyorg.

24. http://wwwsctfcom.

25. Fryer G. Teaching critical thinking in osteopathy – integrating craft knowledge and evidence-informed approaches. Int J Osteopath Med. 2008;11:56–61.

26. Gevitz N. The DOs: osteopathic medicine in America. Baltimore, MD: Johns Hopkins University Press; 2004.

27. Chikly B, Quaghebeur J. Reassessing cerebrospinal fluid (CSF) hydrodynamics: a literature review presenting a novel hypothesis for CSF physiology. J Bodyw Mov Ther. 2013;17(3):344–54.

28. Nelson KE, Sergueff N, Glonek T. Recording the rate of the cranial rhythmic impulse. J Am Osteopath Assoc. 2006;106(6):337–41.

29. Nelson KE. The primary respiratory mechanism. Am Acad Osteopath J. 2002;12(4):25–34.

30. Nelson KE, Sergueef N, Glonek T. The effect of an alternative medical procedure upon low-frequency oscillation in cutaneous blood flow velocity. J Manipulative Physiol Ther. 2006;29:626–36.

31. Littlejohn JM. The physiological basis of the therapeutic law. J Am Osteopath Ass. 1902;2:42–60.

32. McPartland JM, Mein EA. Entrainment and the cranial rhythmic impulse. Altern Ther Health Med. 1997;3(1):40–5.

33. Wirtz DC, Schiffers N, Pandorf T et al. Critical evaluation of known bone material properties to realize anisotropic FE-simulation of the proximal femur. J Biomech. 2000;33: 1325–30.

34. Belingardi G, Chiandussi G, Gaviglio I. Development and validation of a new finite element model of human head. In: Proceedings of the 19th ESV (Enhanced Safety on Vehicles) 2005.

35. Gabutti M, Draper-Rodi J. Osteopathic decapitation: why do we consider the head differently from the rest of the body? New perspectives for an evidence-informed osteopathic approach to the head. Int J Osteopath Med. 2014;17(4):256–62.

36. Iyo T, Maki Y, Sasaki N et al. Anisotropic viscoelastic properties of cortical bone. J Biomech. 2004;37:1433–7.

37. Sasaki N. Viscoelastic properties of biological materials. In: De Vicente J, editor. Viscoelasticity – from theory to biological applications. InTech; 2012. pp. 99–122.

38. Currey JD. Bones: structure and mechanics. Princeton, NJ: Princeton University Press; 2002.

39. Herring SW, Teng S. Strain in the braincase and its sutures during function. Am J Phys Anthropol. 2000;112:575–93.

40. Strait DS, Wang Q, Dechow PC et al. Modeling elastic properties in finite – element analysis: how much precision is needed to produce an accurate model? Anat Rec A Discov Mol Cell Evol Biol. 2005;283:275–87.

41. Motherway JA, Verschueren P, Van der Perre G et al. The mechanical properties of cranial bone: the effect of loading rate and cranial sampling position. J Biomech. 2009;42:2129–35.

42. Madeline LA, Elster AD. Suture closure in the human chondrocranium: CT assessment. Radiology. 1995;196:747–56.

43. Burr DB. Muscle strength, bone mass, and age-related bone loss. J Bone Miner Res. 1997;12:1547–51.

44. Schönau E, Werhahn E, Schiedermaier U et al. Influence of muscle strength on bone strength during childhood and adolescence. Horm Res. 1996;45:63–6.

45. de Jong WC, Korfage JAM, Langenbach GEJ. The role of masticatory muscles in the continuous loading of the mandible. J Anat. 2011;218:625–36.

46. Ross CF. Does the primate face torque? Primate Cranio-fac Funct Biol. 2008:63–81.

47. Chalk J, Richmond BG, Ross CF et al. A finite element analysis of masticatory stress hypotheses. Am J Phys Anthropol. 2011:145:1–10.

48. Herring SW, Rafferty KL, Liu ZJ et al. Jaw muscles and the skull in mammals: the biomechanics of mastication. Comp Biochem Physiol Part A Mol Integr Physiol. 2001;131:207–19.

49. Rice D. Craniofacial sutures – development, disease and treatment. Basel: Karger; 2008.

50. Sutherland WG. The cranial bowl. Mankato, MN: Cranial Academy, reprinted 1947 and 1986 by Free Press Co.; 1939.

51. Herring SW, Teng S. Strain in the braincase and its sutures during function. Am J Phys Anthropol. 2000;112(4):575–93.

52. Markey MJ, Marshall CR. Linking form and function of the fibrous joints in the skull: a new quantification scheme for cranial sutures using the extant fish *Polypterus end-. licherii*. J Morphol. 2006;268 (1):89–102.

53. Ross CF. Does the primate face torque? Primate Cranio-fac Funct Biol. 2008:63–81.

54. Hartman SE. Cranial osteopathy: its fate seems clear. Chiropr Osteopat. 2006;14:10.

55. Downey PA, Barbano T, Kapur-Wadhwa R et al. Craniosacral therapy: the effects of cranial manipulation on intracranial pressure and cranial bone movement. J Orthop Sports Phys Ther. 2006;36(11):845–53.

56. King H. Research in support of the cranial concept. 2005. wwwcranialacademyorg/pdf/PRMresearchpdf.

57. Lee RP. The living matrix: a model for the primary respiratory mechanism. Explore. 2008;4(6):374–78.

58. Yang PF, Brüggemann GP, Rittweger J. What do we currently know from in vivo bone strain measurements in humans? J Musculoskelet Neuronal Interact. 2011;11(1):8–20.

59. Devulder A, Aubry D, Puel G. Two-time scale fatigue modelling: application to damage. Comput Mech. 2010;45(6):637–46.

60. Frost HM. New targets for fascial, ligament and tendon research:a perspective from the Utah paradigm of skeletal physiology. J Musculoskelet Neuronal Interact. 2003;3:201–9.

61. Turner CH. Bone strength: current concepts. Ann N Y Acad Sci. 2006;1068:429–46.

62. Adams MA, Stefanakis M, Dolan P. Healing of a painful intervertebral disc should not be confused with reversing disc degeneration:implications for physical therapies for discogenic back pain. Clin Biomech. 2010;25(10):961–71.

63. Doblare M, García J, Gomez M. Modeling bone tissue fracture and healing: a review. Eng Fract Mech. 2004;71(13–14):1809–40.

64. Mulvihill BM, Prendergast PJ. Mechanobiological regulation of the remodeling cycle in trabecular bone and possible biomechanical pathways for osteoporosis. Clin Biomech (Bristol, Avon). 2010;25(5):491–8.

65. Cowin SC, Doty SB. Tissue mechanics. New York: Springer; 2007.

66. Mikos AG, Herring SW, Ochareon P et al. Engineering complex tissues. Tissue Eng. 2006;12(12):3307–39.

67. Wang Q, Wood SA, Grosse IR et al. The role of the sutures in biomechanical dynamic simulation of a macaque cranial finite element model: implications for the evolution of craniofacial form. Anat Rec Hob. 2010;295(2):278–88.

68. Strait DS, Wang Q, Dechow PC et al. Modeling elastic properties in finite-element analysis: how much precision is needed to produce an accurate model? Anat Rec A Discov Mol Cell Evol Biol. 2005;283(2):275–87.

69. Hamm D. A hypothesis to explain the palpatory experience and therapeutic claims in the practice of osteopathy in the cranial field. Int J Osteopathic Med. 2011;14(4):149–65.

70. Lucas N. Clinical guidelines, adverse events and SQUID. Int J Osteopathic Med. 2009;12(2):47–8.

71. Becker RE. The stillness of life. Portland, OR: Stillness Press; 2000.

72. Sorokin L. The impact of the extracellular matrix on inflammation. Nat Rev Immunol. 2010;10(10):712–23.

73. Morwood SR, Nicholson LB. Modulation of the immune response by extracellular matrix proteins. Arch Immunol Ther Exp. 2006;54(6):367–74.

74. Pienta KJ, Coffey DS. Cellular harmonic information transfer through a tissue tensegrity-matrix system. Med Hypotheses. 1991;34(1):88–95.

75. Pienta KJ, Hoover CN. Coupling of cell structure to cell metabolism and function. J Cell Biochem. 1994;55(1):16–21.

76. Bassett A. Electrical effects in bone. Scientific Am. 1965;213(4):18–25.

77. Ferreira AM, Noris-Suárez K, Lira-Olivares J et al. Collagen piezoelectric effect induce bone healing. Acta Microscopia. 2007;16(1–2): 122–3.

78. Marino A, Becker R, Soderholm S. Origin of the piezoelectric effect in bone. Calcified Tissue Int. 1971;8(1):177–80.

79. Fukada E, Yasuda I. The piezoelectric effect of bone. J Phys Soc Jpn. 1957; 12(10):1158.

80. Pischinger AA, edited by H. Heiner. Matrix and matrix regulation: basis for a holistic theory of medicine. Brussels:Haug International; 1991.

81. Ettlinger L, Doljanski F. On the generation of form by the continuous interactions between cells and their extracellular matrix. Biol Rev Camb Philos Soc. 1992;67(4):459–89.

82. Ingber DE. Tensegrity: the architectural basis of cellular mechanotransduction. Annu Rev Physiol. 1997;59:575–99.

83. Wang N, Butler J, Ingber D. Mechanotransduction across the cell surface and through the cytoskeleton. Science. 1993;260(5111):1124–7.

84. Charles AC, Merrill JE, Dirksen ER et al. Inter-cellular signaling in glial cells: calcium waves and oscillations in response to mechanical stimulation and glutamate. Neuron. 1991;6(6):983–92.

85. Rubin K, Gullberg D, Tomasini-Johansson B et al. Molecular recognition of the extracellular matrix by cell surface receptors. In: Comper W, editor. Extracellular matrix. Vol. 2: Molecular components and interactions. Amsterdam: Harwood Academic Publishers; 1996. p. 295.

86. Berridge MJ, Rapp PE. A comparative survey of the function, mechanism, and control of cellular oscillators. J Exp Biol. 1979; 81:217–79.

87. Hess B. Periodic patterns in biology. Naturwissen-schaften. 2000;87(5):199–211.

88. Strumwasser F,Vogel JM. Cellular oscillators and biological timing: the role of proteins and Ca2. In: Jaasse J, Dulis R, Tilders F, editors. Progress in brain research. Amsterdam: Elsevier Science Publishers; 1992.

89. Marlowe RL, Hoppe A, Rupprecht A et al. Mediation of a phase transition in hyaluronate films by the counter-ions Li, Cs, Mg, and Ca as observed by infrared spectroscopy, optical microscopy, and optical birefringence. J Biomol Struct Dyn. 1999;17(3):607–16.

90. Nordenstrom BE. Biologically closed electric circuits. Nordic Medical Publications; 1983.

91. Fraser JR, Laurent TC. Hyaluronan. In: Comper W, editor. Extracellular matrix. Vol. 2: Molecular components and interactions. Amsterdam: Harwood Academic Publishers; 1996.

92. Vercruysse K, Ziebell M, Prestwich G. Control of enzymatic degradation of hyaluronan by divalent cations. Carbohydr Res. 1999;318 (1–4):26–37.

93. Johanson C. The choroid plexus. In: Adelman G, editor. Encyclopedia for neuroscience. Boston: Birkhauser; 1999. vol. 1, pp. 384–87.

94. Davson H. Formation and drainage of the cerebrospinal fluid. In: Shapiro K, editor. Hydrocephalus. New York: Raven Press; 1984. pp. 3–40.

95. Davson H, Welch K, Segal MB. Physiology and pathophysiology of the cerebrospinal fluid. Edinburgh: Churchill Livingstone; 1987.

96. Pollay M, Curl F. Secretion of cerebrospinal fluid by the ventricular ependyma of the rabbit. Am J Physiol. 1967;213(4)1031–38.

97. Weller RO, Kida S, Zhang ET. Pathways of fluid drainage from the brain: morphological aspects and immunological significance in rat and man. Brain Pathol. 1992;2(4):277–84.

98. Weiss MH, Wertman N. Modulation of cerebrospinal fluid production by alterations in cerebral perfusion pressure. Arch Neurol. 1978;35(8):527–9.

99. Marakovic′ J, Oreskovic′ D, Rados M et al. Effect of osmolarity on cerebrospinal fluid volume during ventriculo-aqueductal and ventriculo-cisternal perfusions in cats. Neurosci Lett. 2010;484(2):93–7.

100. Oreškovic′ D, Klarica M. A new look at cerebrospinal fluid movement. Fluids Barriers CNS. 2014;11:16.

101. Vladic A, Klarica M, Bulat M. Dynamics of distribution of 3H-inulin between the cerebrospinal fluid compartments. Brain Res. 2009;1248:127–35.

102. Bulat M, Klarica M. Recent insights into a new hydro-dynamics of the cerebrospinal fluid. Brain Res Rev. 2011;65(2):99–112.

103. Iliff JJ. A paravascular pathway facilitates cerebrospinal fluid flow through the brain parenchyma and the clearance of interstitial solutes, including amyloid β. Sci Transl Med. 2012;4(147):147ra111.

104. Weed LH. The dual source of CSF. J Med Res. 1914;26:91–113.

105. Weed LH. Forces concerned in the absorption of the cerebrospinal fluid. Am J Physiol. 1935;114(1):40–45.

106. Johnston M. The importance of lymphatics in cerebrospinal fluid transport. Lymphat Res Biol. 2003;1(1):41–4.

107. Johnston M, Zakharov A, Papaiconomou C et al. Evidence of connections between cerebrospinal fluid and nasal lymphatic vessels in humans, nonhuman primates and other mammalian species. Cerebrospinal Fluid Res. 2004;1(1):2.

108. Erlingheuser RF. The circulation of cerebrospinal fluid through the connective tissues system. Academy of Applied Osteopathy Yearbook 1959.

109. Bradbury M, Cole D. The role of the lymphatic system in drainage of cerebrospinal fluid and aqueous humour. J Physiol. 1980;299:353–65.

110. Wiig H, Keskin D, Kalluri R. Interaction between the extracellular matrix and lymphatics: consequences for lymphangiogenesis and lymphatic function. Matrix Biol. 2010;29(8):645–56.

111. Glonek T. Applications of 31P NMR to biological systems with emphasis on intact tissue determinations. In: Stec WJ, editor. Phosphorus chemistry directed towards biology. New York: Pergamon Press; 1980. pp. 157–74.

112. Hara K, Nakatani S, Ozaki K et al. Detection of B waves in the oscillation of intracranial pressure by fast Fourier transform. Med Inform. 1990;15(2):125–31.

113. Pittman-Polletta BR, Scheer FA, Butler MP et al. The role of the circadian system in fractal neurophysiological control. Biol Rev Camb Philos Soc. 2013;88(4):873–94.

114. Huisman SA, Oklejewicz M, Ahmadi AR. Colorectal liver metastases with a disrupted

circadian rhythm phase shift the peripheral clock in liver and kidney. Int J Cancer. 2015;136(5):1024–32.

115. Bode-Boger SM, Boger RH, Kielstein JT et al. Role of endogenous nitric oxide in circadian blood pressure regulation in healthy humans and in patients with hypertension or artherosclerosis. J Investig. 2000;48(2):125–32.

116. Henley CE, Ivins D, Mills M et al. Osteopathic manipulative treatment and its relationship to autonomic nervous system activity as demostrated by heart rate variability: a repeated measures study. Osteopath Med Prim Care. 2008;2:7.

117. Cevese A, Gulli G, Polati E et al. Baroflex and oscillation of heart period at 01 Hz studied by alpha-blockade and cross-spectral analysis in healthy humans. J Phisiol. 2001;531(1):235–44.

118. Crandall CG, Engelke KA, Pawelczyk JA et al. Power spectral and time based analysis of heart rate variability following 15 days head down bed rest. Aviat Space Environ Med. 1994;65(12):1105–9.

119. Moskalenko YE. Regional cerebral blood flow and its rest and during increased functional activity. In: Ingvar DH, Lasen NA, editors. Brain Work, Alfred Benzon Symposium VIII, Munksgaard, Copenhagen; 1975. pp. 343–52.

120. Guyton AC, Harris JW. Pressure-receptor-autonomic oscillation: a probable cause of vasomotor waves. Am J Physiol. 1951;165:158–66.

121. Bertram D, Barres C, Cuisinaud G et al. The arterial baroreceptor reflex of the rat exhibits positive feedback properties at frequency of Mayer waves. J Physiol. 1998;513 (1):251–61.

122. Elghozi JL, Laude D, Girard A. Effects of respiration on blood pressure and heart rate variability in humans. Clin Exp Pharmacol Physiol. 1991;18(11):735–42.

123. Julien C. The enigma of Mayer waves: facts and models. Cardiovasc Res. 2006;70(1):12–21.

124. Nelson KE, Sergueef N, Lipinski CM et al. Cranial rhythmic impulse related to the Traube-Hering-Mayer oscillation: comparing laser-Doppler flowmetry and palpation. J Am Osteopath Assoc. 2001;101(3):163–73.

125. Nilsson H, Aalkjaer C. Vasomotion: mechanisms and physiological importance. Am Soc Pharmacol Exp Ther. 2003;3(2):79–89, 51.

126. Semien CP, Goudeau CA, Dongaonkar R et al. Venomotion: do venules pump blood? Prairie View A&M University Biology Symposium Proceedings, 1996. p.16.

127. Cavallini L, Coassin M, Borean A et al. Prostacyclin and sodium nitroprusside inhibit the activity of the platelet inositol 145-triphosphate receptor and promote its phosphorylation. J Biol Chem. 1996;271(10):5545–51.

128. Zacharia J, Zhang J, Gil Wier W. Ca2+ signaling in mouse mesenteric small arteries: myogenic tone and adrenergic vasoconstriction. Am J Physiol Heart Circ Physiol. 2006;292(3):H1523–32.

129. Fujii K, Heistad DD, Faraci FM. Ionic mechanisms in spontaneous vasomotion of the rat basilar artery in vivo. J Physiol. 1990;430:389–98.

130. Kim Y, Conover D, Lotz W et al. Electric field-induced changes in agonist-stimulated calcium fluxes of human HL-60 leukemia cells. Bioelectromagnetics. 1997;19(6):366–76.

131. Colantuoni A, Bertuglia S, Intaglietta M. The effects of alpha- or beta-adrenergic receptor

agonists and antagonists and calcium entry blockers on the spontaneous vasomotion. Microvasc Res. 1984;28(2):143–58.

132. Colantuoni A, Bertuglia S, Marchiafava PL. Phentolamine suppresses the increase in arteriolar vasomotion frequency due to systemic hypoxia in hamster skeletal muscle microcirculation. Auton Neurosci. 2001;90(1–2):148–51.

133. Schmidt-Lucke C, Borgstrom P, Schmidt-Lucke JA. Low frequency flowmotion/(vasomotion) during pathophysiological conditions. Life Sci. 2002;71(23):2713–28.

134. Wilkin JK. Periodic cutaneous blood flow during post-occlusive reactive hyperemia. Am J Physiol. 1986;250(5):H765–8.

135. Schechner JS, Braverman IM. Synchronous vasomotion in the human cutaneous microvasculature provides evidence for central modulation. Microvasc Res. 1992;44(1):27–32.

136. Rogers JS, Witt PL, Gross MT et al. Simultaneous palpation of the craniosacral rate at the head and feet: intra-rater and interrater reliability and rate comparisons. Phys Ther. 1998;78(11):1175–85.

137. Bollinger A, Hoffmann U, Franzeck UK. Evaluation of flux motion in man by the laser Doppler technique. Blood Vessels. 1991;28(1):21–6.

138. Bollinger A, Yanar U, Hoffmann U et al. Is high frequency flux motion due to respiration or to vasomotion activity? Progr Appl Microcirc. 1993;20:52–8.

139. Hill CE, Eade J, Sandow SL. Mechanisms underlying spontaneous rhythmical contractions in irideal arterioles of the rat. J Physiol. 1999;521(Pt 2):507–16.

140. Griffith TM, Edwards DH. Ca2+ sequestration as a determinant of chaos and mixed-mode dynamics in agonist-induced vasomotion. Am J Physiol. 1997;272(4):1696–709.

141. Griffith TM, Edwards DH. Fractal analysis of role of smooth muscle Ca2+ fluxes in genesis of chaotic arterial pressure oscillations. Am J Physiol. 1994;266(5):1801–11.

142. Chaytor AT, Evans WH, Griffith TM. Peptides homologous to extracellular loop motifs of connexin 43 reversibly abolish rhythmic contractile activity in rabbit arteries. J Physiol. 1997;503(1):99–110.

143. Schmidt-Lucke C, Borgstrom P, Schmidt-Lucke JA. Low frequency flowmotion/(vasomotion) during pathophysiological conditions. Life Sci. 2002;71(23):2713–28.

144. Borgstrom P, Schmidt JA, Bruttig SP et al. Slow wave flow motion in rabbit skeletal muscle after acute fixed-volume hemorrhage. Circ Shock. 1992;36(1):57–61.

145. Schmidt JA, Breit GA, Borgstrom P et al. Induced periodic hemodynamics in skeletal muscle of anesthetized rabbits studied with multiple laser Doppler flow probes. Int J Microcirc Clin Exp. 1995;15(1):28–36.

146. Lee PR. Interface mechanisms of spirit in osteopathy. Portland, OR: Stillness Press; 2005.

147. Porges SW. The polyvagal theory: phylogenetic substrates of a social nervous system. Int J Psychophysiol. 2001;42(2):123–46.

148. Stoddard A. Manual of osteopathic practice. 2nd ed. London: Hutchinson Medical Publications Ltd.; 1993.

149. Vos WK, Bergveld P, Marani E. Low frequency changes in skin surface potentials by

skin compression: experimental results and theories. Arch Physiol Biochem. 2003;111(4):369–76.

150. McDonald F. Electrical effects at the bone surface. Eur Orthod. 1993;15(3):175–83.

151. Silver FH, Siperko LM, Seehra GP. Mechanobiology of force transduction in dermal tissue. Skin Res Technol. 2003;9(1):3–23.

152. Yao H, Gu WY. Physical signals and solute transport in cartilage under dynamic unconfined compression: finite element analysis. Ann Biomed Eng. 2004;32(3):380–90.

153. Charman R. Complementary therapies for physical therapists. Oxford: Butterworth-Heineman; 2000.

154. Korr IM. The emerging concept of the osteopathic lesion. J Am Osteopath Assoc. 1963;100(7):449–60.

155. Korr IM. The neural basis for the osteopathic lesion. Am Osteopath Assoc. 1947;47(4):191–8.

156. Shi X, Rehrer S, Prajapati P et al. Effect of cranial osteopathic manipulative medicine on cerebral tissue oxygenation. Am Osteopath Assoc. 2011;111(12):660–6.

157. Payne P, Crane-Godreau MA. Meditative movement for depression and anxiety. Front Psychiatry. 2013;4:71.

158. Dugailly PM, Fassin S, Maroye L et al. Effect of a general osteopathic treatment on body satisfaction global self perception and anxiety: a randomized trial in asymptomatic female students. Int J Osteopath Med. 2014;17(2):94–101.

159. Tozzi P. Fascial unwinding. In: Chaitow L, editor. Fascial dysfunction: manual therapy approaches. Edinburgh: Handspring Publishing; 2014. ch. 10.

160. Berlucchi G, Aglioti SM. The body in the brain revisited. Exp Brain Res. 2010;200(1):25–35.

161. Schleip R, Jager H. Interoception: a new correlate for intricate connections between fascial receptors emotion and self recognition. In: Schleip R, Findley W, Chaitow L et al., editors. Fascia: the tensional network of the human body. Edinburgh: Elsevier; 2012. pp. 89–94.

162. Anderson RE, Seniscal C. A comparison of selected osteopathic treatment and relaxation for tension-type headaches. Headache. 2006;46(8):1273–80.

163. Cutler MJ, Holland BS, Stupski BA et al. Cranial manipulation can alter sleep latency and sympathetic nerve activity in humans: a pilot study. J Altern Complement Med. 2005;11(1):103–8.

164. Delmonte MM. Electrocortical activity and related phenomena associated with meditation practice: a literature review. Int J Neurosci. 1984;24(3–4):217–31.

165. Solberg EE, Halvorsen R, Sundgot-Borgen J et al. Meditation: a modulator of the immune response to physical stress? A brief report. Br J Sports Med. 1995;29(4):255–7.

166. Bizzarri M. La mente e il cancro. L'Aquila: Frontiera Ed; 1984. p. 45.

167. Kanas N, Horowitz MJ. Reactions of transcendental meditators and nonmeditators to stress films. A cognitive study. Arch Gen Psychiatry. 1997;34(12):1431–6.

168. Michaels RR, Parra J, McCann DS et al. Renin, cortisol and aldosterone during transcendental meditation. Psychosom Med. 1979;41(1):50–4.

169. Walton KG, Pugh ND, Gelderloos P et al. Stress reduction and preventing hypertension: preliminary support for psychoneuroendocrine mechanism. J Altern Complement Med. 1995;1(3):263–83.

170. Infante JR, Peran F, Martinez M et al. ACTH and beta-endorphin in transcendental meditation. Physiol Behav. 1998;64(3):311–5.

171. Mills PJ, Schneider RH, Hill D. Beta-adrenergic receptor sensitivity in subjects practicing transcendental meditation. J Psychosom Res. 1990;34(1):29–33.

172. Degenhardt BF, Darmani NA, Johnson JC et al. Role of osteopathic manipulative treatment in altering pain bio-markers: a pilot study. J Am Osteopath Assoc. 2007;107(9):387–400.

173. Henley CE, Ivins D, Mills M et al. Osteopathic manipulative treatment and its relationship to autonomic nervous system activity as demonstrated by heart rate variability: a re-peated measures study. Osteopath Med Prim Care. 2008;2:7.

174. Gallois P, Forzy G, Dhont GL. Hormonal changes during relaxation. Encephale. 1984;10(2):79.

175. Jevning R, Wilson AF, Smith WR. The transcendental meditation technique, adrenocortical activity and implications for stress. Experientia. 1978;34(5):618–9.

176. Korotkov K, Shelkov O, Shevtsov A et al. Stress reduction with osteopathy assessed with GDV electro-photonic imaging: effects of osteopathy treatment. J Altern Complement Med. 2012;18(3):251–7.

177. Still AT. Philosophy of osteopathy. Kirksville MO: Author 1899, reprinted by the American Academy of Osteopathy, Indianapolis; 1971. pp. 234–49.

178. Zink JG 1973 Applications of the osteopathic holistic approach to homeostasis. Am Acad Appl Osteopath Yearbook. 1973; pp. 37–47: 42.

179. Zink JG, Lawson WB. An osteopathic structural examination and functional interpretation of the soma. Osteopath Ann. 1979;7:12–19.

180. Zink JG. Respiratory and circulatory care: the conceptual model. Osteopath Ann. 1977;5(3):108–12.

181. Pope RE. The common compensatory pattern: its origin and relationship to the postural model. Amer Acad Osteopath J. 2005; 14:19–40.

182. Tozzi P. Does fascia hold memories? J Bodyw Mov Ther. 2014;18(2):259–65.

183. Tozzi P. Selected fascial aspects of osteopathic practice. J Bodyw Mov Ther. 2012;16 503–519.

184. Willard FH, Fossum C, Standley PR. The fascial system of the body. In: Chila A, editor. Foundations of osteopathic medicine. 3rd ed. Philadelphia , PA: Lippincott Williams and Wilkins; 2010. ch. 7.

185. Ortley GR, Sarnwick RD, Dahle BS et al. Recording of physiologic changes associated with manipulation in healthy subjects. J Am Osteopath Assoc. 1980;80:228–9.

186. McPartland JM, Giuffrida A, King J et al. Cannabimimetic effects of osteopathic manipulative treatment. J Am Osteopath Assoc. 2005;105(6):283–91.

187. McEwen BS. Biomarkers for assessing population and individual health and disease related to stress and adaptation. Metabolism. 2015;64(3 Suppl 1):S2–10.

188. Previc F. A general theory concerning the prenatal origins of cerebral lateralization in

humans. Psychological Review. 1991;98(3):299–334.

189. McManus I, Bryden M. Geschwind's theory of cerebral lateralization: developing a formal causal model. Psychological Bulletin. 1991;110(2):237–53.

190. Carreiro J. Pediatric manual medicine: an osteopathic approach. Edinburgh: Churchill Livingstone Elsevier; 2009.

191. Swanson RL 2nd. Biotensegrity: a unifying theory of biological architecture with applications to osteopathic practice education and research – a review and analysis. J Am Osteopath Assoc. 2013;113(1):34–52.

192. Tadeo I, Berbegall AP, Escudero LM et al. Biotensegrity of the extracellular matrix: physiology, dynamic mechanical balance and implications in oncology and mechanotherapy. Front Oncol. 2014;4:39.

193. Chaitow L. Understanding mechanotransduction and biotensegrity from an adaptation perspective. J Bodyw Mov Ther. 3013;17(2):141–2.

194. Gabbiani G. Evolution and clinical implications of the myofibroblast concept. Cardiovasc Res. 1998;38(3):545–48.

195. Hinz B, Pitter P, Smith-Clerc J et al. Myofibroblast development is characterized by specific cell-cell adherens junctions. Mol Biol Cell. 2004;15(9):4310–20.

196. Schleip R, Klingler W, Lehmann-Horn F. Active fascial contractility: fascia may be able to contract in a smooth muscle-like manner and thereby influence musculoskeletal dynamics. Med Hypotheses. 2005;65(2):273–77.

197. Klingler W, Schlegel C, Schleip R. The role of fascia in resting muscle tone and heat induced relaxation. J Bodyw Mov Ther. 2008;12(4):389.

198. Staubesand J, Li Y. Zum Feinbau der fascia cruris mit besonderer Berucksichtigung epiund intrafaszialer nerven. Man Med. 1996;34:196–200.

199. Myers T. Anatomy trains. Edinburgh: Churchill Livingstone; 2000.

200. Schabrun SM, Jones E, Kloster J et al. Temporal association between changes in primary sensory cortex and corticomotor output during muscle pain. Neuroscience. 2013;3(235):159–64.

201. Tsao H, Galea MP, Hodges PW. Reorganization of the motor cortex is associated with postural control deficits in recurrent low back pain. Brain. 2008;131(8):2161–71.

202. Schleip R. Fascial plasticity: a new neurobiological explanation. Part 2. J Bodyw Mov Ther. 2003;7(2):104–16.

203. Cantu R, Grodin A. Myofascial manipulation. Gaithersburg: Aspen Publications; 1992.

204. Chaitow L. Terapia manuale dei tessuti molli. Principi e tecniche del positional release. Milan: Elsevier; 2009. p.171.

205. Upledger J, Vreedevoogt J. Craniosacral therapy. Seattle, WA: Eastland Press; 1983.

206. Sahar T, Shalev AY, Porges SW. Vagal modulation of responses to mental challenge in posttraumatic stress disorder. Biol Psychiatry. 2001;49(7):637–43.

207. Gevitz N. Center or periphery? The future of osteopathic principles and practices. J Am Osteopath Assoc. 2006;106(3)121–9.

208. Schwerla F, Kaiser AK, Gietz R et al. Osteopathic treatment of patients with long-term sequelae of whiplash injury: effect on neck pain disability and quality of life. J Altern Complement Med. 2013;19(6):543-9.

209. Henley CE, Ivins D, Mills M et al. Osteopathic manipulative treatment and its relationship to autonomic nervous system activity as demonstrated by heart rate variability: a repeated measures study. Osteopath Med Prim Care. 2008;2:7.

210. Hensel KL, Pacchia CF, Smith ML. Acute improvement in hemodynamic control after osteopathic manipulative treatment in the third trimester of pregnancy. J Altern Complement Ther Med. 2013;21(6):618-26.

211. Giles PD, Hensel KL, Pacchia CF. Sub-occipital decompression enhances heart rate variability indices of cardiac control in healthy subjects. J Altern Complement Med. 2013;19(2):92-6.

212. Patterson MM. Touch: vital to patient-physician relationships. J Am Osteopath Assoc. 2012;112(8):485.

213. Esteves JE, Spence C. Developing competence in diagnostic palpation: perspectives from neuroscience and education. Int J Osteopath Med. 2013;17(1):52-60.

214. McMakin CR, Oschman JL. 2013 Visceral and somatic disorders: tissue softening with frequency-specific microcurrent. J Altern Complement Med. 2013;19(2):170-7.

# Lymph palpation: hypothesis or frontier?

Osteopathic cranial manipulative medicine (OCMM) describes the primary respiratory mechanism (PRM) as a polyrhythm generated by different factors, one of the intracranial components of which is the cerebrospinal fluid (CSF). We now know that the CSF is related to another extracranial biological fluid, the lymph, with the latter representing 50% of the intracranial fluid outflow.[1] The great importance of the lymphatic system was recognized by Still, who saw in this apparatus a source of both life and death,[2] as well as by Sutherland, who describes the importance of drainage in removing toxins from the cerebral tissue.[3]

Relative to the lymphatic system in the body, the old doctor used to say:[2]

Where is the body? ... Where is it not? No space is so small as to lack connection with the lymphatic system; with their nerves, and their secretory and excretory ducts. So the lymphatic system is complete and universal throughout the body ... along the course of all the nerves and blood vessels, muscles, glands and in all other organs, from the brain to the foot ... and its function is to combine all the impurities of the body and definitely eject them ...

So, the pioneers of osteopathy considered the lymphatic system as being present in all body areas and therefore a possible ally in osteopathic treatments, from the skull to the toes.

## Is the lymphatic stream palpable?

The elements of the lymphatic system include the lymphatic capillaries (or initial lymphatic), with no real valves or muscle units, which carry the interstitial fluid to the pre-collectors. On the fluid inlet site, endothelial cells are leaf-shaped, with the two flaps overlapping so as to leave openings of about 2 μm.[4] The pre-collectors convey the fluid to the lymph collectors, which have a diameter of 100–600 μm and mainly consist of muscle chains of units separated by bicuspid valves, called lymphangions.[5,6] Their contractility was initially objectively evaluated in humans as early as 1979 and 1980.[7,8] These small "lymph hearts" work in the same way as the pacemaker cells of the body, contracting regularly throughout the lymphatic system (lymphangio-motility) and moving the lymph in peristaltic waves.[9,10]

From the *tunica media* to the *tunica externa*, these muscle units receive extensive innervation by the autonomic nervous system,[11] which allows the intrinsic contractility of human lymphatic vessels.[12] This rhythm, phased, synchronized, having peristaltic contraction, and independent of breathing, has a rate of approximately 4–5 cycles/min.[13]

This lymphatic phased contraction, defined as lymphangio-motility:

- seems ideal for the propagation of an action potential at a great distance[14]

- is coordinated by smooth muscle units[11]

- is regulated by the autonomic nervous system, which determines the coordination and motor synchronization.[15] Vagotomy, for example, will cause the lymphatic contraction rhythms and the valve movements to "become irregular and incoherent."[16]

It was also observed that the lymphatic vessels have specific anchoring filaments, called Leak fibers. These filaments are placed on the outer leaflet of the lymphatic endothelium and extend for long distances in the adjacent connective tissue.[17] This complex of fibers connects the lymphatic vessels to the surrounding elastic fibers and is continuous with the dermis.[18] It is therefore plausible that the lymph vessels' phased rhythm waves can be perceived by human mechanoreceptors and transmitted to the skin by the continuity of the surrounding elastic fibers. The lymphatic vessels are located just below the dermal–epidermal junction, which is why the flow within them is potentially palpable.[18]

External manual compression may increase the contractility by stimulating the external lymphatic receptors for stretching.[19] Human mechanoreceptors are extremely sensitive. In this hypothetical model, one of the features that the practitioner should palpate is the effect of "change in diameter" created by the contraction of lymph vessels and transmitted to the skin by the anchoring filaments.[20] The change of the lymphatic vessel diameter during the diastole/systole cycle is of the order of 40–80 μm for a lymphatic vessel of 100 μm in diameter.[9,10] A recent study has also established that human tactile discrimination extends to the nanometer scale.[21] The lymphatic vessels' phased and coordinated contractions, which are transmitted to the surrounding dermal layer by an elastic structure, evoke a signal that human mechanoreceptors could potentially perceive.

However, that does not make the lymph stream immediately "palpable." In osteopathy, as well as in other manual approaches, specific training is needed, without which it would be impossible to identify the precise vectors of lymphatic circulation among the different skin signals. The physiological characteristics of lymphangio-motility reinforce the hypothesis that it would be possible to differentiate between different vessels (blood-lymphatic), or other structures. At the same time, training in perceptual palpation may allow the discernment of the lymphatic flow from other streams. People can train themselves to hear a single instrument in an orchestra during a concert, taking all other instruments "behind the scenes" in their perception, especially if the instrument has a specific sound or rhythm. It is reasonable to consider that training in selective attention palpation may help the discernment of the lymphatic flow from that of other biological fluids.

Chickly and colleagues[22] have recently published a prospective study in which they observed and confirmed the ability of osteopaths to palpate the superficial lymph stream. For this work the sole of the foot was chosen, as it is one of the most difficult areas in which to palpate the lymphatic flow, because of having one of the thickest epidermal layers. The operators said they perceived lymph "signals" that converge on specific terminal lymphatic regions (e.g., armpits and inguinal zone, etc.), operating at a slow rate of about 3 seconds of going forward and 3 seconds of return (about 0.1 Hz ), and a slight pressure of about 15, 30 g/cm$^2$ (measured with a scale). These data suggest that the lymphatic stream detected on palpation by Chickly and colleagues represents the interstitial lymphatic stream. Lymph vessels absorb the surrounding interstitial fluid, following a physiological rhythm, similar to that palpated by these professionals.

The flow directions indicated by the investigators match what one can expect to find in the traditional lymph anatomical maps (see Figure). This result confirms the hypothesis that properly trained professionals are able to provide perceptual palpatory results of lymph streams, consistent with the maps described in the literature. Palpation of lymphatic flow is therefore possible for a practitioner who has "coached his or her mechanoreceptors" to "hear" and differentiate "specific signals" sent by the contraction of lymphatic vessels' smooth muscles, rather than from other structures such as blood vessels or the fascia, etc. Chickly noted that the lymph stream is palpable in the podalic area;[22] we then ask whether this palpation is also possible at a cranial level. Some osteopaths have wondered why colleagues treat the cranial area differently from the rest of the body.[23]

Gabutti and Draper-Rhodes observed how, through palpation and cranial treatment, it is possible to detect physiological parameters of tissue mechanics. The latter, because of the evolution in biomechanics, does not show different patterns between the head and the rest of the body.[23] However, in the case of lymph in the cranial area, we must remember the commonly shared idea that one of the characteristics of the central nervous system is the lack of a classic lymphatic drainage system.[24] Although it is now accepted that the central nervous system is under constant immune surveillance that takes place inside the meningeal compartments, the mechanisms that regulate the entry and exit of the immune cells of the central nervous system remain poorly understood. The search of the "doors" by means of which T cells move in and out of the meninges has led to the discovery of functional lymphatic vessels that line the dural sinuses[24] (see Fig. 3.4).

These structures that express the entire molecular characteristics of lymphatic endothelial cells are capable of transporting fluids and immune cells from the cerebrospinal fluid and are connected to the deep cervical lymph nodes. The unique location of these vessels may have prevented their discovery thus far, thus contributing to the idea, long shared, of the absence of lymphatic vasculature in the central nervous system. The discovery of a lymphatic system in the central nervous system may require a reassessment of the basic assumptions in neuroimmunology, in addition to shedding new light on the etiology of neurodegenerative and neuroinflammatory diseases linked to immune system dysfunction.[24]

Regarding the application of these scientific discoveries in osteopathy, contemporary colleagues,[25] paraphrasing the teachings of Still, have conceptualized lymphatic models on the basis of the PRM, and on this basis they structured osteopathic treatments for drainage of the neuraxis, applicable in conditions such as chronic fatigue syndrome. This model allows considering different applications of osteopathic treatment; the influence of fluid-based osteopathy on neurological, endocrine, metabolic, and immunological systems[25–28] allows us to consider osteopathy as one of the approaches that serve as adjuncts of elective therapies in multiple medical clinical conditions.

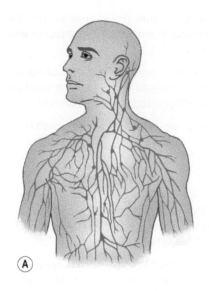

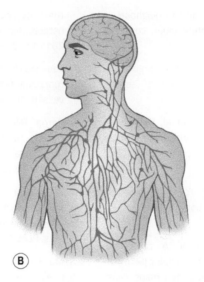

(A) (B)

New map of the lymphatic system. (**A**) The old map reproduced as commonly described in textbooks. (**B**) The updated map graphically described, according to the findings of the Department of Neurosciences of the University of Virginia Health System. (Modified from: Louveau A, Smirnov I, Keyes TJ et al. Structural and functional features of central nervous system lymphatic vessels. Nature. 2015;14432. [Epub ahead of print].

## References

1. Chen L, Elias G, Yostos MP et al. Pathways of cerebrospinal fluid outflow: a deeper understanding of resorption. Neuroradiology. 2015;57(2):139–47.

2. Still AT. Philosophy of osteopathy. Indianapolis: American Academy of Osteopathy; 1971. ch. 6.

3. Sutherland WG. Teachings in the science of osteopathy. In: Wales AL, editor. Teachings in the science of osteopathy. Fort Worth, TX: Sutherland Cranial Teaching Foundation; 1900.

4. Baluk P, Fuxe J, Hashizume H et al. Functionally specialized junctions between endothelial cells of lymphatic vessels. J Exp Med. 2007;204:2349–62.

5. Mislin H. Zur funktionsanalyse der lymphgefassmotorik. Rev Suisse Zool. 1961;68:228–38.

6. Mislin H, Rathenow D. Influencing the spontaneous rhythm of the mesenteric lymph isolated (lymphangion) through various maceuticals. Helv Physiol Pharmac Acta. 1961;19:87.

7. Olszewski WL, Engeset A. Intrinsic contractility of leg lymphatics in man. Preliminary communication. Lymphology. 1979;12:81–4.

8. Olszewski WL, Engeset A. Intrinsic contractility of prenodal lymph vessels and lymph flow in human leg. Am J Physiol. 1980;239:H775–83.

9. Zawieja DC, Davis KL, Schuster R et al. Distribution, propagation, and coordination of contractile activity in lymphatics. Am J Physiol. 1993;264:H1283–91.

10. Zawieja DC. Contractile physiology of lymphatics. Lymphat Res Biol. 2009;7:87–96.

11. McHale NG. Lymphatic innervation. Blood Vessels. 1990;27:127–36.

12. Kinmonth JB, Taylor GW. Spontaneous rhythmic contractility in human lymphatics. J Physiol. 1956;133:30.

13. Szegvári M, Lakos A, Szontágh F et al. Spontaneous contractions of lymphatic vessels in man. Lancet. 1963;281:1329.

14. Thornbury KD. Tonic and phasic activity in smooth muscle. Ir J Med Sci. 1999;168:201–7.

15. Mignini F, Sabbatini M, Coppola L et al. Analysis of nerve supply pattern in human lymphatic vessels of young and old men. Lymphat Res Biol. 2012;10:189–97.

16. Fang Y, Ding Z, Bi Y et al. Effect of vagotomy on dynamics of mesenteric lymphatic vessels in the rat. Chin J Physiol. 2007;50:89–92.

17. Leak LV, Burke JF. Ultra structural studies on the lymphatic anchoring filaments. J Cell Biol. 1968;36:129–49.

18. Solito R, Alessandrini C, Fruschelli M et al. An immunological correlation between the anchoring

filaments of initial lymph vessels and the neighboring elastic fibers: a unified morphofunctional concept. Lymphology. 1997;30:194–202.

19. Gashev AA, Zawieja DC. Hydrodynamic regulation of lymphatic transport and the impact of aging. Pathophysiology. 2010;17:277–87.

20. Akl TJ, Nepiyushchikh ZV, Gashev AA et al. Measuring contraction propagation and localizing pacemaker cells using high speed video microscopy. J Biomed Opt. 2011;16:026016.

21. Skedung L, Arvidsson M, Chung JY et al. Feeling small: exploring the tactile perception limits. Sci Rep. 2013;3:2617.

22. Chickly B, Quaghebeur J, Witryol W. A controlled comparison between manual lymphatic mapping (MLM) of plantar lymph flow and standard physiologic maps using lymph drainage therapy (LDT)/osteopathic lymphatic technique (OLT). J Yoga Phys Ther. 2014;4:173.

23. Gabutti M, Draper-Rodi J. Osteopathic decapitation: why do we consider the head differently from the rest of the body? New perspectives for an evidence-informed osteopathic approach to the head. Int J Osteopath Med. 2014;174:256–62.

24. Louveau A, Smirnov I, Keyes TJ et al. Structural and functional features of central nervous system lymphatic vessels. Nature. 2015;14432. [Epub ahead of print]

25. Perrin RN. Lymphatic drainage of the neuraxis in chronic fatigue syndrome: a hypothetical model for the cranial rhythmic impulse. J Am Osteopath Assoc. 2007;107(6):218–24.

26. Walkowski S, Singh M, Puertas J et al. Osteopathic manipulative therapy induces early plasma cytokine release and mobilization of a population of blood dendritic cells. PLoS One. 2014;9(3):e90132.

27. Mueller DM. The 2012–2013 epidemic influenza and the role of osteopathic manipulative medicine. J Am Osteopath Assoc. 2013;113(9):703–7.

28. Anglund DC, Channell MK. Contribution of osteopathic medicine to care of patients with chronic wounds. J Am Osteopath Assoc. 2011;111(9):538–42.

# 2 | The osteopathic models

## SECTION

*Paolo Tozzi*

## INTRODUCTION

In the early 1980s, the Educational Council on Osteopathic Principles (ECOP), one of the supporting councils of the American Association of Colleges of Osteopathic Medicine (AACOM), developed five conceptual models in the practice of osteopathic medicine, related to patient evaluation, operation and management: the structural, neurological, respiratory and circulatory, metabolic, and behavioral models.[1] Each of these models is based on the principles of anatomy, physiology, biochemistry, and psychology, and provides a specific lens through which the patient can be interpreted and treated. However, the musculoskeletal system remains the primary interface between the models, guaranteeing communication and integration among the basic functions of the body, as well as the ability to adapt to multiple allostatic loads, thus supporting the patient's health.[2]

On the one hand, osteopathic treatment is aimed at facilitating the natural mechanisms of self-healing, approaching areas of somatic dysfunction, i.e., of tissue alteration, which may impede normal neural, vascular, and biochemical mechanisms.[3] On the other hand, from an osteopathic perspective, which is focused on health and globality, it is essential that we refrain from an exclusive focus on the area of dysfunction. With this in mind, the practical application of salutogenic concepts[4] and holistic-osteopathic principles was described by the five models of structure–function relationship, namely five physiological modalities of the individual's adaptive response to any internal or external disturbance, in order to restore and maintain health (Fig. 1).

These five physiological activation forces can be facilitated and supported in order to boost exponentially the individual's capabilities in the physical, mental, and spiritual spheres. In fact, while every human body encompasses the same components and their related functions, each individual develops his or her own biomechanical, neural, fluid, metabolic, and behavioral adaptations in response to physical, chemical, emotional, and psychological events that could destabilize it. The osteopath, therefore, through the five models, turns the principles of osteopathy into a multidimensional approach centered on the individual and on individuality, acting in some cases as a facilitator of the healing process.[5] The five models are usually used in combination to provide a substrate to the subjective and objective clinical data interpretation. The choice of which models to combine is appropriate to the patient's differential diagnosis, comorbidity, and any other ongoing therapeutic regimens.[6]

## THE BIOMECHANICAL MODEL (Chapter 4)

This model interprets the body as an integration of somatic components, mostly musculoskeletal. The emphasis is on skeletal, capsular, ligament, tendon, aponeurotic, muscle, and fascial constituents in constant static and dynamic equilibrium for maintaining a given posture. Proprioception plays a key role in this postural adaptation; this is evidence of the profound physiological and anatomical integration between mechanical and neurological systems. Stress or biomechanical imbalances affect structural dynamic function, resulting in a greater energy expenditure, altered proprioception, postural imbalances, musculoskeletal pain, changes in joint structure, impediments of neurovascular function, and alterations in metabolism.[6]

The osteopath who is going to use this model, both diagnostically and therapeutically, will be interested in testing the body dynamically, carrying out active movement tests, or tests of passive mobility, looking for any restrictions and/or asymmetries, whether positional or functional, instability, and hypermobility, depending on the musculoskeletal load.[7] Similarly, treatment will use structural techniques, such as thrust or articulatory techniques; muscular techniques, such as those in muscle energy; ligamentous techniques, such as balance of ligamentous tension; and/or myofascial release techniques, all with specific mechanical and postural impact, with the ultimate goal of restoring the efficiency of musculoskeletal components,[8] structural integrity, posture, balance, and symmetry.

## THE NEUROLOGICAL MODEL (Chapter 5)

According to the neurological model, the body is a complex system of neural networks, used for receiving and processing multimodal sensory information, and their integration with the efferent, neuromuscular, neuroendocrine, and neurocirculatory control systems.[9]

At the basis of this mechanism, according to Greenman,[7] there are three coexisting subsystems: autonomic, pain relief, and dynamic stability. The first is based on activity and equilibrium between the ortho- and parasympathetic systems. The second, between the central and peripheral nervous systems, is intended for the management of both acute and chronic pain. The third is for postural control and joint dynamic stabilization, through the interdependent relationship of active (muscular), passive (articular-ligamentous), and neuromuscular functions. In this integrated system there are complex reflex activities, which regulate the delicate physiological balance of the organism, but which are also the basis of osteopathic assessment and treatment. In fact, the body is examined in order to identify any area with alteration or aberration of such reflexes (somatovisceral, viscerosomatic, etc.) as a distinctive phenomenon of spinal facilitation as a basis for somatic dysfunction.[10]

Signs of central and peripheral sensitization, of direct and indirect influences of nociception on bodily functions, such as edema, thermal changes, or changes in muscle tone, are all of primary interest in this model. The dermal-visceral Jarricot reflexes, neurovisceral-lymphatic Chapman reflexes, or any tests based primarily on the neural reflex arc and its effects at the tissue are examples of the application of this model in osteopathic evaluation. In the therapeutic sphere, this model aims towards normalizing dysfunctional reflexes, restoring autonomic balance, eliminating nociceptive afferents, reducing pain, intervening in command structures or neurological control complexes, ganglia, neural nuclei, peripheral and cranial nerves, typically by means of counterstrain, cranial, Chapman, or neural inhibition techniques,[11] or treatment of musculoskeletal structures, but taking advantage of the reflex arc as the mechanism of action for the maneuver (suboccipital inhibition, muscular energy, etc.).

## THE RESPIRATORY-CIRCULATORY MODEL (Chapter 6)

In Chapter 6 the main emphasis is on fluids and their freedom of movement, as well as on tissue oxygenation and respiratory mechanics. Any factor disturbing cellular gas exchange or arterial supply and venous-lymphatic-interstitial fluid drainage is a threat to the homeostatic capacity of the organism.[12] The pressure equilibrium between the body cavities, controlled and modulated by the diaphragm's rhythmic action, is of absolute primacy. Areas of edema, congestion, and impaired gas exchange are of primary interest for this model. Osteopathic evaluation aims to identify any disturbance in respiratory efficiency, with particular attention paid to the ribcage, thoracic spine, mediastinum, and cardio-circulatory-respiratory apparatus, including the activities of the four diaphragms (tentorium/superior thoracic/thoracoabdominal/pelvic) and of the lower limbs, as the main engines of the fluid pump.

Treatment aims to restore the pressure equilibrium, where compromised, with techniques for the diaphragmatic structures and central myofascial patterns, to open the muscular-connective tissue paths for fluid passage. Treatment may include lymphatic and osteopathic cranial techniques, techniques of effleurage, petrissage, pumping, and visceral techniques on organs such as the heart, lungs, kidneys, intestines, all with specific fluid and respiratory impact.[13]

## THE METABOLIC-ENERGETIC MODEL (Chapter 7)

This model focuses on the energetic economy, or rather on the dynamic equilibrium between production, distribution, and energy expenditure, from the cellular level to the whole organism, with impact on the activity of the immune and reproductive systems; an equilibrium, moreover, that is under constant adjustment by the neuroendocrine axis and its messengers, such as hormones, immunoregulators, and neuromodulators.[14,15] Hypothalamus, pituitary, pineal gland, thyroid, pancreas, adrenal glands, ovaries, and testes are among the primary organs of interest in this model, in both the evaluation and the therapeutic phases. But the model also includes the autonomic control centers, from the vagal nuclei and the vagus nerve to the splanchnic nerves, the locus coeruleus to the autonomic ganglia and abdominal plexuses. In osteopathic evaluation we focus on detecting areas with excessive energy-metabolic expenditure or deficit, created and maintained by dysfunctional neural–humoral interactions; in reality, any process that interferes with the local or global homeostasis has the potential to increase the body's energy expenditure.[16]

Fatigue, infections, toxicity, and poor tissue repair capabilities are signs that suggest the application of this model. Similarly, treatment will be oriented toward restoring homeostasis thanks to the optimal allocation of resources in order to meet energy demands, the regularization of digestion and absorption of nutrients, and their elimination, through balanced neural and endocrine activity. Lymphatic and visceral techniques are among the most used tools for this purpose, having high immune system impact, supplemented by nutritional counseling and individualized physical activity.[17]

## THE BEHAVIORAL-BIOPSYCHOSOCIAL MODEL (Chapter 8)

Here the individual is seen in the psychosocial context, with all the possible interactions with family, work, and social environment, including heredity, gender, nutritional, cultural, economic, religious and geographical components. But above all, this model analyzes the ways in which such a breadth of relationships can influence the individual's health, and influence his or her perception of pain, illness or disability.[18,19] In other words, particular emphasis is placed on the relationship between the patient's internal environment and the external environment, including the healing process, the individual's psychological nature, and the social environment. Environmental and chemical pollution, physical inactivity, emotional or social trauma, and drug or alcohol abuse are of primary interest for this model.

The evaluation process uses different strategies for approaching the patient, including the physical, mental, spiritual, and social context, determining their effects on the patient's constitution, and also determining how the patient's constitution influences his or her behavioral and psychosocial interactions. Therefore, constitutional and biotypological templates can be applied to the patient's situation and pathology, and can also be used to select and administer the best techniques for tissue-specific action.[20] This model also includes the conscious and appropriate use of the (verbal and non-verbal) relationship between therapist and patient, as well as the accountability of the latter for his or her own healing process,[21] through education – not only of the individual person, but also of his or her family – towards a healthy lifestyle.

## CONCLUSIONS

It is now necessary to point out that the five osteopathic models are intended as purely conceptual models: archetypal strategies of assessment and treatment of the individual and the individual's homeostatic and adaptation potential. However, each archetype, though conceptually strong, puts a particular emphasis on a specific component or function of the organism, or of some of its relationships. This represents not only a conceptual approach, but also a view of overarching applicability.

For example, head and spine would be of primary interest for the neurological model; chest and diaphragm for the respiratory-circulatory model; the abdominal and pelvic region for the metabolic model; the trunk and extremities with their muscular chains for the biomechanical model; lifestyle and social and environmental factors for the behavioral model.[22] However, in practice, it is impossible to think of acting exclusively on specific structures and functions without producing an effect on the others and on the entire organism.

What can be done for the nervous system, without engaging the connective tissue and the surrounding fluids, or influencing the glands and the adjacent target or functionally related organs, and without causing effects on the individual's mental state? This question is valid for every level in which it intervenes. Our body is, in fact, a complex system of integrated functions, based on networks of multi-modal and multisystemic relationships, existing in a network of reciprocal tension through tensegrity architecture, immersed in an informational multi-faceted field of fluid and bioelectrical content, integrated in a unique and unrepeatable social context.

It would be dramatically simplistic and unrealistic to associate an osteopathic treatment with merely selecting a biomechanical, metabolic – or whatever – button to push to cause corresponding reactions in a patient. Rather, the osteopathic models are intended as strategies for the activation of specific body forces, forces of physiological adaptation, which the operator chooses to engage, with a particular emphasis on musculoskeletal system efficiency,[21] to produce the maximum response from the self-regulating forces, with the lowest risk and energy expenditure for the individual. They are the keys, the routes of entry into a system, as well as guides to specific therapeutic targets, to stimulate certain physiological reactions and maximize the effectiveness of the manipulative treatment.[23]

However, the interaction, integration, and combination of multiple models, even within the same session, is almost inevitable. The ultimate goal remains the restoration of health, its maintenance, and its strengthening, and thus the prevention of disease. The removal of pain, though a goal of the osteopathic intervention, acquires a secondary importance when compared to the need to restore function where it is compromised and to support homeostatic mechanisms. It is also true that pain is increasingly recognized as a complex phenomenon, deeply connected with the overall health/disease status of the individual.[24]

This is especially true in patients with chronic illnesses, where pain perception is engaged in a multidimensional environment (genetic, chemical, biomechanical, neurophysiological, psychological, social, etc.), where each component can play a significant role in the pathological framework.[25] Hence the need to use a team approach, from the nutritionist to the psychologist, from the dentist to the orthopedist, the neurologist to the podiatrist, but

above all the patient's active and shared participation in his or her own healing process,[26] by providing correct education regarding postural, ergonomic, supportive, occupational, nutritional, and other factors. In other words, the approach to the individual's health requires a multidimensional approach, most of the time multidisciplinary,[27] which cannot be limited to the elimination of stressors, but must extend to a wider scope.

The first five chapters of Section II of this book will explore the corresponding osteopathic models

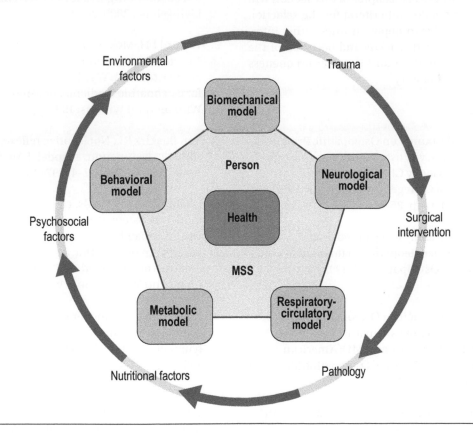

**Fig. 1**
The interaction and integration of the five person-health-centered osteopathic models, through the musculoskeletal system (MSS) interface. They represent the adaptation of five different physiological forces of body, mind, and spirit to stressors of various types: physical (trauma, interventions, etc.), chemical (nutrition, medicines, etc.), psychosocial (family, professional, etc.) and environmental (pollution, radiation, etc.).

in all their expressions and applications, while also offering a discriminating test of structure–function dominance for each model, with the aim of distinguishing: (1) a general adaptation syndrome (GAS), in which the alteration of general function is dominant over any single dysfunctional structure, or (2) a local adaptation syndrome (LAS), in which the single dysfunctional structure is dominant over global function. Using this differential, it will be possible to guide the implementation of the chosen model toward either a global (maximalist approach), or a local (minimalist approach) intervention. Finally, the last chapter of this section will explore the rationale and criteria for the selection of models, in order to apply an osteopathic intervention targeted to the needs and potential of the person being treated, in all his or her uniqueness and multidimensionality.

## References

1. Educational Council on Osteopathic Principles (ECOP). Glossary of osteopathic terminology usage guide. Chevy Chase, MD: American Association of Colleges of Osteopathic Medicine (AACOM); 2011. pp. 25–6.

2. Hruby RJ. Pathophysiology models and the selection of osteopathic manipulative techniques. J Osteopath Med. 1992;6(4): 25–30.

3. Educational Council on Osteopathic Principles (ECOP). Glossary of osteopathic terminology usage guide. Chevy Chase, MD: American Association of Colleges of Osteopathic Medicine (AACOM); 2011. p. 53.

4. Antonovsky A. Health, stress and coping. San Francisco: Jossey-Bass; 1979.

5. Mead N, Bower P. Patient-centeredness: a conceptual framework and review of the empirical literature. Soc Sci Med. 2000:51(7):1087–110.

6. World Health Organization (WHO). Benchmarks for training in traditional/complementary and alternative medicine: benchmarks for training in osteopathy. Geneva: WHO; 2010. pp. 4–5.

7. DeStefano LA. Greenman's principles of manual medicine. 4th ed. Baltimore, MD: Williams and Wilkins; 2011. pp. 48–9.

8. Gibbons P, Tehan P. Manipulation of the spine, thorax and pelvis: an osteopathic perspective. 3rd ed. Edinburgh: Elsevier Churchill Livingstone; 2009. ch. 2.

9. Willard FH, Mokler DJ, Morgane PJ. Neuroendocrine-immune system and homeostasis. In: Ward RC, editor. Foundations for osteopathic medicine. Baltimore, MD: Williams and Wilkins; 1997. pp. 107–35.

10. Van Buskirk RL. Nociceptive reflexes and the somatic dysfunction: a model. J Am Osteopath Assoc. 1990;90(9):792–4, 797–809.

11. DiGiovanna EL. Goals, classifications, and models of osteopathic manipulation. In: DiGiovanna EL, Schiowitz S, Dowling DJ, editors. An osteopathic approach to diagnosis and treatment. 3rd ed. Philadelphia, PA: Lippincott Williams and Wilkins; 2005. p. 670.

12. Degenhardt BF, Kuchera ML. Update on osteopathic medical concepts and the lymphatic system. J Am Osteopath Assoc. 1996;96(2):97–100.

13. Kuchera ML. Lymphatics approach. In: Chila A, editor. Foundations of osteopathic medicine. 3rd ed. Philadelphia, PA: Lippincott Williams and Wilkins; 2011. ch. 51.

14. Pert CB. Molecules of emotion: the science behind mind-body medicine. New York, NY: Touchstone, Simon and Schuster; 1997.

15. Felten DL. Neural influence on immune responses: underlying suppositions and basic principles of neural-immune signaling. Prog Brain Res. 2000;122:381–9.

16. Loo M. Integrative medicine for children. St. Louis, MO: Saunders Elsevier; 2009. p. 26.

17. Hendryx JT. The bioenergetic model in osteopathic diagnosis and treatment: an FAAO thesis, Part 1. Am Acad Osteop J. 2014;24(1):12–20.

18. Quintner JL, Cohen ML, Buchanan D et al. Pain medicine and its models: helping or hindering? Pain Medicine 2008;9(7):824–34.

19. Flor H, Hermann C. Biopsychosocial models of pain. In: Dworkin RH, Breitbart WS, editors. Psychosocial aspects of pain: a handbook for health care providers, progress in pain research and management. Seattle: IASP Press; 2004. pp. 47–76.

20. Parsons J, Marcer N. Osteopathy: models for diagnosis, treatment and practice. Edinburgh: Elsevier Churchill Livingstone; 2006. ch. 5.

21. Rogers FJ, D'Alonzo GE, Glover J et al. 2002. Proposed tenets of osteopathic medicine and principles for patient care. J Am Osteopath Assoc. 2002;102(2):63–5.

22. Seffinger MA, King HH, Ward RC et al. Osteopathic philosophy. In: Chila AG, editor. Foundations of osteopathic medicine. 3rd ed. Philadelphia, PA: Lippincott, Williams and Wilkins; 2011. p. 4.

23. Greenman PE. Models and mechanisms of osteopathic manipulative medicine. Osteopath Med News 1987;4(5):1–20.

24. Gatchel RJ, Peng YB, Peters ML et al. The bio-psychosocial approach to chronic pain: scientific advances and future directions. Psychol Bull. 2007;133:581–624.

25. Kuchera ML. Osteopathic manipulative medicine considerations in patients with chronic pain. J Am Osteo Assoc. 2005;105:29–32.

26. Ballard-Reisch DS. A model of participative decision making for physician-patient interaction. Health Communication 1990;2:91–104.

27. Golden, BA. A multidisciplinary approach to non-pharmacologic pain management. J Am Osteopath Assoc. 2002;102(suppl 3):S1–S5.

# The biomechanical model

*Christian Lunghi*

# 4

## Synopsis

The biomechanical model traditionally analyzes the relationship between bodily attitudes and gravity, as well as the organization of static and dynamic chains in relation to antigravity mechanisms, spinal and vestibular reflexes. In this sense, postural abnormalities involve a substantial asymmetry of body volumes and kinetic functions, with a resulting re-elaboration of the body schema, mediated by the sensory rehabilitation of specific neurophysiological mechanisms. They are found in the loss of harmonious relations between skeletal segments in the three planes of the body, as well as in joint mechanics and alterations of muscular synergies that affect/modify the application of muscular strength and load distribution to skeletal segments.[1]

The biomechanical approach to the processes of care includes different disciplines that address ways to make improvements to any deviations from the ideal posture. These disciplines include those that deal with normalizing biomechanical, compressive, and structural aspects of the body. This is attainable through the correct use of compression, counterweights, and tension in efforts to achieve equilibrium. Perfect posture has been considered to be the state in which the mass of the body is distributed so that the muscles can maintain their normal tone and the ligamentous tensions can neutralize the forces of gravity.[2] In attempting to explain the emphasis on Still's medicine and other manipulative approaches for the spine and musculoskeletal system, Irvin Korr has repeatedly referred to the musculoskeletal

system as "the primary machinery of life," where one can sometimes find causal and maintaining factors of different pathological states.[3]

Efficient posture and good mobility of the entire musculoskeletal system have always been the central focus of the biomechanical model. Osteopaths, chiropractors, and posturologists have given different explanations for body structure misplacements, thus developing different treatment approaches. In osteopathy, somatic dysfunction normalization is considered central in restoring the normal mobility and functionality of the entire musculoskeletal system.[4] Therefore, in the biomechanical model description, in both medicine and osteopathy, different authors have spoken about optimum posture.[5,6] Osteopaths who, until a few years ago, while being anchored to the ideal posture concept, described how difficult it was to identify the clinical reality,[7] now assert that in the presence of a well-compensated body, regardless of any asymmetry and postural adaptations the body presents, it can objectively be said that it functions properly.[8]

This chapter, starting with a discussion on the evolution of the concept of posture, will explore whether, and by how much we now need to step away from the concept of ideal posture, and how we achieve this.[9] In recent years, there have been discussions on the importance of osteopathic principles in defining the unique characteristics of osteopathy. Within these discussions, much attention is given to how much some approaches, such as the biomechanical-postural-structural

## Synopsis continued

model, have been overestimated in the past[10] and to what extent they need to be revised.[11]

In order to critically assess these arguments, the *Journal of Bodywork and Movement Therapy* invited five leading experts in the world of manual medicine, osteopathy, chiropractic, and physiotherapy to address the issue,[12] in particular to meet the argument that, according to Lederman, we cannot justify the use of manual techniques to readjust, correct, and rebalance misaligned structure.[10] The authors argue that as long as postural balance, mobility, strength, and endurance have not recovered, normal functionality without pain can be much more difficult to obtain through rehabilitation strategies. Therefore it is necessary to consider osteopathic manipulative

treatment in terms of holistic approaches intended to integrate body structures and postural function.[12,13]

In discussing posture in osteopathy, we decided to raise the concept of posture and the criticisms of different authors regarding the biomechanical postural model. The intention is also to make a proposal: the multifactorial nature of biomechanical adaptations cannot but lead the osteopath to a global approach that takes into consideration the evaluation of integration between structure and function of an area related to it, and to observing how this relationship can affect the individual's allostatic load and posture, including the ongoing postural response of connective/fascial aspects of the body to internal and external stimuli that place a burden on the person.

## Introduction

When applying the biomechanical model, the osteopath observes the body as an integration of somatic components related to posture and balance mechanisms. Stress or imbalances of any kind within this mechanism will have an effect on dynamic function, causing increased energy expenditure, altered proprioception, changes in joint structure, impediments of neurovascular function, and alterations in metabolism.[14] All levels of human mechanical organization studied so far demonstrate that the human body is a tensegrity structure in which the movement of even a single part involves the whole organism; moreover, this movement includes input from many of the informational exchange functions between cells and molecules, leading to constant changes in biochemistry, distribution, and mechanical energy regulation. Tensegrity systems should be considered as systems of high mechanical complexity.

The science of complexity that now provides the most advanced study models for the understand-

ing of natural phenomena has highlighted some emerging features common to all complex systems, which we also find in a tensegrity mechanical system. The primary characteristic, probably the most important, as the maximum expression of complex systems, is their network topography. They constitute networks, in this case biomechanical, which transmit internal forces which follow a non-linear logic. These depend on the initial condition and the differentiated sensitivity that each constituent element possesses. The differentiated sensitivity means that the received stimuli, both from the external and interior environment, are not processed in the same way by the various constituent elements.

The latter are subject to variability and thus their responses will be partly predictable and partly not: predictable in modality, but not in topography. Within osteopathy there are different approaches to posture, muscular chains, and so on. In this chapter, different postural models will be considered, along with contemporary evidence, to propose observational methods for individual adaptive capacities, through the evaluation of general and local biomechanical organization.

The goal of osteopathic treatment within this model is to restore the most optimal posture that can be achieved by the person at that moment, through the efficient and balanced use of neuromusculoskeletal-fascial components. Posture is observed by the osteopath in its multifactorial nature, through an evaluative process that integrates structure and function. It has been noted that this relationship can influence the individual's adaptive capacity. The treatment proposed in this chapter focuses on the neuro-osteo-myofascial aspects related to abnormal postural responses to stimuli that the body receives, to foster their interoceptive and proprioceptive integration.

## Historical background

The practice of dysfunction resolution by means of spinal manipulation occurs in many native cultures,[15] from Balinese,[16] Hawaiian,[17,18] Japanese, Chinese and Indian cultures[19] to those of Central Asian shamans,[20] Mexican sabodors,[21] Nepali "bonesetters,"[22,23] and the native cultures of Russia and Norway.[24] Concerning the use of manipulation in ancient Western civilization, the Mediterranean area is certainly the place where the foundations for this practice were laid,[25] from the exercises of Hippocrates and traction association[26] to the manipulative techniques described by Galen.[27]

Over the centuries, manipulation was primarily supported by two of the leading complementary health care systems – osteopathy and chiropractic – founded in the second half of the 19th century, in response to deficiencies in allopathic medicine that were detected at that time. Osteopathy and chiropractic care instituted two systems of care based on the biomechanical concepts described by Still, the "lightening bone setter," and Palmer, the "natural healer."[25] In osteopathy, many authors have tried to understand the biomechanical functioning of the body structure through theoretical-visual-empirical modes, developing theories which, although they were not based on scientific evidence, continue to be taught even today. This is probably related to the fact that these modalities were tested from an educational point of view, proving to be effective in providing students with a first interpretation of, for example, spine functioning, giving them the opportunity to acquire a simplified three-dimensional view of biomechanics.[28]

The analysis of spinal biomechanics was pursued by Littlejohn with a global perspective, and with particular observation of the articular and muscular circumstances that can interact with adaptive processes such as scoliosis.[29] Although he thought of himself as "osteopathy's mechanic," John Martin used his attention to the body's overall functionality, introducing an interesting thought pattern in which the lines of force, curves, and functional arches of the spine provide explanations to understand the relationship between postural patterns and somatic dysfunction.[30] He proposed a thorough structural and functional evaluation of the spine's pivots, based on the observation of biomechanical force distribution lines (anterior-posterior, posterior-anterior, anterior-central and posterior-central) and of the body's division into three functional units (craniocervical-thoracic, thoracoabdominal, abdominopelvic). From his teachings emerged global approaches which, through articulatory, rhythmic, and oscillatory routines, aimed to integrate the dysfunctional areas by stimulating the physiological lines of force: this is the general osteopathic treatment and total body adjustment developed in Europe by J. Wernham.[31]

In the same geographical area, England, on the basis of the same principles enunciated by Littlejohn, a minimalist approach was developed that addresses treatment of the positional component of the dysfunction, considered by T. Dummer as being caused by an excessive local accumulation of a traumatic force.[32] Fryette, instead, has described the behavior of individual vertebrae both from the physiological and dysfunctional point of view.[33] These procedures are now used by many osteopaths to conceptually support somatic dysfunction (SD) diagnosis, although there is conflicting evidence in this regard. While the first and the third law of Fryette seem to be generally accepted, there is a wide debate on the second law. Indeed there is evidence to support the coupling of the movements of side-bending and rotation of the cervical spine (i.e., they occur to the same side), while the evidence on the coupled motion in the lumbar vertebral column is inconsistent. Consequently, Fryette's laws may be useful to predict coupling behavior in the cervical spine, but greater caution must be used for the thoracic and lumbar areas of the spine.[34]

Sutherland tried to understand the impact of the craniosacral mechanism on the entire body, observing the synchrony between cranial flexion, thoracic inhalation and external rotation of the whole body, and vice versa between cranial extension, thoracic exhalation and body internal rotation.[35] Magoun described a pattern of flexion movement associated with external rotation and abduction, and a pattern of extension related to internal rotation and adduction.[36] Richter and Hegben, referring to this model, report that when the extension chain dominates bilaterally, the spine is elongated, while the head and limbs are in flexion, external rotation, and abduction of the limbs. The dominance of a flexor chain increases the spine's curvature; the skull is extended and internally rotated, with the arms abducted. The presentation of asymmetrical dominance would allow for the emergence of a pattern of flexion in one half of the body and one of extension in the other half.[37] Other authors have emphasized the treatment of SD of myofascial origin, suggesting treatment models designed to reduce muscle hypertonia related to the dysfunctional area: this is the case of resistive rhythmic induction techniques described by Ruddy and of muscle energy techniques developed by Fred Mitchell.[38]

Different osteopaths and manual therapists have therefore tried to explain joint and periarticular structure dysfunctions through myofascial imbalances.[39] Struyff-Deniss considers the shape of the articular surfaces and the disposition of multiarticular muscles at the base of the spiraling movements which determine the general body schema and related myofascial chains. In this model the shape and movement of these chains are considered to be related to the person's emotional state (see Chapter 8). Myers[39] uses the metaphor of rail transport to describe tissue continuity through myofascial lines that cross their "tracks" in the bony insertions of muscles, representing, as central train "stations," areas of high importance for movement. Busquet[39] describes five muscle chains responsible for the body's movements; they integrate the cranial and extracranial membranes and include the connection between the abdominal organs and the trunk, through the suspensory system of mesenteries, omentums and ligaments. Chaffour[39] describes chains and related points where the fascias are inserted in the skeleton; he considers these anchors as fulcrums of mechanical lines that promote physiological movement. The model described by him allows for research and treatment of dysfunctional areas, considered as abnormal anchor points within the chains.

In osteopathy, the concept of "perfect posture" has evolved over time, moving from the idea of dependence on continued compression of biomechanical structures[7] to concepts that consider myofascial viscoelastic intrinsic properties and their baseline level of passive tension, and resilience on elongation, as leading factors in maintaining postural stability.[40]

## Objectives

In discussing the application of the biomechanical model in osteopathy, the author intends to make a proposal focused on the multifactorial nature of biomechanical and allostatic adaptations. The term posture includes, inevitably, the idea of movement, of fluidity, of action and reaction, integration, reciprocity, tensegrity, of economy, of self-organization, adaptation, complexity, and multisensory factors. This complicates the concept of posture and obligates us to analyze it from a systemic perspective. In posture we observe the same features that are found in complex systems, the object of study in every field of science, from nonlinear thermodynamics to the ecology of autopoietic systems.[41]

This multifactorial nature cannot but lead the osteopath to a global approach that addresses:

- the evaluation of integration between structure and function of an area related to it

- observation of how much this relationship might influence the individual's allostatic load and its reflection on posture

- the neuromyofascial aspects inherent in the continuous postural response to internal and external stimuli that the body receives and integrates through interoceptive and proprioceptive sensation

- the biopsychosocial aspects that through the memory and psychoemotional load of the given person makes the adaptive response so individual and unique.

The biomechanical model frames the patient from a structural or mechanical point of view. The structural integrity and the function of the musculoskeletal system are interactive and interdependent with the patient's neurological, respiratory-circulatory, metabolic and behavioral functions. Therefore, alterations of postural mechanisms of movement and quality of connective tissue, regardless of etiology, often affect vascular, lymphatic, and neurological function. In fact, this model considers that a structural/functional impairment that causes, or is caused by, a muscle dysfunction, joint and/or connective tissue can impair vascular or neurological structures, and thus influence the metabolic processes associated with them and/or behavioral manifestations.

The individual's ability to adapt, to regain functioning following insults and stressors, to prevent further damage, becomes further compromised. The biomechanical point of view leads the operator to assess SD in relation to musculoskeletal structures and the patient's posture. The neuromyofascial stimulus of SD, through the application of osteopathic manipulative treatment, allows the person to regain the associated structural, vascular, neurological, metabolic, and behavioral functions. The goal is to optimize the patient's adaptive potential, through the recovery of structural and functional integrity.

## Indications, contraindications, and unwanted effects

Osteopathic manipulative treatment (OMT) focused on the biomechanical model is indicated for the improvement of pain, function, and skeletal muscle performance in subjects who show postural abnormalities, as in the case of patients with nonspecific low back pain,[42] painful shoulder,[43] or carpal tunnel syndrome.[44] OMT can benefit older subjects who, although they may have osteoporosis,[46] show improvement in dysfunctional pain syndromes,[45] as well as young and athletic subjects, who can improve their performance[47] and prevent injuries.[48]

Some evidence suggest the possibility of improving dysfunctional postural patterns, through the application of osteopathic manipulative treatment.[49,50] However, all authors state that more research is needed before certain hypotheses can be advanced.[51] It is, however, not appropriate to apply the procedures in this chapter to a patient who refuses to be touched or treated with manual techniques, such as patients with psychiatric disorders.[52] It is also contraindicated to manipulate an SD when there is a more urgent and life-threatening condition, such as hemorrhage, vascular thrombosis, or other high priority emergency.[53]

Obtaining written informed consent from the patient is prudent, and in some countries compulsory, prior to taking a history, making the diagnosis, and proposing a treatment plan, wherein the osteopath would explain possible side effects, especially if high-velocity low-amplitude (HVLA) techniques are to be used, and in particular on the upper cervical and lumbar spine.[54] Complications in the clinical application of other procedures of this model have not been identified in the literature. Some experts suggest that invasive techniques, such as HVLA applied on the cervical area of the subjects with symptoms, should be referred to a specialist for evaluation before beginning OMT.[54]

Although the occurrence of complications may have been underestimated, these procedures have been used and taught for years without major consequences. However, it has been proposed that complications after OMT are poorly reported or omitted in the osteopathic scientific literature.[55] Side effects of the techniques, if performed correctly, are minimal and self-limiting within 24/48 hours (see Chapter 9, Box 9.1). The side effects are as follows:

- Myalgia and arthralgia, pain and fatigue

- Erythema of the soft tissues due to increased circulation of fluids

- Occasional headache or dizziness following HVLA techniques of the upper cervical area

- Bruising or ecchymosis following the administration of direct myofascial techniques (may occur in patients under anticoagulant treatment or coagulation disorders). Side effects can often be minimized by applying heat or cold to the affected area for 20 minutes after the procedure[56] (see Chapter 9, Box 9.1).

## Principles and methods of assessment

In the biomechanical approach classically described in osteopathy, we globally observe the posture of the patient in standing, supine, and prone positions.[57] We note postural asymmetries, as well as muscle tension and tissue changes. We observe the patient's natural posture in the standing position. While the patient is in the standing position, we apply the general mobilization test, to evaluate the characteristics of the mobility of different regions of the body. By changing the patient's basic balance, the postural pattern is forced to show its response.

For example, in the supine position the gravity factor is limited, so it is assumed that the motor schema that emerges is a manifestation of muscle imbalances resulting in dysfunctions. We evaluate the gait, which sometimes, because of office space limitations, is simulated by the monopodalic support and coordinated movements of the hips and shoulders. In the biomechanical model, the Zink test is intended to evaluate the organism's ability to adapt to gravity; however, it is often used as a regional test, i.e., to detect the non-alternation of two transition areas, for example thoracoabdominal and abdominopelvic. The osteopath then searches for SD through the use of specific tests in the corresponding areas.

In the muscle chains model described by Richter and Hegben great importance is given to the muscles, intended as flexion and extension chain generators that form the basis of cranial patterns (cranial flexion corresponds to an extension of the skull). These authors,[57] beyond some compensation schemes described by Zink, use visual inspection and anterior-posterior and lateral-lateral palpation of the tissue related to different chains, confirmed by passive mobility tests, to understand the transition area at the level of which the rotation/preferential inclination pattern is manifested most clearly, and then determine if the ventral or dorsal muscles are maintaining it; for example, in the case of the cervicothoracic transitional area correlated with the C1–C3 segments, are the suboccipital or the upper/inferior hyoid muscles maintaining the tissue tension?[57] Or in the case of a positive test for high allostatic load (i.e., more non-alternated transition areas), which myofascial chain maintains the failure or decompensation – the flexion or the extension chain?[57]

The regional tests that use active mobilization lead to the observation of the areas in which the limitations of movement are more pronounced. In the flexion test of lateral inclination and trunk extension in the standing/orthostatic position, we look for harmonious execution of movement, or we detect any interruptions or ambiguous movements. The flexion test can provide information about the presence of any dominant chain in the legs or spine. The hip drop and pelvic shift tests can provide information about the position and mobility of the pelvis, the sacrum, and the lower lumbar spine.

If areas with alteration of active mobility are noted, these will then be examined in more detail through passive local tests of the area. In the supine position we observe the hips, legs, and pelvic rotation. Traction tests are performed for the head and legs, to assess any "dominant" side, i.e., the likely presence of SD in the side where the traction/rotation is "less easy."[57] During the execution of local tests for the detection of the dominant dysfunction we also consider the impact on posture, which is assessed through the selection of the "lesion" that persists in all positions (orthostatic, supine or sitting).

In the biomechanical model proposed in this text, the individual is observed considering that "the body is a unit" and describing the adaptations of the latter as a tensegrity system, in which even a small change in one region of the body can make biomechanical, tension, and ergonomic changes throughout.[58] Tensegrity here means the property of the musculoskeletal system to apply elements in continuous tension and in discontinuous compression in order to maximize efficiency and comfort. The failure or decompensation of this relationship can consistently affect the function of all the other physiological systems. The fascia and connective tissue can serve as a *trait d'union*, linking all these elements, performing the role of integration of the mechanical forces in the whole body.[59] To prove the existence of such a meta-system would then change our basic understanding of physiology.[60] In osteopathy we accept the con-cept of a postural pattern, provided that palpatory tests of tissue preference may provide a "quick look" at the existing interrelationships between body, mind, and spirit and the allostatic load of an individual.[61]

It is believed that fascial compensation represents a useful, beneficial, and functional response, in the absence of obvious symptoms, by the musculoskeletal system. For example, as a result of the development of allostatic overload, of structural asymmetries, such as a shorter lower limb or its excessive use, postural decompensation, describes the same phenomenon with the difference that the changes brought about by adaptation are dysfunctional and symptomatic, and highlight the failure or decompensation of homeostatic mechanisms.[62] According to Zink, by exploring the fascial compensation scheme, the operator is able to glimpse signs of the functions and dysfunctions in anatomical, physiological, and psychosocial elements.

By applying this model, the osteopath "prepares" the neuromyofascial system so that it can respond to postural realignment.[63] Posture is thus considered to be the result of the constant and dynamic interaction of two groups of forces: forces of gravity and the body's reaction to the environment. Postural deterioration indicates the "loss of ground" of the individual's forces in relation to gravity. A key role is played by the anatomical transition areas, both during the period of development and in adult life. These regions (lumbopelvic, thoracolumbar, cervicothoracic, and craniocervical) play a major role, not only in the definition of group curves, but also for their role in the regional compensatory scheme (see Chapter 6).

Respecting the rules of economy, comfort, and no pain, perfect posture for a given individual at a given chronobiological moment will be the best attempt that that body will make at sensory information integration and the best distribution of body mass. This results in minimal muscle energy expenditure, better posture, and harmonization of compression forces on the intervertebral discs through ligamentous tension.

If the body presents structural changes, the osteopath will check whether this change is subjected to an increase in energy demand, or manifests pain. In that case we might define "postural imbalance" as sensitive soft tissues are subjected to pain and affected by anomalies and/or structural changes, such as SD. This will facilitate the disturbances coming from gravity overload, causing various symptoms such as fatigue, back pain, headaches, and so on.[64] The argument that the perception of one's body, the environment, the emotions, and the psyche affect posture[65] is integrated into the biomechanical model.[64]

Individuals with psychological disorders, such as depression and manifested aggression, show rigid and decompensated postural patterns, while in a healthy individual, the posture tends toward soft characteristics and good body flexibility. This implies good adaptability and homeostasis. The osteopathic-postural evaluation process should tell us in the first place if the patient is able to respond positively to a postural treatment in terms of time, cost, and effectiveness. Then the individual's posture:

- plays a role within the given clinical framework

- represents a significant risk factor for pain, dysfunction, or future diseases

- is the result of, and the best adaptation possible for, dysfunctional pathogenic causes and noxious stimuli at the neuromyofascial level

- is the manifestation of a local, segmental and/or global disharmony of the interdependent relationship between structure and function.

The biomechanical model selection procedure (see Chapter 9) leads the osteopath to the detection of the eventual postural overload of the adaptive capacity, in addition to the selection of biomechanical-postural activation forces to use in treatment (Box 4.1).

**Box 4.1**

### Biomechanical model selection procedure

The relationship of trust established through effective communication facilitates the operator during the process of biotypologic constitutional observation (see Chapter 8), clinical and osteopathic assessment aimed at model selection, seeing the situation both as overload domination of the adaptive capacity and as activating force to evoke in the treatment. The elements emerging from the synthesis of medical history and clinical and osteopathic evaluation that lead the osteopath to the selection of the biomechanical model are: disorders such as myalgia, tendonitis, capsulitis, arthralgia, chondropathies, and so on; overloaded structure, such as the musculoskeletal system in general, and in particular the axial and appendicular fascia,[1] ectoskeletal components,[2] antigravity tonic musculature, the "boundaries" described by Irvin as postural boundaries, such as the feet and the sacrum;[3] overloaded function, such as that inherent in motor postural control, i.e., the correlation between muscle coordination, motor control[4] and HRMT.[5]

The unique fascial compartment assessment of the biomechanical model is performed through the axial-appendicular-ectoskeletal fascia test (see Chapter 1); the detection of a dysfunctional area is accomplished with osteopathic tests for somatic dysfunction (see Chapter 2). Adaptive capacity (compensated/decompensated) assessment is achieved through the FCS test (see Chapter 3). The assessment of constitutional observational data, history, and clinical data, data related to the fascial compensation scheme, as well as mobility tests results and dysfunctional area stiffness, unique to biomechanical postural function, provides the limits within which this is maintained. This allows for focusing the treatment approach as either:

- minimalist, mediated by access to the previously detected area, seen to be dominant and clinically relevant for the person, or

- maximalist, favored by the (biomechanical) force typically responsible for activation of the model.

### References

1. Willard FH, Fossum C, Standley PR. The fascial system of the body. In: Chila A, editor. Foundations of osteopathic medicine. 3rd ed. Philadelphia: Lippincott Williams and Wilkins; 2010. ch. 7.

2. Benjamin M. The end of the limbs and back – a review. J Anat. 2009;214(1):1–18.

3. Irvin RE. The origin and relief of common pain. J Back Musculoskelet Rehabil. 1998;11(2):89–130.

4. Winters J, Crago P, editors. Biomechanics and neural-control of posture and movement. New York: Springer; 2000.

5. Masi HV, Nair K, Evans T et al. Clinical, biomechanical, physiological and translational interpretations of human resting myofascial tone or tension. Inter J Ther Massage Bodyw. 2010;3(4):16–28.

In the evaluation process of the individual (Fig. 4.1) and his or her postural adaptations, the biomechanical model in osteopathy requires: participation of the individual in the OMT; overall test; regional and local tests; inhibition test of structure/specific function of the biomechanical model.

### Preparing the patient for OMT

In this phase the operator proceeds through a differential evaluation and an objective examination. In pathology and orthopedics, for example, the osteopath needs to assess the underlying causes in order to understand the influence that the disease has on energy levels and on vertebral mechanics at various levels. Some diseases may majorly influence posture at specific levels and have specific sequelae. An example would be a spondylolisthesis at L5–S1, which mainly affects the sagittal plane, having as a postural effect an anterior displacement of the load, resulting in strain of the iliolumbar ligaments, as well as exacerbation of low back pain and compression of the nerve roots. In such a situation, it may be prudent to refer the patient to his or her doctor (see Chapter 9).

### Global tests

To confirm the information derived from the history and physical examination, one can perform the axial-appendicular-ectoskeletal fascia test, particularly considering the fascial component of the biomechanical model (see Chapter 1). The osteopath verifies the presence of postural adaptations, using fascial compensation schemes (FCS) tests[61] (see Chapters 3 and 6). In the observation phase we can also use the scoliometer and/or plumb line.[66] Tissue preference tests (tension/laxity) in the different areas of transition aid in the detection of a compensated, decompensated, or neutral FCS (see Chapter 3).

If the FCS is neutral or compensated, the osteopath proceeds with the assessment of somatic dysfunctions by examining their clinical correlation with the patient's presenting complaint. Signs and symptoms of gravitationally induced pathophysiology become apparent after compensatory mechanisms are overwhelmed.

If, in phase 2 of the global tests, one detects a decompensated FCS, an index of high allostatic load, the osteopath proceeds in treatment planning with a maximalist approach,[67] moving away from the choice of specific and direct approaches, considered in these conditions as possible further stress to an already compromised system.[68] We will proceed, for example, with standard techniques for the transition areas, in particular considering indirect approaches such as positional release[69] or techniques using fluids and involuntary rhythms (see Chapter 3).

The osteopath then correlates this information with a comprehensive medical history and evaluation of the dynamics of fluids and involuntary rhythms, possibly detecting an allostatic overload that guides him toward a maximalist approach. The decompensated FCS, however, may sometimes also occur in only two of the four areas of transition.

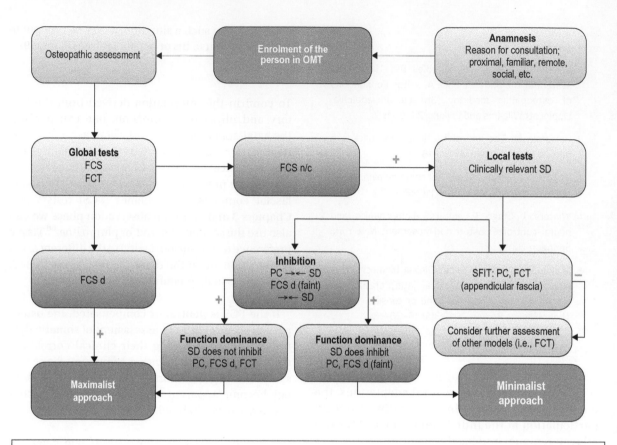

**Fig. 4.1**

Evaluation process of the biomechanical model. The osteopath develops a clear picture of the overall and biomechanical postural condition of the patient through the application of a process of evaluation and selection of the approach and techniques. FCS: fascial compensation scheme; n: neutral; c: compensated; d: decompensated; SD: somatic dysfunction; SFIT: structure/function inhibition test; FCT: fascial compartments test; PC: postural control; +: positive test; -: negative test.

This guides the osteopath to the likely presence of a dysfunctional structure or a component of the impaired postural function between the two diaphragms. To evaluate the possible choice of minimalist or maximalist approaches aimed at reducing the allostatic load on the altered postural function, we should question the presence and type of the dysfunctional postural condition.

If the decompensated FCS has been detected between the craniocervical and upper thoracic transition areas, we could use a structure/function inhibition test, performed, for example, on the stoma-tognathic apparatus. The Zink test is repeated by closing or opening the mouth. A detected improvement (non-alternating, less marked tissue preference) may direct the osteopath toward an integrated approach to the temporomandibular area with techniques that act on fluids and involuntary rhythms, such as balanced ligamentous tension techniques (see Chapter 3).

### Regional and local tests

Through the specific regional and local osteopathic tests (see Chapter 1) we can verify the presence of somatic dysfunctions, including articular/joint or soft tissue (viscera, connective tissue, muscles) dysfunctions, which alter the interrelationship between structure and function involving the postural scheme of the individual. Somatic dysfunction is described as a tissue adaptation local syndrome, which is expressed as the altered position of a body part (asymmetry), free or limited movement direction (mobility restriction), hyperesthesia or tenderness provoked by palpation, and alteration of tissue structure.

The TART (tissue texture abnormality, asymmetry, restriction of motion, tenderness) acronym, is used by osteopaths to describe the palpation of this altered tissue resilience, which today is well described by tissue mechanical parameters, such as viscoelasticity, thixotropy, the ability to resist a deformation as a result of the application of a compressive or tension force, namely stiffness.[40] The osteopathic examination consists of a screening aimed at identifying the region of the body where there is a somatic dysfunction, a detailed visual inspection (scanning) to identify the location in that region, and a local palpatory investigation (perceptual palpation) to define the specific type of dysfunction.

As in other palpatory assessments, the osteopath has to consider that sometimes classically described procedures must be compared and integrated with the available evidence, without being distorted. The palpation procedure used by the osteopath foresees the use of some palpatory tests commonly used in ambulatory care, in which some studies have demonstrated interoperator reliability in SD detection if examiners undergo specific training.[70] These are therefore used to test active, passive, segmental, respiratory and oscillatory mobility, mobility of pressure, tensional mobility, mobility of local listening and of reflex type, which allow the operator to identify the dysfunctional joint, fascial, visceral, etc., areas (see Chapter 2).

### Structure/function inhibition test of the specific biomechanical model

#### Basic test

This is a further global screening tool, which indicates the current levels of functionality and can be repeated to assess progress. This tool consists of the postural control test (Fig. 4.2), i.e., the assessment of balance standing on one leg with

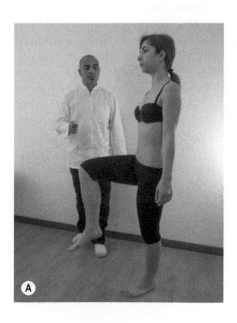
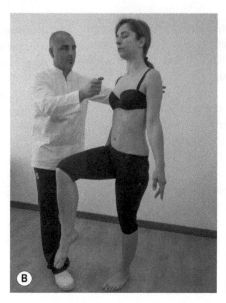

**Fig. 4.2**
Test of postural control. The patient is in the upright position, standing on one foot. The osteopath is positioned beside the patient ready to provide support if necessary and, equipped with a chronometer, records the balance-holding time both with open (A) and with closed (B) eyes, for 30 seconds.

opened and closed eyes. This provides an indication of the neurological integration between interoceptive and exteroceptive input, as well as the central processing and motor control efficiency:[71] in other words, the muscle tone and reflexes ratio. The single leg stance balance evaluation collects information with respect to postural control functioning, which, correlated with muscle coordination, motor control[72] and base myofascial tone,[40] is expressed through a complex relationship between balance and sensory interoceptive, proprioceptive, and exteroceptive mechanisms. They involve somatic and visceral motor efferents.[73]

The basic test consists of the following phases:

1. The patient is asked, while in the orthostatic position in bare feet, to lift one foot (the foot raised should not be placed to support the limb). The knee must be raised up as far as possible within comfort limits.

2. The patient is required to maintain balance for 30 seconds with open eyes.

3. The test is then repeated with the contralateral limb.

4. Once the test is performed with opened eyes, the patient, with eyes closed, is asked to locate and focus a point in front of him, to then try to remain in balance for 30 seconds.

The operator attaches a score corresponding to the amount of time the patient was able to maintain balance, i.e., the time of the occurrence of one or more of the following conditions:

- The raised foot touches the ground or leans toward the other

- The tested limb jumps, moves, or the fingers are raised

- The hands touch things other than the body.

**N.B.** The test can also be recommended as a daily exercise, sometimes using proprioceptive tables, physiological footwear or barefoot shoes, in order to increase the equilibrium time with eyes closed.

### Inhibition phase

In accordance with the principles of the inhibitory pressure technique,[74,75] the operator performs the inhibition phase. This phase of the test aims to evaluate the different tissues in SD areas, after the administration of stresses imposed on postural adaptability, tested with the postural control tests. In fact, after stimulating the tissue-articular barrier of the SD area first with direct and then indirect vector parameters, the operator repeats the same procedure with the basic test. Depending on the response the osteopath can come to the following conclusions:

1. *Dominance of structure*, i.e., of SD, over function (balance/postural control, reflexes) in influencing health, when after the stimulus on the SD, the repetition of the postural tests gives better results. This means that the score obtained for the patient increases, since the equilibrium is maintained for a longer time compared to previous performances. It is noted in this case that structure is dominant over function in influencing health, or that the detected somatic dysfunctions affect the function being examined (postural control), because when we temporarily inhibit the disturbing influence, we get a temporary improvement of the related function (balance). This situation, in terms of choice of therapeutic strategy, may suggest applying a minimalist approach[67] (Fig. 4.3), of specific structural impact, to produce the best global functional response. A further indication is provided by the test response according to the type of stimulus applied, namely direct and indirect. If improvement of the postural tests has occurred as a result of a direct stimulus on the SD, this may mean that it is more appropriate to apply direct techniques to normalize the dysfunction itself (e.g., specific adjustment technique, Fig. 4.4).

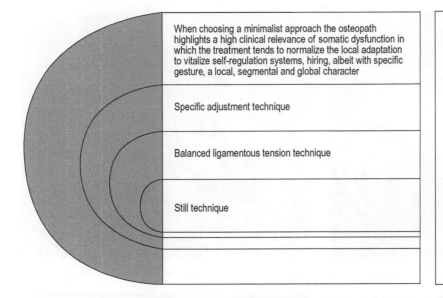

When choosing a minimalist approach the osteopath highlights a high clinical relevance of somatic dysfunction in which the treatment tends to normalize the local adaptation to vitalize self-regulation systems, hiring, albeit with specific gesture, a local, segmental and global character

Specific adjustment technique

Balanced ligamentous tension technique

Still technique

**Fig. 4.3**
Examples of osteopathic techniques; biomechanical model. Minimalist approach.

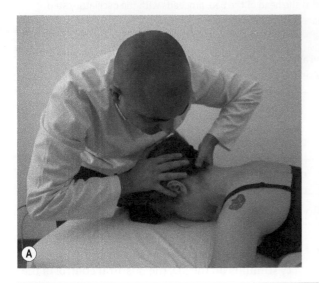

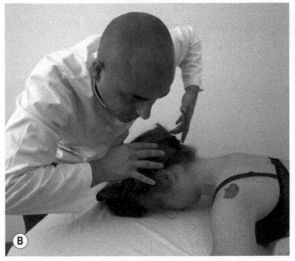

**Fig. 4.4**
Specific adjustment technique (SAT). The techniques are applied to the dominant somatic dysfunction, which in palpatory detection presents an asymmetry as a unique positional parameter. The osteopath approaches the dysfunctional area with the SAT method, by applying harmonic oscillations or rhythmic pressure (A-C), with the goal of detecting, with dynamic modalities, the vector where the stresses become neutral. The operator proceeds with a thrust impulse or toggle at high speed and very little force (B-D) directed to the neutral vectors acquired with the intention to overcome the tensions stored in the tissue.

*Example: upper cervical specific adjustment*

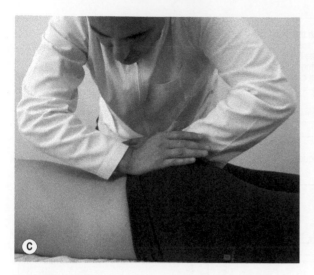
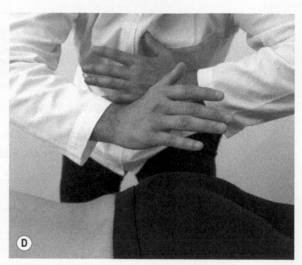

**Fig. 4.4. continued**

The patient is in the prone position. The osteopath, positioned at the head of the bed, proceeds with the oscillatory step (A). The osteopath, still positioned at the head of the bed, proceeds with the adjustment phase (B).

*Example: sacral toggle specific adjustment*

The patient is in the prone position. The osteopath, positioned at the side of the bed, proceeds with the rhythm step of tensioning the soft tissue (C), and then with the adjustment phase (D).

*Example*: in the local test one detects an SD in the vertebral segment T7, with right unilateral flexion dysfunctional parameters. The patient is asked to perform the postural tests. Then the osteopath applies a direct stimulus, i.e., a tissue induction toward the restrictive barrier, through a temporary compression of the left transverse process of the vertebra. Immediately after, the operator repeats the test of postural control, while re-evaluating a possible increase in the maintenance of equilibrium time, compared to that obtained with the first test. If so, direct treatment using direct techniques is indicated. If the basic test remains unchanged after direct stimulation of the SD, we proceed with an indirect stimulus. If the basic test provides improvement in the maintenance of equilibrium time, then the osteopath will be directed toward the use of indirect techniques (e.g., balanced ligamentous tension technique, Fig. 4.5). Sometimes, during the execution of indirect techniques, the operator, in accordance with the tissue viscoelastic responses, can proceed with an articulatory phase, using a combined technique (e.g., Still technique, Fig. 4.6).

2. *Dominance of function* (balance/postural control, reflexes) over structure (SD) in influencing health is demonstrated when, after the inhibitory stimulus on the SD, the postural control of the test pattern does not vary or worsen (for example, the patient fails to maintain balance with closed eyes for more than 6 seconds, both before and after the inhibition on SD). We infer that the postural control exercises a dominant influence on tissue-related dysfunction. In this case, an extreme approach is recommended[67] (Fig. 4.7) to restore the global function, through the use of biomechanical activation forces, as in the case of the "general osteopathic treatment" (GOT).[31]

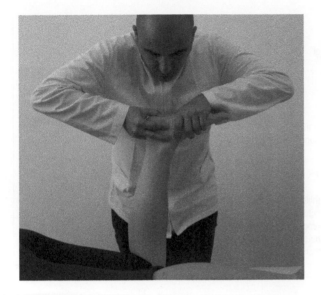

**Fig. 4.5**

Balanced ligamentous tension (BLT) technique.

*Example: approach to the plantar fascia*

The BLT indirect technique requires an initial disengagement of the stretched tissue, through a compressive force applied by inches (in this example) on the plantar fascia. This phase is often followed by an exaggeration of the somatic dysfunction vectors, through distractive forces of the thumbs, until the achievement of a neutral point in the elastic barrier tension. Movements related to tissue remodeling, such as vasomotion, emerge while stress and neurological information is processed, until the release of the capsule-ligament tensions and somatic dysfunction (SD) normalization.

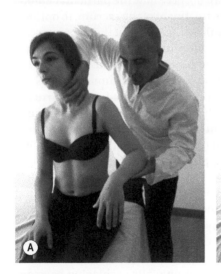
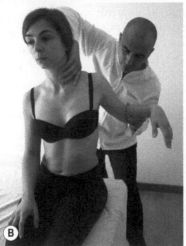
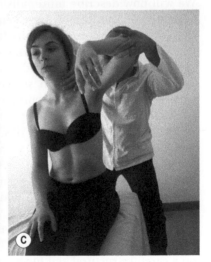

**Fig. 4.6**

Still's technique.

*Example: first rib inhalation dysfunction, patient seated*

(A) Positioning phase in which the osteopath makes contact with the anatomical landmarks. (B) Phase of exaggeration of dysfunctional vectors and linkage between the two hands of the operator through a compression (in this case) or traction phase (C). Articulatory phase of liberation of dysfunctional parameters through achieving the optimal glide of fascial planes that carries the articular restrictions.

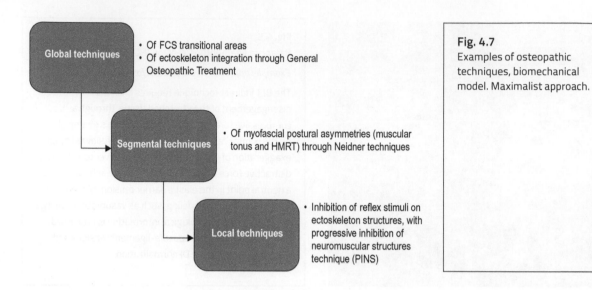

Global techniques
• Of FCS transitional areas
• Of ectoskeleton integration through General Osteopathic Treatment

Segmental techniques
• Of myofascial postural asymmetries (muscular tonus and HMRT) through Neidner techniques

Local techniques
• Inhibition of reflex stimuli on ectoskeleton structures, with progressive inhibition of neuromuscular structures technique (PINS)

**Fig. 4.7**
Examples of osteopathic techniques, biomechanical model. Maximalist approach.

## Principles and methods of treatment

We will now describe minimalist and maximalist approaches. The former are intended to improve the local adaptation conditions that disrupt postural balance. If, after the decision-making process has taken place, there is a need to use more delicate approaches, the osteopath selects indirect techniques that are most appropriate to the case, for example, among osteopathic fascial techniques.[59] According to Irvin, there are postural boundaries (force management stations), such as the feet and the sacrum, that resist daily forces, such as acceleration; mobility evaluation of these areas provides the limits within which postural function is stable.[13]

One of the minimalist approaches proposed is the specific adjustment technique (SAT),[76] which is based on a careful structural and functional assessment of the pivot of the spine, according to the force lines of the biomechanics described by Littlejohn, and articulated on the body's division into three functional units: lumbofemoral, craniocervical, thoracoabdominal. These units would be the result of interaction between sorting lines (anterior-posterior, anterior-central, posterior-anterior, posterior-central) of the gravity forces between feet and the head through the sacral "hub".[77]

While thinking about the characteristics of this method, we can observe how the particular emphasis given to the treatment of the sacrum, to optimize the biomechanical alignment of the person, retraces the concept of boundaries described by Irvin, as related to the postural and causal adaptations of SD.[13] We also know that traumatic stress and mechanical actions are reflected on the articular cartilage and their receptors, by altering the aqueous component of the matrix.[78-80] Also we know that body fluid (euhydration-under hydration) may influence body physiology[81,82] (see Chapter 6).

In 2012, Parker and colleagues noted in their study that osteopathic HVLA technique is more effective under euhydration conditions.[83] It is therefore plausible that the reduction of traumatic lesional parameters through techniques such as thrust or toggle comes about only after achieving harmonic oscillating accord with the tissues and in particular a vibrational coherence with fluids.[59]

The study by Bialosky and colleagues in 2010 suggests new ideas on the neurophysiological mechanisms inherent to the application of the HVLA techniques in musculoskeletal disorders with central sensitization. They propose that hypoalgesia following technique administration is mediated by Aδ pain-reliever fibers, regardless of the production of the characteristic sound of the thrust. However, if during the execution of the technique, as provided for by the SAT, there is an audible sound, we will have better results on the temporal summation of postsynaptic potentials.[84]

The osteopath who approaches with SAT seeks to improve the viscoelastic quality of the tissue in order to then normalize the interoceptive aspects: a passage from classic biomechanical concepts to those related to tissue mechanics. In the maximalist approaches, we usually use global adaptogenic techniques; however, sometimes the operator can use an integration of different approaches from the global segmental focus, in order to reduce allostatic overload. The latter is represented in this model by postural overload.

The author therefore proposes a mix of approaches: one of local focus directed to normalize neuromyofascial reflexes; a segmental approach in order to improve myofascial postural asymmetries; and a global approach to optimize integration between the ectoskeleton and exoskeleton.[85] The ectoskeleton is a soft tissue skeleton for muscle insertions, organized in a particular way by tendons, pulleys, retinacula of the limbs, such as the palmar fascia, plantar fascia and the fascia lata, in communication with the thoracolumbar fascia.

## Examples of minimalist approaches

### Specific adjustment technique

One of the developments of the biomechanical model proposed by Littlejohn is the interesting treatment method known as specific adjustment technique (SAT). In the 1950s, Parnall Bradbury, chiropractor and osteopath, had to deal with a huge amount of patients at his clinic, following an influenza epidemic. Having little time to devote to each patient, he decided to manipulate only the dominant dysfunctional segment in each of them, by applying one of the Still's teachings: "find it, fix it and leave it alone." Bradbury, and later Tom Dummer, identified, with a direct technique, the segment "in positional injury," that is, the dominant somatic dysfunction (particularly the cervical and sacral), which during the palpatory examination presented positional asymmetry as a particular parameter, often following traumatic events.[77] With SAT direct manipulation we do not use the closing of the vertebral segments, but we detect the point, within the motion amplitude allowed by the tissue, in which the perception of dysfunctional tension disappears.

In the author's clinical experience, during this phase there is a more harmonious perception of fluid dynamics. During this kind of adjustment method, the achievement of the neutral point set in the floating field is used as a starting point to reverse the traumatic force vectors stored in the tissue, via a thrust or a toggle at high acceleration and with very little force. The patient then rests for 10–15 minutes to allow for therapeutic input processing, elaboration, and full reintegration of the SD with the rest of the body.[78]

### Balanced ligamentous tension technique

The indirect technique of balanced ligamentous tension (BTL) requires an initial disengagement of the tissue, followed by an exaggeration of the somatic dysfunction vectors, until one reaches a neutral tensional point of the ligamentous barrier. This point is retained while the tensional and neurological information is processed until one achieves the point of fluid balance, the release of the capsular-ligamentous tensions, and the alleviation of SD[59,86] (see Chapter 3).

### Still technique

Still's combined technique first requires the evaluation of the restrictive barrier in a given area of dysfunction. Subsequently, the tissues are moved to a position of greater tension in order to exaggerate these parameters and engage the physiological barrier. Finally, compression or traction is introduced and maintained, while following the tissue in its "untwisting path" to and through the restriction barrier.[59]

## Examples of maximalist approaches

The osteopath proceeds with a routine composed of different approaches, to finalize segmental effects on the neuromyofascial reflexes and on myofascial postural asymmetries and to induce global effects to optimize the integration between the ectoskeleton and exoskeleton. Hyperactive reflex stimuli could be detected and treated, for example using the progressive inhibition of neuromuscular structures (PINS) technique[87] (Fig. 4.8).

## Progressive inhibition of neuromuscular structures technique

Dowling defines this approach as very versatile, especially for the clinician who has a good grasp of anatomy. It can be used alone or in combination with other approaches. PINS is definitely indicated in the treatment of soft tissue or muscles that manifest reflected hyperactivity associated with SD. This technique proposes to address alterations of the basic tone of neuromyofascial structures related to postural balance.

The goal of this phase of the maximalist approach is to reduce the reflex overload in different segments of the ectoskeleton, such as the plantar fascia, Achilles tendon, iliotibial band, thoracolumbar fascia, or palmar fascia.[85] PINS tends to be a very safe approach; it rarely produces adverse effects and can be applied away from dysfunctional areas of high impact on the patient's energy. Nevertheless, the operator who selects this technique within the maximalist routine must keep in mind that overloading the person further is unwise, and must therefore be very careful in deter-

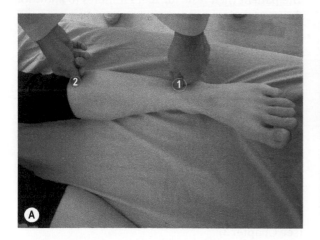

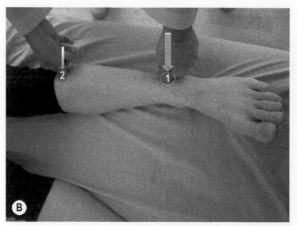

**Fig. 4.8**

Progressive inhibition of neuromuscular structures (PINS) technique.

*Example: interosseous membrane of the lower limbs*

The operator proceeds by detecting two sensitive points in a segment of the ectoskeleton through a test of provoked sensitivity/pain, in this case, on the interosseous membrane (A). After we establish which point is primary (1) and which is secondary (2), according to the degree of sensitivity, we apply a pressure to evoke the sensitivity of the two points by gradually increasing the pressure on the most sensitive spot, until the disappearance of the sensitivity or pain (which occurs within a few seconds to a few minutes) (B).

mining the amount of pressure needed to produce inhibitory effects on the reflex hyperactivity borne by the soft tissue skeleton. The operator proceeds to:

- detect a sensitive point in a segment of the ectoskeleton, through a test of provoked sensitivity or pain on the plantar fascia, Achilles tendon, iliotibial band, the thoracolumbar fascia, or palmar fascia

- detect a distal or proximal point along the same segment

- establish the primary and secondary areas, according to the degree of sensitivity.

The patient is then placed in a position of maximum comfort. The operator applies equal pressure on the two points – just enough to evoke sensitivity. The pressure on the less sensitive point is maintained constant, while the pressure on the most sensitive point is gradually increased, but never to the point of causing pain. After the initial increase in intensity, there should follow a decrease and then disappearance of the sensitivity or pain (occurring within a few seconds to a few minutes).

The operator then proceeds to look for any other ectoskeleton sensitive points. If during the treatment the patient should report higher sensitivity in the secondary point, the major pressure has to be applied on this point.

### Neidner's techniques

The osteopath can approach the regions of postural asymmetry, with muscular and fascial tone alterations, using, for example, Neidner's techniques (Fig. 4.9). William Neidner, a student of Sutherland, was seeking useful treatments for muscular dystrophy. Looking at the entire fascial system, he found that healthy people have hourly

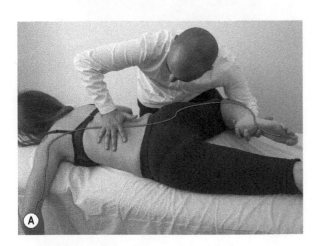
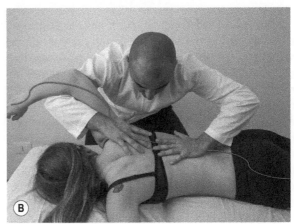

**Fig. 4.9**
Neidner's techniques.

*Example: segmental approach to the axial-appendiceal region*

The operator uses long levers of the lower (A) and upper (B) limbs of the patient to overcome, in a direct manner, the fulcrum corresponding to the thoracolumbar fascia, through which it is possible to perceive the kinematics of ectoskeletal movement. Tension is maintained until tissue restrictions are released.

fascial twisting schemes (like a corkscrew) and that treatment through an approach using the upper and lower limbs as levers could release the fascial twist with a global effect on tissue mismatching.[88] The body regions classically treated with this approach are:

- the craniocervical and upper thoracic region, through the long levers of the upper limbs

- the thoracic region, abdomen, and pelvis, through the long levers of the lower limbs.

Anatomical dissections reveal significant intersections of collagen fibers in the fascial tensile structures of the trunk, lumbar region, and pelvis, highlighting, for example, lateral to apophyseal joints of the ninth and tenth thoracic vertebrae, a convergence of lateral-lateral tractions of the proximal part of the two large dorsal muscles, longitudinal traction of the long dorsal muscle, and oblique traction of the trapezius inferior fibers, that are combined with the opposite thoracolumbar fascia.[89]

Abnormal tension at the intersection is redistributed with resulting asymmetries of related structures. Based on these observations, the author proposes that kinetic tests be performed in order to evaluate the vector forces of the movement restriction between the upper limbs, thoracolumbar fascia, and lower limbs (see Fig. 1.6). Should an asymmetry that involves the entire axial fascia of the appendix be detected, then the upper and lower limbs of the patient are used to engage, with long levers and direct modalities, the thoracolumbar fascia fulcrum, through which we can perceive the kinematics of the ectoskeletal movement. The tension is maintained until the tissue restrictions are released.

### General osteopathic treatment

The maximalist approach could also include the application of a contemporary approach that is inspired by total body adjustment, namely general osteopathic treatment (GOT),[90] which is aimed at achieving an integration of the exo- and ectoskeleton (Fig. 4.10). John Martin Littlejohn firmly believed that

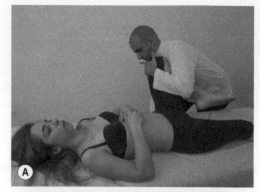

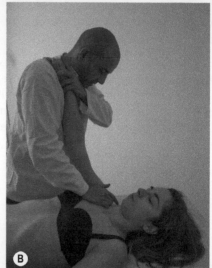

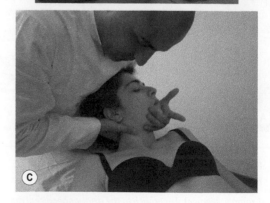

**Fig. 4.10**
General osteopathic treatment (GOT): example of a routine with the patient in the supine position. GOT is

**Fig. 4.10 continued**
interpreted in this work as an articulatory, rhythmic
and oscillatory routine with long levers using a fulcrum
in exoskeletal bony tissue such as the sacroiliac joints
(A), shoulders/clavicles (B), cervical vertebrae (C), and
engages the ectoskeleton (soft tissue) to facilitate
coordination and correlation of somatic dysfunction
with surrounding tissues and with the rest of the body.

every osteopathic treatment had a physiological aim, given that the body is a living thing and not merely a biomechanical machine. He taught that at the basis of a functional change, or physiological pathology, there was an atomic change at the cellular and tissue levels. In order to correct the somatic dysfunction in relation to the surrounding tissues, he proposed a system using long levers and a routine for the coordination and correlation of the somatic dysfunction with the rest of the body. This is the principle of total body adjustment. John Wernham,[150] his heir and successor, continued to practice this approach with amazing results until the age of 99, applying the principle that it is sometimes necessary to treat the part by treating the whole and act locally, segmentally, and globally, through an approach based on 10 laws: routine, rhythm, rotation, mobility, motility, joint integrity, stability, coordination, correlation, and laws of mechanics. He aimed to create and strengthen a line of major resistance, in a battle between vitality of the somatic dysfunction and balance.[90]

Swanson suggests that examples of biotensegrity can be applied at cellular, tissue, organ, and system levels, and even the molecular level, considering elements of tension and corresponding compression. The junction of the tension elements (tie rods) with a compression-resistant element can be seen as a model of complex focal adhesion within the cell, which provides the vital link between the extracellular matrix and the biotensegritive system of the cytoskeleton.[58]

The approach with GOT can be interpreted today as an articulatory, rhythmic, and oscillatory routine, with long levers, using a fulcrum on bony

tissues (vertebrae, iliacs, shoulders/clavicles) to engage the ectoskeleton (soft tissue) to foster the coordination and correlation of somatic dysfunction with the surrounding tissues and with the rest of body. In choosing the treatment plan, techniques and dosage, the osteopath has to take into account different factors, both clinical and constitutional, as well as the age of both the operator and the patient (see Chapter 9). For example, the application of manipulative treatment to postural asymmetries in neonatal or pediatric patients obviously involves different measures than those adopted in the evaluation plan described above (Box 4.2).

## Rationale, mechanisms, and evidence

From the osteopathic perspective, "perfect posture" has been described as a perfect distribution of body mass around the center of gravity, represented by a balanced configuration of the body, depending on the normal arch of the foot, the vertical alignment of the ankles and horizontal orientation of the sacral base.[7] This concept describes how the compressive forces applied on the spinal discs are balanced by the tension of the ligaments, with a low energy demand on the postural muscles.

---

**Box 4.2**

### Biomechanical model in pediatrics

Test selection, as well as the selection of techniques, possible variations in the execution, and the amount of force to be applied, is dependent on clinical, constitutional, and age factors of both operator and patient (see Chapter 9). For example, the application of manipulative treatment to postural asymmetries in neonatal or pediatric patients obviously involves different measures than those adopted in the evaluation plan described above. In the event that the young patient has come to the osteopath's clinic with a particular condition, for example nonsynostotic plagiocephaly, the operator will proceed with an osteopathic evaluation of the child's general condition in terms of asymmetries and postural defects.[1]

To this end, the operator proceeds with FCS test application, which allows for evaluation of whether the impact of childbirth in terms of stress is expressed by a tendency to asymmetry that is not confined only to the skull, but is also expressed in other bodily areas. Obviously in this case the operator cannot apply the postural control test previously described. Compared to the regional test, the operator can proceed through an attraction or fascial listening test, while the use of the step test may not be appropriate. The evaluation the local adaptations require is performed according to SD diagnostic procedures which evaluate, exclusively through passive tests, the parameters described by the acronym TART (see Chapter 2).

The operator, usually standing at the newborn's bedside, evaluates the cranial area, continues with the spine and pelvis, upper and lower limbs, and ends with the ribcage and the viscera.[1] The operator then evaluates the dominant SD, while the "structure/function inhibition test" guides the selection of maximalist or direct/indirect minimalist approach. If the inhibition test leads to a maximalist approach, the operator will proceed in the first session with a general osteopathic treatment[2] that, as described in the literature, reduces the allostatic load and allows a local approach in a second session, without causing any additional stress to the newborn. The minimalist approach provides for SD resolution that may contribute to the maintenance of cranial bone distortion from distant areas; the cranial dysfunctional structures are also treated.

The most used direct techniques are: intraosseous decompression, release of the sutures, intraosseous modeling, sphenobasilar synchondrosis strain correction, and normalization of the occipital condyles.[3] Indirect techniques described in literature are those of balanced membranous and ligamentous tension.[1] Treatment planning obviously requires the participation of the parents and newborn at home; this consists of encouraging the infant's symmetrically use of the cervical muscles, avoiding the infant always lying down on the more convex side of the head, and so on.[4]

**References**

1. Cerritelli F, Martelli M, Renzetti C et al. Introducing an osteopathic approach into neonatology ward: the NE-O model. Chiropr Man Therap. 2014;22:18.

2. Waldman M, Batten C. The classical osteopathic treatment of the infant and child [3 DVDs]. Horsham, UK: Institute of Classical Osteopathy; 2010.

3. Lessard S, Gagnon I, Trottier N. Exploring the impact of osteopathic treatment on cranial asymmetries associated with nonsynostotic plagiocephaly in infants. Complement Ther Clin Pract. 2011;17: 193–8.

4. Carreiro J. Pediatrics: an osteopathic manual medicine approach. The perfect companion to an osteopathic approach to children by Carreiro. Edinburgh: Churchill Livingstone, Elsevier; 2009.

The structural and functional stresses of the body, however, may prevent the achievement of optimum posture, producing homeostatic compensation in the effort to create the best postural function for the individual structure.[7] In the description of postural alignment, Kuchera, albeit anchored to a concept of "perfect posture," reports how hard is to detect it in clinical reality. The idea behind this posture definition shows a concept anchored to biomechanical-structural aspects of the body in continuous compression. Today we can say that if an organism is well compensated from the postural point of view, this organism can work properly, regardless of the asymmetries and the adjustments present. Man's adaptation to gravitational forces and the upright posture (postural control) would therefore seem possible through the relationship between neurological evolution mechanisms and adaptation of musculoskeletal tissues, in order to improve stability.[9]

Normal muscle tone keeps the body standing upright with a minimum increase of energy costs compared to the supine position, and often for prolonged periods, without causing fatigue. It is inferred that this happens because of polymorphic changes in normal myofascial tone. Modern research suggests that the human muscle tone at rest is connected with the passive tone of the fascial tissue. This follows from intrinsic muscular viscoelastic properties: the basic myofascial tone, defined by Masi and colleagues as human resting myofascial tone or tension (HRMT).[40] The HRMT would represent the basal level of passive tension and resilience, which contributes to maintaining postural stability. Conversely, the contraction of muscle is an active neuromotor control, which provides more tone levels (and energy expenditure) for a greater stabilization.

Functionally, the HRMT is integrated with other passive tensional fascial and ligamentous networks of the body to form a biotensegrity system. Through the principle of biotensegrity, the body is able to integrate different stimuli of mechanical forces, which are distributed in nonlinear mode through the tensegrity structure, and then transduced into biochemical signals, to maintain the functional and structural integrity of the system.[58]

From molecules to cells, to tissues and organs, each level can be understood as a biotensegrity structure, intimately connected in a hierarchical organization. This helps us to understand how the forces applied by an osteopath on tissues can have effects both at the cellular level, in terms of gene expression changes,[91] and at the global level, in terms of postural adaptations.[92,93] The principles of biotensegrity can then be used to bridge the gap between basic science researchers and clinical osteopaths, as well as to assist in the search for the mechanisms of action of osteopathic manipulative medicine.

In fact, mechanotransduction (i.e., the process of conversion of mechanical energy into chemical energy, through specific cellular and molecular transducers) could represent one of the mechanisms of interaction between manual intervention and the response of tissue cells. The work done by the muscular contractile proteins during acceleration, deceleration, or maintaining the position of different skeletal elements requires an efficient power transmission through the superficial membranes of the fibers. The most studied of the stress transmission sites are the ends of muscle fibers, where they contact both connective and epithelial tissues. In most animals, irrespective of the phylum, the ends of muscle fibers are typically folded, producing a junctional interface that mostly allows cutting movements, so as to significantly reduce the absolute value of the tension applied to the cellular membrane.[94] This ensures that the main vector of stress on the cellular membrane responds with respect to the tension, by minimizing stress concentrations.

The morphological and molecular similarities of muscle–tendon junctions in animals suggest that the problem of creating a strong adherent junction between a muscle fiber and a tissue of dissimilar physical properties is essentially the same for all muscles, and that the solution has emerged precociously during evolution. The evidence suggests that the transmission of the tensions is a general property of the muscle cell surface and that the specific junctional morphologies are the result of dynamic interactions between the muscle cells and the tissues to which they adhere.[94] The musculoskeletal resting tone would seem therefore to be an intrinsic tensional viscoelastic property, which is expressed in the kinematic chains of the body, organized in a tensegritive fashion. The tone works inseparably from the fascial component and the correlated tendinous-ligamentous structures. The HRMT is thus a passive myofascial function that operates inside the tensional networks of tissues. This tension is a passive element independent of the central nervous system and results from intrinsic molecular interactions of actin-myosin filaments in union with sarcomeres and myofibroblasts.

Muscle contractions, however, activated by the central nervous system, generate much higher tensions, supplied by fascial elements.[95] Therefore, the myofascial tissues activate layers and integrated networks of passive and active tensional forces, which provide stabilizing support and control of movement in the body. The passive myofascial tension that is present in the body, independent of the central nervous system, provides a stabilizing basal level component to help maintain balanced postures.

The HRMT complex analysis is realized during the evolution phase through electromyographic measurements, which have identified silent signals from the lumbar muscles during maintenance of a relaxed upright posture. The HRMT model is now in a new assessment phase through clinical relevance reported by many therapists. The HRMT passive role in helping to maintain balanced position is based on the biomechanical principles of elasticity, tension, stress, stiffness and myofascial tensegrity. However, more research is needed to determine the molecular basis of HRMT in sarcomeres, the transmission of tension between the fascial elements that envelop the micro- and macro-anatomical structures involved, and the way in which the "myofascia" helps maintain an efficient passive postural equilibrium in the body.

Significant deficiencies or excesses in postural HRMT can predispose to symptomatic or pathological musculoskeletal disorders. For example, axial myofascial hypertonicity has been suggested as a predisposing factor for ankylosing spondylitis.[40] This deforming condition, often progressive in the vertebrae and the sacroiliac joints, is characterized by stiffness and bony lesions localized in the osteotendinous joints. These characteristics imply excessive concentrations and transmissions of forces, resulting in tissue micro-lesions and maladaptive reparative reactions. Considering the evolution of the concept of posture in the historical definitions set forth above and, consistent with these, the role HRMT could play on postural equilibrium, we can capture different aspects probably woven in ensuring postural control.

The "postural control" term classically refers to the control of the body orientation and its various segments (postural orientation), in both static and dynamic conditions. It includes:

- postural reflexes

- postural tone, which today can be interpreted as the ratio between muscular tone and HRMT.

It is therefore evident and important that there may be a mechanism for storage of a response in the fascial tissue for individual postural control.[96] A dysfunctional memory may be imprinted through the development of fibrous infiltration and cross-links between collagen fibers, in the nodal points of fascial bands, together with a progressive loss of elastic properties.

Consequently, these changes in the myofascial tissue can alter the activity of the related higher centers, responsible both for proprioceptive and interoceptive sensory integration, and motor control and posture.[97,98] Thus emerges a new model of posture that today in theoretical and scientific terms transcends references exclusively compressive, static and linear. Yet, the observation of the work of many osteopaths seems to be closely tied to the classic biomechanical model, although for many authors of scientific articles that have reflected on this topic, this approach would not be supported by sound fundamentals, and would hardly be based on holistic thinking.

In this regard, Professor Eyal Lederman, osteopath and PhD, is one of the authors critical of the biomechanical model, which he defined as postural-structural-biomechanical. Using back pain as an example, he said that the postural-structural-biomechanical model does not work, as there is no proven relationship between back pain and credible structural, postural and biomechanical configurations. Consequently, attempts to treat and normalize these configurations are meaningless and a waste of time and resources. We will analyze, then, the reasoning of Lederman and give an account of the debate that followed, to lay the foundations of a new biomechanical model based on neuromyofascial and postural biotensegrity concepts.

Lederman says that we cannot yet justify the use of manual techniques to readjust, correct, and stabilize the misaligned structure. The suggestion is that a multidisciplinary rehabilitative strategy that includes physical rehabilitation approaches, methodologies centered on behavior, psychological approaches, cognitive and therapeutic exercise, is the best tool to solve and prevent dysfunctional states such as back pain. Manual techniques have, at best, short-term effects and are highly redundant.[10] We may, on the contrary, argue that manual techniques allow the recovering of strength and resistance, mobility and postural balance. This action makes it easier to obtain correction of pain-free function, through multidisciplinary rehabilitation strategy.[12]

Lederman's statements question the methods of many manual therapists, such as osteopaths. In fact, he calls into question the very basis of much of what is practiced by the majority of operators of manipulative methods of treatment and prevention currently in use. Lederman actually suggests expanding the postural-structural-biomechanical model, proposing an individualized treatment for each case, on the basis of identification of the processes that generate the current state of the patient, followed by the provision of incentives that will support, assist, and facilitate the change. All this is what Lederman defines as "approach to the process."

This argument in itself is not controversial, as it suggests that a passive manual treatment, without the subject being involved in a cognitive, proprioceptive, and interoceptive way, has a small value in the healing and recovery process. The *7th Interdisciplinary World Congress on Low Back & Pelvic Girdle Pain* in 2010 included reports that in many ways have echoed and supported Lederman's position. There have also been reports that highlighted alternative routes, for example the report by O'Sullivan, who proposed a biopsychosocial approach to back pain with cognitive and re-educational strategies, paying particular attention to the underlying mechanisms that can lead to painful alterations[99] (see Chapter 8).

In order critically to assess these arguments, the *Journal of Bodywork and Movement Therapy* invited five leading experts in the world of manual medicine, osteopathy, chiropractic, and physical therapy to discuss Lederman's thesis:[12] Gary Fryer says that although there is a lack of direct evidence that relates posture to low back pain, there is a strong theoretical rationale for why posture can generate pain. An asymmetric posture can create overload on ligaments and other structures, and may contribute to the depletion of reserves of individual compensation, which results in tension and pain. Fryer concludes that the biomechanical model has been overestimated in the past, but it is good to consider the multidimensional nature of pain in order to achieve a holistic approach centered on the patient.

Hannon says that the patient's psychological aspect is considered crucial to the individual's care. This is demonstrated by the effectiveness of traditional massage, during which, thanks to the use of upholstered and heated beds, a more prolonged duration of treatment, and therefore a higher level of relaxation by the patient, is able to obtain immediate results in the relief of pain. He believes that manual therapy should not be based solely on the commitment of the operator to find a diagnosis, but should combine the patient's psychological aspect with the treatment itself, thus uniting art to engineering in order to make each individual an active, not a passive part of the treatment. The "massagers," in conjunction with the diagnostic concept of the tissue causing a disturbance, work directly on well-being, approaching the psyche of the subject in a decisive manner.

Dr. Irvin provides a more complex postural pattern based on three fundamental systems: the feet, the sacrum, and the central nervous system. In the case of an imbalance of one of the three systems one can verify a change of the entire posture and consequent pain onset. It is not always possible to demonstrate a direct relationship between the biomechanical model and the presence of pain, but the tissue changes following poor posture can maintain or aggravate the existing imbalance. The biomechanical model should therefore not be considered to be in decline, thanks to research that is in constant development, review, and integration.

Dr. Lee says that low back pain cannot be classified according to a single etiology. The cause of back pain is to be sought through a more global approach that takes into account the experience and history of each individual patient. In this scheme it is not possible to frame a biomechanical model that is the same for every patient with low back pain.

Dr. McGill, finally, strongly criticizes Lederman's approach to the biomechanical model, stating that a subject as vast as that of back pain cannot be summarized in a report. Each individual will need a therapeutic dose and a personalized approach. Studies reported by Lederman are not fully applicable, as they address this issue with a one-dimensional vision. In addition, the studies do not take into account the evolution of back pain, disc dehydration, changes in the function of the facet joints and the consequent shift from disc pain to facet joint pain. Central sensitization will affect the bonds between pain, mechanical/functional factors and the patient's corrections in order to reduce the neuronal response. Thus, the links between pain and biomechanical factors are variable within the natural history of low back pain. McGill believes that Lederman has omitted important details of the studies cited in his article, details that are rather in favor of the possible relationship between a biomechanical model and the likely development of low back pain, such as neuromuscular asymmetry that anticipates a possible episode of low back pain. Lederman seems to have addressed this issue without considering multiple aspects inherent to back pain such as poor posture, the mechanism of therapeutic exercise and its effectiveness, the kinematics and the kinetics of movement, static anatomical structure, dynamic joint function, neurological function, the mechanisms of pain, different types of damage to the spinal column, patient classification, the load on tissues, and so on. He does not consider, therefore, that an appropriate job has been carried out, but believes that this debate could initiate more thorough and precise scientific studies. However, these studies do not seem to have been actualized in the clinical practice of manual therapists and osteopaths, who are committed to the correction of misaligned or asymmetri-

cal structures. Nevertheless, a more modern idea of posture identifies the latter with the strategy adopted by the neuromyofascial system to react to gravity and afferent proprioceptive and interoceptive stresses.

What to do then? Must we turn away from the concept of "perfect posture?"

The knowledge and evolution of the principles enunciated by Still[100] are a long way from the concept of "ideal" and approach the concept of "individual." Recalling the indivisibility of the body, they lead to an evaluation of integration between structure and function in order to understand the junction where two people with the same dysfunction can advance in their journey by taking different roads: compensation and/or adaptation or failure and/or difficulty of adjustment.

The human body is able to adapt to a wide variety of environmental and internal stressors, maintaining the stability of physiological systems and the oscillatory interdependence between structure and function to restore balance and to minimize internal effects.[101,102] From this follows the nonlinear, unpredictable, but observable complexity with which this adaptation occurs. This, in the opinion of the author, is the evolution necessary today to ensure the survival and development of the biomechanical model. The complex relationship between inputs (afferent receptors) and outputs (postural compensation and adaptations) is realized in the myofascial tone[40,95] constantly looking for new dynamic equilibrium.

The new biomechanical model therefore views a posture as an efferent (musculoskeletal) epiphenomenon as a result of an underlying afferent (neuromyofascial) complexity. For example, in the case of surgery we may notice a reduction of the movement of an ankle because of adhesions that, independently from the surgical procedure used, are traceable in the underlying layers (from the skin to the bone, from the fascia to the nervous tissue). The information from the scar area derives not only from the skin but from all the tissues affected by trauma and involved in the intervention.

The same alteration will be observed in the efferent system, when the information returns to the ankle and the entire mechanical system, consequently altering global postural responses. During the course of gathering a variety of information, there may emerge a symptom, probably in the area less capable of "compliance,"[103] as, for example, in the area for spinal control of the ankle, which may become symptomatic, with relative hypertonia of the paraspinal muscles, and painful to palpation. When stimulated in this way, the sympathetic nervous system can produce a local vasoconstriction of the ankle and disturb postural balance again.[104,105]

The patient may feel pain even when there is only a small aesthetically acceptable scar, because adhesions can create an entrapment in the course of the nerve, for example the peroneal nerve in the case of the ankle. The entrapment is not only of mechanical origin, but will also be a response to afferent stress which induces local and segmental involuntary contractions in the fine postural control system.[106,107] As a result of constant stimulation of pain, the central and peripheral nervous systems adapt and change their structure, creating a vicious cycle.[108,109]

Even visceral nociceptive and interoceptive stimulus, conveyed by C fibers, produces the same effect, since central sensitization is established in the subcortical level and does not need to become conscious.[110] The same events occur, for example, in syndesmotic joint lesions, such as the interosseous membranes or the small dental gomphosis. Therefore traumas, scars, and adhesions at this level can alter gait dynamics, chewing, and proper load distribution.[111,112] A scar on the elbow can cause postural problems affecting cervical and lumbar pain.[103-115]

The treatment made possible by the new biomechanical model in osteopathy is therefore not only a treatment for the efferent (motor) arch,

but also the afferent (sensory) arch, with the aim of identifying (perturbation) and treating (normalization) the somatic dysfunction that caused the postural alteration.[9] Neurologists, who work with prolotherapy and neural therapy, recognize the same altering mechanism of the afferents originating in a scar, which may constitute the basis for more severe organic and postural disorders.[116] Furthermore, some authors speculate that the presence of a vertebral dysfunction results in painful symptomatology, due to an abnormal increase in muscle tone and the distribution of loads, with consequent postural alteration.[117,118]

This dysfunction is attributable to an efferent autonomic pathway and is influenced by electrical and biochemical afferents. It has been suggested that the afferents are able to elicit physiopathological reflexes with the autonomic efferent pathway and consequently to modify the posture that depends on the fascia[119] and the myofascial tissue. The latter is to be considered as a tissue continuum, which, from the limbs, communicates with the rest of the body, in particular through the thoracolumbar fascia,[85] a structure recognized as one of the areas involved in back pain, or abnormalities of the shoulder arthrokinematics.[120] In fact, when the fascia is not in its normal physiological condition, the fascial receptors, as free ends,[119] can become nociceptors and promote the onset of a complex symptomatology.[85,119]

In this regard, Wood Jones[121,122] showed that the muscles and tendons that have a wide insertion on the fasciae use these extended sheets as a functional counterpart of the invertebrate exoskeleton: a soft tissue skeleton for muscle attachments called the ectoskeleton. Tendon networks are a particular feature of the hand and foot. On the back of the hand, for example, there is a whole series of flattened extensor tendons, which expand from under the extensor retinaculum to head toward the fingers. The tendons are connected together by a highly variable set of fibrous fascias known as juncturae tendinum.[123] Together with the tendons and their associated fascia, those fibrous bands contribute to the formation of a complex network of tendon tissue on the back of the hand, which was probably developed from a single embryonic blastema.

The bands are likely to be important in controlling the spacing of the extensor tendons and, by channeling the forces between them; they coordinate the extension of the fingers.[124] This structure is a key to the extensor surface of the hand, thanks to the integrated operation of the entire network of tendons, so that any particular function of its individual elements is subservient to this primary role. Contemporary anatomists use the term "super-tendons" to describe a network of tendons and closely related structures (joint capsules, tendon sheaths, pulleys, retinacula, fat pads, and bags), in which the function of the complex is higher than that of individual members.[125] Recently, the complex interaction of various digital tendons was evaluated in the context of the co-evolution of the brain and body, leaving out the principle of "non-neural somatic logic" underlying the functioning of the cellular networks.[126]

In osteopathy, since the 1920s, direct techniques known as Neidner techniques, or fascial twist, have been in use.[88] These techniques, probably through twisting forces applied to the "super-tendons" of the extremities (palmar fascia, plantar fascia, fascia lata), aim to restore fascial balance and symmetry of transition areas in the spinal column and the postural compensation scheme. The complex nonlinear nature of the biomechanical adaptations leads the contemporary osteopath to observe the integration between the structure of an area and the function related to it and to choose an evaluation and treatment approach suitable for the individual's allostatic load and the reflection of it on the continuous adaptive response of the connective-fascial aspects to environmental stimuli and posture.

But have the osteopathic approaches, classically described in the biomechanical field, been subject to careful examination? Do we have current scientific evidence for these approaches?

In this age where there is a strong focus in health care on evidence-based practice, it is interesting to note that, relative to musculoskeletal disorders, there is still no evidence-based research that supports, for example, lumbar pain surgery,[127] while only 13% of medical practice is considered beneficial, with another 23% considered probably beneficial.[128] Traditional practices taught in postgraduate medical education still rely primarily on expert opinion. Similarly, for over 100 years, osteopaths, as well as chiropractors, have provided manual therapies in accordance with the techniques taught in training programs and considered useful in clinical practice. However, despite the limited resources, we can now say that the professions that use manual therapies have produced a basic test for the treatment of musculoskeletal disorders.

Osteopathy, and more generally, manual therapy, has managed to gain recognition by scientific and governmental entities for clinical applications for patients who suffer from musculoskeletal pain, which is the most common reason why a person seeks medical care in the United States.[129] Before describing an ideal research project for evaluation and validation of the biomechanical model, the author believes that it may be of interest to explore the current state of research on manual therapy for musculoskeletal disorders. Licciardone and colleagues[130] conducted a systematic review and meta-analysis of randomized controlled trials of OMT applied to patients with chronic low back disorders.

This analysis was favorable for the OMT benefits in those patients. Mainly based on chiropractic research, the guidelines published in 1994[131] accept the clinical use of spinal manipulation for treating back pain, if there are no contraindications. Contraindications include the presence of tumors, infections, or conditions around the spinal column, such as cauda equina syndrome, which can lead to a compression of L3–S2 nerve roots, making spinal manipulation too dangerous. A Cochrane Review group[132] reported that in some subjects spinal manipulation is more effective in reducing pain and improving the ability to perform everyday activities compared to placebo treatments. However, it was no more or less effective than pain medications, physical therapy, exercises, back school, or the treatment prescribed by general practitioners.

Other systematic reviews have reported observations in relation to the matter. Cherkin,[133] for example, concluded that spinal manipulation has few clinical benefits, equivalent to those achieved by common therapies. Following these reviews, other clinical studies have been reported on manual therapy applied to patients with back pain. Geisser and colleagues[134] reported a single-blind, controlled, and randomized clinical study of manual therapy for lower back pain with adjunctive exercises. In this study, patients did not know whether they received true or sham therapies; even those who collected the data were blinded to the patients' treatments. The researchers found that patients who received manual therapy with specific exercises had significant improvement in pain.

No significant change was observed in disability, which in fact was higher in the group of patients receiving the sham treatment after 6 weeks. Based on the above results, the medical literature on primary care included manual therapies in back pain management plans.[135] The structure–function osteopathic concept may have the greatest importance for health care benefits when considered in relation to the spine and the neurovascular structures. However, there are well-designed studies that show the benefits of manual therapy on musculoskeletal problems not necessarily related to spine dysfunctions.

Knebl and colleagues[45] conducted a randomized controlled trial, which showed a significant improvement of elderly patients' functions when OMT is applied specifically to dysfunctional shoulders. This study confirms many clinical cases which reported similar benefits. In a series of studies, Sucher and colleagues[136–138] showed a decrease in the pain of carpal tunnel syndrome and increased joint movement of the wrist after OMT application. Gamber and colleagues[139] conducted a clinical study in patients with fibromyalgia and found that most OMT traditional treatments produce significant relief of pain compared to usual care alone. The Knebl and Sucher studies[45,136–138] have also illustrated the structure–function osteopathic concept, in which OMT was formulated specifically to treat muscle and fascial restrictions in the shoulder and wrist with limited mobility.

This brief review focuses on evidence-based research supporting the benefits of manual therapy, in some musculoskeletal conditions, particularly those of the lumbar pain. According to reports in the latest available treatises on the topic,[140] it is necessary to do further research that supports the benefits of manual therapy in a variety of musculoskeletal dysfunctions mainly based on the structure–function relationship, i.e., between anatomical structures and functions of the nerves and vessels, potentially influenced by structures in dysfunction. Some authors have investigated the biological mechanisms that underlie the direct and indirect techniques used in the studies described above,[141] highlighting the interaction of these with the pain–spasm–pain cycle.

Musculoskeletal pain causes an increase in nociceptive input levels when tissues such as muscles, tendons, and bones are damaged or affected by dysfunction. The increased nociceptive input excites the $\gamma$ motoneurons; the result is an increase in the excitability of muscle spindles, also related to the elongation or variation of the muscles. Higher levels of nociceptive input and afferent activity transmit an exciter input to $\alpha$ motoneurons; there is a resulting unintentional activation (i.e., spasm) or inadvertent discharge of $\alpha$ motoneurons caused by low levels of excitatory inputs from other sources (for example, descending input). Manual therapies seem to mitigate the nociceptive input, or reduce the excitatory input to $\gamma$ motoneurons, and normalize the excitability of the stretch reflex.

Indirect myofascial release techniques reduce the discrepancy between the activity of the intra- and extrafusal muscle fibers: the expression of pro-inflammatory cytokines is reduced; there is a balancing of the transcapillary blood flow and interstitial fluid pressure, with reduction of pain, muscle tension, and improved mobility.[142]

## Case study

### General data of the patient

Male, 63, retired (former airline pilot), normal weight, former smoker.

### Chief complaint

Right lower back pain, which extends to the buttock, for 2 months, with afternoon onset; aggravated by movement, relieved by rest. He also reports difficulty in breathing.

### Past history

Basically healthy. He relates: recurrent sprains of the right foot over the past 10 years; scaphoid fracture of the right hand about 5 years ago; ragweed hay fever starting about 35–40 years ago, but disappeared after homeopathic treatment; pneumonia about 7 years ago.

### Social and occupational history

Pensioner, with a good lifestyle, no economic problems, plays golf twice a week and does Nordic walking 3 times a week. He is also a sailor and occasionally participates in winter racing, while also spending the summer on a boat.

### Differential diagnosis

- Myofascial syndrome.

- Costal microfracture from stress.[143]

### Objective examination

- Compression and costal percussion tests: negative.

- Schepelmann test: positive.

- Evaluation of sensitivity: there were no signs of superficial allodynia, but deep right subscapularis allodynia was detected.

- Evaluation of posture:[144] kyphotic upper spine and lumbar hyperlordosis, resulting in moving the axis of the body forward so that the center of gravity, rather than being located at the medial part of the plantar arch level, shifts toward the toes, causing hypertonicity of the paraspinal muscles to stop the anterior displacement of the center of gravity.

- Evaluation of breathing:[144] the patient experiences a breathing pattern similar to that of a hemithorax, which might suggest the replacement of the normal skeletal tissue of the chest wall by a retracting scar tissue. This may preclude normal inspiratory excursion, but being concomitant to pain may have musculoskeletal or neurogenic origin through irritation of the intercostal nerves.

- The patient reported pain equal to 8/10 on a VAS scale.

- Costal microfracture was ruled out and the working diagnosis is myofascial syndrome.

### Osteopathic evaluation

- The Zink test detects one offset scheme with alternating rotations and inclinations.

- We detect:

  - lumbar SD M99.03 (left L1 FRS)

  - thoracic SD M99.02 (T4 bilateral extension)

  - thoracic soft tissue SD M99.08, or an ileocostal trigger point of the chest, just medial to the corner of the shoulder blade.[145]

## Case study continued

- Tests of postural control (monopodalic balance): with open eyes the patient loses balance after 10 seconds on each leg, with closed eyes, after 4:07 seconds.

- The inhibition test performed by directly tensioning the thoracolumbar fascia:

  - improves the T4 mobility restriction and pain caused by palpation

  - improves the L1 mobility restriction

  - inhibits the pain reported in the right buttock

  - improves respiratory chest excursion

  - improves the postural control test, with the patient maintaining balance for 14 seconds with opened eyes and 16 seconds with closed eyes.

### Treatment

1st session

We proceed with a maximalist approach: PINS, Neidner techniques, GOT techniques.

The patient demonstrates improved mobility for the active tests of flexion, inclination, and standing extension; improves in the postural control tests, managing to maintain balance for 20 seconds on both sides of monopodalic support. The patient reports no longer feeling pain and reports pain equal to 4/10 at the right subscapularis level immediately after treatment. The patient is advised to perform the test of postural control (monopodalic balance) at least once a day, with the goal of maintaining balance for at least 30 seconds.

### 2nd session (after 2 weeks)

The patient has improved front posture and breathing; reports having engaged in Nordic walking, and feeling a disturbance in the right anterior leg, and to having done the monopodalic support exercise with closed eyes, reaching the expected 30 seconds. He reports sensitivity to palpation of the ileocostal trigger point. During osteopathic palpation a SD of the anterior right astragal joint (M99.06) is noted. The following treatment was performed: a local technical release directed to the area adjacent to the myofascial ileocostal trigger point of the chest; a segmental fascial unwinding technique, using a double fulcrum alternating between the right shoulder and the posterior aspect of the right foot; a global technique of harmonic oscillation, first with a right scapular fulcrum and then with general oscillatory coherence. The patient reported improvement in sensitivity to palpation of the tender points. During a phone call a week later the patient reported that he was able to return to playing golf.

### Patient education

The patient was been informed of the publication of studies related to stress fractures to the ribs in golfers,[143] including amateur golfers, and urging him to pay attention to his athletic movement during training and matches. A telephone call to the patient's coach revealed that the coach observed abnormal posture in the patient while golfing. The coach advised the patient to consult a naturopath for auricular therapy sessions, considered useful in assisting in reorganization of posture.[146]

## Conclusions

In summarizing this discussion on the biomechanical model, we can point out what has been historically claimed concerning the effects of postural and biomechanical factors in improving the patient's ability to compensate for stress or disease factors.

The proposed treatment involves different techniques at each treatment to allow for improving the movement of the various layers of the connective tissue, osseous and neural systems, improving afferent input in the case of malfunction. However, even in this model, in order to better understand the manual approach, to consciously choose the therapeutic technique to be used, to adapt the treatment to the specific needs of the patient, one must understand the integration between structure and function in the tissue that needs treatment. The fascial continuum can be considered a sense organ of human mechanics, which, if altered, determines postural patterns during daily activities.[147]

Fibroblasts represent one of the bases of the fascial system. These cells have the ability to contract, to communicate quickly with each other, and play a key role in the transmission of the tension produced by the muscles and in the management of interstitial fluids. The connective tissue is also a source of nociceptive and proprioceptive information, useful for the correct operation of the body systems.[93] The fascial system is electrically activated, as shown in some neuronal models, by virtue of the different embryonic origins of fibroblasts located in the connective tissue.[93,148] Information that affects the fascial electric current also affects the behavior of structures involved with the fascia and the interdependent relationship with functions such as posture, and can be palpated by an osteopath.[93,149]

The author has confidence in the good sense of the operator when he or she applies historically shared osteopathic postulates. A critical review of these postulates, in light of available evidence, and integration with the art of osteopathy, allows our thinking and our practices to evolve from the 19th century to today, in line with the procedures described by the "old doctor," by which he or she has often reminded us to keep it pure.

## References

1. Herman R, Mixon J, Fisher A et al. Idiopathic scoliosis and the central nervous system: a motor control problem. The Harrington lecture 1983. Scoliosis Research Society Spine. 1985;10(1):1–14.

2. Kappler RE. Postural balance and motion patterns. J Am Osteopath Assoc. 1982;81(9):598–606.

3. Korr IM. The collected papers of Irvin M. Korr. Vol 2. Indianapolis, IN: American Academy of Osteopathy; 1997.

4. Seffinger MA, King HH, Ward RC et al. Osteopathic philosophy. In: Chila AG, editor. Foundations of osteopathic medicine. 3rd ed. Philadelphia PA: Lippincott Williams and Wilkins; 2011. p.14.

5. Charpentier A. Postural tonic activity. Discussion by doctors Baron Nasse and Gagey (Paris). J Belge Med Phys Rehabil. 1979;2(1):13–29.

6. Gagey PM, Weber B. 2010 Study of intra-subject random variations of stabilometric parameters. Med Biol Eng Comput. 2010;48(8):833–5.

7. Kuchera ML. Postural considerations in coronal horizontal and sagittal planes. In: Ward RC, editor. Foundations of osteopathic medicine. 2nd ed. Philadelphia: Lippincott Williams and Wilkins; 2002. pp. 603–32.

8. Kuchera ML. Postural consideration in osteopathic diagnosis and treatment. In: Chila

A, editor. Foundations of osteopathic medicine. Philadephia, PA: Lippincott Williams and Wilkins; 2010. ch. 36, p.437.

9.  Zavarella P, Asmone C, Zanardi M. Le asimmetrie occluso-posturali. Rome: GLM editore; 2002. vol. 2.

10. Lederman E. The fall of the postural-structural-biomechanical model in manual and physical therapies: exemplified by lower back pain. J Bodyw Mov Ther. 2011;15(2):131-8.

11. O'Sullivan P. Diagnosis and classification of chronic low back pain disorders: maladaptive movement and motor control impairments as underlying mechanism. Man Ther. 2005;10(4):242-55.

12. Chaitow L. Is postural-structural-biomechanical model within manual therapies viable? A JBMT debate. J Bodyw Mov Ther. 2011;15(2):130-52.

13. Irvin RE. The origin and relief of common pain. J Back Musculoskelet Rehabil. 1998;11(2):89-130.

14. Hruby RJ. Pathophysiologic models and the selection of osteopathic manipulative techniques. J Osteopath Med. 1992;6(4):25-30.

15. Schiotz EH, Cyriax J. Manipulation: past and present. London: William Heinemann Medical Books; 1974.

16. Connor L, Asch P, Asch T. Jero Tapakan: Balinese healer. Cambridge, UK: Cambridge University Press; 1986.

17. Handy ESC, Pukai MK, Livermore K. Outline of Hawaiian physical therapeutics. Bernice P Bishop Mus Bull. 1934.

18. Anderson R. Traditional Europe: a study in anthropology and history. Belmont CA: Wadsworth; 1971.

19. Anderson R. Hawaiian therapeutic massage. World Wide Rep. 1982;24(5):4A.

20. Anderson R. The shaman as a healer: what happened? Amer Back Soc Newsletter. 1989;6(2):9.

21. Anderson R. The treatment of musculoskeletal disorders by a Mexican bonesetter. Soc Ser Med. 1987;24(1):43-6.

22. Anderson R. An orthopedic ethnography in rural Nepal. Medical Anthrography. 1984;1:45-59.

23. Darkin-Langley S. Ayurveda in Nepal: a medical belief system in action. Unpublished PhD thesis, University of Wisconsin, Madison, WI, 1982.

24. Anderson R. Spinal manipulation before chiropractic. In: Haldemann S, editor. The principles and practice of chiropractic. 2nd ed. Norwalk CT: Appleton and Lange; 1992. pp. 3-14.

25. Pettman E. A history of manipulative therapy. J Man Manip Ther. 2007;15(3):165-74.

26. Withington ET. Hippocrates, with an English translation. Cambridge, MA: Harvard University Press; 1928.

27. Renander A. 1960 Om sjukdomarnas. Swedish translation of Galenus C. Vol. IV. Venice, Italy: Delocis affectis Libre 1-6; 1960.

28. Parsons J, Marcer N. Osteopathy: models for diagnosis treatment and practice. Edinburgh: Elsevier Churchill Livingstone; 2006. ch. 3 pp. 43.

29. Littlejohn JM. The pathology of the osteopathic lesion. Maidstone College of Osteopathy. Indianapolis, IN: American Academy of Osteopathy Yearbook 1977.

30. Littlejohn JM. The physiological basis of the therapeutic law. J Am Osteopath Ass. 1902.

31. Parsons J, Marcer N. Osteopathy: models for diagnosis, treatment and practice. Edinburgh: Elsevier Churchill Livingstone; 2006. p.243.

32. Parsons J, Marcer N. Osteopathy: models for diagnosis, treatment and practice. Edinburgh: Elsevier Churchill Livingstone; 2006. pp. 225–6.

33. Fryette HH. Principles of osteopathic technique. Carmel, CA: Academy of Applied Osteopathy; 1954.

34. Gibbons P, Tehan P. Spinal manipulation: indications risks and benefits. J Bodyw Mov Ther. 2001;5(2):110–19.

35. Sutherland WG. Teaching in the science of osteopathy. Fort Worth, TX: Sutherland Cranial Teaching Foundation; 1990.

36. Magoun H. Osteopathy in the cranial field. Fort Worth, TX: Sutherland Cranial Teaching Foundation; 1997.

37. Richter P, Hebgen E. Trigger points and muscle chains in osteopathy. New York: Thieme; 2009. ch. 4.

38. Nicholas AS, Nicholas EA. Atlas of osteopathic techniques. Philadelphia, PA: Lippincot Williams and Wilkins; 2008. ch. 10.

40. Richter P, Hebgen E. Trigger points and muscle chains in osteopathy. New York: Thieme; 2009. ch. 2.

41. Masi AT, Nair K, Evans T et al. Clinical biomechanical and physiological translational interpretations of human resting myofascial tone or tension. Inter J Ther Massage Bodyw. 2010;16;3(4):16–28.

42. Zhang X, Zhang Z, Zhao H et al. Extracting the globally and locally adaptive backbone of complex networks. PLoS One. 2014:17;9(6):e100428.

43. Franke H, Franke JD, Fryer G. Osteopathic manipulative treatment for nonspecific low back pain: a systematic review and meta-analysis. BMC Musculoskelet Disord. 2014;15:286.

44. Tsertsvadze A, Clar C, Court R et al. Cost-effectiveness of manual therapy for the management of musculo-skeletal conditions: a systematic review and narrative synthesis of evidence from randomized controlled trials. J Manipulative Physiol Ther. 2014;37(6):343–62.

45. Schreiber AL, Sucher BM, Nazarian LN. Two novel nonsurgical treatments of carpal tunnel syndrome. Phys Med Rehabil Clin N Am. 2014;25(2):249–64.

46. Knebl JA, Shores JH, Gamber RG et al. Improving functional ability in the elderly via the Spencer technique, an osteopathic manipulative treatment: a randomized controlled trial. J Am Osteopath Assoc. 2002;102(7):387–96.

47. Papa L, Mandara A, Bottali M et al. A randomized control trial on the effectiveness of osteopathic manipulative treatment in reducing pain and improving the quality of life in elderly patients affected by osteoporosis. Clin Cases Miner Bone Metab. 2012;9(3):179–83.

48. Brolinson PG, Smolka M, Rogers M et al. Pre-competition manipulative treatment and performance among Virginia Tech athletes during 2 consecutive football seasons: a preliminary retrospective report. J Am Osteopath Assoc. 2012;112(9):607–15.

49. Brumm LF, Janiski C, Balawender JL et al. Preventive osteopathic manipulative treatment and stress fracture incidence among collegiate cross-country athletes. J Am Osteopath Assoc. 2013;113(12):882-90.

50. LeBauer A, Brtalik R, Stowe K. The effect of myofascial release (MFR) on an adult with idiopathic scoliosis. J Bodyw Mov Ther. 2008;12(4):356-63.

51. Brooks WJ, Krupinski EA, Hawes MC. Reversal of childhood idiopathic scoliosis in an adult without surgery: a case report and literature review. Scoliosis. 2009;15;4:27.

52. Posadzki P, Lee MS, Ernst E. Osteopathic manipulative treatment for pediatric conditions: a systematic review. Pediatrics. 2013;132(1):140-52.

53. Osborn GG. Manual medicine and its role in psychiatry. Am Acad Osteopath J. 1994;4(1):16-21.

54. Stephenson C. The complementary therapist's guide to red flags and referrals. Edinburgh: Elsevier Churchill Livingstone; 2011.

55. Cicconi M, Mangiulli T, Bolino G. Onset of complications following cervical manipulation due to malpractice in osteopathic treatment: a case report. Med Sci Law. 2014;54(4):230-3.

56. Vick DA, McKay C, Zengerle CR. The safety of manipulative treatment: review of the literature from 1925 to 1993. J Am Osteopath Assoc. 1996;96(2):113-5.

57. Seffinger MA Hruby RJ. Evidence-based manual medicine. Philadelphia, PA: Saunders Elsevier; 2007. pp. 217.

58. Richter P, Hebgen E. Trigger points and muscle chains in osteopathy. New York: Thieme; 2009. pp. 101-5.

59. Swanson RL. Biotensegrity: a unifying theory of biological architecture with applications to osteopathic practice education and research – a review and analysis. J Am Osteopath Ass. 2013;113(1):34-52.

60. Tozzi P. Selected fascial aspects of osteopathic practice. J Bodyw Mov Ther. 2012;16(4):503-19.

61. Langevin HM. Connective tissue: a body-wide signaling network? Med Hypotheses. 2006;66(6):1074-7.

62. Zink JG, Lawson WB. An osteopathic structural examination and functional interpretation of the soma. Osteopath Ann. 1979;7:12-9.

63. Chaitow L. Terapia manuale dei tessuti molli. Principi e tecniche di positional release. 3rd ed. Elsevier Masson; 2009. pp. 16.

64. Dunnington WP. A musculoskeletal stress pattern: observations from over 50 years' clinical experience. J Am Osteopath Assoc. 1964;64:366-71.

65. Irvine WG. New concepts in the body expression of stress. Can Fam Physician. 1973;19(7):38-42.

66. Sypher FF. Pain in the back: a general theory. J Int Coll Surg. 1960;33:718-28.

67. Parker N, Greenhalgh A, Chockalingam N et al. Positional relationship between leg rotation and lumbar spine during quiet standing. Stud Health Technol Inform. 2008;140:231-9.

68. Parsons J, Marcer N. Osteopathy: models for diagnosis, treatment and practice. Edinburgh: Elsevier Churchill Livingstone; 2006. p.179.

69. Chaitow L. Terapia manuale dei tessuti molli. Principi e tecniche di positional release. 3rd ed. Elsevier Masson; 2009. box 21, p.18.

70. Chaitow L. Terapia manuale dei tessuti molli. Principi e tecniche di positional release. 3rd ed. Elsevier Masson; 2009. ch. 7.

71. Degenhardt BF, Johnson JC, Snider KT et al. Maintenance and improvement of interobserver reliability of osteopathic palpatory tests over a 4-month period. J Am Osteopath Assoc. 2010;110(10):579–86.

72. Bohannon RW, Larkin PA, Cook AC et al. Decrease in time balance test scores with aging. Phys Ther. 1984;64(7):1067–70.

73. Winters J, Crago P, editors. Biomechanics and neural control of posture and movement. New York: Springer; 2000.

74. Charney DS, Deutch A. A functional neuroanatomy of anxiety and fear: implication for the pathophisiology and treatment of anxiety disorders. Crit Rev Neurobiol. 1996;10(3–4):419–46.

75. Chauffour P, Prat E. Mechanical link: fundamental principles, theory and practice following an osteopathic approach. Berkeley, CA: North Atlantic Books; 2002. pp. 38–40.

76. Barral JP, Croibier A. Manual therapy for the peripheral nerves. Edinburgh: Elsevier Health Sciences; 2007. pp. 119–20.

77. Parsons J, Marcer N. Osteopathy: models for diagnosis treatment and practice. Edinburgh: Elsevier Churchill Livingstone; 2006. ch. 11.

78. Richter P, Hebgen E. Trigger points and muscle chains in osteopathy. New York: Thieme; 2009. ch. 55.

79. Aoki T, Watanabe A, Nitta N et al. Correlation between apparent diffusion coefficient and viscoelasticity of articular cartilage in a porcine model. Skeletal Radiol. 2012;41(9):1087–92.

80. Milentijevic D, Torzilli PA. Influence of stress rate on water loss matrix deformation and chondrocyte viability in impacted articular cartilage. J Biomech. 2005;38(3):493–502.

81. Torzilli PA, Grigiene R, Borrelli J et al. Effect of impact load on articular cartilage: cell metabolism and viability and matrix water content. J Biomech Eng. 1999;121(5):433–41.

82. Montain SJ, Smith AS, Mattot RP et al. Hypo-hydration effects on skeletal muscle performance and metabolism: a 31P-MRS study. J Appl Physiol (1985). 1998;84(6):1889–94.

83. Judelson DA, Maresh CM, Farrell MJ et al. Effect of hydration state on strength power and resistance exercise performance. Med Sci Sports Exerc. 2007;39(10):1817–24.

84. Parker J, Heinking KP, Kappler RE. Efficacy of osteopathic manipulative treatment for low back pain in euhydrated and hypohydrated conditions: a randomized crossover trial. J Am Osteopath Assoc. 2012;112(5):276–84.

85. Bialosky JE, Bishop MB, Robinson ME et al. The relationship of the audible pop to hypoalgesia associated with high velocity low amplitude thrust manipulation: a secondary analysis of an experimental study in pain free participants. J Manipulative Physiol Ther. 2010;33(2):117–24.

86. Benjamin M. The fascia of the limbs and back – a review. J Anat. 2009;214(1):1–18.

87. Tozzi P. Balanced ligamentous tension technique. In: Chaitow L, editor. Fascial dysfunction: manual therapy approaches. East Lothian, UK: Handspring Publishing; 2014. ch. 11.

88. Dowling DJ. Progressive inhibition of neuromuscular structures (PINS) technique. J Am Osteopath Assoc. 2000:100(5):285–6, 289–98.

89. Chila A, editor. Foundations of osteopathic medicine. Philadephia, PA: Lippincott Williams and Wilkins; 2010. p. 683.

90. Stecco L. Manipolazione fasciale per le disfunzioni interne. Padova: Piccin Nuova Libreria; 2012. p. 83.

91. Parsons J, Marcer N. Osteopathy: models for diagnosis treatment and practice. Edinburgh: Elsevier Churchill Livingstone; 2006. ch. 10.

92. Maas H, Sandercock TG. Force transmission between synergistic skeletal muscles through connective tissue linkages. J Biomed Biotech. 2010:575672.

93. Cao TV, Hicks MR, Campbell D et al. Dosed myofascial release in three-dimensional bioengineered tendons: effects on human fibroblast hyperplasia hypertrophy and cytokine secretion. J Manipulative Physiol Ther. 2013;36(8):513–21.

94. Bordoni B, Zanier E. 2014 Understanding fibroblasts in order to comprehend the osteopathic treatment of the fascia, evidence-based complementary and alternative medicine. Hindawi Publishing Corporation; 2014. Article ID 860934.

95. Trotter JA. Functional morphology of force transmission in skeletal muscle: a brief review. Acta Anat (Basel). 1993;146(4):205–22.

96. Masi AT, Hannon JC. Human resting muscle tone (HRMT): narrative introduction and modern concepts. J Bodyw Mov Ther. 2008;12(4):320–32.

97. Tozzi P. Does fascia hold memories? J Bodyw Mov Ther. 2014;18(2):259–65.

98. Schabrun SM, Jones E, Kloster J et al. Temporal association between changes in primary sensory cortex and corticomotor output during muscle pain. Neuroscience. 2013;3(235):159–64.

99. Tsao H, Galea MP, Hodges PW. Reorganization of the motor cortex is associated with postural control deficits in recurrent lowback pain. Brain. 2008;131(8):2161–71.

100. O'Sullivan P. Diagnosis and classification of chronic low back disorders. Proceedings of the 7th Interdisciplinary World Congress on Low Back and Pelvic Pain; 2010. pp. 160–77.

101. Rogers FJ, D'Alonzo GE, Glover JC et al. Proposed tenets of osteopathic medicine and principles for patient care. J Am Osteopath Assoc. 2002;102(2):63–5.

102. Selye H. The stress of life. New York: McGraw-Hill; 1956.

103. Schulkin J. Rethinking homeostasis: allostatic regulation in physiology and pathophysiology. Cambridge, MA: MIT Press; 2003.

104. Bordoni B, Zanier E. Anatomic connections of the diaphragm: influence of respiration on the body system. J Multidiscip Healthcare. 2013;6:281–91.

105. Macefield VG. Physiological characteristics of low-threshold mecha-noreceptors in joints, muscle and skin in human subjects. Clin Exp Pharmacol Physiol. 2005;32(1–2):135–44.

106. Mouchnino L, Blouin J. When standing on a moving support cutaneous inputs provide sufficient information to plan the anticipatory postural adjustments for gait initiation. PLoS One. 2013;8(2):e55081.

107. Gilbey MP. Sympathetic rhythms and nervous integration. Clin Exp Pharmacol Physiol. 2007;34(4):356–61.

108. Raju S, Sanford P, Herman S et al. Postural and ambulatory changes in regional flow and skin perfusion. Eur J Vasc Endovasc Surg. 2012;43(5):567-72.

109. Zwerver J, Konopka KH, Keizer D et al. Does sensitisation play a role in the pain of patients with chronic patellar tendinopathy? Br J Sports Med. 2013;47(9):e2.

110. Day JA, Copetti L, Rucli G. From clinical experience to a model for the human fascial system. J Bodyw Mov Ther. 2012;16(3):372-80.

111. Jänig W. Functional plasticity of dorsal horn neurons. Pain. 2013;154(10):1902-3.

112. Skraba JS, Greenwald AS. The role of the interosseous membrane on tibiofibular weightbearing. Foot Ankle. 1984;4(6):301-4.

113. Harrison JW, Siddique I, Powell ES et al. Does the orientation of the distal radioulnar joint influence the force in the joint and the tension in the interosseous membrane? Clin Biomech (Bristol Avon), 2005;20(1):57-62.

114. Leijnse JN, Rietveld AB. Left shoulder pain in a violinist related to extensor tendon adhesions in a small scar on the back of the wrist. Clin Rheumatol. 2013;32(4): 501-6.

115. Stecco A, Masiero F, Macchi V et al. The pectoral fascia: anatomical and histological study. J Bodyw Mov Ther. 2009;13(3):255-61.

116. Stecco A, Macchi V, Masiero F et al. Pectoral and femoral fasciae: common aspects and regional specializations. Surg Radiol Anat. B. 2009;31(1):35-42.

117. Clark GB. Building a rationale for evidence-based prolotherapy in an orthopedic medicine practice. J Proloth. 2011;3(2):664-71.

118. Brumagne S, Janssens L, Knapen S et al. Persons with recurrent low back pain exhibit a rigid postural control strategy. Eur Spine J. 2008;17(9):1177-84.

119. Shirzadi A, Drazin D, Jeswani S et al. Atypical presentation of thoracic disc herniation: case series and review of the literature. Case Rep Orthop. 2013:621476.

120. Kumka M, Bonar J. Fascia: a morphological description and classification system based on a literature review. J Can Chiropr Assoc. 2012;56(3):179-91.

121. Willard FH, Vleeming A, Schuenke MD et al. The thoracolumbar fascia: anatomy function and clinical considerations. J Anat. 2012;221(6):507-36.

122. Wood Jones F. The principles of anatomy as seen in the hand. London: Ballière Tindall and Cox; 1944.

123. Wood Jones F. Structure and function as seen in the foot. London: Ballière Tindall and Cox; 1944.

124. von Schroeder HP, Botte MJ. Functional anatomy of the extensor tendons of the digits. Hand Clin. 1997;13(1)51-62.

125. von Schroeder HP, Botte MJ. Anatomy and functional significance of the long extensors to the fingers and thumb. Clin Orthop Relat Res. 2001;(383):74-83.

126. Benjamin M, Kaiser E, Milz S. Structure-function relationships in tendons: a review. J Anat. 2008;212(3):211-28.

127. Valero-Cuevas FJ, Yi JW, Brown D et al. The tendon network of the fingers performs anatomical computation at a macroscopic scale. IEEE Trans Biomed Eng. 2007;54(6/2):1161-6.

128. Palmer R, Patjin J. Thoughts regarding evidence based medicine. Federation Internationale de Medicine Manuelle; 2009. http//fimm-onlinecom.

129. BMJ. How much do we know? BMJ Clinical Evidence Centre; 2009. http://clinicalevidencebmjcom/x/index.html.

130. United States Bone and Joint Decade. Burden of musculoskeletal desease in United States. United States Bone and Joint Decade; 2009. http://www.boneandjointburdenorg/pdfs/BMUS_IntroPrefaceForeword.pdf.

131. Licciardone JC, Brimhall A, King IN. Osteopathic manipulative treatment for low back pain: a systematic review and meta-analysis of randomized controlled trial. BMC Musculoskelet Disord. 2005;6:43–54.

132. Bigos SJ, Bowyeret OR, Braen GR et al. Acute low back problems in adults: assessment and treatment. Agency for Health Care Policy and Research. Clin Pract Guidel Quick Ref Guide Clin. 1994;(14):iii–iv 1–25.

133. Assendelft WJ, Morton SC, Yu EI et al. WITHDRAWN: Spinal manipulative therapy for low-back pain. Cochrane Database Syst Rev. 2013;31;1:CD000447.

134. Cherkin DC, Sherman KJ, Deyo RA et al. A review of the evidence for the effectiveness, safety and the cost of acupuncture, massage therapy, and spinal manipulation for low back pain. Ann Intern Med. 2003;138(11):898–906.

135. Geisser ME, Wiggert EA, Haig AJ et al. A randomized controlled trial of manual therapy and specific adjuvant exercise for chronic low back pain. Clin J Pain. 2005;21(6)463–70.

136. Patel AT, Ogle AA. Diagnosis and management of acute low back pain. Am Fam Physician. 2000;61(6):1779–86, 1789–90.

137. Sucher BM. Myofascial manipulative release of carpal tunnel syndrome: documentation with magnetic resonance imaging. J Am Osteopath Assoc. 1993;93(12):1273–8.

138. Sucher BM, Hinrichs RN. Manipulative treatment of carpal tunnel syndrome: biomedical and osteopathic intervention to increase the length of the transverse carpal ligament. J Am Osteopath Assoc. 1998;98(12):679–86.

139. Sucher BM, Hinrichs RN, Welcher RL et al. Manipulative treatment of carpal tunnel syndrome: biomechanical and osteopathic intervention to increase the length of the transverse carpal ligament: part 2. Effect of sex differences and manipulative priming. J Am Osteopath Assoc. 2005;105(3):135–43.

140. Gamber RG, Shores JH, Russo DP et al. Osteopathic manipulative treatment in conjunction with medication relieves pain associated with fibromyalgia syndrome: results of a randomized clinical pilot project. J Am Osteopath Assoc. 2002;102(6):321–5.

141. King H, Janig W, Patterson M. The science and clinical application of manual therapy. Edinburgh: Churchill Livingstone Elsevier; 2010.

142. Clark BC, Thomas JS, Walkowski SA et al. The biology of manual therapies. J Am Osteopath Assoc. 2012;112(9):617–29.

143. Cao TV, Hicks MR, Standley PR. In vitro biomechanical strain regulation of fibroblast wound healing. J Am Osteopath Assoc. 2013;113(11):806–18.

144. Bugbee S. Rib stress fracture in a golfer. Curr Sports Med Rep. 2010;9(1):40–2.

145. Orlandini G. La semeiotica del dolore: i presupposti teorici e la pratica clinica. 2nd ed. Rome: Antonio Delfino editore; 2005.

146. Simons DG, Travell GJ, Simons LS. Travell & Simons' Myofascial pain and dysfunction: the trigger point manual. Vol. 1: Upper half of body. 2nd ed. Baltimore: Lippincott Williams and Wilkins; 1999.

147. Bergamaschi M, Ferrari G, Gallamini M et al. Laser acupuncture and auriculotherapy in postural instability a preliminary report. J Acupunct Meridian Stud. 2011;4(1):69-74.

148. Stecco C, Gagey O, Belloni A et al. Anatomy of the deep fascia of the upper limb. Second part: study of innervation. Morphologie. 2007;9(292):28-43.

149. Langevin HM. Connective tissue: a body-wide signaling network? Med Hypotheses. 2006;66(6):1074-7.

150. Findley TW, Shalwala M. Fascia research congress evidence from the 100 year perspective of Andrew Taylor Still. J Bodyw Mov Ther. 2013;17(3):356-64.

# The neurological model

*Giampiero Fusco*

# 5

## Synopsis

In the last century, different neural propagation mechanisms related to somatic dysfunction (SD) were explored, from the first studies on somatovisceral effects,[1,2] the investigation on the peripheral and central effects of spinal facilitation,[3] to somatic and neuroendocrine-immune adaptation due to centrifugal and centripetal nociceptive activity.[4,5] These studies have paved the way for the latest insights on the neurogenic origin of the maintaining of tissue inflammation and/or the perception of somatic pain that can generate central sensitization and long-term potentiation mechanisms.[6–8] In addition, the complex interactions inherent in the neuroendocrine-immune system, such as local adaptation responses generally described in the previous chapters, explain how a nociceptive input can affect the whole body through metabolic reactions.[9]

In the presence of traumatic conditions, cross-talk phenomena may be identified between the sympathetic system and afferent neurons, due to α-adrenergic receptors,[10] showing how the sympathetic system would play a major role in maintaining the somatic dysfunction (SD). Afferent input from different areas of the body can accumulate and further activate an autonomic response,[11] so that even a subliminal stimulus can generate various effects if combined with stimuli from other areas. In the neurological model we will describe the neurophysiological mechanisms underlying SD and its palpatory characteristics, as well as the principles and rules for the application of the model in osteopathic practice, paying particular attention to the potential interconnections of the neural network with all the other body systems. The "lens" of the neurological model represents a fundamental tool of the osteopath who intends to identify and normalize SD, appealing to the intrinsic strength of the neural network, including global effects and the restoration of a stable and lasting health.

## Introduction

The neurological model interprets the patient's symptoms and signs in terms of aberration or impairment of neural functions that cause or are caused by pathophysiologic reactions of structure or of the respiratory-circulatory, metabolic, and behavioral functions. More specifically, the neurological model considers the impact of spinal facilitation, of proprioceptive, motor, neural autonomic and nociceptive function on the individual's health. This model operates on the control, coordination, and integration of body functions, as well as on defense and perception mechanisms.[12] In this sense, of particular importance is the relationship between the somatic, autonomic, and visceral systems.

The neurological model pays particular attention to conditions with chronic and/or acute pain by searching for origins at the musculoskeletal, visceral, autonomic reflex, emotional, and neuro-bio-psychological level. In our clinical practice, we often hear of patients who report not experiencing any improvement from a manual therapeutic approach, and sometimes even a worsening, often not proportional to the administered therapeutic input. This category includes the sensitized patients or those patients in whom the neural network responds in an amplified way to a physical, chemical, or psycho-emotional stimulus. The literature provides two definitions to distinguish the type of pain: acute pain and chronic pain.

Acute pain, also called physiological pain or eudynia, occurs when there is a noxious stimulus, be it chemical, mechanical, or thermal. The pain in the area where the noxious stimulus occurred can lead to primary hyperalgesia (increased sensitivity to pain). Although the peripheral nerves, spinal cord regulation patterns, brainstem, and forebrain can sensitize and intensify this activity, the pain should disappear at the end of tissue repair. In some cases, such as the simultaneous presence of multiple stressors, there can occur secondary hyperalgesia (increased pain sensitivity in areas adjacent to the harmful stimulus, but not directly causative). The secondary hyperalgesia can trigger a closed loop that amplifies the pain due to different reflex neurobiochemical mechanisms, such as the dorsal root reflex (DRR),[13] a phenomenon that can generate peripheral sensitization (PS).

Chronic pain, also called surgical pain or maldynia, is the pain that is still present 3–6 months after the natural healing of damaged tissue. Chronic pain represents a dysregulation in normal sensitization systems present in peripheral nerves, spinal cord, brainstem, and forebrain and often can include central sensitization (CS), defined as the increased responsiveness of central neurons to input of unimodal and polymodal receptors[14] and includes multiple factors:

- Alteration of the central sensitive processes[15]

- Dysfunction of the descending anti-nociceptive mechanisms[16]

- Increased activity of the descending dolorific facilitative pathways

- Temporal summation of secondary pain or wind-up (literally "wrapping load," i.e., more stimuli "charge up" the system and predispose the latter to subsequent sensitization)[17]

- phenomena of long-term potentiation (LTP) in the anterior cingulate cortex.[18]

LTP is a synaptic plasticity phenomenon that consists of increasing the efficacy of a synapse as a result of a particular type of stimulation or endogenous activity. Furthermore, in the central nervous system, LTP is the synaptic substrate for memory and learning.[19]

In the case of CS, the pain is therefore "learned" by the patient who then is able to experience pain and suffering in the absence of peripheral stimuli. CS therefore includes ascending, learning, and descending mechanisms, which cause an increase of responsiveness to various types of stimuli (mechanical, chemical, physical, thermal, etc.), with consequent reduction of body tolerance to stressful loads. In other words, long-term peripheral tissue damage can secondarily cause a pain reinforcement mechanism of central hyperexcitability. We should therefore clarify that CS is a different phenomenon from central neuropathic pain (or central pain), because central pain originates from the abnormal activity of the central neurons due to anatomical damage or primary dysfunction of these neurons.[20]

## The nociceptive system

The nociceptive A-$\delta$ and C fibers (primary afferent nociceptors – PAN) have an important role in understanding the adaptive and maladaptive mechanisms of the neural network, the object of interest of the neurological model. The PAN fibers terminate peripherally in the extracellular matrix, which among other functions seems to take on a key role in the context of nociception[21] and, at the central level, they terminate in the ipsilateral dorsal horn, or with regard to the trigeminal region, in the trigeminal nuclei of the brainstem.

In the spinal cord, the fibers reach the neurons present in lamina I, II, and V and in the medullar gray portion around lamina X. A portion of these fibers is superimposed in a variable manner to touch stimuli, or when subjected to increasing stimulus, the sensation of pain. Unlike the neurons in lamina I, lamina V provides integration between the nociceptive, low-threshold mechanical cutaneous and proprioceptive input. Most of the neurons present in this lamina are of the WDR (wide dynamic range) type, since they are able to respond in a gradual manner to stimuli coming both from the exteroceptive/proprioceptive system and the somatic/visceral nociceptive system, allowing response to increasing nociceptive stimuli, as in the case of wind-up.[22] It is thus an important area of broad spectrum integration (Fig. 5.1).

The PAN fibers can therefore conduct both visceral and somatic input.[23,24] Communication on various levels of the spinal cord within Lissauer's tract[25] and the relation with the visceral nervous system through the intermediate-lateral columns permit a noxious stimulus to propagate both in the tissues and in the viscera through plurisegmental communication.[26] In the case of spinal facilitation, a visceral input can activate circuits that have previously had low activation threshold. The pain of visceral origin related to a somatic area and supplied by local or neighboring spinal segments has been the subject of numerous studies in osteopathy, as well as detection through palpatory examination of the existence of viscerosomatic reflexes.

Of particular osteopathic interest are studies by Head relating to referred pain, a visceral pain that is reflected in some areas of the body (Head zones) rather than in the organ affected by the disease.[27] These studies have been interpreted on the basis of a law named after the researcher. Citing Head's law, when a painful stimulus is exerted on the side with reduced sensitivity, which is in close connection with a side with increased sensitivity, the produced

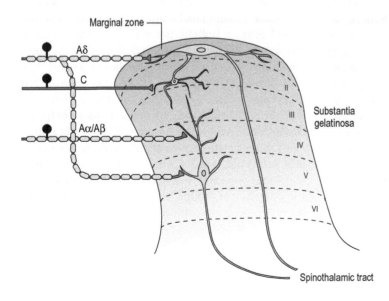

**Fig. 5.1**
Connections in the spinal cord, including lamina V, that provide an integrative system between nociceptive, muscular, and visceral input. Modified by: Benarroch EE. In: Benarroch EE. Basic neurosciences with clinical applications. Philadelphia, PA: Butterworth-Heinemann, Elsevier; 2005. fig. 14-4, p. 399.

pain is felt more in the most sensitive part, rather than in the least sensitive part, where the painful stimulus was directed.[28]

This means that the sympathetic nerves that supply internal organs have, through their central connections (reflex arc), a relationship with the spinal nerves that innervate the muscles and skin areas. Therefore, a patient with liver disease may feel pain or cutaneous dysesthesia on the right side of the ribcage and on the right shoulder through the reflex arc carried by the phrenic nerve to the nociceptive afferents at the C3–C5 levels. As soon as the feelings change, trophic changes also occur in the somatic area of reference. Thus, what disturbs the body "from within" is manifested "externally" and vice versa, which is also one of the fundamental concepts of the osteopathic profession, concepts that were later organized and rationalized in the 1950s by Irvin Korr (see Chapter 2 and the "historical background" section in this chapter). Beal,[29] in describing viscerosomatic reflexes, indicates how the somatic manifestation of the visceral pathology is an integral part of the pathological process rather than a simple sign or symptom.

The terms "referred pain" and "viscerosomatic reflex" were often used interchangeably to define a phenomenon that includes cutaneous hyperalgesia, vasomotor changes, and striated muscle hypercontractility. The concept of the spinal cord central excitatory state is based on the assumption of the existence of referred pain of visceral origin. The visceral afferents will initiate the central excitatory state, and can be facilitated by cutaneous and muscular somatic afferents, or by supraspinal stimuli. Once the excitatory state is created, the activity of this state can be increased and supported by subsequent stimulation of visceral, somatic and higher centers.

A cyclic neuronal pattern is created, through medullar connections, which can be maintained for long periods, even under conditions in which the initial stimuli cease their activity, with resulting continuous cutaneous hyperalgesia and striated-muscle hypercontractility. The visceral referred pain is common with the symptoms experienced by acute conditions of the cardiovascular and gastrointestinal systems, but the variability of the SDs, which can manifest and be related, should be explored in the individual adaptability and variability of innervation of the autonomic nervous system.

## Neurogenic inflammation

The nociceptive network represents a "convergence" system, as it can convey noxious stimuli coming from different tissues, but also "divergence," as it can propagate them elsewhere. In fact, when a branch of the nociceptors is stimulated, the action is directed not only centrally but also toward other terminal branches of the same neuron. On all of the central and peripheral terminations activated, the action potential allows the release of peptide neurotransmitters, including substance P and probably somatostatin. These neurotransmitters act peripherally as vasodilators and attraction agents of macrophages and lymphocytes in tissues.

These nociceptors also stimulate the release of pro-inflammatory synergistic agents such as histamine, serotonin, kininogens, and complement activators that in turn produce vasodilatation and stimulate phagocytosis and inflammatory chemotaxis.[4] From a holistic point of view, the nociceptive system is used to "predict" situations that may lead to further worsening of the patient's condition. This "predictive" system, called feedforward, has a peculiar characteristic that differentiates it from the feedback system, which is that it does not have a predetermined retroactive control point (set point). Consequently the PANs, if subjected to an excessive stimulus, are capable of triggering feedforward reactions that initiate the processes in which the body has to "adapt" to new loads, changing the biochemical composition of the tissues in order to ensure the individual's survival.

This process, called allostasis, represents the "stability through change" and is able to influence the detection of noxious stimuli and the perception of pain.[30] All this has a cost that we can perceive osteopathically, such as changes in regulatory mechanisms and homeostatic control. In this context, neurogenic inflammation could be the pathophysiologic rationale that underlies the neural network imbalance observed through the lens of the neurological model. According to this hypothesis, once the central, peripheral, and autonomic nervous systems are disturbed, pain from the persistent hyperexcitability of nociceptors becomes a pathogenic intermediate category between the tissue and neuropathic pain, supported by antidromic conduction in the C fibers. This can cause neurosecretion of substances responsible for vasodilation and maintenance of the sensitization of the C fibers, initially only locally in the tissue dysfunction, but then eventually in the surrounding areas, and finally, through spinal pathways, up to previously sensitized remote areas. Eventually, a vicious circle would be created, maintaining the pain due to axonal reflexes.[13]

## The interaction with the autonomic nervous system

Regarding the involvement of the autonomic nervous system, it is not yet clear how the increase in sympathetic activity can produce hypersensitivity and pain, since it seems that the explanation based on vasoconstriction and subsequent tissue ischemia is not satisfactory. However, the pathogenic assumptions of CRPS-I (complex regional pain syndrome type I), once called reflex sympathetic dystrophy (RSD), suggest that the pain can be supported by sympathetic hypertonia and that the resulting circulating norepinephrine directly excites the nociceptors, but on condition that they have become hypersensitive to noradrenaline itself, thanks to the formation of $\alpha$1-receptors on nociceptors.[31]

Under these conditions, the sympathetic activity could determine a continuous excitation of the nociceptors which, in turn, would sensitize the WDR neurons enough for the input from low-threshold mechanoreceptors to evoke pain. The allodynia could therefore be supported both by the extreme sensitization of nociceptors, so as to make them also excitable by habitually ineffective tactile stimuli, and thus be C-mediated, and by central hyperexitability, and therefore be Aß-mediated. In addition, the reflex sympathetic activity could have local and distant effects, such as, for example, vasoconstriction of the skin and viscera, vasodilation in striated muscles, increased heart rate and blood pressure, and decreased gastric motility.

The activity of nociceptors indirectly affects the immune system, due to the sympathetic innervation of postganglionic autonomic neurons in the thymus, spleen, lymph nodes, and lymphoid tissues level. This activity seems to modulate the T-independent response and the antibody response mediated by B lymphocytes. The immune cells also possess β2 receptors that bind the serum catecholamines. The activation of these receptors decreases phagocytosis by macrophages, the release of lysosomal enzymes and hydrolytic enzymes from the polymorphonuclears, the formation of T-dependent antibodies, and cellular cytotoxicity mediated by antibodies. Thus, a high activation of the sympathetic nervous system, mediated by nociceptors, may decrease the function of the immune system (immunosuppressive response to stress).[4]

## The global impact of pain

Nociceptive inputs are continuously reformulated by the central nervous system, through the inhibitory descendent pathways related with cognitive and affective factors. The balance between the ascending nociceptive pathways and descending inhibitory system has in recent years been the subject of numerous studies aimed at understanding what mechanisms might lead to a reduction or inhibition of the analgesic mechanisms inherent in the human body.[32] The integrity of these mechanisms is essential in order not to interfere with the dynamic stability of the musculoskeletal system. The body's biomechanical equilibrium requires a powerful neuromuscular system, where we find even predictive mechanisms (feedforward), aimed to "prepare" the body against any unexpected disruptions, as in the case of an injury or an unusual joint movement.

As suggested by Panjabi,[33] the dynamic stability of the musculoskeletal system depends on the interdependent relationship of the active (muscular), passive (joint/ligament), and neuromuscular system: a systemic triad to which osteopathy over the years has directed special attention and research in the development of appropriate techniques. The ability to feel pain, therefore, is no longer seen today as a specific way which individually involves a specific cortical area, but a "matrix system" based on countless interconnections of different brain areas that respond to noxious stimuli and involve feelings and emotions.[34]

Modern research also reveals that the central nervous system "maps" the different sensitive and interoceptive stimuli, by storing them and adapting the body to the environment that surrounds it. Converging evidence suggests that primates have a distinct cortical image inherent to homeostatic afferent activity, which reflects all aspects of the physiological conditions of the body tissues.[35,36] This interoceptive system, associated with autonomic motor control, consists of integrated anatomical pathways, but distinct from the exteroceptive system to the guide somatic motor activity. In human beings, a meta-representation of the primary interoceptive activity is generated in the right anterior insula, which seems to provide the basis for the personal image of the self, i.e., emotional awareness.[37]

The characteristics of pain, the related emotions and perceptions are all aspects of an integrated matrix pain and, in addition to the above-mentioned areas, always involve different brain cortical areas simultaneously. The focus that we must therefore bear in mind is that the functions are integrated and have no "well marked" but functionally variable boundaries. As Selye still reminds us, these mechanisms can centrally activate a generally adaptive complex systemic response, also metabolic, due to the neuroendocrine-immune system[9] (Fig. 5.2).

## The MINE system

Summarizing the concepts described above, it is important for the osteopath to understand the network behind the development and management of aberrant neural reflexes, found in acute and chronic pain conditions. The operator must bring them to mind and subsequently to the hand, and perceive them through the reciprocal connections between structure and function. Elkiss and Jerome[38] remind us that this interdependence is manifested by the interactions of the musculoskeletal (M), immune (I), neurological (N) and endocrine (E) systems, grouped together in a "supersystem" in response to nociception, referred to as the MINE system.

These authors primarily describe the psychophysiological model of Chapman and colleagues,[39] which proposes the human systemic response to pain, due to an immune (I), neurological (N), and endocrine (E) mutual interaction. Elkiss and Jerome define the concepts underlying the Chapman model (INE), consistent with the principles of osteopathic thinking and the work of Denslow and Korr, by demonstrating the biological mechanisms underlying anatomical and physiological human functions. In summary, the INE system described by Chapman is a nest system which in turn is inserted in a larger and more complex system, from which it is fed and which feeds it in turn; namely the neuromusculoskeletal system, which allows us to interact with the external environment and express our needs. Therefore, these are the mutual interactions of the four musculoskeletal, immune, neurological and endocrine systems, and how they interact in response to nociception, to form the MINE super-system that continually adjusts the input received from the internal and external environment (Fig. 5.3).

In response to nociceptive input, the INE system will participate in the modulation of pain through:

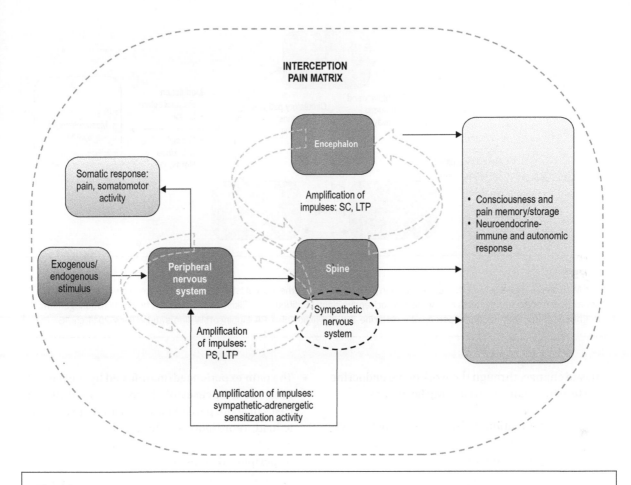

**INTERCEPTION PAIN MATRIX**

Encephalon

Amplification of impulses: SC, LTP

Somatic response: pain, somatomotor activity

Exogenous/ endogenous stimulus

Peripheral nervous system

Spine

Sympathetic nervous system

Amplification of impulses: PS, LTP

Amplification of impulses: sympathetic-adrenergetic sensitization activity

- Consciousness and pain memory/storage
- Neuroendocrine-immune and autonomic response

**Fig. 5.2**
The adaptation of the neural network to exogenous and endogenous stimuli. Note the two amplification areas of aberrant pulses (dashed circular arrows), the first between the peripheral nervous system (PNS) and the spinal cord – which can generate peripheral sensitization (PS) – and the second between the brain and spinal cord for central sensitization (CS). Note also the sympathetic feedback toward the PNS that, in the case of sympathetic-adrenal-sensitivity, may represent a sensitizing nociceptive factor. The figure also shows the somatic responses, neuroendocrine-immune, long-term potentiation (LTP), and the overall interoceptive capacity of the system connected to the genesis of the pain matrix.

- migration of cytokines, which trigger the immune system

- modulation of the endocrine and endocrine-immune system, by the actions of circulating hormones

- modulation of the nervous system, due to neurotransmitters

- neuroendocrine-immune activation, at the hands of the autonomic nervous system in the neurocirculatory pathway.

In response to nociceptive stimulation, in the musculoskeletal system we will have:

- communication mediated by cytokines, through the fluidic fascial system

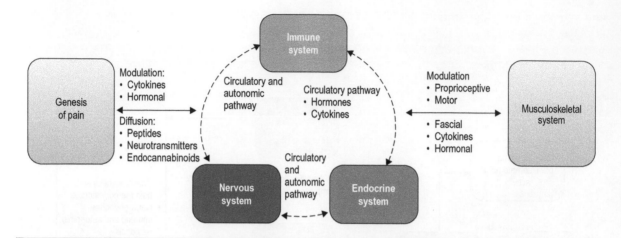

**Fig. 5.3**
The MINE super-system. Note the communication pathways made by the musculoskeletal system to interact with the immune, nervous, and endocrine systems in response to nociceptive input. Modified from: Elkiss ML, Jerome JA. Chronic pain management. In: Chila A., editor. Foundations of osteopathic medicine. 3rd ed. Philadelphia, PA: Lippincott Williams and Wilkins; 2011. ch. 16.

- tissue change, through the work of the endocrine system by means of circulating hormones

- nervous modulation of the motor predictive systems, at the hands of the motor output and of the proprioceptive afferents.

The pain expression is therefore closely linked to the condition of the musculoskeletal system, which acts as a bridge between body and mind, a two-way pathway that allows the emerging activities in the mind to influence the physical neuromusculoskeletal conditions, and vice versa. Therefore, it is the correct integration of the stimuli, through feedforward and feedback mechanisms, which allows the "balance" of the neural network. The nervous system mediates the majority of the inputs that are searched during osteopathic treatment, because the integration given from the neural network, formed by the central nervous, peripheral, and autonomic system, allows the body to adjust various functions and to "coordinate" the health of the somatic and visceral system. From these observations, we can draw very important conclusions in osteopathy:

- The pain experienced/manifested by the patient, in general, in cases of chronic pain but also in cases of acute pain in patients with high allostatic load, represents an altered neuronal activity, more than a simple nociceptive activity triggered by peripheral "generators."

- Most patients suffer lengthy periods of pain, and more may trigger awareness mechanisms, thus making it more difficult to manage, given the difficulty in improving the clinical situation.

## Osteopathic intervention implications

The health-oriented and person-centered osteopathic philosophy offers a unique opportunity to help patients suffering from chronic pain, or where aberrant activities of the neural network deserve special attention. In this context, osteopathic treatment must take into account not only the pathophysiological basis underlying this clinical picture, but also the different biomechanical, genetic, neurophysiological, and psychological processes, each capable of contributing to the clinical manifestation and symptoms. The OMT rationale must take into account the principles of body unity, integrated palpation and the use of appropriate techniques to "desensitize" the system under excessive allostatic load, so as to reduce tissue insults.

Depending on the specific situation and the pathophysiological mechanisms involved, we will assess the role of somatic dysfunction (SD) as a factor that "generates" pain in the tissues.[40] We will try to understand, through a comprehensive, segmental, and local approach, the conditions that undermine salutogenesis, creating a nociceptive load that disturbs or perturbs the autonomic nervous system in a direct or indirect way, thus affecting the neuromusculoskeletal, vascular, and lymphatic elements.

## Historical background

In 1901, Dain Tasker reported in *The Osteopath* magazine of the Pacific College of Osteopathy in Los Angeles the effects of vagus nerve stimulation on the heart. The first studies in neurophysiology began in the early 1900s at the A. T. Still Research Institute of Chicago, where the research was done by Wilborn J. Deason,[41] but experienced greater development when Louisa Burns became the director. Dr. Burns is one of the historical pillars of osteopathic research. In her career she wrote four books, a collection of works and many articles. Burns began to study the effects of SD (at that time spinal lesion) on a laboratory model (rabbit).[42] The myofascial tissues associated with an SD showed thickening, edema, inflammation, and extravasation.

These alterations were later substantiated by Wilbur Cole, who in collaboration with Burns, investigated injuries in different areas of the spine, obtaining histological findings on visceral changes. The results confirmed the hypothesis that the effects of osteopathic lesions were mediated via vegetative reflexes.[43] The autopsy was a survey method used in the first 50 years of osteopathic research, to investigate vasomotor disturbances associated with facilitated segments. From 1939 to 1969, John Stedman Denslow headed the research program in Kirksville.

He postulated that osteopathic research had to be done by scientists after adequate training in research principles and osteopathic methods. Denslow conducted numerous studies that quantified and documented the variations of the muscular and autonomic reflexes in areas of SD, through correlation between palpation and electromyography (EMG).

Denslow developed the concept of spinal facilitation and proposed the use of a standard terminology.[44-46] He began a collaboration and coordination of research activities with the "second great philosopher" of osteopathic medicine, Irvin Korr, who took the anatomical foundations expressed by Still and scientifically elaborated them by correlating them to physiological functions. In addition, he promoted as a research paradigm the complete patient/osteopath interaction. Studies performed by Korr[47,48] in collaboration with Denslow document:

- the variation of skin galvanic resistance due to disorders of the autonomic function in skin areas in which there were associated SDs, detected by palpation

- axoplasmic flow of proteins and trophic functions of the nerves

- facilitation of spinal segments

- sympathicotonia.

Over the years several clinical research studies have been performed to identify the somatic components associated with visceral disease, and the effectiveness of OMT in the resolution of somatic disorders associated with dysfunctional processes. Although some studies were deficient in describing the tests used to identify somatic components, they represent a milestone in the evolution of osteopathic research. In the double-blind study of Kelso,[49] lasting 5 years, 5,000 hospitalized patients were examined, and somatic dysfunctions associated with their medical diagnoses were reported.

Kelso concluded that most of the visceral diseases seem to have more than one region with increased segmental response frequency, while a single organ seems to have increased response in the tissue on one side, with the number of spinal segments involved related to the duration of the disease. In a second report, Kelso[50] observed an increased incidence of palpatory findings in the cervical spine in patients with sinusitis, tonsillitis, esophagus and liver dysfunction. The upper thoracic spine, however, seemed to be involved in patients with bronchitis, coronary heart disease, or other heart disease. Significant somatic dysfunctions in the T5–T12 spinal segments were found in patients with gastritis, duodenal ulcer, pyelonephritis, chronic appendicitis, and cholecystitis.

Beal used a compression test to examine soft tissue texture variation and resistance to segmental joint movement. Somatic dysfunctions were observed at T1–T5 and associated with heart disease, and SD of the T5–T12 segments was associated with gastrointestinal dysfunction. In a blind study of 25 patients he differentiated patients with cardiac or gastrointestinal dysfunctions with an accuracy of 76%.[51]

William Johnston developed the osteopathic approach known as functional technique.[52] Since Still's time, many osteopaths have began to get results with techniques other than direct techniques. In practice they realized that, although not reaching the restrictive barrier, but treating the motor "function," they could restore freedom of tissue movement. In line with the concepts of the neurological model, the goal of the functional method is to resolve SD through an indirect approach, i.e., an afferent input to the central nervous system, which processes this input by sending a corrective response to the triggering neural alteration.

Johnston attempted to establish a scientific basis for functional techniques through reliability studies and verification of corrections by alleviating viscerosomatic reflexes. In a blinded study focused on the palpatory responses of the rib, vertebral and tissue motor dysfunction, the results showed a statistically significant increase in incidence of palpatory findings in the T7–T12 region in patients with renal dysfunction, compared to patients with hypertension or normal blood pressure.

Palpatory responses were associated with increased skin temperature.[29] In general, we can say that the evolution of osteopathic techniques was led by palpation that monitors and corrects continuously in response to the data provided by the tissues, as in the case of balanced ligamentous tension (BLT), facilitated positional release (FPR) or progressive inhibition of neuromuscular structures (PINS) techniques. Some techniques have "modeled" the system that could describe the results obtained, such as, for example, the nociceptive model of Van Buskirk,[4] which correlates the thought of Still to techniques used by him, such as the Still technique.

Theoretically, the Still technique can be applied to all body tissues, since at the basis of SD there is a complex interaction between the neural elements (particularly nociceptors and the central nervous system), reprogramming of nervous patterns, myofascial repair mechanisms and elastic memory, immunological, inflammatory and vascular changes.[4] Osteopathic cranial manipulative medicine (OCMM) is one of the most used systemic, and in some aspects controversial, approaches in osteopathy, but as described in this text, the treatment by operator/patient connection with the dynamics of fluids and involuntary rhythms (DyFIR) is a homeostatic approach, useful to intervene in the general adaptation syndrome, which in this model is related to a systemic disturbance of neural networks.

Developed by William Sutherland, a student of Still, OCMM has as its goal the normalization of nerve function and the reduction of stress factors that can act on neural networks through fluids, fascia, and the autonomic nervous system.[53]

Although the therapeutic mechanisms have not been fully demonstrated, some research on the application of this technique, such as the work of Cutler, showed the effect of compression of the fourth ventricle (CV4) on sleep latency and reducing sympathetic nervous activity.[54]

## Objectives

The neurological model is concerned with the nervous matrix; therefore, assessment and treatment using this model will put special emphasis on the autonomic and sensorimotor neural network through: (1) global DyFIR evaluation; (2) segmental evaluation for the verification of aberrant reflex activities; and (3) local evaluation aimed at SD detection and assessment of the correlation of SD with the possible overload of the neural network, and central or peripheral sensitization associated with signs of acute and chronic pain.

The therapeutic application of the neurological model focuses on the elimination of nociceptive stimuli, and the equilibration of neural inputs and the reduction of excessive mechanical hyperactivity. The goal is to restore normal (optimal) neural function. Restoring or optimizing neural functions of integration and regulation will improve the efficiency of the associated structural, vascular, metabolic, and behavioral functions. This will help to maximize the patient's potential to adapt and regain optimal health.[4]

In light of these considerations, the integration of neural systems allows nociceptive stimuli to be reflected in the neuromusculoskeletal system. The objective is, therefore, to act on the communication between the peripheral nociceptive input and central cortical remodulation through the restoration of tissue viability and therefore the reduction of sensitizing and/or activating substances of nociceptors. This produces a local and distant reflex response of the autonomic nervous system as well as a balancing action on the motor predictive system and remodulation of the nocifensive reflexes.

## Indications and contraindications

In general, osteopathic manipulative treatment (OMT) focused on the neurological model is indicated for the relief of pain in patients who show overload of the neural network and/or central or peripheral sensitization related to signs of acute and chronic pain. Some examples are:

- nonspecific chronic lumbar pain

- chronic disorders associated with whiplash

- myofascial syndromes

- chronic muscle tension headache.

OMT can also be used as a supplement to medical treatment for musculoskeletal dysfunctions that can occur in patients diagnosed with rheumatologic, orthopedic, and neurological diseases, such as:

- fibromyalgia

- osteoarthritis

- rheumatoid arthritis

- chronic fatigue syndrome

- irritable bowel syndrome.

*Contraindications*: in addition to the general contraindications given in Chapter 1, we must mention bone marrow syndromes related to myelitis or spinal tumors, or extrinsic conditions such as trauma and fractures, as well as active infectious processes such as herpes zoster.

## Principles and methods of assessment

### Premise

Prior to performing the osteopathic assessment using the neurological model, it may be necessary to conduct a general clinical examination of the nervous system and any possible deficits, such as the examination of sensitivity, motility and reflexes.

We can also apply specific tests of the meningeal or peripheral root component, such as the valsalva, Lasègue and Wasserman maneuver and neuro-biomechanical tests.[55] Qualitative, quantitative, and affective assessments can help to understand pain from the organic point of view.

During the osteopathic evaluation in this model we must keep in mind the three primary aspects contingent of the neural networks, namely:

1. the burden of nociceptive stimuli as an allostatic load source

2. the viscerosomatic and somatovisceral correlations as propagation of spinal facilitation

3. the influence they can have on the stability of the movement dynamic predictive system or vice versa.

The observation of posture can help us understand if there are musculoskeletal areas that can disrupt the nervous system through excessive nociceptive and/or proprioceptive load. The osteopath will assess and consider these characteristics during the postural and articular evaluation, searching for and identifying the structural factors that may be associated specifically to peripheral or central sensitization, or that can nurture such neural processes.

The osteopath will then evaluate each arthrodial, myofascial, and skeletal SD that can serve as a nociceptive load through the lymphatic, vascular, and nervous systems. If found, the primary specific correlation must be sought in the tissues, such as likely pain generators, identifying the eventual relationship between the presentation of pain and neurological, myotomal, and sclerotomal patterns. Kuchera,[40] writing about the osteopathic management of patients with chronic pain, shows the importance of the recognition of dysfunctions caused by sclerotomal and myotomal patterns, described among others in the *Glossary of Osteopathic Terminology*.[56] The author describes how some somatic responses have been well documented in some persistent pain syndromes in which SD may have causative, reactive, or perpetuating characters, or a combination of these pathophysiologic mechanisms.

Therefore, musculoskeletal SDs could, over time, result first in peripheral (PS) and subsequently in central (CS) sensitization, if they persist. Trigger points are often found in the hypertonic antigravity muscles, which, when subjected to overload, can create referred pain in tissue patterns detected by palpation.[57,58] In response, the antagonist muscles may be weak in strength tests. These phenomena have been related to the presence of segmental spinal facilitation. So the presence of several altered peripheral inputs may produce a downward adaptive response influencing pain in the peripheral pattern, like the somatosomatic reflex.[40] If during assessment the primary nociceptive load is of biomechanical postural order, the tests described in Chapter 4 will be the preferred choice, as well as the integration of the biomechanical model with the neurological model.

## Useful clues during history taking

The signs detected during the history and physical examination allow correlating a musculoskeletal disorder to the sensitization phenomenon. Nijs and colleagues[59] have clearly established the parameters to be detected in sensitized patients. In fact, they proposed the association between some clinical disorders and increased risk of central sensitization, which can be useful to the osteopath during the assessment phase. In his study Nijs has described guidelines to the recognition of the symptoms described by the patient, correlated to the presence of CS, which show high responsiveness to various stimuli, such as mechanical pressure, temperature, stress, emotions, etc., and a low tolerance of the body to any kind of physical, chemical, and emotional stressors.

These guidelines can be extremely useful to the osteopath who faces a clinical picture with probable neural sensitization. Another important clue is the occurrence of a condition of pain threshold decrease during exercise. Physiologically, exercise raises the nociceptive threshold when running and about 30 minutes later with the release of opioids.[60] If the patient reports that during exercise the pain is constant, this could indicate a decrease in non-nociceptive modulation due to the descendant inhibitory pathways.[61] Butler[62] also reminds us that clinical conditions with CS often report:

- hyperalgesia

- allodynia

- pain evoked by emotions

- sudden recrudescence after rest or after being subjected to therapeutic treatments.

It remains clear that even in the presence of any medical diagnosis, or of descriptive symptoms that indicate the presence of CS, it is the osteopath's task to determine the most appropriate treatment plan.

## Model selection

The neurological model selection procedure (see Chapter 9) leads the osteopath to detect neural aberrations that undermine adaptive capacity, as well as the evocation of neurological activation forces to engage during treatment (Box 5.1).

### Box 5.1

Selection of the neurological model

The osteopath selects the neurological model after a review of the information obtained from medical history, clinical and osteopathic evaluation. The operator also observes the constitutional characteristics of the person, for example, an ectomorphic somatotype, in addition to the chronobiological phase and modality in which signs and symptoms present (see Chapter 8). The osteopath takes into account the following elements:

- Changes in sensation (paresthesia, dysesthesia, allodynia, etc.)

- Neuralgias

- Radiculopathies

- Autonomic disorders (hyperthermia, perspiration, etc.)

- Disorders of the sense organs

- Structures subject to fluid overload, such as the meningeal fascia[1]

- The brain, the spinal cord, peripheral nerves, ganglia, and plexuses

- The integumentary system

- Overloaded neural function, particularly in its exteroceptive, proprioceptive, and interoceptive components, components responsible for coordination, levels of nociception and sensitization.

The fascial compartment evaluation of the neurological model is performed through the fascial compartments test (FCT) of the meningeal fascia (see Chapter 3 and Fig. 1.7). Evaluation of the adaptive (compensated/decompensated) capacity is noted through the FCS testing and comprehensive evaluation of DyFIR (see Chapter 3). This information is also integrated with the assessment of dysfunctions (see Chapter 2); these dysfunctions are at the expense of the neural function representative areas (brain nuclei, autonomic ganglia and plexuses, peripheral nerves, etc.). The integration of this information about the person being treated allows targeting the treatment to a maximalist or minimalist focus.

#### Reference

1. Willard FH, Fossum C, Standley PR. The fascial system of the body. In: Chila A, editor. Foundations of osteopathic medicine. 3rd ed. Philadelphia: Lippincott Williams and Wilkins; 2010. ch. 7.

In addition, during evaluation the osteopath will observe the cutaneous vasculature, skin color, and some characteristic signs that may indicate the presence of hypersensitivity of the C fibers or reflex sympathetic hyperreactivity. A skin warmer than normal in the painful area and with thermal sensitivity to heat may indicate hypersensitivity mediated by C fibers, while a greater involvement of the sympathetic system will give signs such as local skin hypothermia, leading to vasoconstriction and reduced local blood flow, sweating, edema, tissue stiffness, trophic disorders of the skin, skin adnexa, and muscles.

Both cases may present hyperalgesia, but not sensory deficits as a sign of frank neuropathic pain. If there is spontaneous pain, it may be the typical neuralgic pain of some post-herpetic neuralgias, or some cases of central pain,[63] which go beyond osteopathic skills are still important to remember, considering that in these pathologies the skin may appear cold due to the reaction of the sympathetic system.

### Table 5.1
Medical diagnoses associated with an increased risk of central sensitization (CS)

| Medical diagnoses that may present CS | Characteristic or plausible signs of the presence of CS |
|---|---|
| • Subacute and chronic disorders associated with whiplash | • Hyperalgesia |
| • Temporomandibular disorders | • Allodynia |
| • Nonspecific chronic low back pain | • Pain evoked by emotions |
| • Chronic muscle tension headache | • Sudden recrudescence after resting |
| • Rheumatoid arthritis | • Sudden recrudescence after being subjected to therapeutic treatments |
| • Fibromyalgia | • Hypersensitivity to: |
| • Osteoarthritis |   – sounds |
| • Chronic fatigue syndrome |   – odors |
| • Irritable bowel syndrome |   – light |
| • Myofascial pain syndrome |   – touch |
| |   – variation of temperature |
| |   – allergens |
| |   – pressure (mechanical) |
| | • Tiredness upon waking |
| | • Sleep disorders and/or nonrestorative sleep |
| | • Fatigue |
| | • Difficulty concentrating |
| | • Sensation of swelling (e.g., leg) |
| | • Numbness |
| | • Paresthesia |
| | • Constant pain during exercise |

Modified from: Nijs J, Van Houdenhove B, Oostendorp RA. Recognition of central sensitization in patients with musculoskeletal pain: application of pain neurophysiology in manual therapy practice. Man Ther. 2010;15(2):135–41.

On palpation the osteopath will assess the tone and tissue texture and the eventual changes that may occur in the upright and/or supine position. In general, the supine position is favored for palpation of the deep tissues.[29] During the evaluation of the tissues we can understand how the detected SDs can affect the neural network. For example, if when applying a pressure less than 4 kg/cm$^2$ on the paraspinal tissues pain is evoked in the symptomatic and in remote areas, there may be CS present, or some other overload of the neural network.[59,64,65] The presence of pain and proprioceptive and muscular alteration without any trauma, indicates the presence of "preparatory" factors of a dysfunctional nature, reducing the adaptive capacity of the neural network, and preparing it for future sensitization. Table 5.1 summarizes what has been described.

## Global tests

### Fascial compartments test (FCT) of the meningeal fascia

This test aims to perceive the longitudinal fluctuation harmony or any changes to the meningeal fascia. The test is described in Chapter 1 and can show reductions or deviations of fascial mobility that directly or indirectly may affect the biomechanical stability, or fluid flow and pressure of the neural network.

### Fascial compensation scheme (FCS) test

As described in Chapters 3 and 6, preferably through the tissue tests (tension/laxity) in the transitional areas (TA), we can evaluate health by looking at the organization of the neutral, compensated or decompensated FCS. The finding of a decompensated FCS, indicating a high allostatic load, if correlated with the patient's history and/or symptoms present in Table 5.1, suggests the presence of a CS. A decompensated FCS, with no alternation of the atlanto-occipital joint/cranial diaphragm and the cervical-thoracic junction/upper thoracic diaphragm can sometimes indicate a neural overload with alteration of the interoceptive processes and directs the osteopath to proceed with local and subsequent tests of structure/function inhibition (see below).

### DγFIR global assessment test (DγFIR GA)

It is of fundamental importance in any therapeutic intervention to be able to recognize the normal functionality, the normal patterns of tension and the normal elasticity or range of movement. This implies feel and the ability to recognize in the patient the different characteristics of intrinsic and extrinsic mobility of different tissues, which allows the osteopath to distinguish between healthy and tissue, including normal and abnormal tension patterns. During the perceptual palpation phase traditionally defined as "generally listening," the osteopath evaluates rhythm fragmentation on the vertical orientation of the perceived body in some areas with latero-lateral fluctuations, in others with inertia and in others with DγFIR "spasm" (see Chapter 3).

### DγFIR local assessment test (DγFIR LA)

This passive listening test is focused on the vitality and the sliding motility of the different connective/fascial planes. This test is used to evaluate the body as a kind of road map for the pursuit of dysfunction. The operator's hand is positioned on areas of the body that he or she considers to be related (directly or indirectly) to pain, or on the tissues which may be involved in excessive allostatic load present in the patient (such as the body cavity formed between two transition areas that were found to be decompensated in the FCS test). By placing his or her hands on the (local) pain-producing areas, the osteopath places himself or herself in an afferent state, and assesses the quality of involuntary rhythms to understand the current state of "health."

The tissue areas that we will detect as having greater diminution will manifest a fragmentation of the rhythm and inertia, also perceived as a "latero-lateral fluctuation." These areas will have priority in the verification of the presence of SD. The osteopath proceeds one area at a time to detect any drag or inertia of perceived movement. In some cases, all the tension patterns at different distances lead to the same point or on two or three major areas of convergence, considered connective/fascial tension indicators. The osteopaths tends to consider as priority areas those where the tissue response manifests increased inertia.[66]

## Segmental tests

### Viscerosomatic and somatovisceral reflex activity

The evaluation of the viscerosomatic reflexes is based on the correlation of the patient's history, which includes the presence of remote or present visceral dysfunctions and the relative palpatory identification of somatic dysfunctions presumably related. The patient is preferably in a sitting position, or lying in a comfortable position. The osteopath can perform the following tests:

- *Red reflex test*:[29,67] this procedure is aimed at identifying the changes in tissue texture, which may be associated with the presence of viscerosomatic reflexes. The osteopath substantially evaluates the vasomotor reactivity as a spinal segmental facilitation index commonly associated with acute SD. This includes mainly the presence of aberrant viscerosomatic reflexes. The osteopath then observes the reduction/whitening time or eventual increase/persistence of redness and notes the time required for the skin to return to normal and whether this occurs in a homogeneous way. In acute SDs there is typically a skin site with persistent reddening, while in chronic SDs the skin tends to whiten (Fig. 5.4).

- *Skin drag test*:[29,67] this procedure is used to assess sudomotor hyper-reactivity, which indicates spinal facilitation and viscerosomatic reflexes associated with SD. The osteopath glides the fingertips lightly over the paraspinal tissues. Areas with sudomotor hyper-reactivity indicative of acute SD will be wetter and will produce more friction to gliding compared to adjacent tissues. The areas with possible presence of chronic SD appear less wet or even dry and provide less friction (Fig. 5.5).

- *Beal's compression test*:[29,67] this is the principal test used by Beal to detect the presence of reflex autonomic hyper-reactivity in the tissues. The test is correlated with sympathetic hyper-responsiveness and in clinical trials performed by Beal is used on the paraspinal tissues of the entire spine, with particular attention to costal-transverse areas of the thoracic spine. Although the following example illustrates the process on the thoracic segments, this test can be applied in each area, given that the autonomic activity is an integrated process that occurs throughout the body.

The patient should be in a supine position to reduce the activity of the superficial muscular layers, but an acutely patient is allowed to choose the position of maximum comfort. Assuming that the patient is in the supine position, the osteopath stands on the side of the paraspinal tissues to be examined. The contact is with the fingertips on the paravertebral tissue, to which a slight upward thrust is applied. Using the principle of layered palpation, the operator evaluates tissues at each level, comparing them with the upper and lower segment. At each level it is possible to simultaneously apply a spring test to identify the presence of mobility restriction of the segment in question.

To examine the other side, the osteopath moves to the other side of the patient. The presence of active viscerosomatic reflexes with high influence on somatic dysfunction can be identified by the perception of an abnormal restrictive barrier, even without positional asymmetry, but which involves more than two adjacent spinal segments. In these segments there will be a tissue texture alteration with hyper-reactivity of the deep muscle tissues (Fig. 5.6).

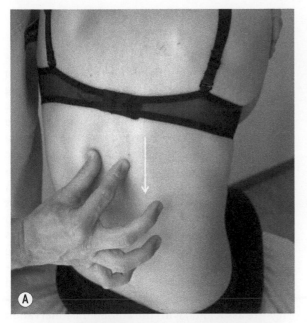

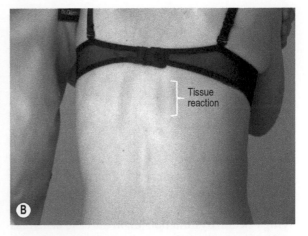

**Fig. 5.4**
Red reflex test. (A) The osteopath rubs the paraspinal tissues three times, and observes the tissue reaction (B).

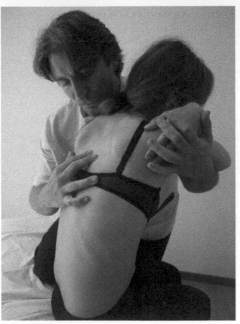

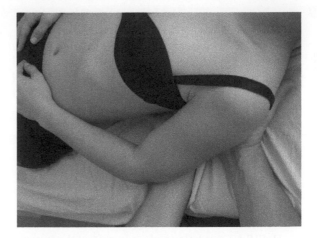

**Fig. 5.5**
Skin drag test. The osteopath slips his or her fingertips lightly on the paraspinal tissues assessing the degree of friction.

**Fig. 5.6**
Beal's compression test. The osteopath is positioned on the ipsilateral side to the paraspinal tissues being tested. His or her hands are placed on the table with palms facing upward, the fingertips contacting the paravertebral tissue to be tested, to which is applied a slight push upward to assess the density, texture, and tension of each layer, comparing them with the paraspinal upper and lower segments.

- *Reflex points*: all areas that are painful to palpation respond to, or are associated with, a certain degree of imbalance, dysfunction or reflex activity, resulting in acute stretching or chronic adaptation in the soft tissue.

Several authors have described reproducible points, but not always correlated with spinal segmental innervation, such as Chapman's points,[68] Jones's tender points,[69] myofascial trigger points,[70] Jarricot's reflex dermalgias,[71] and Head's zones.[72] The presence and identification of reflex points in the tissues offer further confirmation of the underlying visceral dysfunction (or, in the case of myofascial trigger points, of a somatic disturbance that can affect the viscera). The same test can also be applied after the treatment, as confirmation of the resolution. Otherwise, the occurrence of their persistence indicates the priority of this visceral dysfunction or processes that can generate it.

## Local tests: somatic dysfunction detection

The osteopath proceeds with SD evaluation that was considered to be the major priority during global assessment. The tissues in these dysfunctional areas, because they are "anchored" to the neural network imbalance, in addition to the characteristics of the TART (see Chapter 2), may manifest:

- radiation of pain not related to the somatic distribution

- primary hyperalgesia or generalized symptoms

- DyFIR LA not balanced, or inertia of the present movement.

Anatomical and clinical knowledge will allow the osteopath to determine the different correlations between the dysfunctions found and their "weight" in the disorders manifested by the patient. Knowledge of the course of nerves, fascial patterns, muscles and all other facilities will enhance clinical decision-making and help the osteopath to use mobility tests deemed appropriate.

## Test of somatic dysfunction hierarchization: the presence of co-dominance

This test can detect the hierarchical relationship among the identified SDs. This test has been described in Chapter 2 and is a method of correlating viscerosomatic, somatovisceral and somatosomatic SDs; in this model it is used in order to verify the presence of multiple primary dysfunctional areas. We know that somatovisceral and viscerosomatic reflexes are one of the leading integrated mechanisms of body functions that tie closely together, several devices with each other. They are complex interconnections influenced by many factors such as ascending messages, and descending influences from higher centers mediated by processing of the CNS.[73-75] Osteopaths have shown particular clinical interest in the identification of SD associated with organic pathology.[76] The majority of these findings are associated with the autonomic innervation pattern.[77]

However, the nervous system executes and facilitates integrated and dynamic processes, and therefore it is not always possible to relate in a unique way the evaluation of a precise spinal area to a precise visceral area.[78] Nelson and Glonek remind us that in patients in whom visceral disease has been established concomitantly with mechanical dysfunction, it is sometimes impossible (or unnecessary) to discern the primacy between viscerosomatic or somatovisceral dysfunction.[67] Therefore, we recommend using these data and any maps found in many books of osteopathy as an orientation point, but to evaluate and always correlate what is detected.

Moreover, in patients with signs of aberrations of generalized neural input, the body will tend to create primary and adaptive dysfunctions in a different manner. If for example, a dysfunction in the T1–T2 region is identified and visceral palpation identifies a dysfunction in the right iliac fossa, it is advisable to correlate these findings, albeit a direct neuro-segmentary correlation is absent. The focus therefore is on detecting whether the nociceptive input influenced the visceral system, creating organ dysfunction or vice versa. In this case, the osteopath correlates dysfunctional areas that are clinically relevant to palpation. In accordance with the principles described in this model, these may identify primary areas, both somatic and visceral, we cannot necessarily rule out the existence of somatosomatic co-primarities.

The next decision-making process is to determine if there are conditions that will help us to choose between a maximalist or minimalist therapeutic approach.

The test is performed by taking into account two dysfunctions that are primary (whether somatic or visceral). Inhibition is given through a slight tissue pressure on the area being tested,[79] in the following way:

- The osteopath applies inhibitory pressure on the first SD and evaluates possible changes to the second (increase/decrease of the tone, pain, sudomotor activities, tissue texture changes); the same maneuver is performed by inhibiting the second and monitoring the first.

- If during each test, each SD subjected to inhibition results in an improvement of the other's parameters, then we have co-dominance, and the test is positive; in practice, in the presence of CS, the body presents with a high allostatic load that is distributed and propagated through more local adaptations (Fig. 5.7). These adaptations show their multiple "primacy." This test is therefore used in the decisional algorithm of the structure/function interdependence.

## Structure/function inhibition test (SFIT) specific to the neurological model

The sensitization process requires a reworking that uniquely and segmentally engages a tissue area. Although from an osteopathic point of view any peripheral insult still creates a readjustment of the entire body unit, in search of the interaction with

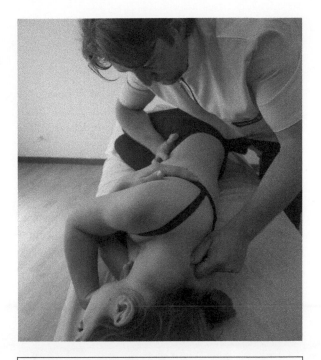

**Fig. 5.7**
Test of somatic dysfunction (SD) hierarchization. In the first phase the osteopath applies gentle inhibitory pressure to the first clinically relevant SD (in the example, the T1–T2 area) and monitors the changes that occur to the second (in this case in the right iliac fossa). The same maneuver is performed by applying inhibitory pressure to the second SD (right iliac fossa) and watching the first (T1–T2).

the person and his discomfort, the osteopath uses both local and global access, knowing that both osteopathic homeostatic approaches, with effects similar to meditation movements,[80] and the specific osteopathic techniques[81] may produce beneficial effects on CS.

The osteopath compares the medical history data that "speak" for the presence of CS and/or PS, with the clues acquired in clinical evaluation as well as from global, segmental, and local tests. In the presence of one or more of the following conditions the solution will be a dysfunctional framework where the three autonomic, nociceptive, and predictive motor systems are compromised:

- FCS decompensated

- DyFIR GA or LA not balanced with the presence of hyperalgesia in many dysfunctional areas detected as primary, both near to and far from the primary area

- Presence of SD that on palpation evokes generalized symptoms

- Presence of tissue changes with persistence of aberrant viscerosomatic or somatovisceral reflexes related to acute and/or chronic clinical pictures.

To select a specific therapeutic minimalist or maximalist approach, the osteopath will perform the SFIT specific to the neurological model. The test is divided in two phases (Fig. 5.8):

1. First, the osteopath assesses nociceptive function, evaluating the clinical signs of CS (Fig. 5.8A). The test assesses the pain threshold to pressure at sites distant from the dysfunctional area. A pressure less than 4 kg/cm$^2$ is applied in areas distant from the symptomatic area. For example, if the dysfunctional area is present in the cervical region, the test can be performed on the lumbar, gluteal, or lower limbs area. The patient is required to give a value on a numerical scale from 0 to 10 to the perceived pain.

2. The osteopath relates the degree of CS (Fig. 5.8B) and the index of stress function load (neural overload of nociceptive input) with identified SD, as follows:

With one hand the osteopath applies direct/indirect vector parameters on the dysfunctional area and with the other applies a pressure of 4 kg/cm$^2$

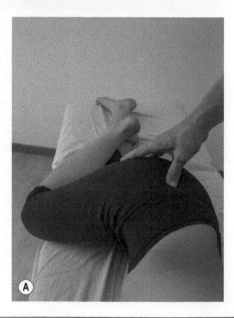
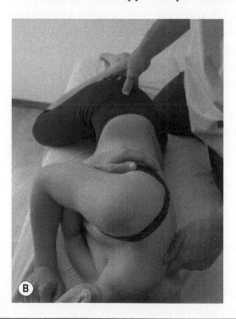

**Fig. 5.8**

SFIT (Specific to the neurological model). (A) A pressure less than 4 kg/cm² is applied in an area separated from the symptomatic area (in the figure the pressure is applied in the right gluteal area) and the patient is required to give the perceived pain a value on a numerical scale from 0 to 10. (B) The somatic dysfunction (SD) selected is inhibited (in the T1 area) and simultaneously the same pressure is applied at a distance, again asking the patient to numerically assess the perceived pain in the right gluteal area.

on distant areas chosen in phase 1. If the patient reports a reduction of the score, this can be interpreted as a reduction of the CS, giving an indication of the structure dominance over function and guiding the osteopath toward a minimalist approach focused on clinically relevant SD.

If the application of direct/indirect vector parameters to the dysfunctional area does not reduce the degree of CS, leaving the score unchanged, we have evidence of function dominance over structure (positive test), which guides the osteopath to a maximalist approach with homeostatic techniques. In the case of co-positive dominance noted during the local test, the SFIT can be performed on individual SDs, and can be considered as supportive.

Figure 5.9 shows the flowchart that summarizes the decision-making process that guided the osteopath in the choice of therapeutic approach.

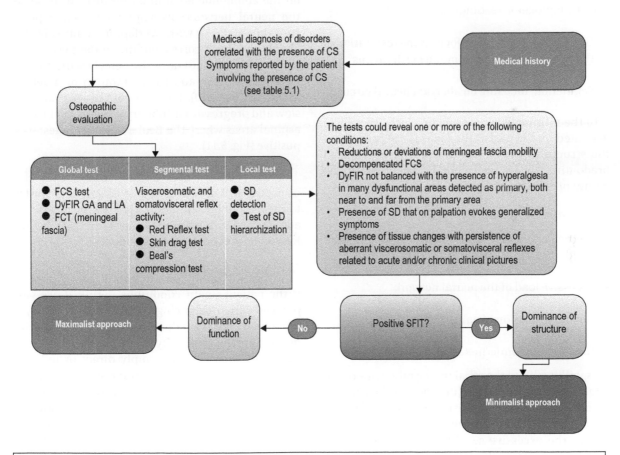

**Fig. 5.9**
The decisional algorithm that allows for making the optimal therapeutic choice between minimalist and maximalist approach. The beginning of the diagram coincides with the history where the osteopath can find clues for the presence of neural network dysfunctions. The osteopath proceeds with the evaluation where, through global, segmental, and local tests, and the evaluations for conditions that may indicate the presence of sensitization, confirmation by the SFIT will assist in making the choice of a maximalist or minimalist approach.

## Principles and methods of treatment

As a result of the decision-making process and the SFIT, the osteopath comes to the choice of the specific therapeutic approach.

In applying the maximalist approach, the aim is to treat "the parts through the whole thing," using a global, segmental, and local focus intended to rebalance the nociceptive, autonomic and predictive-motor systems, preferably through the use of adaptogenic techniques:

- Global/local, where the focus is the restoration of the neural, fluid, and immune mechanisms

- Segmental, focusing on aberrant neural circuits.

In the minimalist approach, in which "the whole is treated by the parts," the focus is the primacy of the structure, where local adaptation is reflected predominantly in the general adaptation of the neural network.

### Maximalist approach

Place the patient in a comfortable position, in order to avoid:

- excessive load of the neural network

- further evocation of pain

- further autonomic/metabolic effort.

This will facilitate the rebalancing processes of the afferent receptor systems (muscle spindles, nociceptors, etc.) and the improvement of the functions related to and coordinated by them. Frequently, due to the excessive sensitivity perceived by the patient, the osteopath cannot perform a technique that uses the evocative area of pain as a fulcrum for access to DyFIR; the osteopath then will choose global techniques of DyFIR to promote a general reflex autonomic response, for example, through the median line technique (see Chapters 3 and 6) or homeostatic techniques, such as CV4, EV4, and/or rolling of the temporals (see Chapters 3 and 6), to produce a global autonomic neural, vascular and immune effect. In the balancing of DyFIR is appropriate to monitor the patient's pain and, if required, the patient can change position to avoid the evocation of pain and decrease nociceptive afferent activity.

Sometimes vibrational techniques may be used on the autonomic abdominal plexuses to balance the neural network. By applying a gentle pressure (bimanual or with overlapping palms) in the abdominal areas corresponding to the plexus, the osteopath waits until he or she perceives the release of tissue tensions and the restoration of inherent motility[82] (Fig. 5.10). The osteopath can also apply a slow and progressive inhibitory pressure in the paraspinal areas where the Beal compression test was positive (Fig. 5.11).

In the presence of a decompensated FCS, the osteopath will normalize it (see Chapter 6) in order to reduce the present allostatic load in the fascial, autonomic, and nociceptive systems (see below, Rationale, mechanisms and evidence).

### Minimalist approach

If the patient's pain conditions permit it, we can proceed with a balancing DyFIR by using the dysfunctional area as a palpatory fulcrum of access. By monitoring the sensitivity caused by palpation and tissue rhythm, we might apply direct or indirect vector parameters to verify improvement of inertia or spasm and rhythm harmonization. This can be perceived as an overcoming of the perception of "latero-lateral fluctuation" and the global harmonic oscillation (longitudinal fluctuations), from which we may see the emergence of the neutral state. By maintaining rhythmic oscillatory contact we wait for the tissue expansion and fluid balancing point which finalize the therapeutic process through a vasomotor, autonomic, and mechanical tissue rebalancing (see Chapter 3).

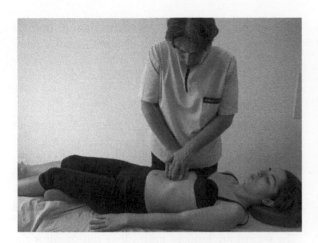

**Fig. 5.10**
Application of a vibrational release technique in the epigastric area.

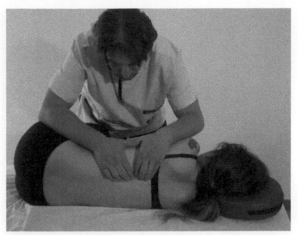

**Fig. 5.11**
Application of inhibitory pressure on the paraspinal tissues, which showed a previously positive Beal compression test. The patient is in the lateral position on the opposite side of the tissue to be treated, the legs are brought down and resting against the osteopath's abdomen, who contacts the area to be treated and, by shifting its center of gravity posteriorly, applies an inhibitory pressure on the tissues.

The variants pressure force, pace, and frequency are the basis of an input that can be administered for stimulation or inhibition of neural and reflex activity. The choice of technique directed to the primary or clinically relevant SD depends on what the tissues allow, but aims at the modulation of the responses of the autonomic system, to reduce the afferent load and resulting reflex efferent responses of the tissues. Generally, although this is not an absolute rule, it is advisable not to use thrust techniques, as they may aggravate the symptoms.[84] The treatment of viscerosomatic and somatovisceral reflexes was developed in osteopathy as a means of reducing neural afferent responses to SD, to stop the reflex circuits, influence the viscera through the stimulation of the somatovisceral effects and vice versa, as well as reduce the preconditioning potential effects of stressors. We can therefore act on autonomic multi-segmental reflexes by treating SDs detected in visceral areas through visceral techniques.[85]

### Driver sensory technique

Sometimes we find co-dominance of musculoskeletal SD and visceral SD (or reflex SD in other soft tissues); therefore, the treatments go beyond the reduction of the paraspinal tissues' reactivity to a remodulation feedback of the spinal mechanisms and medullary interconnections described earlier in this chapter. Once the osteopath has identified a co-primarity between the visceral SD (and reflex SD in other soft tissues) and musculoskeletal SD with peculiar alteration of the paraspinal and costotransverse tissue texture, the treatment can be done with a combined technique, performed with an anterior–posterior approach based on a guided sensory approach called the driver sensory technique (Fig. 5.12): an inhibitory, slow and progressive compression is applied, using a "motor" hand, while a "sensory" hand perceives the change in the treated tissues (both co-dominant SDs).

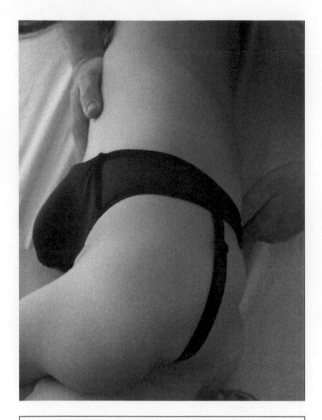

**Fig. 5.12**
Application of driver sensory technique.
Musculoskeletal somatic dysfunction (SD) is present in the T4–T5 paraspinal area, while visceral SD is present in the soft tissues in the epigastric region. The right hand in the epigastric region is the "motor" hand, applying a slow inhibitory and progressive compression, while the left hand is the "sensory" hand that detects the change in the paraspinal tissues.

The procedure is of variable time duration, depending on the condition of the tissues and the permitted load tolerated by the patient. Treatment of the reflex areas will be useful in all acute or chronic conditions where the clinical situation does not allow treatment with articulatory techniques, because of intense pain or poor health conditions. This can happen in the case of a bedridden patient with poor health status and the presence of organic pathologies.[29] Sometimes dysfunctional primacy is detected in areas relating to Chapman's reflex neurolymphatic points. In these instances the osteopath can proceed with direct treatment.[68]

## Functional techniques

Of great usefulness in the minimalist treatment with neurological focus is functional technique.[86] This technique was promoted by Harold V. Hoover in 1969 and reprised by Charles Bowles in 1981, to describe what is achieved when the tissues associated with a joint in dysfunction are placed in a resting position, defined as "dynamic neutral." The technique ignores pain (does not monitor the tissue quality by palpating the tender point) as a guide to the comfort position, and relies instead on the reduction of the palpated tone of stressed tissues (hypertonic/with spasm), while the body (or part thereof) is placed in a position of balance, or harmony, relative to all the potential directions of movement.

In performing the technique, while one hand is the "listening hand" and the other produces movement, the tissues are brought into a position of maximum comfort with respect to all the possible directions of movement (i.e., the dynamic neutral point), in which the various directional components add up in order to get the best possible position. The process of "stacking" can be done by evaluating successively the comfort position relative to the various directions of motion, starting from the point of comfort taken by the previous assessment. After maintaining the dynamic neutral position until the attainment of a feeling of warmth, pulsation, or greater well-being, the entire sequence is repeated at least once more, with variations of the positions of comfort as a result of the changes caused by the first application of the sequence.

Functional technique, as opposed to structural approaches, certainly presents some advantages in the treatment of acute, elderly, bedridden, or postoperative patients, since it can be performed in any position, with minimal traumatic input, and can be repeated without causing reactions. Furthermore, the sensitivity of this technique, given the use of minimum movements, makes it applicable to any part of the body, since it does not rely directly on articular range of motion, but on the tissues and the neuromotor mechanisms. It is also successfully applied in chronic dysfunctions.

## PINS

The local approach can also make use of the progressive inhibition of the neuromusculoskeletal structures (PINS).[87] The PINS technique is a variant of traditional inhibition techniques where, through progressive inhibition, sensitivity/tenderness caused by two co-primary SDs detected on the same body segment (e.g., the skin areas related to the course of a nerve) are normalized.

The operator determines the anatomical path that connects the two co-primary SDs:

- Nervous: through direct connections, the region of innervation or overlaps

- Muscular: through origins and insertions, overlapping and contiguity

- Fascial: through specific tissues (dura mater, fascia lata, and so on), septa, and overlaps

- Ligamentous: through the insertions and the relationship with muscles and nerves

- Articular: by shape and mechanical joint.

The emphasis is on the monitoring, during the procedure, of the tissue changes caused by the SD, which provide the basis for the palpatory evaluation and feedback given by the patient. The patient takes part in the treatment by describing his or her response in terms of sensitivity and quantitative perceived pain, i.e., the changes which occur gradually. The patient is in the comfort position. The treatment begins by palpating the two co-primary SDs and evaluating which of the two is perceived by the patient as more sensitive/painful (primary point) and which less sensitive/painful (terminal point). If, for instance, the co-primary SDs were detected on two cutaneous emergent areas of nervous segments, such as the peripheral nerve, we can find the primary point proximal to the trunk and the terminal point at the end of a branch of the nerve course.

We will therefore perform inhibition with similar purposes to those described by other authors, such as manipulation of peripheral and cranial nerves to promote freedom of movement of the nervous structure, optimal electric conduction, improved arterial-venous intraneural circulation, improved intraneural innervation, and normalized segmental and global response of the individual.[88,89]

If the co-primary SDs were to be detected in a muscle, the primary point would be at the level of the muscle belly and the terminal point in one of its insertions. For a frontal headache, the typical primary point could be the supraorbital foramen and the terminal point might be located in the suboccipital region, and so on. With the fingertips, the osteopath applies pressure simultaneously on the primary and terminal points, with an equal intensity sufficient to elicit an increase in sensitivity reported by the patient.

The patient may report greater sensitivity at the primary point. The osteopath monitors the patient's feelings, reassuring him or her. While maintaining a constant pressure on the terminal point, the osteopath increases the pressure on the primary point and constantly requests the patient's feedback regarding any increasing or decreasing sensitivity. If inhibition is used properly, after a transient increase there follows a decrease in sensitivity until its eventual disappearance. The duration of pressure is variable from seconds to minutes. After this phase, maintaining position and pressure, the osteopath adds a new pressure with another finger simultaneously in a new point (secondary point), about 3 cm away from the primary spot along the predetermined anatomical course in the direction of the terminal point. The osteopath will then apply pressure to the secondary point similar to that which is simultaneously being applied to the primary point.

If in the secondary point the patient experiences sensitivity equal to or greater than the primary point, the osteopath can remove the pressure from the primary point and maintain a constant pressure on the secondary point for about 30 seconds. The secondary point now becomes the new primary point and the osteopath continues in the direction of the terminal point, until the last secondary point, at a distance of 2 cm from the terminal point, has been completely inhibited, while the end point is treated through the constant pressure maintained throughout the therapeutic procedure.

The PINS technique is very suitable for those disorders whose discomfort persists despite various attempts at correction. The application of PINS fully meets the local (as an application) and global (as feedback) therapeutic focus required by the minimalist approach, given its characteristics as perceptual, selective and progressive inhibitory pressure, the monitoring of the tissue hypersensitivity by the neural network, and the feedback given by the patient on what is "felt," as well as the particular use in acute as well as chronic relapsing situations. Moreover, the technique can be used alone during local treatment, or, due to its versatility, can be combined with other techniques. We can, for example, use the strain and counterstrain,[90] facilitated positional release,[91] balanced ligamentous tension,[92] and Still[93] techniques to further reduce the afferent nociceptive load coming from the neuromuscular, fascial and ligamentous structures.

## Articulatory technique (LVHA), high-velocity and low-amplitude thrust (HVLA)

Depending on the accessibility of the SD, we can use articulatory technique, which is a technique that uses low velocity and high amplitude (LVHA), or high-velocity and low amplitude (HVLA) thrust. During the use of LVHA, the pressure-force, rhythm, frequency, and rotation variations, if combined in an optimal manner, can induce an improvement of myofascial restrictions and reduce venous and lymphatic congestion[94] by reducing the presence of nociceptive sensitizing substances. HVLA,[95] used skillfully in the minimalist approach, can restore restrictions of the joint surfaces and capsular mobility, and reduce muscular tension, which is the source of the nociceptive alterations. Experimental evidence[96] indicates that manipulation has a primary impact on the paraspinal tissue afferents, on the motor control system, and on pain elaboration.

## Considerations regarding the clinical course

If the patient reports generalized symptoms in the second session, we must re-verify the presence of sensitization. The osteopathic treatment creates systemic changes; it is a stream where there is a continuous and progressive correlation, moment by moment, between the modifications that the osteopath monitors and the sensations felt by the patient. As a result, it is possible to detect the emergence of new malfunctions or signs that were previously latent, or worsening clinical presentations with generalized signs. In this author's view, patients with complex histories, characterized by various kinds of trauma, surgery, or suffering from chronic illnesses, may show signs of central sensitization at a later time during the course of treatment.

## Rationale, mechanisms, and evidence

It has long been assumed that manual therapy has a biological effect on the nervous system.[97] First and foremost, there is the breaking of the pain–spasm–pain cycle, in which pain leads to muscle hyperresponsiveness (spasm) and the spasm in turn leads to the exacerbation of pain. The scientific knowledge and understanding of muscular and nerve physiology has grown exponentially over the past few decades, with the advent of noninvasive methods of study in vivo. Today, the term "sensory-motor control" highlights the inseparable pair that exists between proprioceptive sensory feedback and motor control. Sensory inputs come from a variety of sources, and muscle spindles are a key input to the development of spinal and cortical sensory information.

There are two hypotheses, both based on the same idea, namely that the major excitatory input to the α-motor neuron pool leads to intense and sustained muscle activity. The rationale of OMT suggested by Korr is that treatment breaks the pain–spasm–pain cycle, reducing the monosynaptic stretch reflex. So far, few studies can confirm this hypothesis. A review by Clark[97] proposed that, in dysfunctional areas, the nociceptive afferents are able to directly transmit to excitatory interneurons and therefore to the α-motor neurons, resulting in greater muscle activation (spasm). However, the hypothesis that muscle spindles act as key anatomical structures involved in a feedforward cycle is analyzed. The cycle begins when the nociceptive fibers send excitatory input to the γ-motor neurons, which increases the sensitivity of muscle spindles.

This increase in the fusal sensitivity intensifies the fusal afferent activity and, consequently, increases the excitatory input to the α-motor neurons, terminating with the increase of muscle activity and pain. Clark, analyzing different studies, suggests that the effect of manual processing is due primarily to the reduction of the nociceptive input and consequent reflex remodulation. Treatment may thus affect the ascending nociceptive pathways (Fig. 5.13), resulting in a cortical remodeling, and the descending inhibitory and motor pathways linked to them. Experimental studies show that a peripheral mobilization takes effect through the involvement of descending inhibitory pathways rather than a local inhibitory reflex.[98] Even the effects of manual treatment on the autonomic nervous system are mediated by the integration of the ascending and descending system with the sympathetic nervous system.[99]

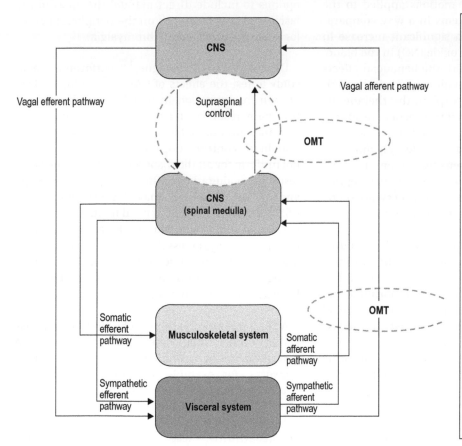

**Fig. 5.13**
Assumptions of the functional effects of manual therapy on nociceptive input attenuation, through the modulation of the spinal and supraspinal afferents. The resulting reduction in the tissue hyperexitability would then be a consequence of the reorganization of the supraspinal circuits. Modified from: King HH, Jänig W, Patterson MM. The science and clinical application of manual therapy. Edinburgh: Churchill Livingstone, Elsevier; 2011. fig. 16.4, p. 291.

The use of OMT can be directed to the modulation of conditions of *hypersympaticotonia* by treating the dysfunctions. Van Buskirk[4] points out that during indirect technique the activity of nociceptors and the subsequent release of substance P are reduced, obtaining a reduction of dysfunctional reflex activity at the spinal level, and a reduction of sympathetic arousal, and therefore minimizing the deleterious effect on vascular and lymphatic vasoconstriction, with a consequent greater nutrition to the tissues and the removal of inflammatory metabolites. The modulation of *hypersympaticotonia* was related to the reduction of pain,[100] the improvement of visceral and somatic functions,[101] and the healing potential.[102] According to Kuchera,[40] these are aspects of OMT that should be taken into account, especially in the osteopathic approach to chronic pain.

It also seems that fluid motions applied to the vascular and nervous systems in a way comparable to OMT[103] can cause a significant increase in the concentration of nitric oxide (NO) in the blood. These results combined with the beneficial effects shown in NO studies[104] provide a dynamic theoretical framework that could explain the therapeutic effects of OMT. Another important aspect resides in the correlation between the fascial system and the autonomic system;[105] the fascia is densely innervated by mechanoreceptors sensitive to manual pressure, and the stimulation of these sensory receptors has been shown to lead to a lowering of sympathetic tone and a decrease of local tissue viscosity.

Fascial inflammation is also proposed as a source of peripheral nociceptive input leading to CS in fibromyalgia.[106] The fascial dysfunction could be due to the insufficient production of growth hormone and dysfunction of the hypothalamic–pituitary–adrenal axis. It has been shown that fibroblasts in the fascial tissue, in response to tissue strain, secrete pro-inflammatory cytokines, particularly IL-6, resulting in a sensitizing effect given the rich fascial innervation. This concept allows us to understand the correlation between decompensated FCS and plausible presence of CS or PS as a mismatch of fascial planes, causing connective restrictions with reduction of

metabolic exchanges and increased allostatic load pertaining to the genesis of the general adaptation syndrome, with subsequent imbalance of the neural networks.

Recent biopsy studies using immune-histochemical staining techniques have found increased levels of collagen and inflammatory mediators in the connective tissue surrounding the muscle cells in patients with fibromyalgia. The inflammation of the fascia is similar to that described in conditions such as plantar fasciitis and lateral epicondylitis, and can best be described as a dysfunctional healing response. This may explain why NSAIDs and oral steroids are not effective in fibromyalgia. Inflammation and/or fascial dysfunction can therefore lead to CS in fibromyalgia. If this hypothesis is confirmed, it could significantly expand the treatment options to include direct manual therapies to the fascia and more research on the peripheral pathological aspects related to fibromyalgia.

Degenhardt and colleagues[107] performed a pilot study to test the effects of OMT on the biomarkers of pain in circulation in people with chronic low back pain, resulting in a decrease in the concentration and duration of biomarkers after OMT, greater than in the control group. The evidence, however, is not uniform for all the disorders that could possibly result in an alteration of the nociceptive processes, and not all conditions may develop compulsory CS.[108] Therefore, we do not need to uniquely associate chronic pain with central alteration processes, but should always assess the patient as a whole. There are, however, some indicators, such as the presence of trigger or tender points in areas of chronic pain, but with no frank structural pathologies.

A similar condition, often referred to as myofascial syndrome, should alert the osteopath to the determination of systemic perturbations of neural networks, for example, chronic muscle tension headaches associated with the possible presence of CS,[109] or, associations with frankly pathological conditions, such as rheumatoid arthritis and/or osteoarthritis. These are all phenomena of local dysfunction which over time can continuously activate polymodal nociceptors, and, secondarily, create central hyperactivation.[64,110] Often these patients can present with chronic orthopedic, rheumatologic, or neuro-musculoskeletal diseases of a chronic nature, and may have already received ineffective treatments. Knowing, therefore, the clinical condition and the presence of co-morbidities may provide useful information for the correct application of the model.

## Case study

Woman, 38 years old, Caucasian, employed, nonsmoker.

### Presenting complaint and past history

For about 5 months, after a collision associated with an attempted theft of the vehicle, she has suffered neck pain that extends from the neck and radiates into the left inferior orbit, to the mid-thoracic spine, occasionally to the shoulder and left arm during abduction or if the elbow rests on the table, but does not extend to the hand. The pain is present during the day, gets worse with movement, and is accompanied at times (such as on the day of the visit) by pain in the lower back, left buttock, and posterior left thigh, but the patient states the pain does not radiate to the lower leg. The pain disturbs sleep during movements in bed and gets worse when the patient wakes up. The pain is alleviated with the use of a cervical collar and ibuprofen. Sometimes there is nausea, blurred vision, dizziness, slow digestion, and postprandial fatigue.

### Hospital report

Distortion of the cervical spine.

### Diagnostic investigations

Cranial CT scan: negative. Cervical spine X-ray: flattening of the cervical spine. Echo Doppler supraortic trunk (TSA): arterial axes regularly explored for size and course bilaterally; regular caliber of the common carotid, with density of the *intima media* in accordance with established norms bilaterally. Left: bulb and bifurcation vessels without significant lesions. Right: findings similar to the left side. Patent vertebral artery with orthodromic flow in VO–V1 and V2 explored bilaterally (dominant left).

### Past medical history

Before the trauma the patient had no muscle disorders. In the past: intermittent stomach pains (no reflux) associated with irregular cycle (5 years before). Occasional premenstrual pain.

### Social and occupational history

Very active during work, but after the trauma is afraid to drive because of the attempted robbery of the vehicle. Played sports (volleyball); good lifestyle; absence of economic problems.

### Differential diagnosis

Disorders associated with whiplash/spinal cord syndrome compression.

### Objective examination

- Sharp–Purser test: negative

- Test of compression of the spine in flexion, extension, rotation, sidebending: negative

- Tests of spinal distraction: positive with cervical and left shoulder pain

- Brudzinski, Kernig, and Romberg signs negative

- Osteotendinous reflex: 2+ (normal)

## Case study continued

- Absence of signs of motor deficits

- Adson test: positive on the left, with the head rotated left

- De Klein test, bilateral SLR test, Nachlas, Manson and Slump test: negative

- Peripheral pulse: 70 bpm, regular.

### Assessment of sensitivity

- Superficial allodynia, left cervical paraspinal tract

- Primary hyperalgesia average in the thoracic spine

- Secondary hyperalgesia buttock and left thigh

- The patient reported pain as 9/10 on VAS scale

- The pain does not change from sitting to standing

- Adverse neurological tests: neurological syndromes are excluded.

### Evaluation of orthostatic posture

- Reduction of the physiological curves with anterior cape

- Right inferior iliac crest

- Inferior right PSIS

- Lumbar convexity to the right, thoracic convexity to the left

- Right shoulder inferior

- Head sidebent left and rotated right.

### Evaluation of breath

Regular breathing (14 per minute) primarily upper thoracic.

### Osteopathic evaluation

#### Global test

- FCT (meningeal fascia): reduction of meningeal fascia mobility

- FCS test: decompensated

- DyFIR GA: not balanced

#### Segmental tests

- Red reflex: positive bilaterally C5–T1 area

- Skin drag: positive T8–T12 area

- Beal's compression test: positive T8–T12 left tract.

#### Local tests

On palpation there is dysfunction of the soft tissues in the muscular area under the neck, with radiation of pain to the left orbital region, insertion of the shoulder elevator reveals ascending left pain, and pain radiating to the left lower back, and to the lumbosacral fascia with radiation of pain to the gluteal area. The patient also reported feelings of anxiety and transient depression. There has been subcutaneous venous and lymphatic flow stagnation in the sacral area:

- SD: Oc-C1 FRlSr

- Joint test for the left shoulder: negative

- Fascial dysfunction in the epigastric area

## Case study continued

- Tests of co-dominance: positive in the epigastric area and soft tissue Oc-C1 region.

### SFIT (specific to the neurological model)

Step 1: the symptomatic left gluteal area is chosen to test for tenderness. With the application of pressure the patient reports a score of 9/10 for tenderness.

Step 2: reveals the links between SD of the soft tissues of the Oc-C1 tract and then the epigastric area, both in relation to the left buttock. The patient perceives the same tenderness when pressure is applied in the left buttock. The test indicates dominance of function over structure; therefore, we opt for a maximalist approach.

## Treatment

Treatment was divided into four sessions, in which we proceeded as follows:

### Session 1

Treatment of disorders of the fascial compensation scheme (see Chapter 3), using the midline technique (see Chapter 6).

### Session 2

Symptomatic area that evokes generalized symptoms (CS): upper thoracic spine:

- Test of SD hierachization reveals presence of co-dominance between SDs: Oc-C1 FRlSr, epigastric area left

- SFIT showed dominance of structure (Oc-C1) over function (CS of the symptomatic area); we opted for a minimalist approach

- OMT: driver sensory technique to the Oc-C1 area vs. left epigastric area; articulatory technique for SD of the Oc-C1 FRlSr.

### Session 3

Symptomatic area that evokes generalized symptoms (CS): the lower thoracic spine:

- Detected SD: paraspinal soft tissue at T8–T12, SD of the left gluteal area in which there is abnormal tissue texture and tenderness

- Dysfunctional hierarchy: dominant SD left gluteal area

- SFIT showed a dominance of structure (left gluteal area) over function (CS of the symptomatic area); we opted for a minimalist approach

- OMT: inhibitory technique to these tissues; PINS technique for a primary point in right parasacral area and a terminal point at the greater trochanter. Connection: piriformis muscle.

### Session 4

Symptomatic area that evokes generalized symptoms (CS): mid-thoracic spine:

- Detected: suboccipital left SD

- SFIT showed dominance of structure (SD frontal-occipital left) over function. We opted for a minimalist approach (CS of the symptomatic area)

- OMT – PINS technique: primary point in the left suboccipital area; terminal point in the supraorbital foramen. Connections: greater occipital nerve, ophthalmic branch of the trigeminal nerve, occipitofrontal muscle.

After four sessions the patient reported disappearance of orbital pain, no soreness in her left shoulder in abduction. The patient could sleep.

## Case study continued

After 3 months the patient reported no further symptoms. There were only two occasions of pain in conjunction with strong emotional stress, but that resolved within 24 hours.

## Patient education

The patient was informed of the effects that a whiplash can have on the body and on the relationship to psychic or emotional stress related to the perceived pain threshold. The patient has learned exercises to relax the diaphragmatic and relax and re-educate the scalene muscles and the thoracic outlet tissues through stretching of the brachial plexus, and active stretch of the scalene muscles.

## Conclusions

The effectiveness of the application of osteopathic models is based on the ability to understand the focus of the models, and how to use them and integrate them in a specific way with each patient. Musculoskeletal pain does not have to be related to processes attributable to sensitization, but this may happen during the therapeutic process, as is often found in patients who exhibit psycho-emotional stress conditions.[59] In these cases, the osteopath, through the use of the criteria described in the biopsychosocial model (see Chapter 8), can understand how to assist the patient in dealing with the causes of such stresses.

In this chapter we outlined how the osteopathic "evaluative and therapeutic lens" of the neurological model can be focused on the expression of the nervous system in tissues. OMT is aimed at promoting the health inherent in the uniqueness of the individual; it consists of body, mind, and spirit. It is important that the osteopath learn to "dose" the treatment, understood as the ability to hear and feel the load which can be tolerated by the individual, since if administered in too large a dose, especially in subjects suffering from chronic pain, it can constitute an additional stress for the patient (see Chapter 9). The nervous system is the anatomical substrate of perceptions, and it is through these perceptions that the osteopath and the patient primarily communicate.

## References

1. Burns L. Studies in the osteopathic sciences. Los Angeles, CA: Occident; 1907. vol. 1.

2. Burns L. Studies in the osteopathic sciences. Cincinnati, OH: Monfort; 1911. vols 2–4.

3. Peterson B, editor. The collected papers of Irvin M. Korr. Colorado: American Academy of Osteopathy; 1979.

4. Van Buskirk RL. Nociceptive reflexes and the somatic dysfunction: a model. J Am Osteopath Ass. 1990;90(9):792–805.

5. Willard FH. Neuro-endocrine-immune network, nociceptive stress and the general adaptive response. In: Everett T, Dennis M, Ricketts E, editors. Physiotherapy in mental health. A practical approach. Oxford: Butterworth-Heinemann; 1995. pp. 102–26.

6. Woolf CJ. Central sensitization: implication for the diagnosis and treatment of pain. Pain. 2011;152(3 Suppl):S2–15.

7. Sandkühler J. Understanding LTP in pain pathways. Mol Pain. 2007;3:9.

8. Baron R, Hans G, Dickenson AH. Peripheral input and its importance for central sensitization. Ann Neurol. 2013;74(5):630–6.

9. Selye H. The stress of life. New York: McGraw-Hill; 1976.

10. King HH, Jänig W, Patterson MM. The science and clinical application of manual therapy. Edinburgh: Churchill Livingstone Elsevier; 2011. p.44.

11. Chung J, Wurster R. Neurophysiological evidence for spatial summation in the CNS from unmyelinated afferent fibers. Brain Res. 1978;153(3):596–601.

12. Seffinger MA, King HH, Ward RC et al. Osteopathic philosophy. In: Chila A, editor. Foundations of osteopathic medicine. 3rd ed. Philadelphia, PA: Lippincott Williams and Wilkins; 2011. p. 6.

13. Howell JN, Willard F. Nociception: new understandings and their possible relation to somatic dysfunction and its treatment. Ohio Res Clin Rev. 2005;15.

14. Meyer RA, Campbell JN, Raja SN. Peripheral neural mechanisms of nociception. In: Wall PD, Melzack R, editors. Textbook of pain. 3rd ed. Edinburgh: Churchill Livingstone; 1994. pp. 13–44.

15. Staud R, Craggs JG, Robinson ME et al. Brain activity related to temporal summation of C-fiber evoked pain. Pain. 2007;129(1–2): 130–42.

16. Meeus M, Nijs J, Van de Wauwer N et al. Diffuse noxious inhibitory control is delayed in chronic fatigue syndrome: an experimental study. Pain. 2008;139(2):439–48.

17. Meeus M, Nijs J. Central sensitization: a biopsychosocial explanation for chronic widespread pain in patients with fibromyalgia and chronic fatigue syndrome. Clin Rheumat. 2007;26:465–73.

18. Zhuo M. A synaptic model for pain: long-term potentiation in the anterior cingulated cortex. Mol Cells. 2007;23(3):259–71.

19. Kandel E, Schwartz JH, Jessell TM, editors. Principi di neuroscienze. 3rd ed. Milan: Casa Editrice Ambrosiana; 2003. ch. 63.

20. IASP (Subcommittee on Taxonomy). Classification of chronic pain: description of chronic pain syndromes and definitions of pain terms. Seattle: ASP Press; 1994.

21. Reichling DB, Green PG, Levine JD. The fundamental unit of pain is the cell. Pain. 2013;154(Suppl 1):10.

22. Benarroch EE. Basic neurosciences with clinical applications. Philadelphia, PA: Butterworth-Heinemann Elsevier; 2005. p. 400.

23. Sato A. Somatovisceral reflexes. J Manipulative Physiol Ther. 1995;18(9):597–602.

24. Sato A, Sato Y, Schmidt RF et al. Somato-vesical reflexes in chronic spinal cats. J Auton Nerv Syst. 1983;7(3–4):351–62.

25. Purves D, Augustine GJ, Fitzpatrick D et al., editors. Neuroscience. 2nd ed. Sunderland, MA: Sinauer Associates; 2001. ch. 10.

26. DeGroat WC. Spinal cord processing of visceral and somatic nociceptive input. In: Patterson MM, Howell JN, editors. The central connection: somatovisceral/viscerosomatic interaction. Indianapolis, IN: American Academy of Osteopathic Medicine; 1992. pp. 47–71.

27. Head H. [1893] On disturbances of sensation with especial reference to the pain of visceral

disease. Brain. 16:1–13. In: Parsons J, Marcer N. Osteopathy: models for diagnosis, treatment and practice. Edinburgh: Elsevier Churchill Livingstone; 2006. ch. 6.

28. Downing CH. [1981] Principles and practice of osteopathy. London: Tamor Pierston. In: Parsons J, Marcer N. Osteopathy: models for diagnosis treatment and practice. Edinburgh: Elsevier Churchill Livingstone; 2006. ch. 6.

29. Beal MC. Viscerosomatic reflexes: a review. J Am Osteopath Assoc. 1985;85(12):786–801.

30. Schulkin J. Rethinking homeostasis. Allostatic regulation in physiology and pathophysiology. Cambridge, MA: MIT Press; 2003.

31. Orlandini G. La semeiotica del dolore I presupposti teorici e la pratica clinica. 2nd ed. Rome: Antonio Delfino editore; 2014. p. 128.

32. Kwon M, Altin M, Duenas H et al. The role of descending inhibitory pathways on chronic pain modulation and clinical implications. Pain Pract. 2013. doi:101111/papr12145 [Epub ahead of print].

33. Panjabi MM. The stabilizing system of the spine. Part I. Function, dysfunction, adaptation and enhancement. J Spinal Disord. 1992; 5(4):383–9.

34. Legrain V, Iannetti GD, Plaghki L et al. The pain matrix reloaded: a salience detection system for the body. Prog Neurobiol. 2011;93(1):111–24.

35. Cauda F, Torta DM, Sacco K et al. Shared "core" areas between the pain and other task-related networks. PLoS One. 2012;7(8):e41929.

36. Jänig W. Neurobiology of visceral pain. Schmerz. 2014;8(3):233–51.

37. Craig AD. Interoception: the sense of the physiological condition of the body. Curr Opin Neurobiol. 2003;13(4):500–5.

38. Elkiss ML, Jerome JA. Chronic pain management. In: Chila A, editor. Foundations of osteopathic medicine. 3rd ed. Philadelphia, PA: Lippincott Williams and Wilkins; 2011. ch. 16.

39. Chapman CR, Tuckett RP, Song CW. Pain and stress in a systems perspective: reciprocal neural endocrine and immune interactions. J Pain. 2008;9(2):122–45.

40. Kuchera ML. Applying osteopathic principles to formulate treatment for patients with chronic pain. J Am Osteopath Assoc. 2007;107(10 Suppl 6):ES28–38.

41. Patterson MM. Foundations of osteopathic medical research. In: Chila A, editor. Foundations of osteopathic medicine. 3rd ed. Philadelphia, PA: Lippincott Williams and Wilkins; 2011. ch. 70.

42. Beal MC. Louisa Burns DO, memorial. American Academy of Osteopathy Yearbook. Indianapolis, IN: American Academy of Osteopathic Medicine; 1994.

43. Cole W. The osteopathic lesion syndrome. American Academy of Osteopathy Yearbook. Indianapolis, IN: American Academy of Osteopathic Medicine; 1951. pp. 149–78.

44. Denslow JS. The central excitatory state associated with postural abnormalities. J Neurophysiol. 1942;5:393–402.

45. Denslow JS. An analysis of the variability of spinal reflex thresholds. J Neurophysiol. 1947;7:207–16.

46. Denslow JS, Korr IM, Krems AD. Quantitative studies of chronic facilitation

in human motoneuron pools. Am J Physiol. 1947;105(2):229–38.

47. Korr IM. The neural basis of the osteopathic lesion. J Am Osteopath Ass. 1947;4784:191–8.

48. Korr IM. Cutaneous patterns of sympathetic activity in clinical abnormalities of the musculoskeletal system. Acta Neuroveg (Wien). 1964;25:589–606.

49. Kelso AF. A double-blind clinical study of osteopathic findings in hospital patients: progress report. J Am Osteopath Assoc. 1971;70(6):570–92.

50. Kelso AF, Larson NJ, Kapler RE. A clinical investigation of the osteopathic examination. J Am Osteopath Assoc. 1980;79(7):460–7.

51. Beal MC. Palpatory testing for somatic dysfunction in patients with cardiovascular disease. JAOA. 1983;82:822–31.

52. Johnston WL. Functional technique. In: Chila A, editor. Foundations of osteopathic medicine. 3rd ed. Philadelphia, PA: Lippincott Williams and Wilkins; 2011. ch. 52d.

53. Magoun HI. Osteopathy in the cranial field. 3rd ed. Boise, ID: Northwest Printing; 1976.

54. Cutler MJ, Holland BS, Stupinski BA et al. Cranial manipulation can alter sleep latency and sympathetic nerve activity in humans: a pilot study. J Altern Complement Med. 2005;11(1):103–108.

55. Butler DS, Jones MA. Mobilisation of the nervous system. Edinburgh: Elsevier Churchill Livingstone; 1991.

56. Educational Council on Osteopathic Principles (ECOP). Glossary of osteopathic terminology. Chevy Chase, MD: American Association of Colleges of Osteopathic Medicine (AACOM); 2009.

57. Travell JG, Simons DG. Myofascial pain and dysfunction. The trigger point manual. Vol. 2. Baltimore, MA: Lippincott Williams and Wilkins; 1992. pp. 168–85.

58. Simons DG, Travell JG, Simons LS. Travell and Simons Myofascial pain and dysfunction: the trigger point manual. Vol. 1: Upper half of the body. 2nd ed. Baltimore, MD: Lippincott Williams and Wilkins; 1999.

59. Nijs J, Van Houdenhove B, Oostendorp RA. Recognition of central sensitization in patients with musculoskeletal pain: application of pain neurophysiology in manual therapy practice. Man Ther. 2010;15(2):135–41.

60. Koltyn KF, Arbogast RW. Perception of pain after resistance exercise. Br J Sports Med. 1998;32:20–4.

61. Whiteside A, Hansen S, Chaudhuri A. Exercise lowers pain threshold in chronic fatigue syndrome. Pain. 2004;109(3):497–9.

62. Butler D. Sensitive nervous system. Adelaide, Australia: Noigroup Publications; 2000.

63. Orlandini G. La semeiotica del dolore. 2nd ed. Rome: Antonio Delfino editore; 2014. p. 90.

64. Yunus MB. Fibromyalgia and overlapping disorders: the unifying concept of central sensitivity syndromes. Semin Arthritis Rheum. 2007;36(6):330–56.

65. Wolfe F, Smythe HA, Yunus MB et al. The American College of Rheumatology 1990 criteria for the classification of fibromyalgia report of the multicenter criteria committee. Arthritis Rheum. 1990;33(2):160–72.

66. Stone CA. Visceral and obstetric osteopathy. Edinburgh: Elsevier Churchill Livingstone; 2007. p. 71.

67. Nelson KE, Glonek T. Somatic dysfunction in osteopathic family medicine. Philadelphia, PA: Lippincott Williams and Wilkins; 2007. ch. 5.

68. Owens C. An endocrine interpretation of Chapman's reflexes. Carmel, CA: Academy of Applied Osteopathy; 1937, reprinted 1963.

69. Jones LH. Strain and counterstrain. Newark, OH: American Academy of Osteopathy; 1981.

70. Travell JG, Simons DG. Myofascial pain and dysfunction: the trigger point manual. Vol. 2. Baltimore: Williams and Wilkins; 1992.

71. Jarricot H. Projections viscero-cutanees. Metameres thoraco-abdominales. Turin: Minerva Medica; 1975.

72. Head H. On disturbances of sensation with especial reference to the pain of visceral disease. Brain. 1893;16:1–132.

73. Eble JN. Patterns of response of the paravertebral musculature to visceral stimuli. Am J Physiol. 1960;198(2):429–33.

74. Schoen RE, Finn WE. A model for studying a viscerosomatic reflex induced by myocardial infarction in the cat. J Am Osteopath Assoc. 1978;78(1):122–3.

75. Cervero F. Visceral and spinal components of viscerosomatic interactions. In: Patterson MM, Howell JN, editors. The central connection: somatovisceral/viscerosomatic interaction. Indianapolis, IN: American Academy of Osteopathic Medicine; 1992. pp. 77–85.

76. Beal MC. Somatic dysfunction associated with pulmonary disease. J Am Osteopath Ass. 1984;84:179–83.

77. Pottenger FM. Symptoms of visceral disease. 5th ed. St Louis, MO: Mosby; 1938.

78. Stone CA. Visceral and obstetric osteopathy. Edinburgh: Elsevier Churchill Livingstone; 2007. p. 43.

79. Chauffour P, Prat E. Mechanical link: fundamental principles, theory, and practice following an osteopathic approach. Berkeley, CA: North Atlantic Books; 2002. p. 38.

80. Payne P, Crane-Godreau MA. Meditative movement for depression and anxiety. Front Psychiatry. 2013;4:71.

81. Bialosky JE, Bishop MB, Robinson ME et al. The relationship of the audible pop to hypoalgesia associated with high velocity, low amplitude thrust manipulation: a secondary analysis of an experimental study in pain free participants. J Manipulative Physiol Ther. 2010;33(2):117–24.

82. Comeaux Z. Harmonic healing: a guide to facilitated oscillatory release and other rhythmic myofascial techniques. Berkeley, CA: North Atlantic Books; 2008.

83. Lederman E. Harmonic technique. Edinburgh: Elsevier Churchill Livingstone; 1990.

84. DiGiovanna E, Kuchera LM, Greenman PE. Efficacia e complicanze. In: Ward RC, editor. Fondamenti di medicina osteopatica. Milan: Casa Editrice Ambrosiana; 1997. ch. 73.

85. Barral JP. Visceral manipulation. Seattle, WA: Eastland Press; 1998.

86. Schiowitz S. Functional techniques. In: DiGiovanna EL, Schiowitz S, Dowling DJ, editors. An osteopathic approach to diagnosis and treatment. 3rd edn. Philadelphia: Lippincott Williams and Wilkins; 2005. ch. 20.

87. Dowling DJ. Progressive inhibition of neuromuscular structures (PINS) technique. J Am Osteopath Assoc. 2000;100(5):285–6, 289–98.

88. Barral JP, Croibier A. Manual therapy for the peripheral nerves. Edinburgh: Elsevier Churchill Livingstone; 2007.

89. Barral JP, Croibier A. Manual therapy for the cranial nerves. Edinburgh: Elsevier Churchill Livingstone; 2008.

90. Glover JC, Rennie PR. Strain and counterstrain approach. In: Chila A, editor. Foundations of osteopathic medicine. 3rd edn. Philadelphia, PA: Lippincott Williams and Wilkins; 2011. ch. 49.

91. Schiowitz S. Facilitated positional release. In: DiGiovanna EL, Schiowitz S, Dowling DJ, editors. An osteopathic approach to diagnosis and treatment. 3rd edn. Philadelphia, PA: Lippincott Williams and Wilkins; 2005. ch. 15.

92. Crow WT. Ligamentous articular strain technique and balanced ligamentous technique. In: DiGiovanna EL, Schiowitz S, Dowling DJ, editors. An osteopathic approach to diagnosis and treatment. 3rd ed. Philadelphia, PA: Lippincott Williams and Wilkins; 2005. ch. 19.

93. Van Buskirk RL. The still technique manual: applications of a rediscovered technique of Andrew Taylor Still, MD. 2nd ed. Indianapolis, IN: American Academy of Osteopathy; 2006.

94. Nicholas AS, Nicholas EA. Atlas of osteopathic techniques. Philadelphia, PA: Lippincott Williams and Wilkins; 2008. ch. 17.

95. Nicholas AS, Nicholas EA. Atlas of osteopathic techniques. Philadelphia, PA: Lippincott Williams and Wilkins; 2008. ch. 11.

96. Pickar JG. Neurophysiological effects of spinal manipulation. Spine J. 2002;2(5):357–71.

97. Clark BC, Thomas JS, Walkowski SA et al. The biology of manual therapies. J Am Osteopath Assoc. 2012;112(9):617–29.

98. Skyba DA, Radhakrishnan R, Rohlwing JJ et al. Joint manipulation reduces hyperalgesia by activation of monoamine receptors but not opioid or GABA receptors in the spinal cord. Pain. 2003;106(1–2):159–68.

99. Sato A. The somatosympathetic reflexes: their physiological and clinical significance. In: Goldstein M, editor. The research status of manipulative therapy. Bethesda, MD: National Institutes of Health; 1975. pp. 163–72.

100. Schwartzman RJ, Maleki J. Postinjury neuropathic pain. Med Clin North Am. 1999;83(3):597–626.

101. Kuchera ML, Kuchera WA. Osteopathic considerations in systemic dysfunction. 2nd ed. Columbus, Ohio: Greyden Press; 1994. pp. 189–203.

102. Kiecolt-Glaser JK, McGuire L, Robles TF et al. Psychoneuroimmunology and psychosomatic medicine: back to the future. Psychosom Med. 2002;64(1):15–28.

103. Salamon E, Zhu W, Stefano GB. Nitric oxide as a possible mechanism for understanding the therapeutic effects of osteopathic manipulative medicine (Review). Int J Mol Med. 2004;14(3):443–9.

104. Garthwaite J. Concepts of neural nitric oxide-mediated transmission. Eur J Neurosci. 2008;27(11):2783–802.

105. Schleip R. Fascial plasticity – a new neurobiological explanation. Part 1. J Bodyw Mov Ther. 2003;7(1):11–9.

106. Liptan GL. Fascia: a missing link in our understanding of the pathology of fibromyalgia. J Bodyw Mov Ther. 2010;14(1):3–12.

107. Degenhardt BF, Darmani NA, Johnson JC et al. Role of osteopathic manipulative treatment in altering pain bio-markers: a pilot study. J Am Osteopath Assoc. 2007;107(9):387–400.

108. Morris VH, Cruwys SC, Kidd BL. Characterization of capsaicin-induced mechanical hyperalgesia as a marker for altered nociceptive processing in patients with rheumatoid arthritis. Pain. 1997;71(2):179–86.

109. Langemark M, Bach FW, Jensen TS et al. Decreased nociceptive flexion reflex threshold in chronic tension-type headache. Arch Neurol. 1993;50(10):1061–4.

110. Yunus MB. Role of central sensitization in symptoms beyond muscle pain, and the evaluation of a patient with widespread pain. Best Pract Res Clin Rheumatol. 2007;21(3):48–97.

# The respiratory-circulatory model

*Paolo Tozzi*

## Synopsis

In this chapter we present the respiratory-circulatory model, beginning with the fundamental principles of the model and proceeding to applications, for both diagnosis and treatment. We also explore the objectives and clinical rationale, as well as the most traditional and contemporary aspects, in the light of the critical analysis of the latest evidence, and including the author's personal considerations and applications. This model represents the gas-fluid model *par excellence* in osteopathic practice, where the activating force resides in the fluids, in all their bodily expressions, but especially in their free circulation and oxygenation. This model focuses on the exchange of gases and nutrients, the removal of metabolites, and chemical-physical communication at different levels, as well as an efficient immune response.

The dynamic equilibrium among the pressure gradients is the main engine/driver of the gaseous and fluid forces; diaphragms are the "guardians" and modulators; the respiratory system is the gas distributor; the cardiovascular and musculoskeletal systems are the action pumps; the venous and lymphatic systems are the discharge and defense mechanisms. However, none of these components work in isolation; on the contrary, they cooperate synergistically in a complex integrated unity of structure and function, in constant motion, to increase exponentially the adaptive capacities and homeostatic potential of the organism. Similarly, osteopathic evaluation and treatment based on this template will respect its global, regional and local expressions, approaching the patient with specific tests and techniques but in a comprehensive and systemic perspective.

Precisely for this reason, as for each of the other five models, as well as for the respiratory-circulatory model, we cannot successfully treat the patient by appealing only to a single component, the fluid component in this case, without exerting an inevitable effect on the others: biomechanical, neurological, metabolic, and psychosocial components. The combination of each of these factors will be the key to better understanding and intervention of any clinical condition we will be facing. However, if, in osteopathic philosophy, fluids really play a supreme role in health as well as in sickness, in the evaluation procedure as well as in treatment, this model is definitely the embodiment of its deepest essence.

## Introduction

The respiratory-circulatory model addresses the maintenance of the extracellular and intracellular environments through the free exchange of oxygen and nutrients and removal of cellular metabolic waste.[1] For the purpose of ensuring such dynamic equilibrium, the model operates on the fluid circulation in each and every form: from the arterial to the venous, from the lymphatic to the interstitial, and the cerebrospinal, including the structures and key organs for the performance of such functions. Although one might think that the arteriovenous system represents the main fluid constituent of the body, in fact, of an average 42 liters of total fluids in the human body, 28 are from the intracellular fluid and 14 the extracellular fluid, of which 11 are from interstitial fluid, and only three are from blood plasma.[2]

The fluids carry nutrients such as oxygen and glucose to all body tissues, and remove waste products such as lactic acid and carbon dioxide. They are also mediators for the humoral communication systems, essential to the body's defenses and the maintenance of homeostasis. For example, the cells of the immune system are conveyed from the vascular system and toward the extracellular matrix, in case of need. Similarly, hormones, neuromodulators, and cytokines are diffused through the fluid system. Because of this function, the fluids can be thought of as the transmission medium of the life force in the body.[3]

However, we should not underestimate the role of support and protection of the fluid system. In fact, this system "fills" the fascial cavities, thus providing structural support, as if it were a hydraulic support system, ensuring an even distribution of forces and reducing the total effect on the body, both locally and globally.[4] At the same time, myofascial tensions are involved in the physiologic alternation of pressure gradients, both intra- and inter-cavity, as a basic function of fluid dynamics. Not surprisingly, the respiratory-circulatory model also relies on the role of the musculoskeletal system, and in particular of the diaphragms, as a pump for the low pressure (venous and lymphatic) circulatory systems.

It is sufficient to say that diaphragmatic excursion may oscillate from a minimum of 0.9 cm in a normal respiration, up to a maximum of 4.7 cm in a forced respiration,[5] thus creating an increase in negative thoracic pressure and compression of the abdominal viscera. Simultaneously, there is an increase of lymph flow[6] and of the blood flow in the superior vena cava, along with a reduction of the blood flow in the portal vein.[7] It is easy to imagine, then, how deficiencies of the muscular and diaphragmatic system cause a slowing of the venous and lymphatic return, leading to accumulation of fluid in the extremities, revealing all the critical aspects of the musculoskeletal function.[8]

Among other things, it is interesting to note that the respiratory rate appears to synchronize and interact with fluctuations in blood pressure,[9] heart rate,[10] and lymphatic system[11] and brain activity,[12] being itself amplified by resonance with these other rhythms.[13] This demonstrates the full interaction and integration with the other functions of the body. But the diaphragms are certainly not the only force to generate a fluid dynamic. Recent evidence suggests that the fascia has contractile properties similar to the smooth musculature,[14] properties perhaps modulated even by the autonomic nervous system.[15] This would strengthen the possibility that the perivascular strata can contribute to fluid dynamics, and assist the known pumping action of the smooth and striated musculature.

However, even the hydrostatic, osmotic, oncotic, osmolar, and electrical gradients play a fundamental role in the movement of fluids[2] by adding to the natural mobility of the cells, tissues, and organs. It is easy to imagine how in cases of somatic dysfunction, which is itself characterized by restriction of mobility and change in tissue texture,[16] we can verify a reduction of local perfusion,[17] resulting in hypoxia and local congestion. The locally altered gradient of pressure can reduce the perfusion of high pressure areas and increase the stagnation in low pressure areas, with alteration of the physiological effects of the fluid: nutrition, communication, removal of metabolic waste products, and so on. Consequently, any noxious factor that interferes with free gas exchange and with the normal circulatory flow represents a threat to tissue homeostasis. This does not exclude postural deterioration, which can affect the balance among the cavities of the body, with a corresponding effect on fluid circulation.[18]

For this reason, the application of the respiratory-circulatory model includes the evaluation of thoracic and respiratory mechanics, circulation, and the flow of body fluids, including the homeostatic response to pathophysiologic processes.[19] This includes central and peripheral processes that are involved in the dynamics of these two prominent functions – breathing and circulation – processes such as central nervous control, cerebrospinal fluid flow, the arterial supply, venous and lymphatic drainage, as well as lung, cardiovascular, kidney, and intestinal function. Similarly, the resolution of any somatic dysfunction occurs through intervention methods that restore fluidic mobility, in particular respiratory-circulatory efficiency, to ensure the proper physical and chemical conditions for the body's self-regulation abilities. Finally, like any other model, this also provides for the interaction between respiratory-circulatory function and musculoskeletal, neurological, metabolic, and behavioral functions, as constituent elements of the adaptive response to allostatic and homeostatic stimuli, i.e., of the global health potential of the individual.

## Historical background

A. T. Still, founder of osteopathy, on several occasions reminded us of the supreme importance of free arterial,[20] venous-lymphatic,[21] and fluid circulation[22] to ensure optimal conditions for healing and health processes. Since 1898, specific osteopathic maneuvers have been described for lymph drainage of organs and structures, with the aim of enhancing the immune response in various pathological conditions.[23] In 1907, Burns performed studies on viscerosomatic and somatovisceral dysfunctional reflexes,[24] which were then followed by specific research on the treatment of lung[25] and heart diseases.[26]

The effectiveness of these principles and manipulative techniques was soon put to the test: between 1917 and 1919, in the United States, approximately half a million people died from Spanish influenza, or complications such as pneumonia;[27] deaths in the rest of the world were around 100 million. However, data collected at that time showed that about 100,000 patients with influenza had a general mortality rate of 0.25% in those treated osteopathically, compared with 5% in those treated medically.[28] Furthermore, of those who developed pneumonia, only 10% of the osteopathic patients died, compared with 30–60% in those treated with standard medical therapy.

It was at that time that vertebral articulatory and rib-raising techniques were conceived, giving optimal results in improving functional respiratory capacity. In particular, a student of Still, Frederick Millard, was the first to develop a physical examination of the lymphatic system[29] and to propose a series of specific techniques for drainage, with a recommended treatment duration of 5–10 minutes.[30] Earl Miller introduced the lymphatic pump technique, and also the thoracic lymphatic pump.[31]

Such techniques were presented as effective for acute, edematous, and congestive infections,[32] capable of reducing blood glucose, uric acid and urea in the blood within 30 minutes after treatment.[33] Another osteopath, Galbreath, described a method of lymphatic drainage of the mandible and the middle ear[34] so that, following the experience derived from the influenza pandemic, the treatment of lung diseases was increased by including a wide range of lymphatic pump techniques,[35] which also proved to have a beneficial effect on immune function and on specific antibody responses,[36-38] although only splenic pump technique was applied, with the technique being performed for 1 to 5 minutes, with a frequency of 21 compressions per minute.

Sutherland, Still's student and Millard's contemporary, called the osteopath the "mechanic of the fluids,"[39] pointing out on several occasions the importance of the diagnosis and treatment of fluids, particularly their fluctuation, especially of the lymphatic, for the maintenance of health. In those same years, another student of Still, Frank Chapman, postulated the diagnostic and therapeutic role of lymph in visceral function, and in particular of neurolymphatic reflexes corresponding to specific visceral structures.[40] Ruddy proposed a muscular pumping system, which he called "rapid rhythmic resistive duction," targeted to the treatment of fluid congestion, especially in the head and neck.[41]

Inspired by the work of Millard, Zink expanded the approach to the integrated function of breathing and circulation,[42] forging another model. He pointed to the thoracoabdominal and pelvic pump as fundamental to good fluid dynamics, and described fascial restrictions as a major obstacle to venous and lymphatic drainage. This gave a strong boost to the osteopathic community in the provision of the best guidelines for the treatment of cardiac and respiratory conditions,[43,44] supported by contemporary evidence on the facilitated reflexes of the somatic dysfunction. Hix[45] demonstrated specific musculoskeletal reactions in response to stimulation of the renal and urinary organs in rats, working in conjunction with Denslow and Korr.

Conversely, Mannino[46] stimulated the T11 vertebral segment through osteopathic manipulative treatment, with the intention of influencing adrenal function, and found a significant reduction in aldosterone levels (but not in blood pressure) in hypertensive patients. Subsequently, Beal cataloged over 100 distinct relationships in patients with overt heart and lung disease and specific vertebral somatic dysfunction, determined by structural examination. He found, for example, a correlation between heart disease and somatic dysfunction of T1–T4,[47] as well as between lung disease and somatic dysfunction at the T2–T7 segmental levels.[48]

The results supported the existence of viscerosomatic interactions as the scientific basis of facilitated reflexes of somatic dysfunction, i.e., the mechanism of action of OMT and other manual therapies. At the same time, investigations began on the effects of treatment of thoracic dysfunction on the residual volume and total lung capacity in patients with chronic respiratory disorders.[49] Not all studies gave the expected improvements in lung function parameters.[50]

## Objectives

Considering the importance of the artery in the "Still's medicine," this model embodies the principles and methods of supreme interest for osteopathic practice. Evaluation and treatment place particular emphasis on fluids in general, aiming for optimization of the capacity and efficiency of respiratory and cardiocirculatory function and the flow of body fluids, in order to maximize the potential for homeostasis and, consequently, the individual's health.[51] The objectives of the respiratory-circulatory model, as described by Kuchera,[52] are to:

- release myofascial paths in transitional areas of the body (atlanto-occipital, cervicothoracic, thoracolumbar, lumbosacral)

- optimize the diaphragmatic movements

- treat target organs to improve arterial, venous, and lymphatic dynamics

- increase pressure gradients and hydrodynamic pumping.

## Indications, contraindications, and selection criteria for the model

Through physical examination, the operator evaluates the presence of any condition by the significant fluid component, to determine the need for a respiratory-circulatory approach (Box 6.1).

The respiratory-circulatory model is one of three instruments at the disposal of osteopathic medicine for the treatment of systemic diseases, in addition to intervention strategies for the orthosympathetic and parasympathetic systems.[52] First, this implies the weighting of the risk:benefit ratio related to osteopathic intervention for a given condition. The use of the respiratory-circulatory model approach to compensating schemes and the use of coordinated and systematic lymph techniques are in fact based on the determination of what the patient would benefit from, compared to the risk of their application.

In general, fluid techniques are indicated for:[1]

- mucosal, lymphatic, venous congestion

- inflammation or infection, especially of the respiratory tract (pharyngitis, bronchitis, pneumonia, ear infections, etc.)

- fluid retention, as in the case of pregnancy or thyroid disorders

- post-surgical or post-traumatic edema

- acute somatic dysfunction.

Fluid techniques are generally contraindicated in:[55]

- fracture, dislocation, severe joint instability

- severe osteoporosis

- organ fragility (e.g., the spleen in mononucleosis)

- hepatitis and splenomegaly

- pneumothorax

- severe heart failure

- aneurysms

- hemorrhage

- thrombosis

---

**Box 6.1**

**Conditions in which the respiratory-circulatory model is indicated**

- Respiratory disorders: e.g., upper respiratory tract infections, sinusitis, bronchitis, pneumonia, asthma, sleep apnea, chronic obstructive pulmonary disease, emphysema.

- Cardiac and arterial disorders: e.g., mild heart failure, high blood pressure, previous heart attack or ischemia, atherosclerosis, pericarditis, endocarditis, arterial disease.

- Venous and lymphatic disorders: e.g., hemorrhoids, varicose veins, phlebitis, venous insufficiency, hypertension, varicocele, hydrocele, lymphedema, lymphangitis, and lymphadenopathy.

- Organ disorders: in particular those that adversely affect liver, kidney, and spleen functions.

- Other conditions: e.g., scoliosis, kyphosis, ankylosing spondylitis, pregnancy, obesity, abdominal or thoracic surgery,[53] or in general any postural or metabolic alterations that directly or indirectly compromise respiratory mechanics and cardiocirculatory efficiency.

---

- open wounds

- malignancies (e.g., lymphoma).

Caution should be maintained in cases of anemia, pregnancy, mild or slight osteoporosis, coagulation disorders, and valvular heart disease; if present, implants, plates, pins, or other types of orthotics; congenital anomalies of the venous or arterial circulation, or antiplatelet or anticoagulant treatment, especially after surgery or an ischemic attack. As regards the application of the model in patients with cancer, the topic remains controversial. Although there is concern that treatment directed toward the improvement of fluid dynamics could favor metastatic spread of the primary tumor, recent animal studies suggest that OMT stimulates an antibody response with specific anticancer action, originating from the gastrointestinal lymphoid tissue.[56] However, further research is needed on the potential effects and possible effectiveness of the respiratory-circulatory model approach in cancer.[57]

As evident from the aforementioned data, there are several clinical conditions that may be the best representatives for the selection of the respiratory-circulatory model. However, even the bioconstitutional (e.g., a mesomorphic biotype) and postural component (see Chapter 8) may suggest the application of this approach, as well as osteopathic tissue evaluation, in the case of evident primary dysfunctional patterns that affect the diaphragms, lymphatic stations, and cardio-circulatory, respiratory, and urogenital systems. In addition, it is possible to carry out a test of the cervical-thoracic portion of the visceral fascia (see Chapter 1), proposed as a fascial compartment of the respiratory-circulatory model, to obtain additional confirmation of the suitability of this model to the individual case.

## Principles and methods of assessment

In accordance with the principles and objectives of the respiratory-circulatory model, the following is a proposed osteopathic evaluation (Fig. 6.1), divided into the following three stages and levels:

- *Global*: identification of myofascial central schemes/analysis of involuntary rhythms, examination of the central tendon, and assessment of the midline (median line)

- *Regional*: examination of the fluid pumping and regional and peripheral patterns

- *Local*: evaluation of correlated somatic dysfunctions.

The first two levels can best be normalized through homeostatic techniques, and the last through specific techniques.

## Overall assessment

### Test of the fascial compensation scheme and involuntary rhythms

Possible causes of fluid flow restrictions can be identified by palpation of the fascial compensation scheme, by performing the tissue preference test (also known as the Zink test) and palpating the involuntary rhythms (fascial). According to Zink,[51] the state of health of an individual coincides with his or her ability to adapt to stressors or compensation of any kind that can affect respiratory and circulatory function. Therefore, the greater the adaptability capacities, the better will be the general state of health.

Now, these capabilities would be explained in myofascial patterns of alternated rotation-inclination[58] in specific areas of transition, i.e., long vector plans that coincide with bodily apertures (tentorial/upper thoracic/thoracoabdominal/pelvic) and around specific myofascial points and biomechanical fulcrums (Fig. 6.2). These correspond to the structural transitional areas of the spine (occipito-atlantal-axial/cervicothoracic/thoracolumbar/lumbosacral). Theoretically, the diaphragms should be aligned and move rhythmically and in a coordinated manner during breathing. However, most commonly they rotate and tilt about their respective vertebral fulcrums, to compensate for various types of stressors.[59]

Therefore, the resulting myofascial alternating rotation patterns would represent a useful model, beneficial and functional (in the absence of obvious symptoms) in response to anomalies, such as a lower limb length discrepancy or a functional overload of a limb. Functional failure, however, describes the same phenomenon, the difference being that the changes brought about by adaptation are dysfunctional and symptomatic, and highlight the failure of homeostatic mechanisms and adaptation.[60] Using tests of tissue preference, Zink and Lawson[58] argue that it is possible to classify three types of schemes (Box 6.2).

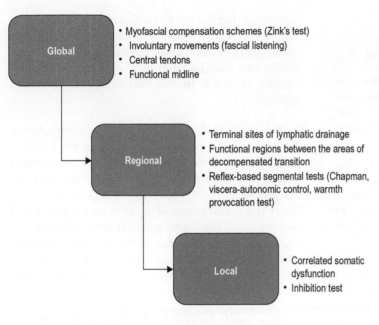

- Global
  - Myofascial compensation schemes (Zink's test)
  - Involuntary movements (fascial listening)
  - Central tendons
  - Functional midline

- Regional
  - Terminal sites of lymphatic drainage
  - Functional regions between the areas of decompensated transition
  - Reflex-based segmental tests (Chapman, viscera-autonomic control, warmth provocation test)

- Local
  - Correlated somatic dysfunction
  - Inhibition test

**Fig. 6.1**
A possible application of the respiratory-circulatory model in osteopathic evaluation, from a global perspective to a regional focus, to a local depth. We must remember that the three levels of exploration can be performed independently (as well as sequentially), according to the diagnostic needs of the operator, the patient's clinical presentation and the intended therapeutic goals.

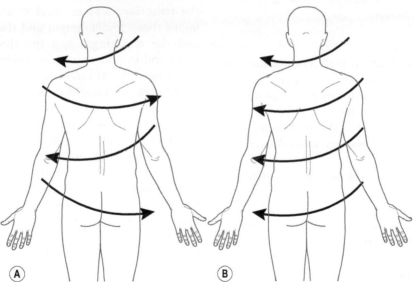

(A)        (B)

**Fig. 6.2**
(A) The physiologic alternation of rotation/inclination of four transitional areas. In this case, with a common pattern of rotation from top to bottom, toward L/R/L/R. However, less commonly, it could also be toward R/L/R/L. (B) An example of severely decompensated scheme with all four transitional areas rotating in the same direction. However, less serious patterns might occur with just two areas that rotate consecutively to the same side. Courtesy of Elsevier Health Sciences,[60] as amended.

### Box 6.2

### Central myofascial schemes

- *Ideal schemes*: in these schemes the alternated rotational tendencies of the transition areas are minimal, and thus the adaptation loads transferred are minimal. However, Zink himself noted the rarity of such schemes in clinical practice.[61]

- *Compensated schemes*: alternate in direction from one area to another and usually have some form of adaptation. Among these are a more common pattern (in 80% of healthy patients), with an alternating rotation of L/R/L/R, and a less common pattern (in 20% of cases) of R/L/R/L.

- *Uncompensated schemes*: the rotations do not alternate and are normally a result of a stimulus/ sudden    trauma    or    microstimulus/repetitive microtrauma, which, among other things, has been recently found in children with cerebral palsy and recurrent ear infections.[62]

To assess the directional preference of the four transition areas, traditionally the patient is in the supine position. The operator induces a rotational motion, alternately to the left and to the right, in each region, sensing which is the qualitatively (not quantitatively) favored direction. We evaluate:

- the tentorium around the occipitoatlantoaxial[60] complex (Fig. 6.3)

- the upper thoracic diaphragm at the cervicothoracic junction (Fig. 6.4)

- the    thoracoabdominal    diaphragm    at    the throacolumbar junction (Fig. 6.5)

- the pelvic diaphragm at the lumbosacral junction (Fig. 6.6).

For each station the operator induces a slight rotation and/or alternating inclination to the left and to the right, as if it were applied on a cylinder, judging which of the two directions is qualitatively

preferred. The operator can also use listening to test the myofascial tissues, intentionally inducing an alternating rotation of the fascial planes. This latter mode can also be used as a confirmation of the results received in the classic mode described above.

The relationship between the diaphragmatic system and the respiratory and circulatory mechanisms of the body is essential. Each diaphragm has a role in modulating the intra- and intercavity pressures of the organism, by adjusting accordingly the pressure gradients of dynamic fluids and oxygenation. Each diaphragm therefore exercises a hydraulic pump function on the arterial supply and the venous lymphatic and interstitial flow return, facilitating gas exchange and ensuring chemical and physical balance.

Attention is focused on the relationship between the tentorium and cerebral venous sinuses, the upper thoracic diaphragm and the thoracic duct, and the diaphragm and the thoracoabdominal aorta and inferior vena cava, including the pelvic diaphragm and arterial-venous plexus of the associated organs. In addition, each aperture suspends or supports organs and viscera of primary importance for the respiratory and circulatory mechanisms of the body, thus facilitating fluid pumping and oxygenation during each breath. It is therefore easy to imagine the deleterious effects that one or more regions with uncompensated schemes can exercise on respiratory-circulatory systemic balance, altering pressure gradients, fluid dynamics and, therefore, tissue oxygenation and removal of metabolic wastes and thus favoring congestion and inflammation, not to mention the influence that all this would have on proprioception, posture, and the joint and mechanical stability of the corresponding regions involved.[63]

In the case of a severely uncompensated scheme, given the consequent reduction of the overall function and adaptive capabilities of the organism, usually a global maximal therapeutic approach (such as GOT) is suggested,

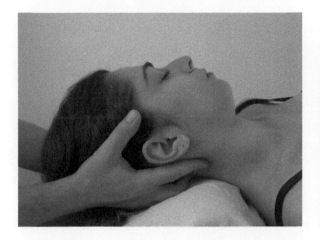

**Fig. 6.3**
The transition test on the first area can be performed by supporting the occiput with both hands and with the tips of the fingers on the posterior processes of C1 and C2. Alternatively, the operator supports the occiput with one hand, monitoring the atlas with a thumb–index finger contact, while with the other hand he or she contacts the front and performs the test after having flexed the head (to better isolate the movements of the C0–C2 complex); or again, supporting the occiput with one cupped hand and the atlas between thumb and forefinger of the other hand. The operator applies a slight traction to the occiput and tests the preferential rotation on both sides.

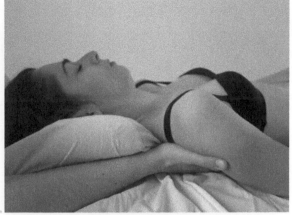

**Fig. 6.4**
The operator, seated at the head of the patient, contacts the shoulders with cupped hands, and applies alternating pressure on the shoulders toward the ceiling, pivoting with his or her elbows on the table, to test the rotational preference of this region. Alternatively, the operator can perform the test while standing, facing the patient, with the thumbs along the clavicles and the third and fourth finger of each hand in contact with the scapular spines.

rather than one of specific and local impact,[64] such as the SAT.[65] This concept reflects a basic principle that the authors of this text propose at several levels: if there is dominance of an altered general function on the individual structural and local dysfunction (GAS), then the treatment is oriented toward a maximalist approach; in the case of a dominant altered local structure over general function (LAS), a minimalist and local approach is preferred. In other words, we try to give an appropriate treatment for the general homeostatic capabilities, although clearly there can be no single approach; rather, there are indications that require custom adjustments for each individual case.

Although the osteopathic world has often proudly supported the concept of holism and focus on health, most of the manual tests used in osteopathic evaluation paradoxically only aim to seek dysfunction. The Zink test, however, is one of the few osteopathic tools that aims to evaluate the individual and his or her homeostatic capabilities, through the analysis of myofascial patterns oriented along diaphragmatic planes, which have high impact on respiratory and circulatory functions. This is also the main test that the authors of this volume propose in order to discriminate among the adaptive responses of the patient to the allostatic load present, making it possible to guide the choice of the type of osteopathic intervention most appropriate to the case (maximalistic or minimalistic).

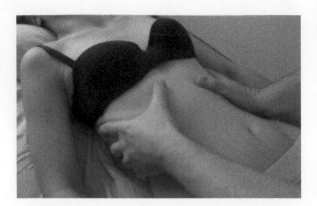

**Fig. 6.5**
The operator stands facing the patient and places the thumbs along the lower costal margin, with the rest of the hands on the lateral sides of the rib cage. Alternatively, the operator's hands contact the posterior inferior portion of the rib cage, with the fingertips directed toward the spinous processes of T12–L1.

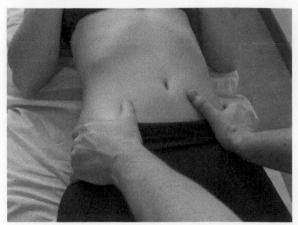

**Fig. 6.6**
The operator stands facing the patient, contacting the ASIS with the thenar eminences and wrapping the fingers around the innominates. Alternatively, the palms of the hands can support the pelvis on both sides, with the fingers pointing toward the PSIS.

However, the test has been used in osteopathic practice to locate the origin and nature of the dysfunctional component, particularly when one finds a slight failure (e.g., only two non-alternating transition areas), not accompanied by other historic and clinical elements which suggest an allostatic overload. Some authors, for example, suggest the use of the Zink test with the patient standing, comparing its results with those obtained in the supine position.[66] This is to determine whether the lower limbs influence the test, and then consider possible ascending dysfunctional patterns from the hips, knees and ankles. In this case, uncompensated patterns in the standing position should improve significantly in the supine position, while descendant primary dysfunctions would show decompensated patterns both in standing and in the supine position. Following the same principle, we can test any dysfunctional interference with the diaphragmatic system by specific functional subsystems, such as mandibular function (asking the patient to open the

mouth during the test), dental occlusion (asking the patient to clench the jaw), lingual function (asking the patient to push with the tongue on the interincisal spot), or ocular function (requiring specific eye movements), and so on.

Clearly, this application of the Zink test to determine the primary dysfunction, by engaging or excluding a specific system to test any interference on the diaphragms, is an extrapolation of the test forced by the context in which it was originally designed and the purpose for which it was traditionally applied. However, it can be useful in some cases, especially if we suspect a disturbing influence of one of the elements of the fine postural system (vestibular, ocular, lingual, occlusal, dental).[67]

Even more specifically, the Zink test can be applied to localize primary dysfunctional areas, which correspond to regions with uncompensated rotational schemes. If, for example, the test revealed that the thoracoabdominal and pelvic transition areas rotate preferentially toward the same side, while the cranial and the upper thoracic alternate in opposite directions, this suggests that the primary dysfunctional area gravitates in the abdominopelvic region, being able to affect "the container" (lower ribcage, dorsal and lumbar spine, pelvis) and/or "content" (viscera, nerves, vessels, etc.) and/or diaphragms themselves, inherently involved. In the latter case, the dysfunction may be classified into three types (Box 6.3).

These dysfunctions of the transition areas are often caused by:

- dysfunctions of viscera or joint/vertebral structures adjacent to the diaphragm involved or functionally linked to it

- traumatic events, both isolated, such as slips and falls, and repetitive, often related to professional or sporting activities

- surgical interventions, such as episiotomy to the pelvic diaphragm or cholecystectomy, which affects the thoracoabdominal diaphragm

- bad posture, especially related to the work ergonomics or sporting activity or hobby

- psycho-emotive shock or prolonged periods of intense stress, considering that most of the diaphragms are anatomically and functionally connected with neurovegetative plexuses or with organs of the neuroendocrine axis

- systemic collagen diseases, such as lupus erythematosus, rheumatoid arthritis, polymyositis, etc., that cause a global structural involvement of the diaphragmatic system and associated connective structures.

The clinical symptoms most commonly associated with dysfunctions of the transitional areas are the:[68]

- cranial area: headache, suboccipital pain, neck pain, nausea, tinnitus, disorientation, irritability, etc.

- upper thoracic area: cervical brachialgia, disorders of the venous and lymphatic drainage of the upper limbs, breathing problems, arrhythmias, etc.

- thoracoabdominal area: respiratory and cardiac disorders, gastroesophageal reflux disease, colitis, rib and dorsolumbar pain, etc.

- pelvic area: hemorrhoids, proctalgia, cystitis, coccydynia, incontinence, sexual activity disorders, disorders of the venous and lymphatic drainage of the lower limbs and so on.

---

### Box 6.3

### Types of diaphragmatic dysfunction

- Local: typical of the diaphragm (or hemidiaphragm) musculature or vertebra-rib-joint anatomically related structures ("container"), or of the organs adjacent to it (viscera, vessels, fascia, ligaments, etc., that constitute the "content").

- Segmental: typical of the metameric unity that physiologically rules the transition area in dysfunction. As a result of spinal facilitation, we would find the involvement of a metabolic area as well as a neurological area, so as to produce skin-somatic-visceral dysfunctions with the associated dysfunctional reflexes (including those of Chapman or Jarricot, with involvement of neurovegetative activity and correspondent vascular circulation).

- Global: typical of the whole fascial compensation scheme or of a section between the transition areas that are decompensated, inharmonious, and destabilized. The physiological reserve of the area between two or more transition areas in dysfunction is significantly decreased (with biomechanical decompensation, pressure imbalance, functional-hormonal-immune imbalances, etc.).

Returning to the classical evaluation of fascial compensation schemes, we must not forget that the transition areas, because of the diaphragm system, are also a physiological system that promotes body realignment to the central line of gravity, by drastically reducing energy waste in achieving stability. In fact, in addition to being connected to the joint junction areas of the spine, the diaphragms are also connected to the entire connective tissue system of the body, arranged in longitudinal tubular compartments such as pannicular, axial-appendicular, visceral, and meningeal fascia.[69]

Therefore, it is plausible that any distortion of these fascias involves a myofascial twist of the entire longitudinal axis. Consequently, their functions, such as body vascular pumping, respiratory efficiency, and corresponding fluid dynamics, will be altered, with consequent increase of mechanical stress on the longitudinal axis. For this reason, the author considers it necessary to integrate the traditional Zink evaluation with the test of the central tendon, if the preferential rotation tests reveal that all four of the transition areas are uncompensated (i.e., they rotate together in the same direction).

## Test of the central tendon

The central tendon is not an anatomical structure in itself, but more like a central connective reference for the body. It is identified as a cervical-thoracic-abdominal-pelvic chain: a set of myofascial structures that connect all the diaphragms, the whole body from the occiput to the foot and the back to the front (vertebrae–sternum), to maintain good posture of the body and, above all, to establish a center line of reference and union of the diaphragms.[70]

The central tendon could coincide with what some anatomists identify as axial fascia,[69] which, in osteopathic practice, also has connections with the viscera (pericardium, kidney, etc.), thus representing the link between the structural component and the deep visceral component of the body.[71,72] It consists of (Fig. 6.7) the:

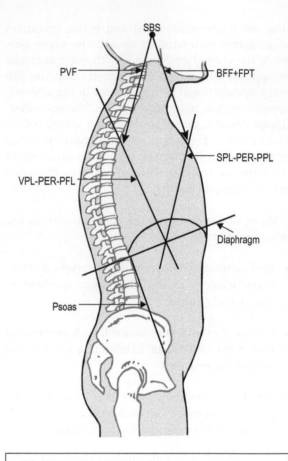

**Fig. 6.7**
The central tendon components and their tension forces: superior-posterior portion, superior-anterior, diaphragmatic and psoas-inferior joints. The PVF (prevertebral fascia) portion originates at the occipital part of the SBS (sphenobasilar symphysis) and extends to T4, and then toward the PER (pericardium), through the VPL (vertebropericardial ligament), and then to the diaphragm with the PPL (phrenopericardial ligament). The BPF (buccopharyngeal fascia) originates at the front component of the SBS and extends to the hyoid bone, and is then continuous with the PTF (pretracheal fascia). This extends to connect with the SPL (sternopericardial ligament), and then with the PER and the PPL. In addition to the cranial base, the two upper portions of the central tendon meet at the diaphragm and continue with the line of force of the psoas, to the lower limbs.

- superior-posterior portion: consisting of the prevertebral fascia, which connects the posterior cranial base with the pericardium (via the vertebro-pericardial ligament) and with the diaphragm (via the phrenopericardial ligament)

- superior-anterior portion: consisting of the buccopharyngeal and pretracheal fascias, connecting the anterior cranial base with the hyoid bone, the sternum and pericardium (through the sternopericardial ligaments), and diaphragm (again by means of the phrenopericardial ligament)

- inferior portion: consisting of the diaphragm and its posterior pillars, which are functionally continuous with the psoas, the transversus abdominis muscle aponeurosis, the iliac fascia and, hence, the hips down to the feet via the myofascial chains of the lower limbs.

If three or four transition areas are shown to be uncompensated in Zink tests, one or more portions of the central tendon may be involved, causing or maintaining the corresponding diaphragmatic failure and/or the entire fascial scheme. In this case, it is appropriate to evaluate all three of the central tendon components:

- Superior-posterior portion (Fig. 6.8): in normal conditions, the position and movement of the sternum should be homogeneous and along the midline. In case of mild dysfunction, however, we perceive a fascial twist of the sternum, with a slight lateral deviation. In severe cases, there is a net lateral deviation.

- Superior-anterior portion (Fig. 6.9): in normal conditions, the position and movement of the manubrium should be homogeneous and along the midline. In case of mild dysfunction, however, we perceive a fascial twist of the manubrium, but if the dysfunction is more severe there will also

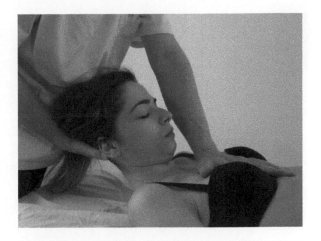

**Fig. 6.8**
The patient is supine; the operator stands at the patient's head. One hand supports the occiput and flexes the patient's head, while the other hand contacts the medial third of the sternum (at the level of T3–T4). This contact corresponds to the origin and insertion of the posterior superior portion of the central tendon. First, the operator generates a slight tensioning of the tissues, by flexing the patient's head while maintaining the pressure on the sternum. Next, the operator asks the patient to take a deep inhalation (while the operator maintains the applied tension), followed by a deep exhalation, while increasing the pressure on the sternum toward the table, keeping the head flexed.

be a slight lateral deviation. In severe cases, lateral deviation will be prevalent.

- Inferior portion (Fig. 6.10): in case of minor dysfunction, we perceive a fascial twist of the sacrum, but if the dysfunction is more severe we see a slight lateral deviation. In cases of severe dysfunction, however, the lateral deviation will be the strongest component.

Usually, we identify only one portion of the central tendon in dysfunction. However, in chronic conditions, it is not uncommon to find two or all three components of the tendon in dysfunction. If this

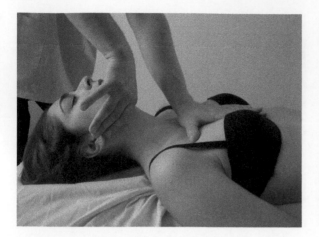

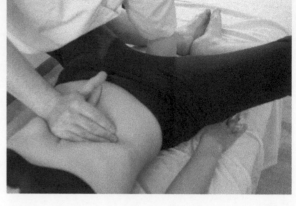

**Fig. 6.9**
The patient is supine with the cervical spine in extension, with the operator standing at the patient's head. One hand contacts the lower edge of the patient's jaw, with a thumb-index arc hold (for adults) or with a V index-medium arc hold (for children). In both cases, the main contact is on the lower jaw and not on the hyoid bone. The other hand is on the manubrium (which corresponds to the insertion of the superior sternopericardial ligament). First the operator generates a slight tensioning of the tissues, by extending the cervical spine further while stabilizing the sternal manubrium, which correspond, respectively, to the origin and insertion of the superior-anterior portion of the central tendon. Next, the operator asks the patient to take a deep inspiration (during which the applied tension is maintained), followed by a deep exhalation, while increasing the pressure on the manubrium toward the table, and maintaining a stable contact on the mandible.

**Fig. 6.10**
The patient is supine with bent legs; the soles of the feet are in contact and also externally rotated as much as possible. The operator stands at the side of the bed facing the patient. One hand contacts the thoraco-abdominal diaphragm, below the xiphoid process; the thenar and hypothenar eminences of the hand are on the lateral edge of the nearest rectus abdominis muscle and the fingertips contact the lateral margin of the opposite rectus. The hand is then closed and slightly curved, creating a pressing effect on the diaphragmatic dome, which should serve as a fixed point for the test. The other hand is cupped on the sacrum, with the arm between the patient's legs. The operator asks the patient to take a deep inhalation, and then, during exhalation, gradually slide the feet toward the bottom of the table, keeping the feet in contact for as long as possible, and then finally extend the legs completely. During this phase, the operator, while maintaining stable contact on the diaphragm with one hand, applies tension toward the sacrum with the other hand, assessing the homogeneous descent along the median line during the extension of the hips. Through the myofascial connection of the lower limbs with the pelvis, the psoas, and the diaphragm, this maneuver tests the compliance of the lower portion of the central tendon.

is the case, following the same principle applied to the fascial compensation (Zink) test and the test of the central tendon, the author suggests further assessment, by testing for any dysfunction at the midline, which represents a central body reference even deeper to the formation of the connective central tendon.

## Tests on the midline

According to some authors,[73–75] the functional midline of the body originates during primordial embryonic development, representing the first expression of a functional central axis around which is arranged the spatial organization of the entire body.

The functional midline refers to a range of structures including the primitive streak, the neural groove, the notochord, the meningeal fascia, the terminal lamina, along with the phases of involuntary expansion and retraction of tissues, such as cranial motion.[76] With embryological and anatomical knowledge, we can intentionally assess any changes in the midline. With the patient in the supine position, the operator sits at the patient's side, viewing the entire midline, first through a monodigital contact on its most extreme points of reference: vertex and coccyx. The operator visualizes and intentionally connects with the midline, focusing on anatomical structures with which the midline is connected (the nuclei of the intervertebral discs, cervical alar ligaments, basilar portion of the occiput and sphenoid body).

Once the operator has identified an area of any alteration of the central line, he or she changes the contacts by choosing the proximal and distal contacts that are closest to the perceived dysfunctional area. Usually the chosen contact points are:[73]

- vertex-sternum

- vertex-umbilicus

- sternum-coccyx

- umbilicus-coccyx.

Alternatively, the operator can evaluate the midline with the patient in the lateral decubitus position, making sure to keep the patient's head in line with the rest of the spine. In this case, the optional contact points are:

- vertex/cervicodorsal

- cervicodorsal/thoracolumbar

- sacrococcygeal/thoracolumbar

- sacrococcygeal/lumbosacral.

In any case, the evaluation is intended to perceive twisting, deviations or even interruption of the median line between the selected contact points.

Therefore, according to the respiratory-circulatory model, the first evaluation phase, the global one, may provide for an analysis of the four transitional areas. If there are three or four decompensated areas, the osteopath examines the three parts of the central tendon. If this evaluation reveals two or three components in dysfunction, the operator may proceed with the evaluation of the midline. The rationale is that one fully assesses the global dysfunctional scheme by engaging the possible origins in reverse order: from simple diaphragmatic-myofascial-joint failure schemes on the transverse plane, to the central connective axis distortions along the longitudinal axis, and finally a search for abnormalities of the functional midline, the central position of which is the reference for the function and embryonic origin of each organ and tissue.

## Regional evaluation

Examination of fluid pumping and the peripheral and regional schemes

This second phase of the evaluation would allow more contact with the specific regional areas, focusing on the areas revealed as more dysfunctional by previous global tests. The evaluation proceeds as follows:

### Evaluation of the lymphatic drainage terminal sites

The evaluation of lymphatic drainage terminals sites[77] aims to identify areas of congestion (Fig. 6.11). The operator observes and palpates the following areas:

- Submandibular region (for mouth and viscerocranium drainage)

- Retroauricular and suboccipital region (for neurocranium drainage)

- Supraclavicular space (for the head and neck drainage)

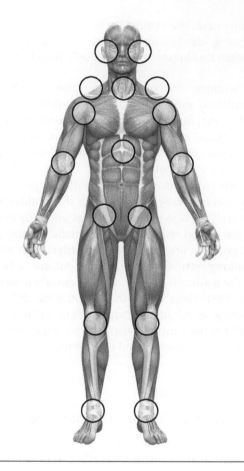

**Fig. 6.11**
Terminal sites of lymphatic drainage to be evaluated to identify areas of congestion.

- Axillary regions (for upper limb drainage)

- Cubital region (for hand and the forearm drainage)

- Epigastric region (for chest and abdomen drainage)

- Inguinal regions (for lower limb drainage)

- Popliteal regions (for leg drainage)

- Achilles regions (for foot and ankle drainage).

In addition, the operator can decide to evaluate regional lymph motility, manually perceptible as a two-phase flow, identifying any areas of altered flow and congestion.[78]

### Observation and palpation of the decompensated diaphragms

The observation and palpation of each functional region between the two uncompensated diaphragms, including the articular structures and adjacent organs, allows for the assessment of restrictions that may limit fluid flow. In the supine position, respiratory movement should be palpable in all body tissues,[79] extending to the pubic symphysis, while the diaphragm should move in synchrony, showing equal tensions in the muscular walls and their insertion points. The operator then palpates and compares the mobility and the tensions of the diaphragmatic domes during respiration, assessing the upper thoracic, thoracoabdominal, and pelvic diaphragms, and evaluates the articular structures on which the diaphragms are inserted.[80] In the case of the tentorium, the operator can evaluate the tension along the insertion line on the occiput, with a two-hand grip on the inferior nuchal line, as well as examine the motility of the temporal bones and the base of the skull.

### Application of specific functional tests

The specific segmental tests aim to provide information for understanding the influence of specific organs or structures on the congested fluid region, via dysfunctional facilitated reflexes. For example, the operator can test, through observation and palpation, the fluid-visceral effects of a congested liver relative to the corresponding vertebral area of sympathetic (T7–T9) or vagal (jugular foramen, C1–C2, esophageal hiatus) control.

A second example could be the evaluation of Chapman's reflexes.[81] These are neurovisceral lymphatic reflexes associated with abnormalities of anterior and posterior tissue texture: small hard and palpable nodules, about 2–3 mm in diameter, located in the deep fascia or periosteum – though not confirmed by biopsy findings[82] – constant in their anatomical location and attributable primarily to corresponding visceral dysfunction. On palpation, the patient usually feels a distinct pain, acute but without irradiation. Although traditionally, osteopathic intervention requires treatment of both reflex points, the anterior ones are usually used for diagnosis while the posterior ones are generally used for the treatment.

Finally, the last example of regional tests is the "warmth provocation test" described by Zink, used to identify areas of spinal somatic dysfunction, significant for preventing venous and lymphatic regional drainage.[83] The test consists of a mild and constant abdominal pressure applied with an open hand at the center of the abdomen, which should give as a response a uniform feeling of warmth. An abdominal area (of a spinal reflex) perceived as warmer when compared with others can be interpreted as an indication of somatic dysfunction, which then requires treatment to maximize fluid performance. The local heat increase could be due to the anastomosis between the spinal venous, epidural and azygos plexus and systemic and abdominal venous and lymphatic circulation, which, in cases of corresponding somatic dysfunction, and via facilitated neurovascular reflexes, would become more congested and then warmer.

## Local evaluation

### Evaluation of correlated somatic dysfunctions

This assessment phase consists of detailed observations, evaluating locally any somatic dysfunction that can affect the respiratory-circulatory system and its general function. The operator focuses on areas where global and regional tests have indicated particular dysfunctional disturbances. The mediastinum, ribcage, sternum, skull base, and sacrum are among the structures of primary interest in this assessment phase, in addition to the high cervical and thoracic spines. Heart, lungs, liver, intestine,

spleen, and kidneys are among the organs of greatest relevance.

This phase of the local screening can be extremely detailed, identifying not only visceral and autonomic ganglionic specific dysfunctions, but also dysfunctions of large or medium caliber arteries, such as the aorta or the vertebral artery.[84] Moreover, one should not underestimate the assessment of scarring or adhesions in the abdomen, pelvis, and lower extremities, which reveal a subcutaneous edema, venous and/or lymphatic congestion in the surrounding area, and limited gliding movement of the connective tissue in at least one of the planes of possible movement[85] (Box 6.4).

Finally, after identifying the most significant local dysfunctions – in terms of tissue texture and motion restriction – it is possible to relate them through an inhibitory or balancing test.[86,87] This test incorporates the concept of inhibition, the basis of many traditional techniques of the osteopathic armamentarium such as PINS,[88] even using it in formulating the differential diagnosis. It allows the operator to establish a possible hierarchical relationship between the identified dysfunctions, discriminating those that are compensatory/adaptive from those that are primary/high priority/causative. The test is performed by contacting the two most significant dysfunctions and applying and maintaining a slight pressure on one of them (by inhibiting it), while the other is tested, listening to any changes in involuntary rhythms or by assessing the changes in tissue texture while applying a slight pressure.

The inhibition test is then applied on the second dysfunction, and the osteopath observes the responses of the first one. The principle of the test is that during the temporary pressure applied (inhibition) on a dysfunction, its disturbing influences on the other are eliminated or reduced temporarily (perhaps by way of the gate mechanism). In that period of time, the dysfunction will reveal an improvement, worsening or maintenance of its restrictive parameters. We can therefore get the following responses (in the author's clinical experience):

- *Ratio of no relationship*: in this case, by alternately inhibiting and disinhibiting a malfunction, the other one does not show changes in its restrictive properties. The test therefore suggests that there is no dysfunctional hierarchical relationship of any kind between the two zones, indicating a probable history of diversity, etiology, severity, and depth. From the therapeutic point of view, therefore, the two dysfunctions can be treated with different modalities and timing, or not, requiring no particular order of preference.

- *Ratio of dominance*: when, by inhibiting one dysfunction, the second gets better, but when inhibiting the second, the first does not change, the first is probably dominant. Indeed, when

---

**Box 6.4**

Osteopathic evaluation of scars

It is appropriate to test adhesions, or scar areas, to assess any restrictions, through the testing of:

- density: pressing vertically along its course

- tension: by pulling the scar longitudinally and transversely along its course

- mobility: testing connective tissue shearing relative to the layers below, superiorly and inferiorly, medially and laterally

- rolling: pinching and rolling the tissue involved

- motility: listening to the involuntary movement and surrounding fascial motility

- dermal-visceral reflex: evaluating changes in the nearest arterial pulse, before and after pressure on the scar area, to test the possible involvement of the corresponding autonomic supply.

---

inhibiting the disturbing influences, the second dysfunction improves in its restrictive parameters. However, the opposite does not occur. In this case, the test suggests that, if action is taken on the dominant dysfunction, one may achieve improvements of the adaptive secondary dysfunction. It must be understood, however, that in some cases, it is possible to observe a worsening of the restrictive parameters of the dominant dysfunction when the secondary dysfunction is inhibited. This often indicates that compensation/adaptation is vital to ensure balance in the system, opposing the destabilizing forces of the dominant dysfunction, which is common when the dysfunction is long-standing, resulting in compensated equilibrium. Therefore, the last thing an osteopath should do in such cases is to treat the compensation in a session and leave the primary dysfunction for the next visit. If this situation occurs, the patient may experience a major decompensation, often a cause of significant problems beyond those of a physical nature.

- *Ratio of co-dominance*: this type of relationship emerges when, by alternately inhibiting one of the two dysfunctions the other improves. In this case, the test suggests that the two areas are in a relationship of co-dominance, probably dictated by a shared etiological factor. It follows that the two dysfunctions should be treated in the same session, possibly via a maneuver that normalizes them simultaneously (as for example, a fascial unwinding).

Finally, the author proposes that, if the evaluation as a whole reveals signs of GAS (i.e., of general impairment of function), such as generalized symptoms (metabolic disorders, asthenia, insomnia, loss of appetite, diffuse myalgia, etc.), seriously decompensated Zink schemes, compromised central tendon, or more altered areas and regions, all without evidence of a clear local dysfunctional focus, the respiratory-circulatory model should be applied in a maximalistic mode. In contrast, when the assessment reveals signs of LAS (i.e., a well-defined symptomatic and local picture with dominance of a specific dysfunctional structure), the Zink pattern being uncompensated in the corresponding zones, with a normal central tendon and midline, with an inhibition test which indicates a clear dysfunctional primacy of a specific structure, then the model should be applied in a minimalistic way.

The fascial compensation (Zink) test is therefore proposed as the main discriminating test for dysfunctional dominance between structure (LAS) and function (GAS) within the respiratory-circulatory model, although it is right to integrate it with all the other information obtained from the evaluation process. From here one deduces indications on which to base the osteopathic intervention, described in the next paragraph.

## Principles and methods of treatment

The respiratory-circulatory model can be applied gradually, going from maximal to minimal, varying the focus in the following three ways (Fig. 6.12):

- *Global*: including the effects of interaction of the dysfunctional area with all the other systems of the patient, including psycho-physical equilibrium. This type of maximal intervention is suggested in cases in which the homeostatic capacity, then the general function, are strongly compromised (GAS), and they have priority on the single dysfunctional local structure.

- *Regional/segmental*: in the metameric unit that physiologically governs the dysfunctional area.

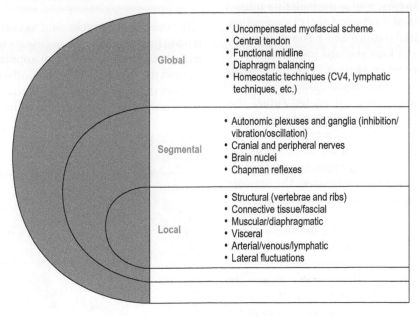

**Global**
- Uncompensated myofascial scheme
- Central tendon
- Functional midline
- Diaphragm balancing
- Homeostatic techniques (CV4, lymphatic techniques, etc.)

**Segmental**
- Autonomic plexuses and ganglia (inhibition/vibration/oscillation)
- Cranial and peripheral nerves
- Brain nuclei
- Chapman reflexes

**Local**
- Structural (vertebrae and ribs)
- Connective tissue/fascial
- Muscular/diaphragmatic
- Visceral
- Arterial/venous/lymphatic
- Lateral fluctuations

**Fig. 6.12**
Some of the possible applications of the respiratory-circulatory model used in osteopathic intervention, through both global and segmental approaches, and including local ones. A global approach is more suitable for general functional failure conditions, while a local one is indicated in conditions of dysfunctional dominance of a single structure over the global function. The choice of the number and the type of the treatment will be at the discretion of the operator, depending upon his or her skills and experience, as well as on the clinical presentation of the patient, for potential homeostatic and general adaptation and, finally, for shared therapeutic targets (see Chapter 9).

- *Local*: in the part most directly affected by the dysfunction, which may or may not coincide with the symptomatic part. This minimalist approach is suggested mostly in cases in which the alteration of the structure is dominant impact over the function, i.e., in which the local dysfunctions have dysfunctional dominance over the general function (LAS).

### Global

The therapeutic application of the global model can be articulated as described below.

#### Uncompensated scheme treatment – central tendon – midline

This treatment allows for restoring a functional and axial equilibrium of the body, a pressure balancing of the diaphragms, and a normalizing impact on the movement of fluids and their oxygenation. The uncompensated pattern can be normalized by treating each of the four stations toward (facilitated positional release) or against (muscular energy technique) the facilitated fascial tissue vectors of the transversal structures and related spinal segments.[64] The treatment generally starts at the pelvic station, treating it in an indirect manner (by seeking a point of balanced tension) or directly (seeking the restrictive barrier and using opposite muscle contraction). Once the release is obtained, the operator evaluates and treats the other three stations.

Sometimes, instead of treating the regions consecutively, it is appropriate to approach them simultaneously, especially in the presence of severe imbalances. In this case, the operator locates the point of balanced tension at each station, starting from the pelvic station and proceeding to the upper thoracic, and maintaining each neutral point through the aid of a wedge, placed below the raised side. Then the operator sits at the patient's head, finds and maintains a neutral point at the cranial and occipital-atlas-axis complex levels. To facilitate the complete and simultaneous release of all four regions, the operator requires the patient to take a deep inhalation, then a full exhalation, and

then maintain the exhalation position for as long as possible. If necessary, the operator can now verify that the diaphragms are now free, synchronous, and harmonic, and eventually balance them through specific techniques.[89] For example, the operator can perform a cranial-abdominal (Fig. 6.13) or abdominal-pelvic synchronization (Fig. 6.14).

In both procedures, it is necessary to increase the myofascial tensions of the two hemi-diaphragms contacted, until a balanced tension point is located. Then, while this point is maintained by the operator, he or she has the patient take a deep inhalation, then a full exhalation, and then maintain the exhalation position as long as possible. The resumption of breathing coincides with the release and the synchronization of the two diaphragms involved. If necessary, the maneuver may be repeated.

If, however, the assessment has also found central tendon impairments, it is necessary to normalize the latter before the operator can approach the pattern. To treat the superior-posterior and superior-anterior portion the operator uses the corresponding holds, previously described in Figs. 6.8 and 6.9.

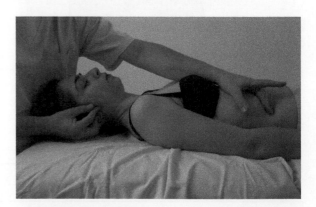

**Fig. 6.13**
The operator is situated at the patient's head while the patient is in the supine position, with a five-finger hold on the dysfunctional side, and the patient's head turned slightly to that side. The operator's other hand is on the ipsilateral thoraco-abdominal hemidiaphragm.

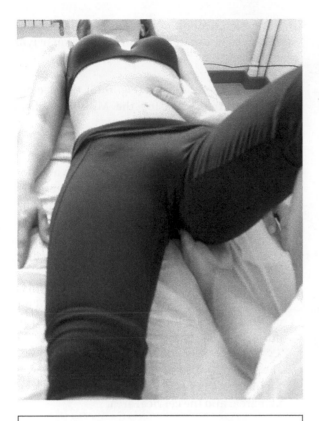

**Fig. 6.14**
The operator is situated at the patient's pelvis while the patient is in the supine position, with the thumb of one hand on the closest pelvic hemidiaphragm, medial to the ischial tuberosity; the other hand is on the corresponding thoraco-abdominal hemidiaphragm.

However, for treatment it is necessary to bring the sternum or the manubrium to the barrier (in the opposite direction to that which is favored and demonstrated by the test). The cranial hold on the occiput or the lower jaw is used as a lever and directed along the correction vector. If, for example, the sternum deviates to the left during the test of the superior-posterior portion, the treatment technique involves one hand moving the sternum to the right and engaging the barrier, while the other hand flexes the occiput and tilts the head to the right to line up along the correction vector. Thus, after

identifying the tissue barrier, this position is maintained during the forced inhalation requested of the patient, followed by a expiratory phase. The maneuver is repeated 3–4 times, crossing many tissue barriers, until full release. For correction of the lower portion of the central tendon, the same test hold is applied as demonstrated in Fig. 6.10, but it requires the patient to perform a full extension of the legs after three consecutive expiratory phases: during inhalation position is maintained, while during exhalation the patient gradually extends the legs by a third; until the third exhalation, in which the patient fully extends the legs on the table, without contact between the soles of the feet. The operator, is located standing on the side opposite the lateral deviation or the sacral torsion. Maintaining the same contacts described in the test, during the inspiratory phases the osteopath locates and maintains the tissue barrier, while, during the expiratory phase, using the forearm on the table, locating the next barrier. Finally, at the end of the third exhalation, the operator has the patient fully extend the legs applies a final impulse maneuver on the sacrum, moving through the last perceived barrier.

If, the evaluation has shown an alteration of the midline, this has priority for treatment, prior to the normalization of the other dysfunctions. In this case, the operator chooses contacts on the two landmarks of the midline that are most proximal and distal to the affected area. For example, if there is alteration of the midline at the lumbosacral level, the proximal and distal contacts for treatment would be thoracolumbar and coccyx, respectively. The operator then "connects" intentionally with the midline and with the anatomical structures that represent it; the parameters (twist, deviation, and so on) are exaggerated, both proximally and distally to the affected area until a neutral point or balanced tension point is identified.

This position is then maintained until the release, which may be encouraged by requiring the patient to take a forced respiration.[90] If instead there is a disruption of the midline, this balancing phase can be enhanced by applying a fluid drive, i.e., a fluid pulse in a superior-inferior direction, toward the disruption. The technique involves an intentional connection of the operator on the fluidic components (liquors, interstitial, etc.), to then direct them from a contact used as the source or the cathode to a second contact point considered as receiving or anode. In the case of the midline, the proximal contact to the cut is the source that appeals to local fluids, intentionally guided by the operator, while the distal contact is the reception point of such fluidic vectorial fluctuation.[91]

## Application of homeostatic techniques

The application of techniques such as compression of the fourth ventricle (CV4), temporal rocking,[92] or the Miller and Dalrymple lymphatic pumps aim to stimulate lymphatic drainage and general immune response. Zink believed that, of all the fluid systems, the lymphatic one was more easily obstructed since it is at low pressure, although it is more receptive to OMT. We can therefore treat this system by treating somatic dysfunctions that represent a significant obstacle to lymphatic flow and via specific lymphatic techniques. These techniques rely mostly on stimulatory-percussive and vibratory – effleurage, petrissage, and pompage[93] – approaches, which aim to create and release temporary pressure gradients within and between body cavities, thereby facilitating the circulation of fluid from areas of major congestion toward those of better drainage.

The general principle is to start centrally and then proceed distally, starting with the thoracic cage (usually at the thoracic inlet), to include the pumping action of the lower limbs.[94] Given that a large part of the lymphatic flow of the body drains into the subclavian venous system, the thoracic inlet is one of the first targets of this phase of intervention. The Miller thoracic lymphatic pump, the Dalrymple lymphatic pedal pump, and Galbreath mandibular drainage are all techniques often applied in this treatment phase, and are included in the glossary of osteopathic terminology published by the Educational Council on Osteopathic Principles.[95] Most of these maneuvers provide for the alternating and

rhythmic application of pressure and traction on strategic regions of the body for stimulation of lymphatic flow:[96]

- After the thoracic inlet (Fig. 6.15) the pectoral region is treated, using the Miller lymphatic pump (Fig. 6.16).

- Treatment can be done from the sternum, identical to the previous technique, but with a double contact on the sternum, with one hand reinforcing the other hand; the thoracoabdominal diaphragm is treated using the redoming technique for myofascial release and consequent impact on the aorta, inferior vena cava, and lymphatic duct.

- At the axillary sulcus one can treat using myofascial release with one hand in the axilla and one on the corresponding arm, using it as a fulcrum during the maneuver.

- The osteopath also assesses and treats to improve drainage of the eustachian tube, the submandibular area, and the cervical area.

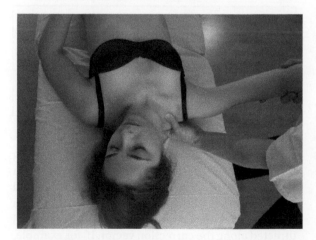

**Fig. 6.15**
The operator is standing at the side of the supine patient, with the patient's arm abducted; one hand is at the thoracic inlet and the other uses the arm as a lever for traction and compression, or for myofascial release of the inlet.

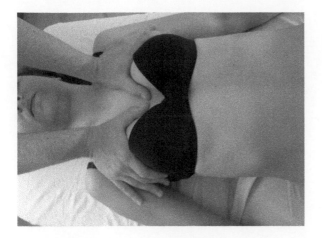

**Fig. 6.16**
The operator stands at the supine patient's head, contacting the pectoral regions bilaterally. The operator applies alternating pressure and release, which uses the natural elastic recovery of the tissues, optionally in synchrony with pulmonary respiration.

- At the popliteal fossa the technique is as follows: the patient is in the supine position with legs extended. The osteopath contacts the center and the lateral margins of the popliteal fossa with both hands.

- From the plantar and Achilles tendon regions, one can use the Dalrymple pedal pump, applicable both from the prone or supine position, at an approximate rate of 120 thrusts per minute for 2 minutes, but contraindicated in cases of deep vein thrombosis.

## Segmental

On a segmental level, the respiratory-circulatory model can be used in a number of ways to treat a dysfunctional fluid area, through action on the corresponding (metameric in some cases) control systems. For example, one can treat the T1–T6 spinal region, because of dysfunctions of the cilia-spinal and cardiopulmonary centers, thus affecting the function of the lungs, bronchi, and myocardium; or the T6–T11 spinal region because of the perturbations of diaphragm, renal plexus, and adrenal and liver function, thus affecting the visceral and vascular function of the intestine, liver, spleen and adrenal gland.[97] They all have specific impact on cardiorespiratory function and body fluid dynamics. Segmental application can be extended to:

- **Plexuses and autonomic ganglia** involved in the modulation of cardiorespiratory function, including vasoconstriction and contraction of vascular bands, thereby regulating fluid pressure. It is possible to work on them through the following techniques:

  - *Pressure/inhibition techniques,*[98] by applying a gradual, moderate and steady pressure on the transverse processes of the thoracic vertebrae corresponding to the ganglia to be normalized. For example, to treat the stellate ganglion, the operator sits at the supine patient's head and makes contact with the thumbs at the transverse processes of T1, while stabilizing the thoracic inlet and clavicle with the rest of the hands and fingers. The operator applies an anterior (toward the ceiling) and lateral gradual and steady pressure with thumbs on the T1 transverse processes, until he or she feels tissue resistance on the two transverse processes (that may not be the same). This barrier is maintained as necessary, requiring occasional respiratory support to accelerate the release. Once the first barrier is released, the operator locates the next, repeating the maneuver until complete release. With some variations, the same principle can be applied to the pterygopalatine ganglion,[99] superior cervical ganglion (at C2), medial cervical ganglion (at C5), or the thoracic paravertebral ganglia (by means of a hypothenar contact on the transverse processes of the corresponding vertebrae of the prone patient). At the sacral level, the operator can apply the same principle through a ligamentous technique directed at the sacroiliac joints, effecting the sacral splanchnic nerves (Fig. 6.17). These types of techniques and their interaction with the autonomic control of the fluid circulation support the validity of the triple combined action (respiratory-circulatory, orthosympathetic and parasympathetic) on systemic diseases.[52]

– *Vibratory techniques* (Fulford percussion) may also be used. It is possible to apply this approach[100] to the abdominal autonomic plexuses, for example, by first treating the myofascial lines of tension of the corresponding abdominal area then applying vibrational pressure to the plexus, until release is achieved. Not infrequently, this stage is accompanied by a somatosensory emotional release.[101] This type of technique is usually applied with the patient in the supine position, with bent legs, soles of the feet on the table and relaxed abdomen. Via a two-hand contact with one hand reinforcing the other, the operator first contacts the abdominal region just below the xiphoid process for the celiac plexus; between the xiphoid process and the navel for the superior mesenteric plexus; at the umbilical level for the inferior mesenteric plexus; and at the suprapubic level for the hypogastric plexus. Then gently, but gradually, as the abdominal tissues release, the operator moves his or her fingertips in a vertical direction toward the patient's spine, following the tissue release and paying attention to the myofascial forces. Finally, the operator applies vibrational pressure at a variable frequency and equal to the "dysfunctional" frequency. The maneuver ends when complete release is perceived in the treated area.

– *Techniques of oscillation* use oscillations on one or more regions of the body to establish a state of tissue "resonance."[102] This state is obtained when the operator reaches the maximum oscillatory mass excursion with the lowest applied oscillatory effort. Once oscillatory resonance is achieved, with or without the use of a lever, the operator can add slight traction to the oscillation, engaging the barrier (direct mode), or slight compression in the direction of the dysfunctional vectors (indirect mode). At the same time, the other hand can be used as a fulcrum for convergence (or divergence) of the oscillations, to obtain release of the congested and edematous area, as well as enhancing the release of the tissue complex and the autonomic ganglia via

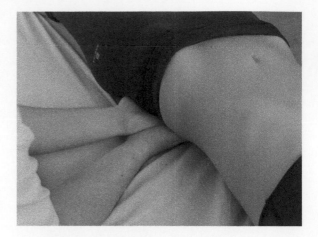

**Fig. 6.17**
With the patient in supine position, the operator, sitting at the patient's pelvis, contacts the nearest buttock, with one hand over the other and the tips of the fingers at the PSIS. Making a fulcrum with elbows on the table, the operator bends the elbows, maintaining wrists and hands stable, thereby applying anterior (toward the ceiling) and lateral (toward himself or herself) traction on the PSIS, and engaging the tissue barrier. This position is maintained until tissue release is felt, after which the operator engages the next barrier. The procedure continues until the operator achieves a full release of the area.

inhibition or local myofascial release. For example, with the patient in the prone position and the operator standing on one side of the patient, the operator can apply oscillations to the spine through contact with the iliac fossa, while the other hand approaches the paraspinal ganglia with a contact on the transverse processes of the corresponding vertebrae. Once the oscillation of resonance is identified, the operator can converge or diverge the oscillations from the dysfunctional area by applying tension or compression from the pelvis, while with the other hand the operator can apply a local treatment to the ganglion dysfunction or even apply a fluid pumping technique to a congestion zone. Finally, the operator can use rhythmic motion as an additional treatment effort. By increasing or decreasing the rhythmic motion, we may rebalance the corresponding autonomic activity or local fluid circulation. This approach can also be incorporated in the evaluation procedure, as dysfunctional and congested areas tend to alter the transmission of oscillations, slowing or diverting the natural path through the body's tissues.

- *Articulatory techniques*[103,104] – vertebral and costal especially – can be used to boost local fluid circulation or its regional control by treatment of the corresponding autonomic regulation centers. A classic example would be the articulatory/joint techniques for the upper costovertebral joints (Fig. 6.18). This can influence the activity of the orthosympathetic paraspinal ganglia of the congested area, as well as exercise a circulatory impact on the corresponding azygos venous system. Similarly, the operator can use the leg as a lever in order to treat the sacral splanchnic nerves, acting on the sacroiliac joints and the sacrum, or on specific organs with circulatory impact such as liver and kidneys, rhythmically applying pressure and traction on them, or to treat the abdominal plexuses that govern the target organs for fluid circulation.

- **Peripheral or cranial nerves,** which control the function of structures and organs of specific respiratory and fluid interest, may also be treated. For example:

- *Phrenic nerve*: can be treated in order to normalize diaphragmatic function, by acting on its vertebral roots (C3–C5), through inhibitory pressure techniques, balanced ligamentous tension technique, facilitated positioning, etc., using access points along its course, such as in front of the anterior scalene muscle or posteriorly to the midpoint of the medial half of the clavicle, or the intersection of the 10th rib and interclavicle line as the access point for abdominal phrenic innervation. At these points we can, for example, apply direct myofascial release or an inhibitory pressure.[105]

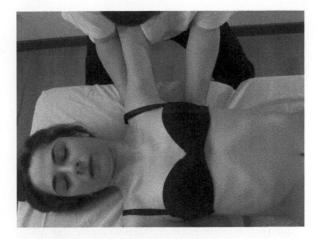

**Fig. 6.18**
The patient is in the supine position, and the operator, standing at the side, contacts the costal-vertebral joints of the same side from T2 to T5 with the fingers of both hands, after having positioned the patient's arm at about 90° of abduction, with the scapula resting on the operator's palms. Using his or her forearms on the table as a lever, the operator can apply an articulatory technique, with variable rate and rhythm, depending on tissue feel and the therapeutic goal.

- *Vagus nerve*: can be treated to improve nerve conduction and optimize lung and heart functions as well as vascular pressure gradients. It is possible for the operator to treat the vagus nerve at the point where it exits the skull, with techniques for the petro-jugular suture,[106] decompression applied to the occipital condyles,[107] on its cervical course, with treatment to the upper cervical area, at the supraclavicular and posterior clavicle levels, before the nerve penetrates into the thoracic cavity, and finally at the abdominal level, by treating the esophageal hiatus though which it passes.[108]

- **Central nuclei:** for example the pneumotaxic and apneustic nuclei, the nuclei of the solitary tract and dorsal motor vagus, mostly at pontobulbar level, which could be approached with a CV4, or EV4,[109] having effects on the cardiorespiratory-vascular global function. Decompression of sphenobasilar synchondrosis and alternated rocking of the temporals could exert a similar effect, by balancing dural–tentorial tensions, ventricular fluctuation, and hypothalamic activity. One can also use a direct approach at the level of specific mesencephalic and pontobulbar brain nuclei.[110]

- **Chapman reflexes:**[40] the anterior points are usually used for diagnosis (confirmed by locating a corresponding sensitive posterior point), while the posterior points are generally used for treatment, which consists of a circular massage of about 20–30 seconds (up to 90 seconds), performed with the fingertip deep into the reflex point, so as to dissipate the local edema. Alternatively, we can treat the corresponding intestinal areas and recheck the Chapman points to evaluate the tissue response.

## Local

Local intervention may provide a number of corrective measures for specific dysfunctional areas, determined during evaluation to be the most relevant to fluid balance and respiratory dynamics. Locally, the respiratory-circulatory model can be applied at the following levels:

- **Structural, particularly costal or spinal:** through articulatory, balanced ligamentous tension, muscle energy, facilitated positional release, lift techniques, etc., on the lower limbs, sacrum, ribs (rib 1-2, rib 7-12), and vertebrae (C2–C5–C6–T2–T4–T6), to improve heart and lung function, by improving the mobility, flexibility, and consequently the efficiency of the entire thoracoabdominal and pelvic cylinder.

- **Connective tissue-fascial,** by applying techniques such as effleurage and petrissage to the soft tissues, techniques for the interosseous membranes, unwinding of fascial restrictions to boost tissue oxygenation, as well as the venous and lymphatic return, especially in the limbs. An example is treatment of the myotendineal-fascial fold of the posterior axilla, referred to by Zink[111] as the "gate" to the upper limb. Myofascial dysfunctions of this area can interfere heavily with the venous and lymphatic drainage of the upper limb and the pectoral region. Consequences of dysfunction in this area[112] may include edema, temporomandibular joint disorders, upper limb dysesthesia, congested sinuses, and tender breasts, because of congestion in the subclavian lymph nodes. Finally, scars or adhesions may be treated with petrissage techniques, direct myofascial and fascial unwinding techniques,[113] loosening or connective tissue thrust techniques; the "cutting" technique of Jarricot,[114] techniques for the normalization of corresponding autonomic regulation centers, isolitic muscular energy[115] (in which the operator overcomes the voluntary muscle contraction of the patient, with the goal of obtaining a fibrolytic effect and realignment of functional collagen fibers), facilitated positional release (in which tissues are tested in their preferred directions of movement, and stacked in these positions of ease, to achieve a dynamic neutral "position,"[116] which is maintained until the tissues release).

- **Diaphragmatic:** for the correction of specific dysfunctions of a diaphragm or of its fascial extensions, both at the muscular domes and on their respective tendon insertions, through direct or indirect myofascial redoming techniques,[117] or muscle energy or functional inhibition often aided by the patient's respiratory effort.

- **Muscular:** through paraspinal muscular inhibition, or voluntary rapid muscle contractions (about 60 per minute), as in Ruddy's technique,[118] of specific muscles or muscle groups surrounding the dysfunctional area. This would favor the fluid circulation along its physiological course, taking advantage of the natural mechanism of myofascial pumping and related neuromuscular reflexes.

- **Visceral:** with treatment of local dysfunctions of target organs such as the lungs, heart, liver, kidneys, spleen, and intestine, for circulatory and respiratory function.[119] For almost all of these organs it is possible to have a treatment effect locally on mobility, with global lift techniques, or specifically on the related suspensory ligaments (especially the mesentery); on motility, by acting on respective involuntary movements; on viscosity-elasticity, observing the compliance of the bowels to compression and tension, and treating any areas for intra-tissue restriction; on the mobility of any serous layers that cover them, freeing, for example, restrictions between the parietal and visceral pericardium; on intra-mobility, treating limitations of gliding between two areas of the same organ (e.g., between the upper and lower lobe of the left lung); on hemodynamics, for example, opening the caval hiatus and then pumping to normalize dysfunctions of a congested liver (also indicated in infections caused by the right lung). The same principle can be applied with splenic pumping (also indicated for left lung infections). Obviously, both of these techniques are contraindicated in the presence of hepato- and splenomegaly, respectively.

- **Venous-lymphatic:** with routine and local techniques of specific for venous circulation release, such as the drainage of intracranial venous sinuses,[120] including frontal and parietal lifts,[121] and techniques for viscerocranium, such as vomer-ethmoid pumping or drainage of the Eustachian tube;[122] or lymphatic drainage techniques such as the Zink pectoral traction[123] or those for the thoracic duct or cisterna chyli.[124] The pumping techniques can be applied in synchronization with respiration, increasing the effect of inspiratory expansion through local application of tensile forces, or

using compressive forces to enhance the expulsive phase of exhalation.

If we want instead to provide a greater incentive for fluid release, we can gradually increase the local pressure on the treatment area during the expiratory phase, and then release the pressure abruptly just before the inspiratory phase. This would create a rapid and elevated pressure gradient in favor of circulatory release. However, if applied to the chest, it is to be avoided in patients with emphysema or chronic bronchitis,[125] since the air forcibly inhaled during the maneuver would remain trapped in the alveolar cavities because of the resistance of the terminal airways. Finally, to facilitate venous and lymphatic return is also possible to apply, during the expiratory phase, some local vibrations in the congested area, with variable frequency and force as needed. Sutherland himself suggested the application of vibrations to the lymphatics,[126] in particular the thoracic duct and the cisterna chyli, to facilitate drainage.

- **Arterial:** using reflex techniques, working on the ganglia and the corresponding autonomic complexes; visceral techniques to free the course of the main arterial routes;[127] or specific techniques for dysfunctions of the fascial and muscular walls of large and medium-sized arteries (aorta, coronary, carotid, brachial arteries, iliac, femoral, etc.), both in myofascial mode[128] and in recoil.[84]

- **Interstitial fluid:** especially for dehydrated and chronically dysfunctional areas, but also for those that are congested and edematous, through effleurage and tapotement techniques.[93] Before applying these techniques one must free the vascular paths through the connective tissue pathway, by using, for example, balanced ligamentous tension techniques[129] or membranous techniques. In addition, by using the fluid drive mechanism it is possible to intentionally connect with the fluid dimension, with one hand in the "source" and the other in the area of dysfunctional "reception," as is usually done with the V-spread technique.[130] Generally, we choose sources that are in opposite anatomical positions to that of the dysfunctional reception (e.g., for an edematous area in the anterior knee, we opt for the popliteal fossa as a posterior source, or, for a lumbar disc dehydrated zone, we opt for a an anterior abdominal source). Interstitial fluid fluctuation can be driven by the operator toward the dysfunction, in the case of chronic dehydration, or away from the dysfunction, as in the case of edema or congestion. Another example, suggested by Sutherland,[131] is fluctuations applied laterally to the forearm (or leg). Here, one must first treat the ulna, the radius, and then finally the wrist (from proximal to distal), possibly including balanced tension of the interosseous membrane, and then applying lateral fluctuation to the forearm.[112]

Finally, in reference to the diagnostic and therapeutic applications of the respiratory-circulatory model, it should be specified that this is not intended to provide a protocol for osteopathic evaluation and treatment, making it a mere sequence of tests, techniques, or procedures. Rather, it should be interpreted as a guideline, with interchangeable and modifiable components, depending on the operator and the patient's needs, in the context of each unique therapeutic interaction. Certainly, the operator can, when necessary, use only one of the presented tests or in different sequences than those listed, or decide whether to approach the patient only globally or only locally. The operator may also perform an evaluation and treatment that uses multiple osteopathic models.

In fact, just as the nervous, cardiorespiratory, mechanical, metabolic, and psychological functions in the body act and interact in an integrated fashion, as a complex unit of structure and function in constant dynamic equilibrium, thanks to a multisystemic connection with multimodal relationships of nonlinear form and nature, so the assessment and osteopathic treatment will have to be flexible and adaptable to the patient being treat-

ed, suitable to the specific complaint, clinical progression, social status and family history, any drug treatment or other forms of concomitant therapy, in constant dynamism and change, together with the tissue responses after application of a test or corrective measures.

The operator does not impose, therefore, an a priori model of respiratory-circulatory type on the basis of certain clinical findings and strict procedural sequences, but rather constantly "models" an intervention of primary fluidic impact based on the adaptive responses of a single and unique patient, in constant functional and structural dynamism, in order to strengthen self-regulation mechanisms and the general state of health.

Regardless of the level of intervention chosen and applied, it is still a good idea to educate the patient to the best lifestyle that can maintain the results achieved by OMT and prevent eventual recurrences. Within the respiratory-circulatory area, for example, recommending regular moderate physical activity may be essential to maintaining good circulation and oxygenation of the fluids; or, one may teach the patient a series of exercises for specific muscle groups, intended to maintain local fluid dynamics.

Cases of cardiorespiratory disease, especially if chronic, require the integration of osteopathic treatment with rehabilitative physiotherapy, through sessions of cardiorespiratory gymnastics, or specific methods for the recovery of respiratory efficiency,[132] in addition to possible pharmacological care, and positional maneuvers, such as reclining at 45° from the supine position. In the case of specific congestion areas, as might happen as a result of trauma or surgery, elevation of the involved area, functional bandaging and kinesio-taping, associated with lymphatic drainage or tissue massage and circulatory gymnastics, could produce excellent results and prepare the tissue for a better response to osteopathic treatment and/or medication.

However, it is always advisable to pay attention to the ergonomics adopted in the workplace or in the performance of sporting and hobby activities. Prolonged standing or sitting positions (as required in many professions) or lying down (as required in many pathological conditions) are nevertheless always to be alternated as much as possible, since they can profoundly affect the circulation of fluids, in particular venous and lymphatic flow. In that case, elastic bands, such as an elastic/compressive stocking, could be of help, as well as the adoption of behavioral changes, such as alternating between sitting and standing during long plane flights.

## Rationale, mechanisms, and evidence

The basic principle of the Zink model is that a good circulation of all body fluids, including drainage and proper nourishment of the tissues down to the cellular level, is the basis for health status and homeostasis.[51] This represents the circulatory part of the method. To achieve this goal, respiratory processes should work correctly, through the action of the "respiratory pump," performed by the thoracic diaphragm, from the chest and from the lungs. This mechanism would work as a "triple" suction pump, by sucking air, venous blood and lymph, in synergy with the cardiac "pressure pump," to ensure the circulation of body fluids.[51] This is the respiratory aspect of the method. There is also another element which, according to Zink, is essential for respiratory physiological mechanisms, namely the primary respiratory mechanism, described by Sutherland[131] as an involuntary rhythm that would spread throughout the body, including fluids, with a probable fluid-lymphatic-interstitial flow as its basis.[133]

Special emphasis has therefore been placed by Zink on the freedom of movement of the pelvic and cranial diaphragms, and in their relationship with the thoracic diaphragm, including the joint mobility of the sacrum between the iliac bones, by highlighting the importance of a cranium–sternum–sacrum system.[134] Primary respiration supports the secondary respiration and its pelvic-thoracic-abdominal pump in constant synergy with the heart. What is certain is that both of these respiratory mechanisms are engaged by the corresponding osteo-pathic model, in order to reduce edema and remove metabolites. For this purpose, manual treatment is traditionally focused on:[52]

- the opening of fascial paths in the four areas of transition, to remove every connective tissue obstacle to the free movement of the fluids

- the optimization and synchronization of the primary and secondary respiration

- the facilitation of venous and lymphatic drainage.

This would ensure an increase in the cellular and tissue health level, and therefore of the homeostatic and adaptation potential of the organism. The medical and osteopathic professions have recognized the importance of the lymphatic system in the maintenance of health,[135] and the homeostatic effect of lymphatic pumping techniques. It appears that their rhythmic action of stimulation on the fluid circulation favors the endothelial release of the nitric oxide synthase enzyme.[136]

This has also been confirmed by recent studies on the effect of isolated lymphatic techniques, such as the Dalrymple pedal pump, which can cause an increase of nitric oxide, equivalent to moderate physical exercise.[137] These data, combined with the overwhelming amount of research on the beneficial effects of nitric oxide,[138] provide a dynamic theoretical framework to explain some of the effects of OMT. What is certain is that many of the fluid techniques make use of oscillatory forces and vibratory percussions during their implementation.

These techniques seem to promote fluid flow among tissue compartments by means of hydraulic mechanisms,[139] with possible effects on endoneural blood flow,[140] spinal excitability,[141] the central nervous system,[142] tissue repair, and vessel regeneration.[143] At the same time, manual techniques such as petrissage and effleurage have been proven to be effective in myalgias, edema, and recovery of muscle function,[144] as well as in the modulation of nociception.[145] If applied with excessive pressure

(70–100 mmHg) they can cause lesions of the peripheral lymphatic vessels, especially in conditions of lymphedema or venous return disorders.[146]

Even more interesting is the effect that fluid techniques, even when isolated, seem to produce both on the general immune response, causing an increase in blood basophils[147] and on the specific antibody response,[148] increasing the reaction speed of the body to antiviral vaccines.[149] In the latter case, the techniques were applied three times a week for 2 weeks, after the administration of the vaccine. Therefore, it is easy to imagine the impact that they can exercise on the efficiency of the immune system, and subsequently on the costs of a nation's health system, especially in light of the demonstrated effects on reducing the use of antibiotics during influenza outbreaks[150] as well as on preventive, protective, and therapeutic results, for both healthy and hospitalized patients, particularly in cases of high emotional or physiological stress, related to the levels of IgA.[151]

However, some studies on the thoracic lymphatic technique did not note a significant increase in either the specific antibody response following administration of influenza vaccines[152,153] or interferons in serum.[154] It became crucial to investigate the effects in the laboratory on non-anesthetized animals, which first showed an increase of flow in the thoracic duct on dogs, after two sessions of 30 seconds of abdominal and chest-pumping,[155] and that increase in lymph flow coincided with an increase in flow and in the leukocyte count.[156]

Subsequent studies demonstrated that the main source of the produced leukocytes is from the gastrointestinal lymphoid tissue.[157] Although these results have so far been found only partially in humans,[158] they will probably suggest a similar mechanism of action. Recent research has shown an intrinsic contractility of the smooth musculature of the lymphatic system,[159] capable of generating the propagation of waves of rhythmic, tonic, and phasic contractions, and consequent pressure gradients,

fundamental for the propulsion of the lymph (systolic blood pressure from 12 to 70 up to 100 mmHg; diastolic blood pressure of 0–5 mmHg).[160]

These contractile properties may be mediated by the autonomic nervous system, supporting the use of osteopathic manipulative techniques aimed at influencing the neurovegetative system to improve lymphatic circulation.[52] A pilot study in 2005 showed the influence of the CV4 on the latency period of sleep and the activity of the autonomic nervous system on a muscular level (MSNA) in healthy individuals.[161] The experimental group showed a decrease in sleep latency, as well as the MSNA, in comparison with the control and sham group (p <0.05). The MSNA, in particular, decreased even more in the experimental group after the still point of the technique, compared to the previous phase (p <0.01), and in a different manner from the control and sham group (p <0.05).

Later, Nelson and colleagues explored the effects of the CV4 technique on the Traube–Hering oscillations of blood flow velocity,[162] mediated by the activity of the autonomic nervous system.[163] They found an increase in the Traube–Hering wave amplitude after application of the technique, thus supporting the influence of the technique on the autonomic nervous system and, consequently, on the bloodstream. To confirm this, a study in 2011 noted that the application of osteopathic cranial techniques causes a statistically significant decrease in oxygen saturation in the prefrontal cerebral lobes, associated with both a reduction in orthosympathetic influence and an increase in the parasympathetic influence on cardiac and systemic circulatory parameters.[164]

In addition, lymphatic techniques seem to be able to modulate orthosympathetic hyperactivities with improvements on different hemodynamic[165] and cardiac[166] functions, while manual techniques seem to exert an influence on the flow of parasympathetic tone with consequent effects on the blood turbulance and shear rate.[17] This once again demonstrates the interaction between the circulatory and nervous systems, requiring an equal integration of corresponding osteopathic models. Research on the effects of fluid techniques was extended to vascular and cardiac functions, first on healthy subjects, demonstrating that lymphatic techniques are able to increase diastolic pressure,[165] while cranial venous drainage techniques result in an increase in vertebral basilar artery perfusion.[167] Second, while studying patients with diseases, OMT applied in cases of peripheral arterial disease has been shown to improve endothelial function and the quality of life, resulting in a significant increase in brachial flow mediated by vasodilatation, the brachial and crural pressure index, the first claudication time, and physical health status and quality of life.[168] In patients with essential hypertension, a 1-year follow-up study has shown that osteopathic treatment for fluid impact is able to improve intima-media vessel thickness and systolic (but not diastolic) blood pressure. These findings suggest a potential benefit of OMT in the management of patients at risk of cardiovascular accidents.[169]

Earlier studies had suggested the potential action of OMT in the treatment of hypertension,[170] identifying the dysfunctional somatic and palpable effects in hypertensive patients.[171] Manipulative treatment is also an effective method in patients suffering from dizziness caused by cervical instability.[172] The effectiveness seems to be related to improvement of blood flow in the vertebral artery, measured by transcranial Doppler, and the restoration of cervical stability (p <0.05), verified by radiography. Finally, studies on surgical patients have proven the hemodynamic effects of OMT immediately after coronary artery bypass.[173] The treatment, which aims to improve respiratory and hemodynamic functions, was performed while the subjects were completely anesthetized. A comparison of measurements taken after the surgery on the treated subjects and the control subjects noted significant differences in the cardiac index (p < or = 0.02) and the mixed venous blood oxygen saturation (p < or = 0.005).

Contemporary research has also shown that the myocardial ischemia induces an increase in paraspinal muscular tone located in the T2–T3 region, detected by palpation.[174] The subjects of the experiments were 15 conscious dogs, instrumentally examined before, during, and after artificially induced ischemia. The operator performed electromyographic analysis and manual palpation assessment of the T2–T3 and T11–T12 spinal segments (control). The results were that the myocardial ischemia is associated with a significantly increased paraspinal muscle tone, localized in the T2–T3 left lateral myotomes – changes which are reversible after left ventricular sympathectomy. This also confirms the validity of palpation as a useful tool to recognize tissue changes in areas with altered autonomic tone.[175]

Over the past two decades, several clinical studies have investigated the effects of vertebrocostal manipulations and lymphatic pump techniques on respiratory efficiency, demonstrating a significant increase in thoracic expansion, total lung capacity, oxygen saturation, and vital capacity.[176,177] Many studies have investigated the effects on lung diseases, particularly in the elderly. With age the compliance of the thoracic cage decreases, as does the vital capacity, while the residual volume increases.[178] Two pilot studies found significant reductions in the use of intravenous antibiotics and hospitalization time on elderly patients suffering from pneumonia,[179,180] suggesting that the mechanism of action of OMT may be related to humoral factors that increase the immune response.[181]

Following these preliminary studies, a multicenter research study was done involving 406 patients with pneumonia.[182] The results showed a significant reduction in hospital stay, administration of antibiotics, cases of respiratory failure, and death in patients who also received osteopathic treatment compared to those who received only conventional treatment. However, the same positive results were also seen in the group which was given treatment in light touch mode, indicating that there may be important questions about the influence of the placebo effect in studies on the effectiveness of OMT, or on the therapeutic potential of the light touch.

In some studies the results were not as positive, although still useful for understanding the mechanism of action. For example, use of lymphatic pump techniques on patients suffering from chronic obstructive pulmonary disease produced an immediate decrease of forced expiratory flow, expiratory reserve volume, and flow resistance in the airways (associated with increased residual volume and total lung capacity). The authors hypothesized that the worsening was caused by alveolar air entrapment introduced by the "active" component of the thoracic lymphatic pump, resulting in an increase in residual volume for the airway resistance in chronic bronchitis.[125] This was also suggested in view of the possible side effects of breathing exercises on patients with chronic bronchitis, which could trigger mechanisms similar to those generated by the application of OMT.[183]

Pilot studies have also investigated the effects of osteopathic techniques with respiratory impact on asthmatic pediatric patients[184] and on patients suffering from chronic asthma,[185] finding in the first case an increase in expiratory peak flow from 7 to 9 L per minute (with a 95% confidence interval), and in the second case a significant increase in forced respiratory excursion (but not the peak expiratory flow and symptomatic complaints). In addition, there was a significant reduction (p = 0.01) in episodes of apnea after two sessions of manipulative techniques on infants suffering from obstructive

sleep apnea,[186] although the differences between these episodes, evaluated by polysomnography, was not significant (p = 0.43) compared to that found in the control group after a follow-up period of 2 weeks.

Mills and colleagues studied the effects of OMT as an adjuvant therapy to the usual treatment of 57 children with recurrent acute otitis media[187]. In 6 months of follow-up, the authors found a reduction in the number of acute episodes and a normalization of tympanograms (but not of audiometric tests) compared to the control group. These results added to the findings in a recent pilot study of 52 patients, aged between 6 months and 2 years.[188] However, a systematic review of studies that have investigated the effects of OMT in pediatrics found serious methodological flaws in nearly all the research so far, applied mostly on very small populations and without follow-up, rarely ensuring control of the placebo effect or blinding of patients, and only occasionally blinding of the examiners.[189]

It has also been speculated that the adverse reactions caused by the OMT have not been adequately reported in scientific studies.[190] For example, the application of too much treatment or of excessively long sessions can result in unwanted effects.[191] We should not forget that osteopathic procedures often involve energy expenditure by the patient which we should not underestimate. This suggests that the therapeutic input should be kept below the individual's physical capacity, for example in the acute phase, and not to expect a complete resolution with only a few applications in the chronic patient[192] (see Chapter 9).

## Case study

A 47-year-old man, divorced, with a daughter, employed full-time and with mesomorphic biotype, presents with a dull, continuous pain in his right ankle, following a mild inversion sprain which had occurred 6 weeks earlier. The pain worsens after about half an hour of prolonged standing or sitting and is relieved by rest. An MRI performed 2 weeks after the event did not report any type of tissue injury, although he noticed a diffuse periarticular edema at the lateral perimalleolar level. The man also suffers chronically from external hemorrhoids, for which he

## Case study continued

underwent surgery 5 years ago. A cholecystectomy was performed 9 years ago, due to gallstones and consequent repeated inflammation of the gall bladder. Finally, from the age of around 10 to 18 years or so he suffered from episodes of severe allergic asthma, with a tendency in the last decade to develop recurrent infections of the upper respiratory tract (especially frontal sinusitis and pharyngitis).

On physical examination, the man has a strong back posture, with the occiput in extension, anterior neck, increased thoracic kyphosis and sternalcostal compression, collapse of the abdominal and pelvic visceral tensions, with overload of the sacroiliac joints and the posterior aspects of the feet. His weight appears majorly transferred to the lower left limb, resulting in translation and rotation of the pelvis to the left. The Zink test, performed in standing position, shows that his myofascial patterns are decompensated at the cervical-upper thoracic level (with rotation to the right) and at the abdominal-pelvic level (with rotation to the left). The latter, however, normalizes when performing the Zink test in the supine position (suggesting one descendant dysfunctional pattern). The central tendon test shows a clear lateral deviation of the right posterior superior component. On palpation, there are Chapman points for the larynx and liver, while among the terminal sites, the supraclavicular areas, the inguinal area, but especially the Achilles tendon and right perimalleolar areas are edematous.

The left pelvic and right upper thoracic diaphragms are clearly dysfunctional, associated with tissue stiffness and hypomobility of the corresponding spinal transitional segments. In particular, the T1–T3 region shows a group dysfunction NSRright with hypertonia of the paraspinal tissues, R>L. The right main bronchus is clearly dysfunctional, with a marked reduction in tissue

compliance to pressure tests and lower lateral distension. Finally, the cholecystectomy scar is active, with consequent alteration of liver mobility in anterior dysfunction. The inhibition test reveals a right bronchus dominance over the T1–T3 vertebral group, a non-relationship between the scar and the right bronchus, and a co-dominance between the scar and the pelvic hemidiaphragm.

There is an evident primacy of the right bronchus, perhaps related to previous asthmatic episodes that may have facilitated the corresponding sympathetic control, compromised the corresponding portion of the central tendon of the diaphragm and upper thoracic drainage terminal sites, and predisposed the patient to venous and lymphatic congestion and infection of the upper airway. Concomitantly, there is a less primary dysfunctional framework, but perhaps more primary toward the current disorder in his right ankle, i.e., a fascial-connective dysfunction at both hypochondric and right hemipelvic levels probably associated with the corresponding surgeries (gallbladder and hemorrhoids) and possibly related to the congestion detected in the lower right limb. The patient's sedentary lifestyle, as well as the lack of appropriate manual treatment or rehabilitation of the ankle after the trauma, may represent a further point against joint functional recovery.

In the *first session* we proceeded with the aim of reducing the symptoms, given that the patient reported the frustrating need to get up often from the workstation due to the pain in his ankle, making it difficult to fulfill his contractual commitments. So, first of all we normalized the posterior-lateral upper portion of the central tendon, and then we approached the hemidiaphragm pelvic dysfunction with direct myofascial techniques. Finally, we simultaneously balanced

## Case study continued

the whole diaphragmatic system, through the use of wedges to maintain balanced tension of each of the four stations. We then applied fascial unwinding to the scar in the right upper quadrant, and finally a pedal pump technique to the lower limbs, particularly effleurage to his right ankle.

In the *second session*, 2 weeks later, the patient reported a marked improvement of symptoms, allowing him greater autonomy in both standing and sitting positions. However, on examination, the swelling persisted in the right ankle (but not in the inguinal region), along with dysfunctional disturbance of the right bronchus, and active Chapman points for the larynx. The Zink test was uncompensated in the first two stations, while the central posterior-superior tendon showed only a twist to the right. We proceeded to inhibit the upper thoracic paraspinal ganglia, then to release the right bronchus by direct technique. This was followed by BLT in the sitting position to release the thoracic inlet, and drainage techniques of the same region. The final phase ended with the normalization of the central tendon and synchronization between the upper thoracic diaphragm and the right pelvic diaphragm.

In the *third session*, 3 weeks after the second, the patient reported the disappearance of the initial symptoms, but reported infra-nuchal tension and widespread heaviness in the head, especially within the last few days, which was aggravated in the evening. The Zink test revealed a slight tendency toward unbalancing the first two stations, with the supra-nuchal and superior cervical terminal sites having major congestion, associated with compression of the cranial base. We performed a CV4 and then the venous sinus drainage technique, after freeing the left thoracic inlet, and finally applied articulatory techniques for the neck and upper chest.

At the first session, the patient was informed about his current condition and instructed to avoid aggravating factors, as well as to pursue activities which alleviated his symptoms. Water gymnastics were recommended for cardiorespiratory function, thus favoring increased venous and lymphatic drainage. Proprioceptive exercises were recommended to optimize neuromotor control of the ankle and reduce the risk of recurrence. Ergonomic advice was provided to the patient to better organize his workstation (type and height of the chair, the computer's position and location, etc.) and manage work hours (with intervals of stretching exercises for the neck area and lower limbs associated with breathing; appropriate use of mouse and phone, etc.).

## Conclusions

The respiratory-circulatory model was created as, and remains fundamentally, a conceptual model, emphasizing assessment and treatment of the fluid component of the body and its oxygenation. Since its origins, it has offered to osteopathic medicine a unique tool of its kind, adaptable on both a global and a local level, with effects on health and disease. The ultimate goal is always the maintenance of the self-regulatory capacity of the body and the person's mental and physical health. Although the essence of the model is purely conceptual, its principles have been organized in diagnostic manuals and treatment procedures, as suggested in this chapter, but also in other texts, with particular emphasis on the lymphatic system approach and on the primary respiratory mechanism.[193,194] Although, to date, fluid techniques remain among those frequently used by modern osteopaths,[195] evidence of their effectiveness, although available, is incomplete, requiring greater exploration, supported by more accurate, reproducible, and objective methods. Finally, the respiratory-circulatory model cannot be separated from interaction and integration with all the other models, requiring application with frequency, duration and dosage compatible with the individual's capacity to respond at the time of consultation.

## References

1. Kuchera ML. Lymphatics approach. In: Chila A, editor. Foundations of osteopathic medicine. 3rd ed. Philadelphia, PA: Lippincott Williams and Wilkins; 2010. p. 793.

2. Hall JE. Guyton and Hall textbook of medical physiology. 12th ed. Philadelphia, PA: Saunders Elsevier; 2010. ch. 25.

3. Lee RP. Interface: mechanisms of spirit in osteopathy. Portland, OR: Stillness Press Llc; 2005.

4. Parsons J, Marcer N. Osteopathy: models for diagnosis treatment and practice. Edinburgh: Elsevier Churchill Livingstone; 2006. pp. 159–64.

5. Boussuges A, Gole Y, Blanc P. Diaphragmatic motion studied by mode ultrasonography: methods reproducibility and normal values. Chest. 2009;135(2):391–400.

6. Riemenschneider PA, Shields JW. Human central lymph propulsion. JAMA. 1981;6;246(18):2066–7.

7. Smith HJ. Ultrasonic assessment of abdominal venous return. I. Effect of cardiac action and respiration on mean velocity pattern cross-sectional area and flow in the inferior vena cava and portal vein. Acta Radiol Diag. 1985;26(5):581–8.

8. Wainapel SF, Fast A. Alternative medicine and rehabilitation: a guide for practitioners. New York, NY: Demos Medical Publishing; 2003. p. 322.

9. De Burgh Daly M. Interactions between respiration and circulation. In: Cherniack NS, Widdicombe JG, editors. Handbook of physiology. Section 3: The respiratory system. Vol II: Control of breathing. Part 2. Bethesda, MD: American Physiological Society; 1986. pp. 529–94.

10. Song SH, Lehrer P. The effects of specific respiratory rates on heart rate and heart rate variability. Appl Psychophysiol Biofeedback. 2003;28(1):13–23.

11. Gashev A. Physiological aspects of lymphatic contractile functions: current perspectives. Ann N Y Acad Sci. 2002;979, 178–87.

12. Busek P, Kemlink D. The influence of the respiratory cycle on the EEG. Physiol Res. 2005;54(3):327–33.

13. Courtney R. The functions of breathing and its dysfunctions and their relationship to breathing therapy. Int J Osteopath Med. 2009;12(3):78–85.

14. Schleip R, Klingler W, Lehmann-Horn F. Active fascial contractility: fascia may be able to contract in a smooth muscle-like manner and thereby influence musculoskeletal dynamics. Med Hypotheses. 2005;65(2):273–7.

15. Staubesand J, Li Y. Zum Feinbau der fascia cruris mit besonderer Berucksichtigung epi- und intrafaszialer nerven. Manuelle Medizin. 1996;34:196–200.

16. DeStefano LA. Greenman's principles of manual medicine. 4th ed. Baltimore, MD: Williams and Wilkins; 2011. p. 47.

17. Queré N, Noël E, Lieutaud A et al. Fasciatherapy combined with pulsology touch induces changes in blood turbulence potentially beneficial for vascular endothelium. J Bodyw Mov Ther. 2009;13(3):239–45.

18. Wernham J, Hall TE. The mechanics of the spine and pelvis. Maidstone, UK: Maidstone College of Osteopathy; 1960.

19. Seffinger MA, King HH, Ward RC et al. Osteopathic phylosophy. In: Chila AG, editor. Foundations of osteopathic medicine. 3rd ed. Philadelphia, PA: Lippincott Williams and Wilkins; 2011. pp. 5–6.

20. Still AT. Autobiography of Andrew T Still, revised ed. Kirksville, MO; 1908.

21. Still AT. The philosophy and mechanical principles of osteopathy. Kirksville, MO; 1892. Reprinted Kirksville, MO; Osteopathic Enterprises; 1986.

22. Still AT. Philosophy of osteopathy. Kirksville, MO; 1899. Carmel, CA: Acadademy of Applied Osteopathy; reprinted 1946.

23. Barber ED. Diseases of the lymphatic system. In: Osteopathy complete. Kansas City, MO: Hudson-Kimblerly Publishing Co.; 1898. pp. 129–32.

24. Burns L. Viscerosomatic and somatovisceral spinal reflexes. J Am Osteopath Assoc. 1907;7:51–7.

25. Burns L. Osteopathic case reports of pulmonary disease: a review. J Am Osteopath Assoc. 1933;33:1–5.

26. Burns L. Principles governing the treatment of cardiac conditions. J Am Osteopath Assoc. 1944;43:231–4.

27. Bowling DJ. Lymphatics. In: DiGiovanna EL, Schiowitz S, Dowling DJ, editors. An osteopathic approach to diagnosis and treatment. 3rd ed. Philadelphia, PA: Lippincott Williams and Wilkins; 2005. pp. 589.

28. Smith RK. One hundred thousand cases of influenza with a death rate one-fortieth of that officially reported under conventional medical treatment. J Am Osteopath Assoc. 2000;100(5):320–3 [reprint of J Am Osteopath Assoc. 1920;19:172–5].

29. Millard FP. A lymphatic examination. J Osteopath. 1922;29:78–81.

30. Millard FP. Applied anatomy of the lymphatics. Kirksville, MO: International Lymphatic Research Society; 1922.

31. Miller CE. The lymphatic pump, its application to acute infections. J Am Osteopath Assoc. 1926;25:443–5.

32. Miller CE. Osteopathic principles and thoracic pump therapeutics proved by scientific research. J Am Osteopath Assoc. 1927;26:910–4.

33. Miller CE. Lymph stasis. J Am Osteopath Assoc. 1928;28:173–4. In: Chikly B. Manual techniques addressing the lymphatic system: origins and development. J Am Osteopath Assoc. 2005;105(10):457–64.

34. Galbreath WO. Acute otitis media including its postural and manipulative treatment. J Am Osteopath Assoc. 1929;28:377–79.

35. Miller CE. The specific cure of pneumonia. J Am Osteopath Assoc. 1924;24:99–101.

36. Lane MA. On increasing the antibody content of the serum by manipulation of the spleen. J Osteopath. 1920;27:361–4.

37. Castilio Y, Ferris-Swift L. The effect of direct splenic stimulation on the cells and the antibody content of the blood stream in acute infectious diseases. Carmel, CA: Academy of Applied Osteopathy; 1934, reprinted 1955. pp. 121–38.

38. Ferris-Swift L. The effects of indirect splenic treatment in normal individuals. J Am Osteopath Assoc. 1936;35:225–9.

39. Sutherland WG. Teachings in the science of osteopathy. Fort Worth, TX: Sutherland Cranial Teaching Foundation Inc; 1990. p. 127.

40. Owens C. 1937 An endocrine interpretation of Chapman's reflexes. Carmel, CA: Academy of Applied Osteopathy; reprint 1963.

41. Ruddy TJ. Osteopathic manipulation in eye ear nose and throat disease. American Academy of Applied Osteopathy Yearbook 1962. pp. 133–40.

42. Zink JG. Respiratory and circulatory care: the conceptual model. Osteopath Ann. 1977;5(3):108–12.

43. Allen WT, Pence TK. The use of the thoracic pump in treatment of lower respiratory tract disease. J Am Osteopath Assoc. 1967;67:408–11.

44. Frymann VM. The osteopathic approach to cardiac and pulmonary problems. J Am Osteopath Assoc. 1978;77:668–73.

45. Hix EL. Reflex viscerosomatic reference phenomena. Osteopath Ann. 1976;4:496–503.

46. Mannino JR. The application of neurological reflexes to the treatment of hypertension. J Am Osteopath Assoc. 1979;79:225–31.

47. Beal MC. Viscerosomatic reflexes: a review. J Am Osteopath Assoc. 1985;85:786–801.

48. Beal MC, Morlock JW. Somatic dysfunction associated with pulmonary disease. J Am Osteopath Assoc. 1984;84:179–83.

49. Howell RK, Allen TW, Kappler RE. The influence of OMT in the management of patients with COPD. J Am Osteopath Assoc. 1975;75:757–60.

50. Miller WD. Treatment of visceral disorders by manipulative therapy. In: The research status of spinal manipulative therapy [monograph]. no 15:295–301. Bethesda, MD: National Institute of Neurological and Communication Disorders and Stroke; 1975.

51. Zink JG. 1973 Applications of the osteopathic holistic approach to homeostasis. American Academy of Applied Osteopathy Yearbook 1973, pp. 37–47.

52. Kuchera ML. Osteopathic manipulative medicine considerations in patients with chronic pain. J Am Osteo Assoc. 2005;105:29–32.

53. Loo M. Integrative medicine for children. St Louis, MO: Saunders Elsevier; 2009. pp. 26–7.

54. Pope RE. The common compensatory pattern: its origin and relationship to the postural model. AAO J. 2003;13(4):19–40.

55. Bowling DJ. Lymphatics. In: DiGiovanna EL, Schiowitz S, Dowling DJ, editors. An osteopathic approach to diagnosis and treatment. 3rd ed. Philadelphia, PA: Lippincott Williams and Wilkins; 2005. ch. 107.

56. Hodge L, Harden L, Pedrueza M et al. Lymphatic pump treatment increases leukocyte trafficking and inhibits tumor formation in the lungs of rats. J Am Ost Assoc. 2010;110(8):478.

57. Opipari MI, Perrotta AI, Essig-Beatty DR. Oncology. In: Ward RC, editor. Foundations of osteopathic medicine. 2nd ed. Philadelphia, PA: Lippincott Williams and Wilkins; 2002. pp. 473–4.

58. Zink JG, Lawson WB. An osteopathic structural examination and functional interpretation of the soma. Osteopath Ann. 1979;7:12–9.

59. Defeo G, Hicks L. A description of the common compensatory pattern in relationship to the osteopathic postural examination. Dynamic Chiropractic. 1993;24:11.

60. Chaitow L. Terapia manuale dei tessuti molli. Principi e tecniche di positional release. 3rd ed. Elsevier Masson; 2009. p. 17.

61. Zink JG, Lawson WB. Pressure gradients in osteopathic manipulative management of the obstetric patient. Osteopath Ann. 1979;7(5): 42–9.

62. Davis MF, Worden K, Clawson D. Confirmatory factor analysis in osteopathic medicine: fascial and spinal motion restrictions as correlates of muscle spasticity in children with ce-rebral palsy J Am Osteopath Ass. 2007;107(6):226–32.

63. Hruby RJ. Pathophysiologic models and the selection of osteopathic manipulative techniques. J Osteopath Med. 1992;6(4):25–30.

64. Chaitow L. Cranial manipulation: theory and practice: osseous and soft tissue approaches. Elsevier Health Sciences; 2005. pp. 370–2.

65. Dummer TG. Specific adjusting technique. Hove: JoTom Publications; 1995.

66. Liem T, McPartland JM, Skinner E. Cranial osteopathy: principles and practice. Edinburgh: Elsevier Churchill Livingstone; 2004. pp. 340–2.

67. Zavarella P, Asmone C, Zanardi M. Le asimmetrie occluso-posturali. 2nd ed. Rome: GLM editore; 2002. vol. 1.

68. Stone C. Science in the art of osteopathy: osteopathic principles and practice. London: Nelson Thornes; 1999. ch. 9.

69. Willard FH, Fossum C, Standley PR. The fascial system of the body In: Chila A, editor. Foundations of osteopathic medicine. 3rd ed. Philadelphia, PA: Lippincott Williams and Wilkins; 2011. ch. 7.

70. Stone CA. Visceral and obstetric osteopathy. Edinburgh: Elsevier Churchill Livingstone; 2007. pp. 12–13.

71. Hebgen EU. Visceral manipulation in osteopathy. Thieme Publishing Group; 2011. ch. 1.

72. Chauffour P, Prat E. Mechanical link: fundamental principles theory and practice following an osteopathic approach. Berkeley, CA: North Atlantic Books; 2002. pp. 15–18.

73. Liem T, McPartland JM, Skinner E. Cranial osteopathy: principles and practice. Edinburgh: Elsevier Churchill Livingstone; 2004. chs 18 and 20.

74. Sills F. Craniosacral biodynamics: the primal midline and the organization of the body. Berkeley, CA: North Atlantic Books; 2003. pp. 19–26.

75. Shea MJ. Biodynamic craniosacral therapy. Berkeley, CA : North Atlantic Books; 2007. vol. 1, ch. 30.

76. McPartland JM, Skinner E. The biodynamic model of osteopathy in the cranial field. In: Chaitow L, editor. Cranial manipulation: theory and practice: osseous and soft tissue approaches. Edinburgh: Elsevier Health Sciences; 2005. p. 106.

77. Kuchera M. Kuchera W. Osteopathic consideration in systemic dysfunction. Columbus, OH: Greyden Press; 1994. pp. 205-7.

78. Chikly B. Silent waves: theory and practice of lymph drainage therapy with applications for lymphedema chronic pain and inflammation. IHH Publishing; 2001.

79. Lewit K. Manipulative therapy in rehabilitation of the motor system. London: Butterworths; 1985. pp. 35-8.

80. Kuchera M, Kuchera W. Osteopathic consideration in systemic dysfunction. Columbus, OH: Greyden Press; 1994. pp. 209-17.

81. Owens C. Chapman's reflexes. Chapman's Reflex Foundation Clinics; 1942.

82. DiGiovanna E. An encyclopedia of osteopathy. Indianapolis, IN: American Academy of Osteopathy; 2001. p. 24.

83. Kuchera ML. Lymphatics approach. In: Chila A, editor. Foundations of osteopathic medicine. 3rd ed. Philadelphia, PA: Lippincott Williams and Wilkins; 2011. pp. 792-3.

84. Chauffour P, Prat E. Mechanical link: fundamental principles, theory and practice following an osteopathic approach. Berkeley, CA: North Atlantic Books; 2002. ch. 12.

85. Lewit K, Olanska S. Clinical importance of active scars: abnormal scars as a cause of myofascial pain. J Manipulative Physiol Ther. 2004;27(6):399-402.

86. Chauffour P, Prat E. Mechanical link: fundamental principles, theory and practice following an osteopathic approach. Berkeley, CA: North Atlantic Books; 2002. pp. 38-40.

87. Barral JP, Croibier A. Manual therapy for the peripheral nerves. Elsevier Health Sciences; 2007. pp. 119-20.

88. Dowling DJ. Inhibition and progressive inhibition of neuromuscouloskeletal structures. In: DiGiovanna EL, Schiowitz S Dowling DJ, editors. An osteopathic approach to diagnosis and treatment. 3rd ed. Philadelphia, PA: Lippincott Williams and Wilkins; 2005. ch. 23.

89. Frymann VM. The core-link and the three diaphragms. A unit for respiratory function. In: The collected papers of Viola M. Frymann DO. 2nd ed. Michigan: Edward Brothers; 2000. pp. 134-40.

90. Kimberly PE. The application of the respiratory principle to osteopathic manipulative procedures. J Am Ost Assoc. 2001:101(7):410-3. Reprinted from J Am Osteopath Assoc. 1949;48(7):331-4.

91. Liem T, McPartland JM, Skinner E. Cranial osteopathy: principles and practice. Edinburgh: Elsevier Churchill Livingstone; 2004. pp. 640-8.

92. DeStefano LA. Greenman's principles of manual medicine. 4th ed. Baltimore, MD: Williams and Wilkins; 2011. pp. 175-8.

93. Wieting JM, Andary MT, Holmes TG et al. Manipulation massage and traction. In: De Lisa JA, Gans BM, Walsh NE, editors. Physical medicine and rehabilitation: principles and practice. Lippincott Williams and Wilkins; 2005. vol. 1, pp. 296-300.

94. DeStefano LA. Greenman's principles of manual medicine. 4th ed. Baltimore, MD: Williams and Wilkins; 2011. p. 50.

95. Educational Council on Osteopathic Principles (ECOP). Glossary of osteopathic terminology usage guide. Chevy Chase, MD: American Association of Colleges of Osteopathic Medicine (AACOM); 2011. pp. 30–2.

96. DeStefano LA. Greenman's principles of manual medicine. 4th ed. Baltimore, MD: Williams and Wilkins; 2011. pp. 87–98.

97. Stone CA. Visceral and obstetric osteopathy. Edinburgh: Elsevier Churchill Livingstone; 2007. pp. 125–30.

98. Kuchera ML, Kuchera WA. Osteopathic principles in practice. Columbus, OH: Greyden Press; 1994. pp. 75–9.

99. Liem T, McPartland JM, Skinner E. Cranial osteopathy: principles and practice. Edinburgh: Elsevier Churchill Livingstone; 2004. pp. 465–7.

100. Comeaux Z. Harmonic healing: a guide to facilitated oscillatory release and other rhythmic myofascial techniques. Berkeley, CA: North Atlantic Books; 2008.

101. Liem T, McPartland JM, Skinner E. Cranial osteopathy: principles and practice. Edinburgh: Elsevier Churchill Livingstone; 2004. ch. 19.

102. Lederman E. 1990 Harmonic technique. Edinburgh: Elsevier Churchill Livingstone.

103. Littlejohn JM. The fundamentals of osteopathic technique. Maidstone, UK: Institute of Classical Osteopathy.

104. Wernham J. The 1956 yearbook. Maidstone, UK: Institute of Classical Osteopathy.

105. Barral JP, Croibier A. Manual therapy for the peripheral nerves. Edinburgh: Elsevier Churchill Livingstone; 2007. pp. 99–104.

106. Liem T, McPartland JM, Skinner E. Cranial osteopathy: principles and practice. Edinburgh: Elsevier Churchill Livingstone; 2004. pp. 151–5.

107. DeStefano LA. Greenman's principles of manual medicine. 4th ed. Baltimore, MD: Williams and Wilkins; 2011. p. 177.

108. Barral JP, Croibier A. Manual therapy for the cranial nerves. Edinburgh: Elsevier Churchill Livingstone; 2008. ch. 22.

109. Liem T, McPartland JM, Skinner E. Cranial osteopathy: principles and practice. Edinburgh: Elsevier Churchill Livingstone; 2004. pp. 54–9.

110. Chikly B. Brain tissue nuclei fluid and autonomic nervous system. Course script. Hamburg, Germany: OSD; 2010.

111. Zink JG, Fetchik WD, Lawson WB. The posterior axillary folds: a gateway for osteopathic treatment of the upper extremities. Osteopath Ann. 1981;9(3):81–8.

112. Kuchera ML. Lymphatics approach. In: Chila A, editor. Foundations of osteopathic medicine. 3rd ed. Philadelphia, PA: Lippincott Williams and Wilkins; 2011. pp. 804–5.

113. Tozzi P. Fascial unwinding. In: Chaitow L, editor. Fascial dysfunction: manual therapy approaches. Edinburgh: Handspring Publishing; 2014. ch. 10.

114. Jarricot H. Stimulo – thérapie – tegumentaire. In: De Dannaiaud J, editor. Paris: Médicine Pratique; 1962.

115. Kuchera ML, Kuchera WA. Osteopathic principles in practice. Columbus, OH: Greyden Press; 1994. pp. 290–1.

116. Dickey J. Postoperative osteopathic manipulative management of median sternotomy patients. J Am Ost Assoc. 1989;89(10):1309–22.

117. Wallace E, McPartland JM, Jones JM. Lymphatic system: lymphatic manipulative techniques. In: Ward RC, editor. Foundations of osteopathic medicine. 2nd ed. Philadelphia, PA: Lippincott Williams and Wilkins; 2002. pp. 1063–8.

118. Ruddy TJ. Osteopathic rhythmic resistive duction therapy. Academy of Applied Osteopathy Yearbook 1961:58–68.

119. Stone CA. Visceral and obstetric osteopathy. Edinburgh: Elsevier Churchill Livingstone; 2007. chs 4 and 9.

120. Ettlinger H, Gintis B. Diagnosis and treatment. In: DiGiovanna EL, Schiowitz S, Dowling DJ, editors. An osteopathic approach to diagnosis and treatment. 3rd ed. Philadelphia, PA: Lippincott Williams and Wilkins; 2005. pp. 575–6.

121. DeStefano LA. Greenman's principles of manual medicine. 4th ed. Baltimore, MD: Williams and Wilkins; 2011. pp. 178–9.

122. Liem T, McPartland JM, Skinner E. Cranial osteopathy: principles and practice. Edinburgh: Elsevier Churchill Livingstone; 2004. pp. 117–9, 629–30.

123. Zink JG, Lawson WB. The role of pectoral traction in the treatment of lymphatic flow disturbances. Osteopath Annals. 1978;6:493–6.

124. Wallace E, McPartland JM, Jones JM. Lymphatic system: lymphatic manipulative techniques. In: Ward RC, editor. Foundations of osteopathic medicine. 2nd ed. Philadelphia, PA: Lippincott Williams and Wilkins; 2002. pp. 1068–9.

125. Noll DR, Degenhardt BF, Johnson JC et al. Immediate effects of osteopathic manipulative treatment in elderly patients with chronic obstructive pulmonary disease. J Am Osteopath Assoc. 2008;108(5):251–9.

126. Sutherland WG. Teaching in the science of osteopathy. Fort Worth, TX: Cranial Teaching Foundation Inc.; 1990. pp. 135–6.

127. Stone CA. Visceral and obstetric osteopathy. Edinburgh: Elsevier Churchill Livingstone; 2007. ch. 8.

128. Barral JP, Croibier A. Visceral vascular manipulation. Edinburgh: Elsevier Churchill Livingstone; 2011.

129. Tozzi P. Balanced ligamentous tension technique. In: Chaitow L, editor. Fascial dysfunction: manual therapy approaches. Edinburgh: Handspring Publishing; 2014. ch. 11.

130. King HH, Lay EM. Osteopathy in the cranial field. In: Ward RC, editor. Foundations of osteopathic medicine. 2nd ed. Philadelphia, PA: Lippincott Williams and Wilkins; 2002. pp. 999.

131. Sutherland WG. Teaching in the science of osteopathy. Fort Worth TX: Cranial Teaching Foundation Inc.; 1990.

132. Chaitow L, Gilbert C, Bradley D. Recognizing and treating breathing disorders: a multidisciplinary approach. 2nd ed. Edinburgh: Elsevier Churchill Livingstone; 2014.

133. Chikly B, Quaghebeur J. Reassessing cerebrospinal fluid (CSF) hydrodynamics: a literature review presenting a novel hypothesis for CSF physiology. J Bodyw Mov Ther. 2013;17(3):344–54.

134. Kuchera ML. Lymphatics approach. In: Chila A, editor. Foundations of osteopathic medicine. 3rd ed. Philadelphia, PA: Lippincott Williams and Wilkins; 2011. p. 787.

135. Degenhardt BF, Kuchera ML. Update on osteopathic medical concepts and the lymphatic system. J Am Osteopath Assoc. 1996;96:97–100.

136. Salamon E, Zhu W, Stefano G. Nitric oxide as a possible mechanism for understanding the therapeutic effects of osteopathic manipulative medicine. Int J Mol Med. 2004;14(3):443–9.

137. Overberger R, Hoyt JA, Daghigh F et al. Comparing changes in serum nitric oxide levels and heart rate after osteopathic manipulative treatment (OMT) using the Dalrymple pedal pump to changes measured after active exercise. J Am Osteopath Assoc. 2009;109(1):41–2.

138. Tota B, Trimmer B, editors. Nitric oxide. Elsevier Health Sciences; 2011.

139. Lederman E. Fundamentals of manual therapy: physiology neurology and psychology. London: Elsevier Churchill Livingstone; 1997. pp. 39–55.

140. Lythgo N, Eser P, de Groot P et al. Whole-body vibration dosage alters leg blood flow. Altern Ther Health Med. 2009;29(1):53–9.

141. Kipp K. Johnson ST, Doeringer JR et al. Spinal reflex excitability and homosynaptic depression after about of whole-body vibration. Muscle Nerve. 2011;43(2):259–62.

142. Coghill R, Talbot J, Evans AC et al. Distributed processing of pain and vibration by the human brain. J Neurosci. 1994;14(7):4095–108.

143. Leduc A, Lievens P, Dewald J. The influence of multi-directional vibrations on wound healing and on the regeneration of blood and lymph vessels. Lymphology. 1981;14(4):179–85.

144. Zainuddin Z, Newton M, Sacco P et al. Effects of massage on delayed onset muscle soreness, swelling and recovery of muscle function. J Athl Train. 2005;40(3):174–80.

145. Lund I, Ge Y, Yu LC et al. Repeated massage-like stimulation induces long-term effects on nociception: contribution of oxytocinergic mechanisms. Eur J Neurosci. 2002;16(2):330–8.

146. Eliska O, Eliskova M. Are peripheral lymphatics damaged by high pressure manual massage? Lymphology. 1995;28(1):21–30.

147. Mesina J, Hampton D, Evans R et al. Transient basophilia following the application of lymphatic pump techniques: a pilot study. J Am Osteopath Assoc. 1998;98(2):91–4.

148. Measel JW. The effect of the lymphatic pump on the immune response: I. Preliminary studies on the antibody response to pneumococcal polysaccharide assayed by bacterial agglutination and passive hemagglutination. J Am Osteopath Assoc. 1982;82(1):28–31.

149. Jackson KM, Steele TF, Dugan EP et al. Effect of lymphatic and splenic pump techniques on the antibody response to hepatitis B vaccine: a pilot study. J Am Osteopath Assoc. 1998;98(3):155–60.

150. Noll DR, Degenhardt BF, Stuart MK et al. The effect of osteopathic manipulative treatment on immune response to influenza vaccine in nursing home residents: a pilot study. Altern Ther Health Med. 2004;10(4):74–6.

151. Saggio G, Docimo S, Pilc J et al. Impact of osteopathic manipulative treatment on

secretory immunoglobulin A levels in a stressed population. J Am Osteopath Assoc. 2011;111(3):143-7.

152. Breithaupe T, Harris K, Ellis J et al. Thoracic lymphatic pumping and the efficacy of influenza vaccination in healthy young and elderly populations. J Am Osteopath Assoc. 2001;101(1):21-5.

153. Dugan EP, Lemley WW, Roberts CA et al. Effect of lymphatic pump techniques on the immune response to influenza vaccine. J Am Osteopath Assoc. 2001;101:472 P02.

154. Paul RT, Stomel RJ, Broniak FF et al. Interferon level in human subject throughout a 24-hour period following thoracic lymphatic pump manipulation. J Am Osteopath Assoc. 1986;86(2):92-5.

155. Knott EM, Tune JD, Stoll ST et al. Increased lymphatic flow in the thoracic duct during manipulative intervention. J Am Osteopath Assoc. 2005;105(10):447-56.

156. Hodge LM, King HH, Williams AG et al. Abdominal lymphatic pump treatment increases leukocyte count and flux in thoracic duct lymph. Lymphat Res Biol. 2007;5(2):127-33.

157. Hodge LM, Bearden MK, Schander A et al. Lymphatic pump treatment mobilizes leukocytes from the gut associated lymphoid tissue into lymph. Lymphat Res Biol. 2010;8(2):103-10.

158. Walkowski S, Singh M, Puertas J et al. Osteopathic manipulative therapy induces early plasma cytokine release and mobilization of a population of blood dendritic cells. PLoS One. 2014;10;9(3):e90132.

159. Muthuchamy M, Gashev A, Boswell N. Molecular and functional analyses of the contractile apparatus in lymphatic muscle. FASEB J. 2003;17(8):920-2.

160. Olszewski WL. Contractility patterns of normal and pathologically changed human lymphatics. Ann N Y Acad Sci. 2002;979:52-63; discussion 76-9.

161. Cutler MJ, Holland BS, Stupski BA et al. Cranial manipulation can alter sleep latency and sympathetic nerve activity in humans: a pilot study. J Altern Complement Med. 2005;11(1):103-8.

162. Nelson KE, Sergueef N, Glonek T. The effect of an alternative medical procedure upon low-frequency oscillations in cutaneous blood flow velocity. J Manipulative Physiol Ther. 2006;29(8):626-36.

163. Akselrod S, Gordon D, Madwed JB et al. Hemodynamic regulation: investigation by spectral analysis. Am J Physiol. 1985;249(4/2):H867-75.

164. Shi X, Rehrer S, Prajapati P et al. Effect of cranial osteopathic manipulative medicine on cerebral tissue oxygenation. J Am Osteopath Assoc. 2011;111(12):660-6.

165. Rivers WE, Treffer KD, Glaros AG et al. Short-term hematologic and hemodynamic effects of osteopathic lymphatic techniques: a pilot crossover trial. J Am Osteopath Assoc. 2008;108(11):646-51.

166. Henley CE, Ivins D, Mills M et al. Osteopathic manipulative treatment and its relationship to autonomic nervous system activity as demonstrated by heart rate variability: a repeated measures study. Osteopathic Med Prim Care. 2008;52:7.

167. Huard Y. Influence of the venous sinus technique on cranial hemodynamics. In: King HH, editor. Proceedings of international

research conference: osteopathy in pediatrics at the Osteopathic Center for Children in San Diego, CA, 2002. Indianapolis, IN: American Academy of Osteopathy; 2005. pp. 32–6.

168. Lombardini R, Marchesi S, Collebrusco L et al. The use of osteopathic treatment as adjuvant therapy in patients with peripheral arterial disease. Man Ther. 2009;14(4):439–43.

169. Cerritelli F, Carinci F, Pizzolorusso G et al. Osteopathic manipulation as a complementary treatment for the prevention of cardiac complications: 12-months follow-up of intima media and blood pressure on a cohort affected by hypertension. J Bodyw Mov Ther. 2011;15(1):68–74.

170. Spiegel AJ, Capobianco JD, Kruger A et al. Osteopathic manipulative medicine in the treatment of hypertension: an alternative conventional approach. Heart Disease. 2003;5(4):272–8.

171. Johnston WL, Kelso AF. Changes in presence of a segmental dysfunction pattern associated with hypertension: part 2. A long-term longitudinal study. J Am Osteopath Assoc. 1995;95(5):315–8.

172. Chen L, Zhan HS. [A transcranial Doppler ultrasonography and X-ray study of cervical vertigo patients treated by manipulation in supine position] Zhong Xi Yi Jie He Xue Bao. 2003;1(4):262–4.

173. O-Yurvati AH, Carnes MS, Clearfield MB et al. Hemodynamic effects of osteopathic manipulative treatment immediately after coronary artery bypass graft surgery. J Am Osteopath Assoc. 2005;105(10):475–81.

174. Gwirtz PA, Dickey J, Vick D et al. Viscerosomatic interaction induced by miocardial ischemia in conscious dogs. J Appl Physiol. 2007;103(2):511–7.

175. Longmire DR. An electrophysiological approach to the evaluation of regional sympathetic dysfunction: a proposed classification. Pain Physician. 2006;9(1):69–82.

176. Sleszynski SL, Kelso AF. Comparison of thoracic manipulation with incentive spirometry in preventing postoperative atelectasis. J Am Osteopath Assoc. 1993;93(8):834–8, 843–5.

177. Pratt-Harrington D, Neptune-Ceran R. The effect of OMT in the post-abdominal surgery patient. Acad Appl Osteopath. 1995;9:9–13.

178. Janssens JP, Pache JC, Nicod LP. Physiological changes in respiratory function associated with ageing. Eur Respir J. 1999;13(1):197–205.

179. Noll DR, Shores JH, Bryman PN et al. Adjunctive osteopathic manipulative treatment in the elderly hospitalizad with pneumonia: a pilot study. J Am Osteopath Assoc. 1999;99(3):143–6, 151–2.

180. Noll DR, Shores JH, Gamber RG et al. Benefits of osteopathic manipulative treatment for hospitalized elderly patients with pneumonia. J Am Osteopath Assoc. 2000;100(12):776–82.

181. Licciardone JC, Buchanan S, Hensel K et al. Osteopathic manipulative treatment of back pain and related symptoms during pregnancy: a randomized controlled trial. Am J Obstet Gynecol. 2010;202(43):1–8.

182. Noll DR, Degenhardt BF, Morley TF et al. Efficacy of osteopathic manipulation as an adjunctive treatment for hospitalized patients with pneumonia: a randomized controlled trial. Osteopath Med Prim Care. 2010;19;4:2.

183. Stiller KR, McEvoy RD. Chest physiotherapy for the medical patient – are current practices effective? Aust N Z J Med. 1990;20(2):183–8.

184. Guiney PA, Chou R, Vianna A et al. Effects of osteopathic manipulative treatment on pediatric patients with asthma: a randomized controlled trial. J Am Osteopath Assoc. 2005;105(1):7–12.

185. Bockenhauer SE, Julliard KN, Lo KS et al. Quantifiable effects of osteopathic manipulative techniques on patients with chronic asthma. J Am Osteopath Assoc. 2002;102(7):371–5.

186. Vandenplas Y, Denayer E, Vandenbossche T et al. Osteopathy may decrease obstructive apnea in infants: a pilot study. Osteopath Med Prim Care. 2008;19(2):8.

187. Mills MV, Henley CE, Barnes LL et al. The use of osteopathic manipulative treatment as adjuvant therapy in children with recurrent acute otitis media. Arch Pediatr Adolesc Med. 2003:157(9):861–6.

188. Steele KM, Carreiro JE, Viola JH et al. Effect of osteopathic manipulative treatment on middle ear effusion following acute otitis media in young children: a pilot study. J Am Osteopath Assoc. 2014;114(6):436–47.

189. Posadzki P, Lee MS, Ernst E. Osteopathic manipulative treatment for pediatric conditions: a systematic review. Pediatrics. 2013;132(1):140–52.

190. Vick DA, McKay C, Zengerle CR. The safety of manipulative treatment: review of the literature from 1925 to 1993. J Am Osteopath Assoc. 1996;96(2):113–5.

191. Kimberly PE. Formulating a prescription for osteopathic manipulative treatment. J Am Osteopath Assoc. 1980;79:506–13.

192. DeStefano LA. Greenman's principles of manual medicine. 4th ed. Baltimore, MD: Williams and Wilkins; 2011. p. 52.

193. Chikly B. Silent waves: theory and practice of lymph drainage therapy. An osteopathic lymphatic technique. 2nd ed. Scottsdale, AZ: IHH Publishing; 2004.

194. Kuchera ML. Lymphatics approach. In: Chila A, editor. Foundations of osteopathic medicine. 3rd ed. Philadelphia, PA: Lippincott Williams and Wilkins; 2011. pp. 798–806.

195. Johnson S, Kurtz M. Osteopathic manipulative treatment techniques preferred by contemporary osteopathic physicians. J Am Osteopath Assoc. 2003;103(5):219–24.

# The metabolic-energetic model

*Christian Lunghi*

7

## Synopsis

This chapter presents the metabolic-energetic model in order to bring to the fore the whole decision-making process, from evaluation to treatment and ongoing management of the person. This will all be delivered with the particular mode of this text, which is to present a comparison between tradition and evidence, and to proceed toward an innovation that must be faithful to first principles. The model is described in all of its forms, from the more typical, related to the biological-metabolic model and visceral osteopathy, whose forerunner was the old doctor who, for example, applied his manipulations to children in cases of fever and dysentery,[1] to the more modern, from the scientific evidence point of view, and related to biological electromagnetism.

From the conventional perspective, therapy requires the elimination of the pathogen; in osteopathy we also search for the cause of the disease or condition, which allows us to provide a specific therapy or local treatment. However, the scheme presented here also suggests an alternative strategy, which is to increase the level of basal energy, through the evaluation of consistency within and between the systems, and, if they are related in unison by a state of resonance of their own electromagnetic fields, would make them resistant to the local production of pathogenic energy.[2] The osteopath who evaluates the patient with the metabolic-energetic approach encourages the efficiency of self-regulatory activity, of procurement systems, metabolism, exchange and storage of energy, through the connective anatomical arrangement of bodily organs and glands by which the autonomic target, nutrients and drainage are so influenced. We will also address issues such as the patient's ongoing management by providing advice related to lifestyle, nutrition, and physical activity.

## Introduction

The focus of this model is the energy balance relative to metabolic and immunological factors. The osteopath evaluating the person with the metabolic-energetic model centers his or her approach on the relationship between supply, management, and expenditure of energy. This approach has been observed by different authors. In their documents, articles, or treatises they have characterized the model as metabolic[3] or energetic,[4-9] emphasizing different facets and sometimes focusing more heavily on metabolic aspects, sometimes on bioenergetics aspects.

However, within osteopathy this dichotomy has been integrated[10] into an approach focused on the relationship between metabolic and immunological factors and the individual's energy supply, in order to influence the individual's adaptation. One of the nonspecific innate adaptive mechanisms is inflammation, the defense system that forms a protective response (following the action of harmful physical, chemical, and biological agents), whose ultimate goal is the elimination of the initial cause of cell or tissue damage, and the start of the healing process. It is a purification process that occurs at the cell, internal organ, and extracellular matrix level, to remove toxins (foreign or produced by the body) through the intervention of defense cells.

The inflammatory process is considered one of the cardiometabolic risk substrates, which today is a leading cause of death.[11] Different authors have observed that people in an inflammatory state, which promotes musculoskeletal pain syndromes such as back pain, are carriers of metabolic conditions such as an increase in adipose tissue and body mass index.[12] Recent studies have established that patients with metabolic syndrome or type 2 diabetes and who are overweight have a higher risk of developing musculoskeletal pain than normal weight individuals. Overweight individuals are more likely to suffer from headaches, fibromyalgia, abdominal pain, and chronic widespread pain.[13]

Although several studies have shown a link between body weight and lower back pain,[14-16] the guidelines for the treatment of low back pain have never recommended attention to lifestyle or dietary guidelines.[17] Despite the association between obesity, diabetes, and cardiovascular diseases reported in literature, the "fat" may erroneously be regarded only as storage of excess calories and not the result of the response of an immune/endocrine organ to a continued overload that can generate chronic inflammation.[18-20] Several studies show that increased allostatic load influences food choices and, conversely, that diet can affect mood and pro-inflammatory responses to stressors.[21]

Following an unbalanced diet consisting of high-calorie meals can lead to an expansion of adipose tissue.[22] With the rise of obesity, there is a fundamental change in the metabolic activity of adipose tissue. In thin individuals, the adipocytes exert an anti-inflammatory function through the release of adiponectin and anti-inflammatory interleukin-10, which promote the health and repair of the body.[23] Adiponectin supports insulin sensitivity and mitochondrial biogenesis in skeletal muscle, while interleukin-10 has analgesic, anti-inflammatory, and immune system modulation properties.[24] The term "adiposopathy" was proposed to distin-guish an overweight condition associated with an inflammatory state from a presentation with no inflammation.[18-20]

In other words, an increase in the adipose tissue does not necessarily coincide with an increase in chronic inflammation. This could be the explanation of the inconsistent relations between the index changes in body mass and low back pain. The interpretation that emerges is that the adiposopathy and the related metabolic syndrome lead to chronic pain, because the non-resolved inflammation is a state that promotes pathophysiological nociception in the damaged/dysfunctional musculoskeletal tissues and prevents healing.[25-27] Chronic inflammation is in fact associated with a variety of seemingly unrelated chronic diseases, such as low back pain, arthritis, atherosclerosis, cancer, chronic obstructive pulmonary disease, asthma, inflammatory bowel disease, neurodegenerative disease, multiple sclerosis, psoriasis, and rheumatoid arthritis.[28,29]

Thus, to understand the nature of inflammation, its correlation with lifestyle, for example nutrition, becomes relevant for the treatment of inflammatory processes[30] of low back pain and other conditions that are treated daily by manual therapists.[12] However, inflammatory disorders, in addition to being associated with lifestyle, manifest alterations in the immune regulation of local and systemic inflammatory processes, in metabolic regulation, in autonomic response, and in the activation of mesenchymal stem cells residing in the extracellular matrix of the connective tissue. The latter is also known for its possible interface with electromagnetic signals capable of generating a resonance effect, namely bioresonance, with living organisms.[31,32]

An acute inflammatory process is started by a stimulus that causes the release of inflammatory mediators with remodeling of the extracellular matrix (ECM) and increase of on-site free charges.[31,32] The inflammatory process may also have systemic effects, with activation of chemical mediators, which causes activation of serum acute phase proteins and neuroendocrine and hematopoietic variations. If the stimulus is suppressed, it follows a phase characterized by fluid and catabolite removal; if the tissue cannot regenerate, it follows the cicatrizing process. The ECM, in this phase, is characterized by increased water, ions and on-site conductivity. If the stimulus persists, it starts the evolution from acute to chronic inflammation.

The transition from acute to chronic inflammation occurs, for example, if in the involved area there occurs an accumulation of fluids and components of the infected plasma, of plasma cells, with tissue damage and repair attempts. The ECM is therefore reshaped and reorganized. In chronic inflammation there is a constant call for macrophages, specific chemotactic factors with proliferation by mitotic division, prolonged persistence, and immobilization of the affected cells in the inflammatory process. We have verified increased conductivity, lower than that found in the acute stage. The persistent presence of the inflammatory agent causes complications of chronic inflammation, namely the activation of the limbic–pituitary–adrenal axis resulting in the release of glucocorticoids and decreased pituitary–adrenal-limbic system response to exogenous stimuli.

For several years the researchers have acknowledged a type of inflammation referred to as the central sensitization phenomenon,[33] often called "silent inflammation."[34] This type of internal inflammation has an insidious nature and is responsible for many chronic ailments such as diabetes, hypertension, and cardiovascular risk.[11] These disorders are mainly caused by improper lifestyle and environmental pollutants, which, by leading to a hormonal imbalance, cause systemic silent inflammation.[35] The extracellular matrix, in both physiological and pathological conditions, is subject to a continuous remodeling, as it plays a very important role in the spread of all biochemical signals that modulate cell proliferation, differentiation, survival, and migration.

The ECM remodeling under physiological conditions follows a biphasic circadian rhythm: a first phase in which it appears as a soluble gelatin (sol state), in which takes place the demolition and dis-posal of metabolic wastes and proteins (disposal stage), and a second phase, in which the ECM appears as a jelly that recondenses (gel state) to facilitate the reconstitution of the matrix and of the proteins (reconstruction phase). This biphasic circadian balance can break down as a result of trauma, viral or bacterial infections, functional insufficiency of the lymphatic system, excessive production of toxins due to incorrect diet, intake of pharmacological substances, and stress conditions.[36]

In these conditions, the organism activates a supplementary state to accelerate the disposal through inflammation. In the presence of an inflammatory process, a series of mechanisms that induce ECM remodeling are activated. Inflammation is a response to tissue damage, whose main roles are removal of damaged tissues and protection against infection. If they are present simultaneously, the agent or damaging stressor, the tissue injury, the healing efforts of the damaged tissue, and the immune response generate a chronic inflammatory state. This coincides with a condition in which the disposal and ECM remodeling are no longer sufficient with respect to the quantitative discard in the extracellular space of organic acids relative to the catabolism of fat mass; thus, the biphasic circadian remodeling of the ECM changes to an absence of circadian rhythm, resulting in a gradual loss of anatomical and functional integrity and relative increase of the percentage of the ECM compared to body mass (increase of catabolites).[36]

In clinical practice, there is a decrease in body cell mass or metabolically active mass, depending on age and nutritional status.[36] This may depend on the reduced muscle mass characteristic of sedentary or obese subjects. Generally, the increase in ECM, extracellular mass, or inert mass is associated with pathological conditions where the extracellular space is expanded. The causes of this phenomenon are numerous, but a decisive role is played by the breaking of the physiological balance between production and elimination by the actions of the antioxidant defense systems of the oxygen reactive species. The latter, through both direct and indirect mechanisms, promote the destruction of, and prevent the synthesis of, matrix proteins, triggering abnormal phenomena of tissue repair and remodeling of the same matrix, with an increase in the percentage of the ECM relative to body mass.

The joints, due to the reduction of the lubricating capacity of the intercellular substance, progressively lose their functionality, with frequent onset of rigidity and destruction of the articular cartilage. Some chronic inflammation in the osteoarticular tract may show forms of ankylosis. The disease most likely to lead to this anomaly is rheumatoid arthritis. There may also be an impairment of the coating structure of the blood vessels and respiratory mucous membranes, gastrointestinal and genitourinary that becomes more sensitive to environmental stressors, with onset of allergies, infections, and immune phenomena. The transport of hormones and neurotransmitters becomes inefficient; cell sensitivity to them is reduced, facilitating the onset of metabolic syndrome and subclinical hormonal alterations.[36]

A substantial body of evidence supports the notion that the imbalance between the activity of the metal-proteinases of the matrix and their inhibitors may contribute to the alteration of vascular remodeling and the pathogenesis of cardiovascular diseases such as atherosclerosis and heart failure progression.[37] In addition, the weak mechanical signals that travel through the extracellular matrix may elicit significant cellular responses, causing gel/sol state transitions and actin–myosin contraction. These mechanical signals may result from alterations of physiological activities, such as heart rate, and harmful stimuli to which tissues respond by rearranging the cytoskeleton of cells and remodeling the extracellular matrix. Such viscoelastic changes also affect the function of nociceptors by modulating the transmission of pain.[38]

All this requires from the body's defense system is a low level chronic and continuous inflammatory intervention, which, if protracted in time, leads to exhaustion of the immune system. In silent inflammation, therefore, the biochemical cascade

progression gives way to chaotic reactions that hinder each other, so much so that sometimes, in susceptible individuals, tissues lose their ability to recognize their own cells, identifying them as invaders, and attacking them.[39] The systemic inflammatory state is fueled by pro-inflammatory cytokines, such as IL-2, IL-6 and TNF-$\alpha$,[40,41] by inflammatory markers such as C-reactive protein, eicosanoids, cortisol, insulin and endogenous opioids.[42,43]

If increased levels of stress and depression are also present there is a greater risk of infection, delayed healing by infectious episodes or wounds, as well as an increase of the processes that can feed production of pro-inflammatory cytokines. The latter may be directly responsible for the inflammatory response even in the absence of injury, and lead to inadequacy of neural-immune-endocrine reaction.[44-55] The person fails to contain and possibly extinguish the inflammation, the result being damage of healthy tissues. If this process continues over time, it can cause great damage to organs, blood vessels, and tissues.

This continuously triggers the immune response, in time even providing the grounds for autoimmune diseases, skin disorders such as atopic dermatitis or psoriasis, forms of chronic pain such as rheumatoid arthritis, rheumatic polymyalgia, fibromyalgia, chronic fatigue syndrome, respiratory tract diseases of allergic and inflammatory nature (allergic rhinitis, asthma forms), atherosclerosis, multiple sclerosis, allergic conjunctivitis.[39,56-60] It is increasingly clear and convincing that the pathogenesis of organic diseases can be attributed to the blockade of the regulative activity of the fundamental substance, the ECM: in acute form, inactive depolarized, excitable; in chronic form, inactive hyperpolarized, inexcitable.

Both undergo alterations of an electric and magnetic type that involve the physiological biological current flow, and are translated into the local lesion current, with an increase in the potential difference, the skin conductance response, and in biochemical/biophysical alterations. The lock status is accompanied by psychofunctional symptoms, in which pain is co-present as the main clinical manifestation.[61] The ECM plays the function of protecting the thermal, pressure and volume integrity of the cells, for the performance of all organic functions within the limits of homeostasis. The maintenance of the water temperature within the range of homeostatic values, which is essential for the operability of ECM/cell unity, depends on conserving the balance of two water phases with different structure: liquid phase, and near-crystalline phase.

The potential difference between the various components of the ECM facilitates the chemical reactions related to the transport of energy and information. The collagen fibrils behave as semiconductors, diodes capable of differentiating the current direction according to the relative arrangement between cells and fibrils. The afferent fibrils conduct to the cells the coherent electromagnetic energy conveyed into the neural network of the ECM; the efferent fibrils would carry energy from the cell to the tissue. Toxins are deposited in the structure of the matrix, where there takes place almost simultaneously millions of chemical reactions, with exchange of electrons, polarity changes, release of energy within an environment in continuous transformation. The ECM assumes the character of a molecular filter along the transit routes between capillaries and cells, and also functions as an energy dissipater.

The endocapillary passage of nutrients to the ECM does not make use only of physical energy, but is also governed by differences in potential created by three factors:

1. The electrical resistance of the arterial and venous endothelial cells (150–200 times greater than that of plasma)

2. The electrical-conductive ability of plasma (blood vessels are similar to electric cables)

3. The closure of the circuit with transendothelial passage of the material into the ECM.[36]

The rhythm of exchanges (increased blood flow) would be linked to the endothelium relaxation for hyperpolarization of the proteoglycans (PGs) and glycosaminoglycans (GAG) in electronegative specific ions. The integrity of the ECM has specific relations with the vascular system, which is responsible for the arrival of substances in the extracellular space. This would depend on a closed system in which the action of the capillaries prevails and which are responsible for the role of suppliers and regulators of the passage of substances. This step must be done in a passive sense, driven by an electric mechanism, and supported by an electrochemical polarization induced by anabolic and catabolic processes.[36] Bioelectricity of the ECM is mediated by the intracapillary circulatory system.[62] A positive charge is generated in a lesional area of the transit pathway. This stabilizes the potential differences in the current, acting as a biological battery that is waiting to be activated.

This bioelectrical charge is "activated" by a modification of the insulating capacity of the capillary membranes. As the membranes become less permeable to the ion flow, the intrinsic bioelectrical flow is forced to pass in a way that opposes a lower resistance, i.e., through the bloodstream. The bioelectrical energy currents, following the increase in blood flow, are directed toward the dysfunctional area. This dysfunctional electrical potential can range from excessive positive polar values (acute or chronic inflammation) to an excess of negative polar values (chronic degeneration) when the anatomical and functional structure of the capillaries undergoes action by vasoactive substances released by the sympathetic or parasympathetic system, which depend on the redox system and the presence of oxidizing or reducing substances. The potential of the lesion would show a fluctuating course (flux and reflux), mainly influenced by the intensity and polarity of the potential differences existing between the injured tissue, with positive hypo-oxygenation, and surrounding tissue, with negative oxygenated.[62]

The potential differences alter the current flow, the free energy and the value of the conductance. The generation of a specific signal, defined as the lesional current, causes another signal that initiates reconstruction. The lesional signal gradually decreases with the progress of the reconstruction process, until it runs out when the process is complete. Thus, in the ECM, areas of pathological tissue and healthy tissue with different polarities are established, which give rise to a potential difference and an electrochemical flow of current between points having different electrical resistance, as if it had generated a real "biological battery."

Even the electromagnetic fields behave and react according to the principle of minimum energy: wave forms with minimal local energy expenditure, with minimal local response and amplified at a distance. This includes the possibility of triggering feedback by means of ordered electrical stimuli. The ECM has a dynamic nonlinear control system which allows the ECM to easily return to its own original state (rhythm), using feedback processes. Its action as molecular filter puts it in a position to undergo mechanical stresses which deform its morphology. The ECM reacts to these stresses as a viscoelastic system, absorbing the shock and dispersing the distortion.

The atoms (ions) of biological tissues move in accordance with the viscosity of the fluid in which the substances inside and outside the cells are immersed (e.g., water). In the currents of biological tissues, the positive and negative ions are mobile, and negative ions carry electrons through the fluid. When applying an electric or magnetic field, electromotive forces are generated as potential differences, and an electric current is induced. The particles with excessive electrons migrate to where there are nearby positive charges, or toward the surface of muscle or nervous tissues that are richly charged. Free particles of electrons migrate to the interior, where the electrons are freely available. Organic components such as hemoglobin, DNA, RNA, as well as collagen, have semiconductor properties.[63,64]

Complementary approaches, including the application of polarized microcurrents, acupuncture, and osteopathy, have an impact on immune and metabolic problems in the electrochemical reactions that take place in the tissue with destructive effect on toxins.[65] Different hormonal and metabolic factors may influence the stiffness of the fascial tissue, playing a possible role in the genesis and maintenance of somatic dysfunction (SD) and fascial compensation schemes (FCS). The osteopathic approach to the fascial tissue related to organs, glands, and systems produces an integrated modulation of energetics and metabolism through effects on the dynamics of the arterial-venous-lymphatic fluids, on the autonomic influences and on the immune-endocrine responses.

## Historical background

The metabolic-energetic model is used by the operator to encourage the efficiency of adaptive responses, orchestrated through positive and negative feedback control systems of the various forms of supply, metabolism, exchange and conservation of energy by which the organs and bodily glands are affected. In osteopathy, the metabolic activity, for example of an organ, has been historically considered as related to alterations of the muscle and tissue tone at rest in areas of the fascial musculoskeletal system, particularly in the myotome, dermatome, and sclerotome of reference. According to Korr's "y loop" hypothesis, this condition, SD would be maintained by orthosympathetic hyperactivity.[66,67]

We also know from the studies of Johansson and Sojka first,[68] and then of Knutson and Owens,[69,70] that this tissue tension is powered via the production of metabolites and in time can facilitate the dorsal root ganglion. More recent research has shown that muscular passive stiffness, elasticity, extensibility, tension at rest, and muscle tone can be influenced by the fascia by virtue of its sensory and contractile properties. The fascia is a means through which superficial lesions, contractions, or tissue constraints could affect epigenetic reactions and, consequently, internal organs. It may thus be one of the systems for which difficulties of organ functioning may be expressed within the organ's walls. Recent research has shown that fibrosis created by a superficial lesion can spread to the internal organs and create the so-called fibro-contractive disease.[71,72]

Epigenetic alterations may also be responsible for the differentiation of myofibroblasts and the accumulation of extracellular matrix in chronic inflammatory conditions and fibrotic disorders.[73,74] The fascial network permeates and extends from the capsules to internal organs and could therefore be involved both in the origin and in the resolution of somatic and metabolic-visceral disorders. Recent work by Finando and Finando[75] suggests that the fascia is the means involved in the effects of acupuncture on organ pathology. When the body is stressed or traumatized, the fascia responds by synthesizing new fibers to provide support to the injured area and "pasting" tissues, organs, and muscles adjacent to each other.[76] The thickening and sticking of fascial layers can persist long after a lesion has healed and leave behind accumulations or non-resilient bands that can be perceived by palpation deep into the tissue.[77]

These palpable densities may correspond to somatic dysfunction, trigger points, and stretched bands described by Travell and Simons,[78] or to inflammatory pockets described as a local expression of adaptation syndrome by Selye[79] (see Chapter 2). Local residual tensions and fascial network adhesions can lead to compensatory tensions that extend throughout the musculoskeletal system. Such compensations may disturb more structures distant from each other, leading to compromised movement schemes, leaving the body more vulnerable to further lesions. These acquisitions are of high importance for the understanding of disorder or somatic and visceral dysfunction. However, if on one hand they help us in rationalizing the long-term responses, which are obtained with the application of osteopathic and complementary techniques, such as acupuncture, on the other hand they do not

explain the immediate improvement responses of tissue texture reported by different studies.[65]

McMakin and Oschman say that such quick reflexes may have an energy basis in specific locations of the fascial network.[65] Therefore, activities that are verified through the metabolic processes and the functioning of the neural-endocrine-immune system, and all internal organs, interact and communicate with musculoskeletal fascial system for self-regulatory purposes, constituting a process that produces energy. This field of energy would also be used for the purpose of information transmission.[80] The study of how different forms and sources of endogenous and exogenous energy influence and manage the living systems and their environment is the prerogative of biophysics, a field little considered by biomedicine. In the field of traditional and complementary medicine, the issue of bioenergy is discussed in many studies.[81–83]

Moreover, the National Center for Complementary and Alternative Medicine searches out and supports research designed to that effect.[84] Bioenergetic concepts have actually been part of osteopathic language and practice since their beginnings, as Andrew Taylor Still, in laying the foundations of our profession, integrated the practice of "bonesetters" with that of the magnetic healers.[85] In his writings we find traces of concepts described at the time by the Theosophical Society, for example, the Biogen,[86] a protoplasmic substance on which the old doctor reported that treatment was focused, and which claimed a training and autoregulatory potential of living matter.[87,88] Still also insisted on the importance of electrical and electromagnetic forces on health.[87]

For Littlejohn, the vibration force was the life force, or the expression of matter and spirit. He noted the existence of different oscillator rhythms in all living tissues and surmised that various levels of "vibrancy" were correlated with normal and abnormal functioning, with health and disease. According to his perspective, the encouragement of balance in the vibrating body is one of the osteopathic treatment goals.[89] In 1903 Hulett said that good health depends on the successful coordination of energy, while disease emerges from a state of impaired coordination of living matter; on this basis he conceived an osteopathic energy model.[90] Sutherland developed osteopathic cranial manipulative medicine in an attempt to explain the rhythmic movement inherent in tissues, called the primary respiratory mechanism, or potency.[91] Magoun referred to the energetic force of this rhythm, by appealing to the hydrodynamic mechanisms and potential positive and negative electrical biological fluids, focusing on the human electro-biological aspects and their relationship with the environment to carry out a continuous transmutation around the body.[92] These concepts were explored and expressed in many osteopathic approaches such as polarity therapy, described by Randolph Stone, and use of the vibropercussor by Robert Fulford.[93] Rollin Becker continued research in the cranial field, deepening the bioenergetic aspects related to the intrinsic biological energy fields, biodynamic and biokinetic, observing the different modes of expression in people in good health and those affected by disease,[94-98] although he did not realize that the concepts expressed by him were unappreciated and difficult to understand for colleagues.[99]

Based on the waveform diagrams and models of vibrational interferences of the tissues produced at the end of the 1980s, Davidson developed the neurofascial release technique, which can be applied to musculoskeletal and visceral dysfunctions with emotional impact.[100] The rationale is very similar to the approaches based on the concept of "emotional cysts" described by Upledger and MacDonald.[101,102] In the 1990s, Holland discussed the colloidal nature of the tissues, and the status transitions from gel to sol, i.e., the viscoelastic and viscoplastic changes of the fractal tissue adaptation in response to energy or physical stress.[103,104] In the late 1990s, O'Connell described the bioelectric fascial activation and release approach that, through holographic palpation and fascial activation energy, aims to support homeostasis, restoring fascial electrical potential and its continuity with the compensation schemes and the environment, concepts that are still present today in her descriptions of the myofascial release technique.[105,106]

In the 2000s, Comeaux described an approach defined as facilitated oscillatory release, which focuses on the mechanical facilitation of coherent vibration in the tissues, resulting in normalization of function. This project is characterized by the fusion of the principles of techniques such as those described by Fulford along with those of myofascial release and muscle energy.[107] In 1939, McConnell reminded colleagues to keep in mind that osteopathic pathogenesis is essentially a starting field of firmly grounded pathological phases of biophysical concepts,[108] and that time saw the dawning of the soundness and completeness of the science of osteopathy, based on foundations that are now raising interest in all areas of medicine.[109]

Over time, approaches were developed that are directed to the metabolic-energetic components based on neuroautonomic foundations. In cases of visceral inflammatory disorders, such as in the treatment of people suffering from irritable bowel syndrome,[110] evaluation procedures and subsequent treatments have been described:

- Dorsal-lumbar spine (T4–L2), to consider the innervation of the sympathetic nervous system

- Superior cervical spine, the skull base and suboccipital area, because it reduces the tension of the tissue surrounding the vagus nerve, since it passes through the jugular foramen. Emphasis is given to the mid-cervical region (C3, C4, C5) to consider relations with the phrenic nerve innervating the thoracic diaphragm

- Pelvic and sacroiliac joints, with interest in the pelvic splanchnic nerves (S2, S3, S4) that innervate the descending and sigmoid colon

- Soft tissue adjacent to the celiac ganglia (superior and inferior mesenteric), to obtain autonomic orthosympathetic responses

- Visceral and glandular dysfunctional areas, which have an impact on the hypothalamic–pituitary–adrenal axis and autonomic nervous system, involving the release of neurotransmitters and hormones such as corticotropin-releasing factor, which may play a role in modulating various regulatory functions

- Parasympathetic innervation, where the therapist focuses on the course of the vagus nerve, which innervates the small intestine and the colon as far as the splenic fissure

- Chapman's reflex points to optimize the lymph flow in organs and endocrine glands.

Other approaches do, however, refer to the connective-tissue origins of dysfunctional processes,[111] and approach the fascial periglandular/visceral component using techniques such as myofascial release, integrated neuromusculoskeletal release, fascial release, and fascial ligamentous release, to have metabolic effects with impact on:

- the removal of metabolic waste from inflammatory conditions, for example affecting the skin, such as the respiratory tract[111]

- the energetics of the impaired person, for example from post-traumatic conditions.[111]

## Objectives

The osteopath emphasizes the concepts of life force or energy flow inherent in the body, the bio-physical-electrical tissue and energetic communication with the environment, to achieve the objective of improving the adaptive homeostatic-allostatic responses, orchestrated from positive and negative feedback systems, as well as the adjustment of the various forms of exchange and conservation of energy that occur through metabolic processes and functioning of the organs.[8] In cases where the decision-making process leads the osteopath to the selection of this approach, his or her work focuses on identifying and handling:

1. FCS, indicators of the balance of the neural, endocrine, and metabolic activity and of the interaction with homeostatic-allostatic systems,

including the connective organization, the dynamics of biological fluids and the electromagnetic field related to it, which may give indications as to the overall energy expenditure of the organism, sometimes suffering from toxicity, digestive difficulties or absorption, infections, chronic fatigue, poor capacity for tissue repair, etc.

2. global techniques for fluid and involuntary rhythms; these techniques are of high immune impact, supplemented by nutritional counseling and individualized physical activity, and are the specific tools used by the operator to cope with conditions of discomfort of the patient

3. SD, as areas that express and are able to influence a condition of excessive or deficient energy-metabolic expenditure, for example to load organs, and their function, maintaining or worsening musculoskeletal conditions.

The specific techniques for lymphatic and visceral areas are among the most popular tools to improve these conditions.

## Indications and contraindications

Through medical history, physical examination, and osteopathic evaluation we observe conditions of a metabolic nature which allow the osteopath to select this model preferentially. In general, this model is indicated for all the painful conditions and musculoskeletal functional disorders associated with metabolic disorders such as fibromyalgia,[112] systemic disorders, metabolic syndrome, diabetes and its complications,[113] as well as symptoms related to disorders such as irritable bowel syndrome,[114] gastralgias and gastroesophageal reflux,[115] colonic inertia,[116] biliary disorders,[117] hypertension,[118] and pain related to the female endocrine axis disorders, such as endometriosis with colorectal involvement.[119] The author's clinical experience, supported by the concepts discussed in the "Rationale, mechanisms, and evidence" section, suggests that we consider the usefulness of the application of this model in cases where the person has easy and frequent fatigue, alterations of sleep rhythm, sweating, immune hypo- or hyperactivity, tissue repair deficiency, appetite changes with weight loss or gain in excessive amounts compared to the energy supply.

We must first assess the risks and benefits of osteopathic intervention on a certain condition. In this model it is important to do an analysis of the signs and symptoms through medical history, clinical presentation, and type and pattern of pain, and to assess the possible presence of characteristic indices of systemic disease. In such a case we do a review of systems, to ensure whether or not we are in the presence of a systemic clinical picture. For example, cutaneous manifestations and joint pain can be characteristic of a systemic disease such as Crohn's disease or psoriatic arthritis or an adverse reaction to medication. Abnormalities of hair and nails, intolerance to heat and cold, and a sense of unjustified fatigue relative to activities carried out by the patient are signs and symptoms associated with endocrine disorders. Variations in the frequency of urination, or in the flow or color of urine indicate urological involvement.

Professionalism is the ability to understand the limits of our knowledge and refer the person to the doctor. Examples of metabolic conditions that require urgent medical attention include:

- anginal pain that does not recede after 20 minutes

- angina associated with nausea, vomiting, and profuse sweating

- bowel/bladder incontinence and/or saddle anesthesia from lesions of the cauda equina, or pain of the cervical spine associated with urinary incontinence

- anaphylactic shock

- symptoms of inadequate ventilation or $CO_2$ retention

- a diabetic patient who appears confused or lethargic

- McBurney's point tenderness or rebound tenderness

- sudden worsening of intermittent claudication correlated with thromboembolism

- chest, back, or abdominal pain that increases with effort, accompanied by a throbbing sensation when lying on the back and in the presence of a palpable abdominal mass attributable to an aneurysm.[120]

Medical advice is needed in the presence of:

- diarrhea, constipation, fever, abdominal pain, decreased appetite, weight loss, nausea, skin lesions, arthritis migrans, joint pain, hip pain (iliopsoas abscess), uveitis and other eye inflammation that may indicate ulcerative colitis or Crohn's disease

- rectal bleeding, hemorrhoids, abdominal pain, pelvic, lumbar or sacral pain radiating to the legs, changes in bowel emptying, which may indicate colorectal cancer

- constipation that progresses to diarrhea with mucus, nausea, vomiting, abdominal distension, weight loss, fatigue and shortness of breath that may indicate advanced stages of irritable bowel syndrome.[121,122]

Conditions that may require precautions or contraindication to treatment include:

- chronic heart failure or uncontrolled pulmonary edema

- infectious myocarditis

- intermittent syncope

- severe dyspnea

- excessive fatigue

- loss of palpable pulse

- patients with diabetes; glucose levels should be stabilized (safe range 70–110 mg/dL; precaution if <100 or >250 mg/dL)

- unexplained or poorly tolerated heart rate at rest >120 or 130 bpm

- unexplained or poorly tolerated systolic pressure at rest >180–200 mmHg

- unexplained or poorly tolerated diastolic pressure >105–110 mmHg.[120]

## Principles and methods of assessment

During an evaluation the osteopath tries to understand any process that interferes with the local or global homeostasis resulting in increased energy expenditure of the organism,[9] observing the association of fatigue conditions, infection, toxicity, impaired tissue repair, associated with the reason for consultation. The first step in the evaluation process is the pattern of signs and symptoms. Safety is paramount and, as noted above, if there are warning signs or "red flags," the patient should be referred to his or her family doctor.[121,122] The model selection procedure in question (see Chapter 9) leads the osteopath to detect evidence of metabolic-energetic overload of the body's adaptive capacity, as well as the selection of the type, amount and duration of treatment to be used (Box 7.1).

---

**Box 7.1**

Selection procedure for the metabolic-energetic model (see Chapter 9)

Having knowledge of constitutional bio-typology (see Chapter 8), the osteopath uses the most effective mode of communication to establish an empathic relationship, which allows the osteopath to structure a medical history, and clinical and osteopathic assessment, aimed at determining any overload

---

of the patient's adaptive capacity, determining the appropriate model, and deciding on the activating forces that can be used during treatment.

The elements that lead the operator to the selection of the metabolic-energetic model are:

- disorders such as fatigue, infections, toxicity, scarce capacities in tissue repair, sleep disorders, thyroid disorders, etc.

- the overloaded structure: this is generally the abdominal-pelvic portion of the visceral fascia,[1] the extracellular matrix of the surrounding regions, the internal organs, and the neighboring tissues of the neuroendocrine axis glands

- the overloaded function: this manifests in the evaluation of the patient's energy balance, the metabolic processes of immune regulation, the levels of inflammation, and in digestion, absorption of nutrients, in the expulsion of metabolic waste, the reproductive capability.

The evaluation of the fascial component of the metabolic-energetic model is performed through the visceral fascia tests (abdominal-pelvic portion) (see Chapter 1); the revelation of any dysfunctional area is noted with the SD osteopathic tests (see Chapter 2); the evaluation of the adaptive (compensated/decompensated) capacity is performed through the FCS tests (see Chapter 3).

The assessment of the constitutional observational data, medical history, and clinical data related to the condition of the fascial compensation scheme, as well as the results of the tests of mobility and stiffness of the dysfunctional areas specific to metabolic-energy function, provides the limits within which this is maintained. This allows focusing the treatment to either:

- a minimalist approach: addressed to the area previously detected as dominant and clinically relevant for the person, or

- a maximalist approach: favored by the metabolic-energy activation force typically used with this model.

## Global tests

The osteopathic examination[123] includes global tests such as the fascial compensation scheme test (FCS) and the dynamics of fluids and involuntary rhythms (DyFIR) (see Chapters 1 and 3), aimed at assessing the state of health of the person. Immunological changes and other stressful or pathogenic agents alter fascial organization in spiral form and modify the intersections of fascial bands, maintaining fascial tension, in turn related to an alteration of the interstitial fluid, blood flow, and of organic functional efficiency. The reason for consultation and the symptoms reported are thus placed in relation with their causal circuits, which may be maintained by metabolic disorders related to neural, autonomic, and endocrine control, and stored in the connective network. The transition areas connect articular junction areas of the spine, transverse diaphragms, and longitudinal tubular compartments such as the axial, the visceral, and the meningeal fascia, and through fascial junction areas that may experience fibrotic adhesions in case of high stressful metabolic, emotional, and neuroendocrine load.

As a result of this consideration, the information obtained from the history and the clinical semeiotic tests are integrated into the osteopathic evaluation. Consistent with this model the osteopath applies, preferentially, a test of what is considered the specific fascial compartment of the model, the visceral fascia test (see Chapter 1). Metabolic alterations and consequent mechanical stresses can undermine one of the functions of the transition area that represents the energy expenditure of the modulation unit with consequent body alignment to the central line of gravity. Visceral fascia is derived from splanchnic embryological tissue that extends from the skull base to the pelvic cavity, surrounding the pleural, pericardial, and peritoneal cavities, and functioning as the body's metabolic functional unit (see Chapter 1). The finding of a decompensated FCS guides the osteopath to the selection of a maximalist model. If the overall test indicates, for example, a decompensated FCS, the operator proceeds with the local test, which will first be regional, then area-specific.

## Regional tests

The step test (see Chapter 1) allows the operator to evaluate regions where he or she is likely to encounter, through specific tests, any pivotal areas that are likely to be present within the cavity delineated by two transition areas. For example, one might determine that the cavity between the thoracoabdominal and pelvic areas has altered cavity pressure resulting in metabolic problems, as well as indicating the likely presence of SD in the region. The osteopath considers that in the ventral cavity the fibrous network participates in organ tropism and organizes the parenchymal tissues by providing support for them. The membranes around the heart, lungs, and abdominal organs are generated during embryonic development. This results in different organ densities "conglomerated" in tissue membranes, tied more or less closely to the vertebral column rather than with each other, mobilized by the movement of the thoracic diaphragm and, to a lesser extent, other body movements, as well as by external forces such as gravity.[124]

During perceptual palpation of the abdominal quadrants, the operator must take into account that the visceral fascia has an extreme variability of fibers and density of orientation[125] (Fig. 7.1). During the evaluation for possible tensions in an area, for example a quadrant of the abdomen, the assumption is that one can also evaluate broader myofascial chains which may include distant areas, both in the longitudinal direction, such as the cervical-cranial or pelvic, and obliquely, like the upper and lower limbs. These "dysfunctional binaries" do not necessarily correlate with the physiological pathways of distribution of the loading forces on the musculoskeletal system, described by other authors as myofascial chains,[126] but represent real flowing lines of tensional forces, in a well-defined circuit inside the connective tissue network, and not altered by physiological events. As the result of the mechanical forces that develop in the tissues subjected to non-physiological metabolic loads, and therefore reshaped in their tensegrity, these lines will develop a new movement pattern in an area, a segment, or

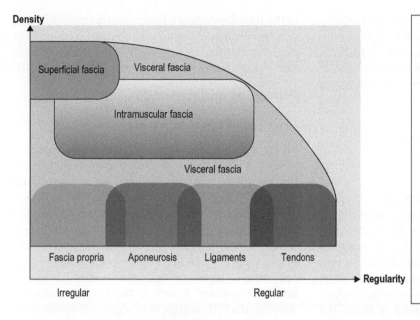

**Fig. 7.1**
Different densities and alignments of fibers in the fascial tissue; the fascial tissues differ in terms of density and directional alignment of collagen fibers. For example, the superficial fascia is characterized by a lower density and presents an irregular alignment of the fibers, while in the tendons or ligaments the fibers are denser and mostly unidirectional. The visceral fascia has an extreme variability of orientation of the fibers and density. Modified from: Schleip R, Müller DG. Training principles for fascial connective tissues: scientific foundation and suggested practical applications. J Bodyw Mov Ther. 2013;17(1):103–15.

sometimes the whole organism. Normally during the performance of regional tests, such as the listening/fascial attraction test (see Chapter 1), these lines allow the operator to perceive a convergence of forces, with amplitude and direction toward the higher density areas of the tissue, indicating the likely presence of SD.

## Local tests

With respect to the areas to be evaluated in a subject whose reason for consultation is some form of chronic inflammation, such as irritable bowel syndrome, in the absence of red flags the literature[110] suggests that the osteopath pay attention to the T4–L2 spinal segments and the related orthosympathetic innervation areas, as well as to the celiac, upper and lower mesenteric ganglia. In reference to the parasympathetic system, for example the vagus nerve, the osteopath should evaluate the upper cervical area, the skull base and cervical musculature, particularly the area of the jugular foramen. A scanning of the mid-cervical area with reference to the phrenic nerve, and of the sacral area with reference to the splanchnic nerves, is also recommended, as well as evaluation of the corresponding Chapman's reflex points.[110,127] Notwithstanding

the importance of the suggestions described in the literature, the author believes that the osteopath should proceed with specific tests of the area, as indicated by the results of the regional tests.

These specific tests assess for the presence of free and limited motion parameters, and TART (see Chapter 2). In this model, particular emphasis is given to the visceral approach, where the palpation of the abdominal quadrants allows the osteopath to assess the plasticity and elasticity of the fascial tissues surrounding the organs in each quadrant, then the continuity that exists between a connective tissue density surrounding the organ and the organ itself. In the diagnostic approach to the abdominal organs, we consider that a regular mobile tissue has a soft consistency that, when slightly compressed, produces a kind of rebound, while a fascial tissue affected by an overload will not return the energy, since the rigidity of its texture prevents the tissue from doing so. The evaluation is confirmed by the same pressure exerted locally, to objectify any rigidity to the pressing and the releasing of an area with respect to the surrounding regions.

The osteopath then proceeds with assessment at the specific visceral level, as described by different authors such as Barral (who codified the mobility of each internal organ),[128] Finet and Williame (who explored the visceral-fascial aspects),[129] Kuchera (who described visceral circulatory approaches),[130] and Chapman (who observed reflexes related to neurolymphatic aspects).[127,131]

## Tests for the assessment of the interdependence between structure and function

As previously described, the osteopath first gathers information about the general adaptation ability of the patient through global tests, for example by observing a decompensated FCS; then, using local tests, detects the presence of areas of adaptation, palpating any deterioration in the mechanical tissue, for example in the right iliac fossa, or a likely clinically relevant SD of the ascending colon; finally the osteopath proceeds, through a structure/function inhibition test, to the selection of the maximalist or minimalist approach by relating the FCS to the SD, or the general adaptation mode of the tissues to the area that has lost resilience as a result of metabolic overload imposed by the environment. The osteopath proceeds then by applying vector parameters in the dysfunctional area, by manually engaging the tissue for a few seconds with direct and indirect mode.

The stimulus induced (in this example) on the ascending colon may inhibit the decompensated FCS, normalizing the response to the tissue preference test or the DyFIR test immediately after being re-executed, giving an indication of the dominance of structure over function, and guiding the osteopath to a minimalist approach focused on the SD.

Conversely, the application of direct/indirect vector parameters to the dysfunctional area may not inhibit the decompensated FCS, leaving unchanged the response to the tissue preference test or to the DyFIR test immediately after being re-executed, giving indication of the dominance of function over structure and leading the osteopath to a maximalist approach, or to the administration of adaptogenic techniques. In this model, the test for the assessment of the interdependence between structure/function can be performed, along with the test of inhibition mode by comparing the result of the visceral fascia test[132] (see Chapter 1) with the clinically relevant SD.

## Principles and methods of treatment

### Example of the maximalist approach

Whenever the osteopathic evaluation process reveals a dominance of function over structure, the treatment that follows will be a maximalist approach. With reference to the selection of different adaptogenic techniques, the clinical experience of the authors, in accordance with information from the first English osteopaths, Littlejohn and Wernham,[133,134] allowed the development of an approach defined as "general metabolic osteopathic treatment" (GMOT). The English pioneers developed a full routine, called general osteopathic treatment, to normalize structure by stimulating physiological function. Using an articulatory approach that follows the individual rhythm of the patient, every structural manifestation of tension, stiffness, swelling, or toxicity is detected and released. This approach also encourages the distribution of fluids and inherent forces, in order to stimulate the coordination and correlation of the body's self-regulating mechanisms. The latter, stabilized and harmonized by the joint integrity that is achieved, will be able to prepare, re-educate, and normalize each local adaptation expressed by SD.

This approach includes the musculoskeletal structure using an articulatory corrective force in order to influence innervation and blood distribution in a specific way.[135] In the clinical observations of the authors of this book, the strength of rhythmic harmonic oscillatory activation can be successfully used if applied to the soft tissues of the visceral relationships in the neck, thorax, and pelvis, especially in conditions where the person evidences pain accompanied by metabolic alterations. The oscillatory movements, like those of a pendulum or a spring, are cyclic, harmonic, rhythmic movement sequences, present in nature and also in man. The movement of the arms during walking is one of the sequences of harmonic and oscillatory movement of the body. Such movement operates within a three-dimensional harmonic movement around the three axes of space. The characteristic of these systems is that they transform, at different stages of movement and in a cyclic way, kinetic energy into potential energy, and vice versa. The oscillatory system can therefore conserve energy and return it. If it were not for the power and mechanical damping effects, the frequency of an oscillating system would remain constant.

In biological systems, the cushioning effects depend on the elasticity of tissues and liquids.[136] During the GMOT procedure, the patient is in the supine position and the osteopath proceeds with an anteroposterior two-handed approach with a focus on the autonomic innervation (Fig. 7.2). For example, for a balancing autonomic influence, one hand is positioned and acts as a pivot in the sacrococcygeal region, while the other hand is positioned with a "C"-shaped contact, with the first and second finger immediately above the symphysis pubis, projecting toward the pelvic urogenital organs, or over the left iliac fossa in the area of the colic flexure (Fig. 7.3A), with the osteopath then inducing an oscillatory stimulus to the tissues. The osteopath then proceeds to a posterior contact on paravertebral masses from T1 to L3, while the anterior hand applies rhythmic oscillatory forces from the cervical (at the upper cervical plexus, middle and lower) to the abdominal and pelvic (at celiac and mesenteric plexus) regions to finalize a hemodynamic stimulus to an autonomic sympathetic target (Fig. 7.3C). Another method for influencing tissues surrounding the parasympathetic innervation involves the osteopath placing one hand in the posterior cervical-occipital area, while the other hand switches between the cervical thoracic-abdominal regions (Fig. 7.3B).

The operator then focuses on the endogenous rhythmic properties of the patient's body, mainly driven by the nervous system and plastic-dynamic tissue properties, also known as the tonic vibration reflex.[137] An alteration, acceleration, or deceleration of the intrinsic oscillatory properties of the body indicate a possible area of dysfunction. Treatment consists of approaching every station of the autonomic

system via an A/P contact, which allows, through harmonic techniques, for acceleration of the rhythm if it has slowed down, or deceleration if it is too fast. During the routine the osteopath engages tissue tensions in a direct fashion, with the aim of integrating the oscillatory rhythm and stress state of the targeted areas with those of the surrounding region and of the whole body, via oscillation. The operator then tries to achieve a single resonance state within the soft tissue of the body cavity. This state of resonance is achieved when the osteopath observes certain parameters when inducing motion in the patient.

The frequency of the induced movement must be as close as possible to the natural frequency of the physiological movement of the segment. To obtain a constant oscillation, it is necessary that the energy fed by the osteopath is at least equal to the energy lost by the cushioning tissue phenomena. When, during the routine that involves the relationship between joints and cervical-thoracic-abdominal-pelvic regions, the osteopath detects an oscillatory slowdown in one area, he or she tries to re-establish resonance, using a force that respects the physiological direction of the motion of the oscillating segment.[137]

This approach of soft tissue and joint mobilization allows the entire body to integrate altered structures through refreshed metabolic function and reduces anxious conditions and related changes in body perception.[138] In addition to the author's suggestion, the osteopath who intends to use a maximalist approach to metabolism and energetics can use different global approaches, including those for the normalization of fascial decompensation, which, through balancing techniques for the transition areas and related diaphragms, are able to obtain a reduction in tension in the thoracic and abdominal cavities. One may also use the classical approaches of cranial osteopathy, as well as those described as specific for the DyFIR field (see Chapter 3).

## Example of a minimalist approach

Where the osteopathic evaluation shows a dominance of structure over function, the osteopath detects one or more clinically relevant disorders

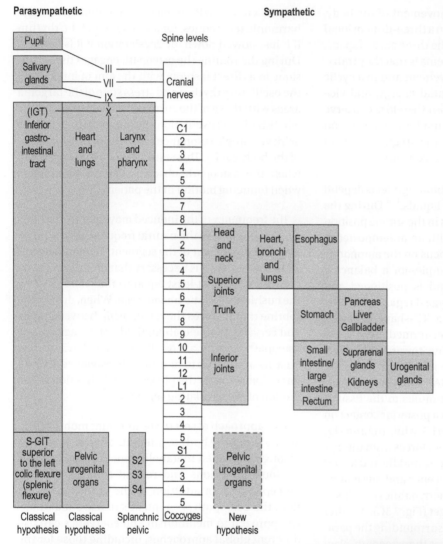

**Parasympathetic**

**Sympathetic**

Spine levels

| | | | |
|---|---|---|---|
| Pupil | | | |
| Salivary glands | III — VII — IX — | Cranial nerves | |
| (IGT) Inferior gastro-intestinal tract | X — Heart and lungs | Larynx and pharynx | C1, 2, 3, 4, 5, 6, 7, 8 |

| Spine | Sympathetic targets |
|---|---|
| T1–5 | Head and neck / Superior joints |
| | Heart, bronchi and lungs / Esophagus |
| T6–9 Trunk | Stomach / Pancreas Liver Gallbladder |
| T10–L2 Inferior joints | Small intestine/ large intestine Rectum / Suprarenal glands Kidneys / Urogenital glands |

S-GIT superior to the left colic flexure (splenic flexure) — Pelvic urogenital organs — S2 S3 S4 — Pelvic urogenital organs

Coccyges

| Classical hypothesis | Classical hypothesis | Splanchnic pelvic | | New hypothesis |

**Fig. 7.2**
Autonomic nervous system; the left side shows outflow of the parasympathetic system; the right side shows the outflow of the sympathetic system. According to Espinosa-Medina et al. (2016) the parasympathetic nervous system receives input from cranial nerves exclusively and the sympathetic nervous system from spinal nerves, thoracic to sacral inclusively (Espinosa-Medina I, Saha O, Boismoreau F, et al., (2016). The sacral autonomic outflow is sympathetic. Science. 354(6314):893–897.) Modified from: Parsons J, Marcer N. Osteopathy: models for diagnosis, treatment and practice. Edinburgh: Elsevier Churchill Livingstone; 2006. p. xv.

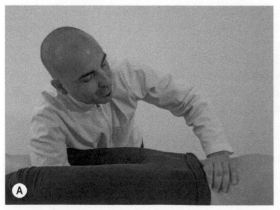

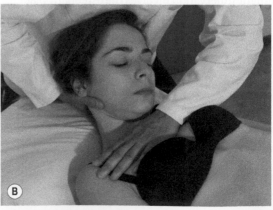

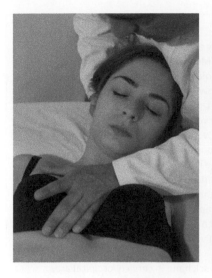
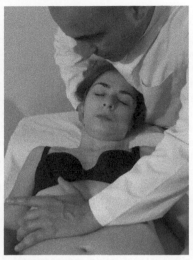
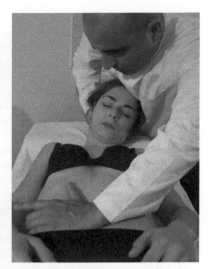

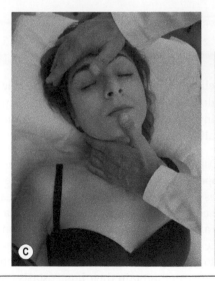
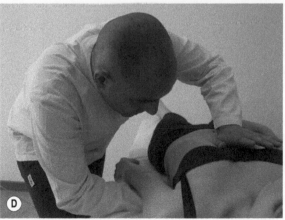

**Fig. 7.3**

The sequence outline of " general metabolic osteopathic treatment." The patient is supine. The osteopath sits at the patient's side and proceeds with an anterior-posterior bimanual approach focusing on the autonomic innervation. For example, for the parasympathetic system, one hand is positioned in the sacrococcygeal region, while the other hand uses a "C"-shaped contact, with the first and second fingers immediately above the symphysis pubis, projecting toward the urogenital pelvic organs (A); or, when the osteopath contacts the posterior cervico-occipital region with one hand, and the other hand alternates between the cervical-thoracic-abdominal areas (B). To influence the sympathetic system, the osteopath proceeds first with rhythmic pressures in the cervical region (C), and then approaches the paravertebral masses of the T1–L3 segments with a posterior contact, while, with the other hand placed anteriorly, applying alternating oscillatory rhythmic thrusts to the thoracic-abdominal-pelvic area, with particular focus on the mesenteric and celiac ganglia (D), and stating on the new hypotesis on sacrum (A).

Fig.7.3 continued

Sacral preganglionic neurons are considered parasympathetic, as are their targets in the pelvic ganglia that prominently control rectal, bladder, and genital functions. Recently, Espinoza-Medina et al. (2016) uncovered 15 phenotypic and ontogenetic features that distinguish pre- and postganglionic neurons of the cranial parasympathetic outflow from those of the thoracolumbar sympathetic outflow in mice. For every single one, the sacral outflow is indistinguishable from the thoracolumbar outflow. Thus, the parasympathetic nervous system receives input from cranial nerves exclusively and the sympathetic nervous system from spinal nerves, thoracic to sacral inclusively. This simplified, bipartite architecture offers a new framework to understand pelvic neurophysiology as well as development and evolution of the autonomic nervous system. Also contextualizing this information in the practice described above, although this does not change in the executive mode, requires several clarifications in defining the rationale of the technique; the GOMT routine is intended to improve a possible generalized visceral overload through an output autonomic balance obtained through an oscillatory tissue manual procedure, which, following the integration of new knowledge, will provide an approach to skin areas in reference to:

- orthosympathetic via a bimanual anterior/posterior approach (front approach soft tissues in the area of the celiac and mesenteric ganglia, and posterior approach in correspondence of dorsal vertebrae 5–9, then ridges 10 and 11, 12 and finally 1 and 2 lumbar and sacrum) (A, C, D)
- parasympathetic through an outlet bimanual anterior/posterior approach (back hand in cervico-occipital area emergency vagus nerve, while the front switches between the cervical-thoracic-abdominal lodges respecting the nerve progress) (B).

Espinosa-Medina I, Saha O, Boismoreau F et al. The sacral autonomic outflow is sympathetic. Science. 2016;354(6314):893–897.

that in individuals with metabolic load are often manifested by changes in the viscosity of the fascial tissue related to viscera and glands, leading to a minimalist approach. An example of a minimalist approach within this context is the visceral osteopathic approach: different approaches to visceral normalization have been emphasized in the osteopathic literature, from the direct method with direct contact with an organ to interact with its mobility, to normalization focused on the organ's inherent motility. However, recent animal studies and human trials with ultrasound suggest that:

- fascial tissue affected with the metabolic load of the organ that it contains loses part of its normal resilience and influences metabolic functions[139]

- peritoneal connective adhesions can be palpated, prevented, and treated with visceral mobilization[139]

- using techniques aimed at reproducing the dynamics of the superficial fascia associated with healthy organs, the osteopath attempts to eliminate all the tensions that restrict the freedom of operation of the visceral-diaphragmatic interconnection, enhance functionality, and alleviate musculoskeletal pain.[140]

Osteopathic visceral normalizations, in the proposed model, are directed toward the fascia that lines the organ, and the organ's reference area within the cervical-thoracic-abdominal-pelvic cavities, with the aim of freeing all the restrictive tensions imposed, for example, on the intra-abdominal organs, and to restore the plasticity and elasticity of those organs, in order to maintain their homeostasis (Fig. 7.4). The purpose of visceral techniques is to restore the homeostasis within the fascial environment of the organ, to affect the organ itself, and within the circulatory, lymphatic and neurovegetative systems which are in an interdependent relationship with the visceral system. When performing a technique, the osteopath can sometimes approach different organ areas using the same single action that focuses on an entire quadrant, for example the iliac fossa, flank, hypochondriac, epigastriac, mesogastrium or hypogastrium. The mesenteric system and the visceral ligaments are seen as

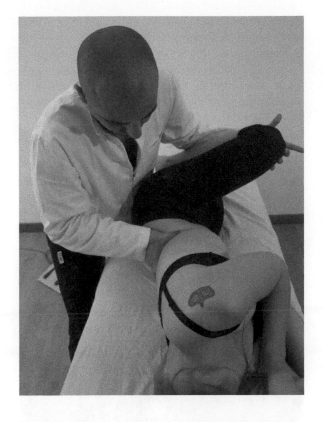

**Fig. 7.4**
Approach to the kidney area. The patient is lying sideways with the uppermost leg flexed; the operator is positioned behind the patient. One hand supports the patient's thigh with the flexed knee. The other hand is in contact with the lumbar region, in the kidney area. Using the patient's thigh as a lever and the hand on the kidney area as a fulcrum, the osteopath performs a tissue correction with the intention of releasing the entire area, which includes the kidneys, psoas muscle, lumbar spine, with resulting improvement in renal-diaphragmatic mobility. Photos courtesy of: Tozzi P, D Bongiorno, Vitturini C. Low back pain and kidney mobility: local osteopathic fascial manipulation decreases pain perception and improves renal mobility. J Bodyw Mov Ther. 2012;16(3):381–91.

interdependent units, beyond the individual constituents of the gastrointestinal tract.

Clinical observations show that there can be great variability among patients regarding the location of their abdominal organs. Thus, with respect to the use of manual treatment, alteration of the structure, represented by altered tissue texture detected in an abdominal quadrant, can thus influence the functioning of the organs of that area. Stated in other terms, visceral techniques can act on the dynamics of an organ and its fascia,[137] as well as on its function.[115,116] The areas where the osteopath will focus in order to enable the energetic-metabolic force are represented by surrounding fascial tissues, organs, and viscera, such as the thyroid, to relieve an overload of the basal metabolism, liver and pancreas in their roles in intermediary metabolism, gonads for their particular activity in reproduction, the adrenal glands in their participation in

the regulation of the stress response, the parathyroid, thymus, etc.

Although the author has proposed an approach directed to the normalization of alterations in stiffness-viscoelasticity-thixotropy of the fascial tissue related to internal organs, viscera, and glands, each operator, based on his or her sensitivity, along with the results of palpation assessment, can focus treatment on the mobility axes or on the ligamentous attachments of an organ, through recoil or inhibition techniques,[128] such as techniques of pressure on tissue reflections that can evoke vascular-lymphatic effects.[130,131]

## Minimalist/maximalist integration: energy techniques

In this discussion, the author describes the osteopathic approach while describing flow diagrams that can guide the operator in the relationship with the patient. However, sometimes the didactic-descriptive boundaries must be exceeded by the operator in a way that artfully relates to the patient. In the case of the energy-metabolic model, for example, the boundary between minimalist and maximalist approach can be transcended in a particular way when we refer to energy approaches, which, by focusing on the piezo-electric nature of local fascial areas, aim at involving the entire body electromagnetic field.[8,9]

These approaches are preferred in cases where, following the maximalist or minimalist approach, selected with the previously described decision-making process, the SD areas maintain a condition of abnormal spasm or inertia of DyFIR, with no apparent remaining findings and slow improvement of the symptoms reported by the patient. One of the energy techniques to which we can refer in osteopathy is the technique described by Hendryx as dynamic strain vector release.[141] The osteopath, having detected an SD, seeks to perceive with one hand the presence of a stress sensitive vector, defined as strain vector, which maintains a condition of spasm or inertia of fluid dynamics and related involuntary rhythms. The sensitive hand follows the most prominent abnormal attractive force emanating from the area of dysfunction.

As already mentioned, the remaining local tensions and fascial network adhesions can lead to compensatory tensions that extend across the musculoskeletal system, occasionally involving distant structures, leading to the emergence of traction forces and compromised movement patterns, palpable by the osteopath, for example, via the "fascial attraction/listening test" (see Chapter 1). The operating hand searches and is positioned in relation to the terminal point of the attraction force of the vector. While the sensory hand focuses on the terminal points of the dysfunctional vector, the operating hand proceeds toward and away from the malfunction, sensing an increased tension between the two hands, as if they were connected by a rubber band, maintaining a maximum energy tension on the dysfunctional vector.

When the point of maximum tension between the two hands is reached, the operator awaits

the emergence of a balance point, a subtle vibration at high frequency, followed by a return of the inherent movement in resonance with the surrounding tissues, thought to be attributable to an autonomic balance of the baroreflex response of vasomotion and tissue mechanics. The sensory hand then detects variations of viscoelastic quality, an increase in temperature and a disappearance of the dysfunctional vector[141] (Fig. 7.5). The fascia combines the properties of a sol-liquid conductor and a liquid crystal system that is intrinsic to the continuum of the matrix, which can generate

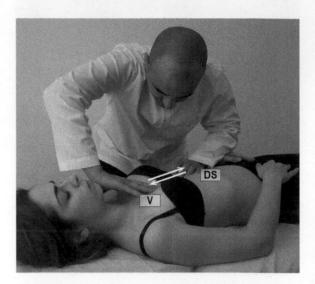

**Fig. 7.5**

Dynamic strain vector release. Abdominal approach: the osteopath has detected a somatic dysfunction (SD) and the sensory hand perceives the presence of a tensional vector, known as a strain vector, between the left hypochondrium area and the sternum. The other hand rests in the terminal point of the vector of the attraction force (V), in this case in the sternal portion of the body, and the operator proceeds with inductions toward and away from the feeling hand, and the points of terminal dysfunctional carrier, sensing an increased tension between the two hands, as if they were connected by a rubber band, until a tensional vector release point is reached, and a balancing of the dynamics of fluids and involuntary rhythms.

and conduct direct current and vibration. The dysfunctional tissue causes an alteration of the electricity perceived by conductors or semiconductors (nerves, fascia) and produces bio-electromagnetic fields.[82] The bioenergetic component of SD can therefore be perceived during osteopathic palpation through the emergence of vectors with attraction forces and amplitude greater than that of the inherent movements perceptible in a normal tissue.[141]

The osteopath can then select the most suitable approach for the case by assessing whether there is a need for:

- a minimalist approach focusing on the dysfunctional area

- a maximalist approach focusing on stimulation or inhibition of the metabolic activation force

- an integration between dysfunctional structure and overloading function, through the treatment of the dysfunctional vector used as a mediator of the vibrational agreement between the electric and electromagnetic fields of the operator and patient; an agreement holographically accessible through a connection with the appropriate vibrational frequency.

## Lifestyle and patient's ongoing management

From the information above there arises a clear concept, at least in terms of principles, for all health professionals and their patients: health maintenance also depends the lifestyle one leads. The osteopath must necessarily engage, through a treatment plan that includes information on lifestyle aimed at reducing the metabolic load, and focusing on nutritional lifestyle, for those people suffering from disturbances related to non-perceptible inflammations related to nutrition.[12] The use of food hygiene regimens and physical activity exercises also allows the operator to fill in the gap that a passive manual treatment (without the patient's cognitive, proprioceptive and interoceptive involvement

in the process) can leave in the healing and recovery process.[142]

### Nutrition advice

The relationship between food, bacterial flora, enterocytes, and immunocompetent cells could affect the health or illness of the patient.[143] An increase of chronic inflammatory diseases is recognized today as diabetes, atherosclerosis, asthma, chronic liver diseases, autoimmune diseases, degenerative diseases, and inflammatory bowel diseases. The increase in chronic inflammatory disorders would be related to the spread of the so-called "Western diet," considered a risk factor for chronic inflammatory diseases and cancer: it is characterized by high levels of red meat, simple carbohydrates (sugars), fats, "refined" grains, and low levels of vegetables, fruit, and fish. It is also becoming increasingly common in developing countries and its consumption is correlated with an increased incidence of chronic inflammatory diseases in the last six decades.[144,145] The damage that this diet leads to is due to the inability of the human genome to adapt to rapid changes in the environment, in particular the same diet.[146] The Mediterranean diet has increasingly been considered the basic salutogenic diet for humans.[147]

Thanks to its richness with olive oil, fruits, vegetables, integral cereals, nuts, and dried fruits in general, as well as the modest consumption of fish and white meat and low intake of red meat and simple carbohydrates, the Mediterranean diet is much closer to the diet of our ancestors than it is the current diet. Not surprisingly, the food pyramid, which summarizes the dietary recommendations of the US Ministry of Agriculture for proper nutrition in order to prevent obesity, is based on the Mediterranean diet: it reduces the risk of cardiovascular disease, cancer, Alzheimer's disease, Parkinson's disease, and premature death in general. The results of very recent studies[148] confirm the superiority of the Mediterranean diet, even in comparison with other diets rich in vegetables and fruits, in the primary prevention of cardiovascular disease events.

It is precisely the nutritional characteristics of the food complexes, rather than individual macronutrients (proteins, carbohydrates, and fats) and micronutrients (minerals and vitamins), that play an important protective role in the effect of the Mediterranean diet.[147]

The Mediterranean diet is rich in fibers and non-absorbable carbohydrates, which play an important role in the prevention of many so-called "modern" diseases. In fact, people who consume adequate or abundant amount of fiber have a lower incidence of chronic inflammatory diseases such as colitis, type 2 diabetes, and even colon cancer, compared to people who consume diets low in fiber.[149] The low incidence of asthma in Japan compared to Australia and the United States, all countries with a high degree of hygiene and urbanization, has been linked to the richness of the Japanese diet of rice, legumes, fermented foods, and fish.[150] In recent years the concept of an anti-inflammatory diet has been developed, which is the diet that can counteract the inflammatory processes and oxidative stress that characterizes many chronic degenerative diseases such as diabetes, cardiovascular diseases, and painful functional disorders of the musculoskeletal system, including those related to intense physical activity and musculotendinous injuries related to sport.

An Italian group[151] has undertaken research to determine the particulars of the antioxidant potential of the main plant foods, fruits, drinks, and oils consumed in Italy, thus creating a database to which we can refer for the preparation of an anti-inflammatory diet. With respect to the anti-inflammatory diet, it is not a single food that is effective, but rather the synergy between foods that brings different antioxidant molecules to counteract the action of free radicals or inflammatory processes that occur, for example, after a muscle injury. For the effective implementation of such food information, the osteopath can make use of a progressive and individualized approach for each patient,[152] but these are more likely to be cases where the professional osteopath refers the patient to a nutritionist. So, in principle, the osteopath can direct the patient toward general guidance and a healthy eating style, as long as there are no specific problems.

We believe that the traditional Mediterranean diet, as represented in the food pyramid (Fig. 7.6), is a sustainable diet, as it has a low environmental impact and is healthier for consumers.[153] It should also be noted that, today, ethical and health choices lead a growing percentage of people toward adopting a vegetarian or vegan diet.[154] Vegetarian diets produce health benefits in reducing the risk of hypertension in type 2 diabetes and certain types of cancer, reduction in body mass, as well as lower mortality from ischemic heart disease.[154] While bioavailability of nutrients may be impaired when diets devoid of animal proteins are consumed without proper attention (nutritional deficiencies were detected in long-term Western vegetarians), vegetarian diets can be nutritionally adequate when appropriately planned. For this reason, the operator who structures a treatment plan for a vegetarian or vegan patient should evaluate with the patient as to whether the diet adheres to the guidelines in the literature (Fig. 7.7).

Recent studies have shown that diets based on the principles of the Mediterranean diet, both the omnivorous type with low meat consumption and the ovo-lacto-vegetarian type, allow a low utilization of foods whose consumption should be moderate for health reasons and which coincide with those with a greater impact in terms of water consumption and $CO_2$ emission.[155] To paraphrase the authors of the food pyramid for Italians: "Is the diet of the past the best diet for our future?"[153]

## Advice on physical activity

It seems now widely known that having an active lifestyle helps to ensure a healthy life. Obviously extreme behaviors, including those in the pursuit of health, such as excessive exercise, or compulsiveness, often associated with eating disorders, bring with them negative consequences, both psychological and physical.[156-158]

Sometimes even athletes of elite teams, despite their training, report painful inflammatory and functional problems, often associated with skeletal or muscular problems, where the ligaments, tendons, joint capsules, and connective tissues have been stressed beyond their limits.[159,160] Up to

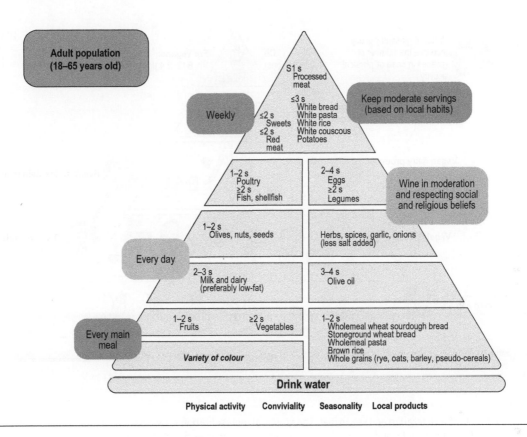

**Fig. 7.6**

The food pyramid. In order to guide people toward healthier eating behaviors, the Italian Ministry of Health gave a group of experts (DM 1/9/2003) the task of developing a reference diet pattern that is consistent with our current lifestyle and with the food traditions of our country. In accordance with Mediterranean traditions, Italian cultural heritage, and scientific evidence, the authors have proposed that only foods made with cereals with low glycemic index and rich in fibers must be placed at the base of the pyramid in the Mediterranean diet, while refined cereals with high glycemic index and starchy foods must be located at the top. Modified from: D'Alessandro A, De Pergola G. Mediterranean diet pyramid: a proposal for Italian people. Nutrients. 2014; 16;6(10):4302–16.

now, most sports training, whether for amateurs or competitive athletes, has emphasized the classic triad of muscle strength, cardiovascular conditioning, and neuromuscular coordination, perhaps leaving out certain aspects related to movement. Some researchers, along with body workers, now suggest targeted training aimed at the fascial network, as it could be of great importance to athletes, dancers, and ordinary people who want to benefit from movement.[125] Schleip and Müller claim that, if the fascial body is well trained, that is to say in such a way as to make it elastic and resilient, then the fascial body can be called into action to achieve an effective performance, with a high degree of prevention of accidents or their recurrence.

In osteopathy one uses exercises directed to the management of local adaptations, for example prevention of the recurrence of musculoskeletal[161] and visceral SD.[162] There are also general exercises directed to individual energy management.[163] We suggest that osteopathic professionals should incorporate the basic principles of fascia-oriented training[125] and apply them within

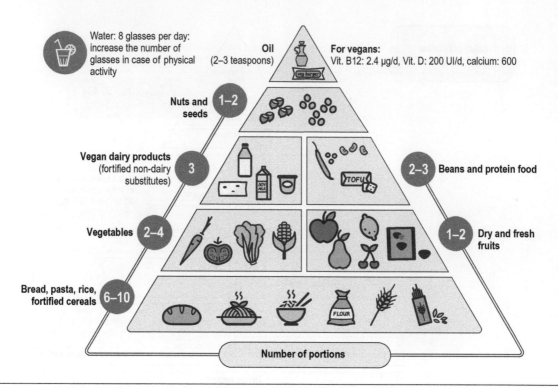

**Fig. 7.7**
The food pyramid of a vegetarian and vegan diet. The graphical representation shows a suitably programmed dietary regime to avoid nutritional deficiencies; this description of the vegetarian-vegan diet adheres to guidelines in the literature. Modified from: Twenty CA, Johnston CS. Modified food guide pyramid for lactovegetarians and vegans. J Nutr. 2002;132(5):1050–4.

specific contexts, especially with the energetic-metabolic model, in which we have observed how central the fascial metasystem is for salutogenesis: the fascial tissue of young people expresses more often a clear bidirectional orientation and a strong interconnectivity of their network of collagen fibers compared to sedentary subjects and elders. The application of proper exercise can induce an organization of such tissue architecture, with an increase in connectivity, when these characteristics are altered. Lack of exercise, however, has been shown to induce a network of multidirectional fibers and a decreased formation of "crimps," i.e., of physical and electrical connections (Fig. 7.8). The central principles of training oriented to the fascia are the following:

- *Fascial remodeling*: in reaction to targeted daily stress, the fascial tissue, with the help of fibroblasts, respond with a constant remodeling in the arrangement of the network of collagen fibers. For example, with the passing of years, half of the collagen fibrils are replaced in a healthy body. The intention of an approach aimed at fascial fitness, performed 1–2 times per week for 6–24 months, is to affect this substitution through specific training activities and to favor a more permanent maintenance of a tensegritive body which is not only strong but allows flexibility and a uniform joint mobility (Fig. 7.9).

- The *mechanism of tissue elastic return (fascial recoil)* is stimulated through targeted exercises, in which

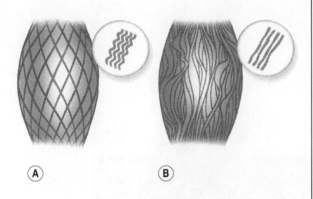

**Fig. 7.8**
Architecture of collagen in response to load. Young people (A) more often express a bidirectional orientation of their network of collagen fibers with strong physical and electrical connections. Lack of exercise induces disorganization of the network with little formation of multidirectional fibers connected between them (B). Modified from: Schleip R, Müller DG. Training principles for fascial connective tissues: scientific foundation and suggested practical applications. J Bodyw Mov Ther. 2013;17(1):103–15.

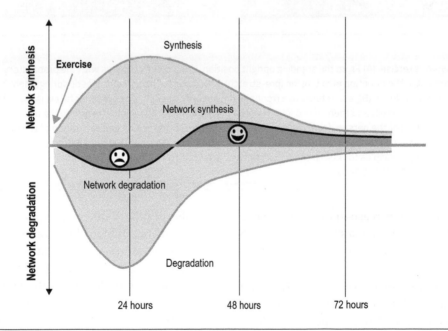

**Fig. 7.9**
Turnover of collagen after exercise. The upper curve shows that the synthesis of collagen in the tendons increases after exercise. However, the stimulated fibroblasts also increase the speed of collagen degradation. Interestingly, during the first few days following exercise, collagen degradation exceeds synthesis; afterwards this situation is reversed. To increase the strength of the tendons with fascial fitness training, the exercises should be performed 1–2 times a week in order to achieve an appropriate tissue stimulation. Modified from: Schleip R, Müller DG. Training principles for fascial connective tissues: scientific foundation and suggested practical applications. J Bodyw Mov Ther. 2013;17(1):103–15.

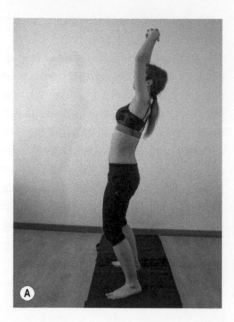
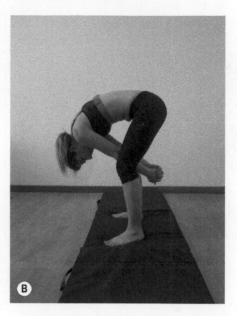

**Fig. 7.10**

"The flying sword" exercise. (A) From the standing upright position, the patient proceeds with the preparatory counter-movement in the direction of extension (pre-stretch), which starts the dynamic elastic spring; then the patient proceeds toward the release (B), and returns to a front and downward direction. The posterior fascia is loaded together with the whole superior part, and then moved into flexion; a harmonic bounce leads to a return to the upright standing position. The attention of the person doing the exercise should be on optimal timing and calibration of the movement to create the most fluid and smooth movement possible. It is also possible to use light weights. Photos courtesy of: Schleip R, Müller DG. Training principles for fascial connective tissues: scientific foundation and suggested practical applications. J Bodyw Mov Ther. 2013;17(1):103–15.

a preparatory phase increases the elastic tension of the fascial body, followed by a stage where the body releases the weight as a catapult (Fig. 7.10).

- *Dynamic stretching oriented to the fascia* (Fig. 7.11): instead of a static stretch position, a more fluid approach is suggested that, if performed long-term and regularly, can positively influence the architecture of the connective tissue by keeping it more elastic.[164]

- With respect to *proprioceptive and interoceptive sensation*, it is interesting to note that the receptors that are found in joint capsules and ligaments have proven to be of minor importance for normal proprioception, since they are usually only stimulated during extreme movements and not during common physiological movements.[125] On the contrary, proprioceptive free nerve endings located in the more superficial fascial layers are called into play by small angular joint and sliding movements. Recent findings indicate that the superficial fascial layers of the body are more densely populated with nerve endings as compared to tissues located more internally.[165] Accordingly, the recommended exercises of "fascial perception" are those where the patient experiences different qualities of movement, for example using extremely slow to very fast movements, micromovements not visible to an observer and large movements that involve the whole body (Fig. 7.12). Such movements are active and

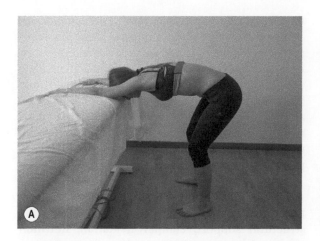
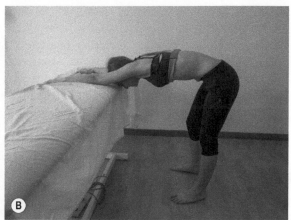

**Fig. 7.11**

"The big cat stretch" exercise. (A) Proceed with a slow elongation movement of the long posterior chain, from the tips of the fingers to the ischial tuberosity, from the heels and the sacrum to the top of the head. Several aspects of the fascial web undergo slow and steady movements to slightly change the angle of flexion. (B) The patient rotates and stretches the pelvis and chest toward one side – in this example to the right. The intensity of the stretch feeling on that entire side of the body is then gently reduced. Photos courtesy of: Schleip R, Müller DG. Training principles for fascial connective tissues: scientific foundation and suggested practical applications. J Bodyw Mov Ther. 2013;17(1):103–15.

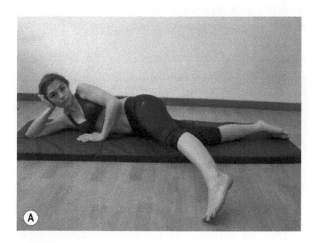
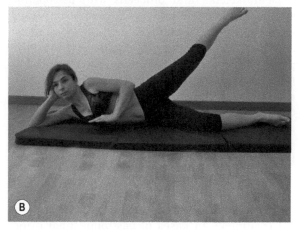

**Fig. 7.12**

"Octopus tentacle" exercise. With the image of an octopus's tentacle in mind, the patient explores in slow motion a multitude of extension movements through the whole leg. The tensional fascial proprioception is activated through the creation of changes in muscle activation patterns. This feature goes hand in hand with a deep myofascial stimulation that aims to reach not only the fascial sheaths, but also the septa between the muscles. Photos courtesy of: Schleip R, Müller DG. Training principles for fascial connective tissues: scientific foundation and suggested practical applications. J Bodyw Mov Ther. 2013;17(1):103–15.

specific and can have effects that are not possible with larger movements. In making these fascial coordinated movements, it seems possible to specifically deal with adhesions, e.g., between deep muscle septa in the body. Furthermore, these small and specific movements can be used to bring awareness to perceptually neglected areas of the body, i.e., those that are interoceptively compromised.[166]

## Rationale, mechanisms, and evidence

This model searches for energy balance by maintaining the adaptation to metabolic and immunological stresses. We know how a silent inflammation associated with metabolic conditions such as the increase of adipose tissue and body mass index, promotes, maintains and worsens pain and musculoskeletal function.[167,168] This unphysiological state promotes nociception in the dysfunctional musculoskeletal tissues, prevents healing, and is associated with a variety of chronic diseases.[28,29] The osteopath recognizes this type of patient after observing the metabolic nature of the inflammation, for example musculoskeletal, and proceeds with osteopathic approaches directed to SD that have been proved effective in the literature.[169] These minimalist approaches, especially visceral techniques, have proven to be useful in improving painful and dysfunctional systemic conditions linked to alterations of neurotransmission,[170,171] such as colic.[116] Other studies have reported improvement of painful abdominal conditions associated with disorders such as constipation or diarrhea, and related to biliary dyskinesia.[117]

Some authors recommend the inclusion of osteopathic manipulative treatment with standard medical treatments in cases of gastrointestinal disorders and musculoskeletal pain related to bacterial infections.[172] Osteopathic manipulative treatment also represents a potential means to reduce fatigue and self-perceived stress in a population of healthy subjects.[173] OMT application in a population of students resulted in improved physiological parameters (maximum force of closed fist, fatigue time of the forearm flexor muscles, heart rate, and peripheral vascular flow) and an improvement in performance in school.[174] Some researchers have noted an improvement in symptoms associated with myalgic encephalomyelitis and chronic fatigue syndrome (fatigue, memory disorders, pain in the cervical and axillary lymph glands, muscle aches, headache, non-restorative sleep, etc.), with muscle fatigue reduction if the affected patients receive OMT, compared to untreated patients.[175,176]

In this chapter, we discussed how the fascia performs many functions in the body, including structural support, compartmentation, nutrition support, immunity, tissue repair, and communications. We proposed ways in which the extracellular matrix and body fluids can modulate both function and cellular pathophysiology, showing changes in bio-resonance.[80,82] The fascia is a connective tissue organized as a three-dimensional network that surrounds, supports, maintains, protects, connects, and divides the muscular, skeletal, and visceral components of the body. Studies suggest that the fascia will reorganize along imposed tension lines or those expressed naturally by the body, with effects that can cause repercussions or contractures on the whole body. This can potentially create stress on each shape surrounded by the fascia itself, resulting in mechanical and physiological effects.[137] Recent studies have suggested global adaptogenic approaches, described in the osteopathic literature,[177] to improve the immunological structure and better address the complications of influenza-like illness.[178] In addition to being able to stimulate the immune system, which makes them indicated in cases of infections, these approaches produce a redistribution of inflammation mediators.[179]

From an osteopathic perspective, adaptogenic techniques described in this chapter focus on the fascial aspects of visceral-somatic connections, as in the case of "internal general osteopathic treatment," as well as the rhythmic bioelectric components inherent to the extracellular matrix and body electromagnetic field, such as the dynamic strain vector release. These techniques aim to release these tensions, relieve pain, and restore function altered by excessive allostatic load. The mechanism underlying osteopathic techniques that target the fascia is based on several studies that take into account the plastic, viscoelastic, and piezoelectric properties of the connective tissue, and after the application of these techniques show effects such as:

- neuromuscular,[137] or neural and tissue physical stress input diminution. The application of force vectors can remove load from the muscle spindles, and probably adds load to the Golgi bodies. This can change the pattern of sensory inputs in the spinal cord in the treated area, inhibiting the nociceptors and decreasing the release of substance P which produces local edema. A slow rhythmic oscillation causes an inhibitory effect on the vestibular nuclei, causing muscle relaxation and inhibition of motor neuron excitability. The oscillations may also facilitate the flow of fluids through intercompartmental hydraulic mechanisms, as well as a possible modulatory effect of the gate mechanisms of pain in the spinal cord

- structural,[137] in that the collagen matrix in the dermis can be changed by a manual approach in areas of the body suffering from chronic pain. The changes reflect the differences in tension, smoothness, and regularity that can be palpated before and after treatment. Myofascial release techniques have shown persistent changes in fascial thickness for at least 24 hours, observable by ultrasound

- viscoelastic,[137] with transformation of the substance from its basal dense state (gel) into a more solid state (colloidal). This change in viscosity seems to increase the production of hyaluronic acid and, along with the flow within the fascial tissue, improves the drainage of inflammatory mediators and metabolic waste, decreases the chemical irritation of the autonomic nervous system terminations and the nociceptive stimuli to the somatic terminations, thus eliminating somatovisceral and/or viscerosomatic aberrant reflexes

- fluidic,[137] with increase in the flow of interstitial fluids and stimulation of the proliferation of fibroblasts, their differentiation into myofibroblasts and collagen organization, contributing to fibrogenesis and fascial repair. The moment the blood and lymph flow are optimized and the oxygenation returned to normal levels, the nutrients are brought to appropriate concentrations in the cells, while toxins and inflammatory products are removed

- cellular,[137] since the manual stimulus of the fascia can cause changes through the activation of the fibroblast response and the different receptors in the fascial tissue and lead to hypertonicity corrections and abnormal cross-linking of collagen in the tissues

- analgesic,[137] through an effect on the endocannabinoid anandamide system. The activation of the endocannabinoid system following fascial treatment decreases nociception and pain, reduces inflammation in the myofascial tissues, and plays a role in fascial reorganization. The pain reduction is also correlated with the modulation of sympathetic hypertonia and parasympathetic tone, with an improvement in a variety of somatic and visceral functions

- immunological and adaptogenic: the evidence suggests that manual therapy applied twice weekly to myofascial tissues could cause persistent modulation effects on the function of the hypothalamic–pituitary–adrenal axis and on immune function.[180,181] An increase of oxytocin and a decrease of ACTH as a result of manual treatments were detected.[180] Hormonal changes with reduction of cortisol and arginine vasopressin levels were maintained for up to 4 days, while changes in cytokines and increased levels of oxytocin persisted for up to 8 days[180]

- reparative, as the benefits of osteopathic manipulation, including myofascial work, were observed to be related to an increase in blood concentration of nitric oxide.[182] This process could promote the synthesis of collagen, improving tissue repair, clinical symptoms, and the recovery of functions after injury,[183] and may promote relaxation of smooth muscles, angiogenesis,[184] improved neurotransmission,[185] and increased response to immunogens[186]

- epigenetic, as suggested by a recent review of the literature, in which a possible epigenetic effect related to manipulative approaches was reported.[187] The mechanical forces applied during treatment of the fascial field could contribute to the reduction of DNA methylation, by activating epigenetic cell adjustment, affecting the composition of the extracellular matrix, the levels of inflammation, angiogenic activity, the activity of fibroblasts and differentiation, and the repair of tissues.[188]

### Applied vibrational mechanical signals

Fibroblasts in culture were seen as an epigenetic factor in the microenvironment regulation of ECM.[189] In particular, they produce significant increases in glycosaminoglycans and decreased collagen, thus providing a basis for reducing tissue adhesions and improving the function of the connective tissue.[190]

Some of the free nerve endings in the interstitial myofascial tissue were defined as interoceptors because they give information about the brain's physiological tissue conditions, such as temperature, pH, and visceral variations.[191] In particular, "C-tactile fibers" have recently been discovered in human subcutaneous connective tissue. While C-fibers are classically described as nociceptors or chemoreceptors, these tactile C-fibers are low-threshold mechanoreceptors, part of an alternative warning system in humans.[192]

It seems that the activation of these sensory myelinated fibers during therapies that use a gentle touch sends signals to the insular cortex, the medial prefrontal cortex, and the anterior cingulate cortex, resulting in an integration of sensory and affective information,[193] resulting in peripheral effects on psychoendocrine function, the immune system, autonomic regulation, and modulation of pain.[194]

## Case study

### General patient data

A 40-year-old woman, entrepreneur, sedentary, overweight, smoker, nulliparous.

### Present medical history

The reason for consultation is a headache in the occipital base region, accompanied by muscle tension and cervical and mid-thoracic pain. The headache pain occasionally extends to the posterior orbital area, and is improved by taking non-steroidal anti-inflammatory drugs (NSAIDs) recommended by the doctor. The patient states that the headache is of variable onset, reporting sporadic episodes during the morning and more frequent and more intense episodes in the afternoon or early evening. The latter occurring on a daily basis during the 6 months prior to the consultation. She does not report symptoms such as vomiting, fever, chills, blurred vision, or photophobia.

### Past history and family medical history

The patient reports having experienced, for about 2 years, intermittent nausea and swelling that worsens after eating. She reports intestinal spasms, heartburn (alleviated by taking antacids), fatigue, and insomnia. She has had no gastroenterological investigations in the

## Case study continued

past, nor at the time of consultation. Refers to a car accident resulting in whiplash that occurred about two and a half years prior to consulting. Penicillin allergy. Reports a family history of hypothyroidism, hypertension, glaucoma.

### Social and occupational medical history

Reports that all of the symptoms are related to a stressful period when she was unable to maintain a good lifestyle, because of heavy work commitments;

Although her symptoms are often improved by taking NSAIDs, the patient, recommended by acquaintances, wants to try osteopathic manipulative treatment, believing that it can also help alleviate the symptoms.

### Differential diagnosis

- Cervicogenic headache

- Biliary dyskinesia

- Gastritis/gastric infections. For this condition a consultation with a gastroenterologist is recommended. A specialist close to the patient's workplace is sought, and an appointment is made for the following day.

### Objective examination

Palpation of the abdomen showed swelling and distension. McBurney's point is painless, while the epigastrium is sensitive, but not explicitly painful.

### Osteopathic evaluation

- The FCS test detected a mild decompensated scheme, with non-alternated rotations and inclinations in the cervicothoracic and thoracoabdominal transition areas. The visceral

fascia test showed tension in the abdominal portion of the visceral fascia. Although the global tests were positive, confirming the high allostatic load reported in the patient's narrative, rather than proceed with a maximalist approach, we proceeded with local tests.

- The step test (see Chapter 1) confirmed the presence of an area of tension and hypomobility in the abdominal cavity, during the performance of the simulated movement by the patient.

- Specific local tests clearly showed a thoracic SD (M99.02) (T6 bilateral extension). It also showed an SD of the soft tissue in the abdominal area (M99.09) (left upper quadrant).

- The inhibition test, performed by stimulating the somatic dysfunction detected by both direct and indirect methods, did not improve the T6 mobility restriction or pain on palpation. It did not improve the mobility restriction or the alteration of the abdominal area, and did not improve the failure of the fascial scheme, and also appeared to alter the dynamics of fluids and involuntary rhythms especially in the abdominal area.

### Treatment

During the *first session* a maximalist approach was used, using the metabolic-energetic model, and specifically a "general metabolic osteopathic treatment." During the immediate evaluation after treatment, we detected a non-balanced dynamic of fluids and involuntary rhythms, with spasms of the perceived rhythm in the left hypochondrium, while a considerable inertia was present both in the thoracic and in the cranial regions. We then proceeded with a dynamic strain vector release technique by approaching the area of correspondence of the stomach, until a local tissue release, corresponding to a uniform

## Case study continued

rhythm of the fluid dynamics in the cranial, thoracic and abdominal areas, was achieved (Fig. 7.13).

At the *second session* (2 weeks later), the patient reported an immediate improvement of all painful cranial and cervicothoracic symptoms. The patient also had not experienced any further gastric symptoms and reported improved sleep with no more nighttime awakenings, but was still having difficulty falling asleep.

The patient reported having been to a gastroenterologist who diagnosed infection with *Helicobacter pylori* and, given the impossibility of using antibiotic therapy, recommended taking the probiotic bacteria *Lactobacillus reuteri*, usually used in combination with sequential therapy to eradicate the bacterium,[195] along with individualized dietary advice. The "internal general osteopathic treatment," associated with an approach to the central tendon (see Chapter 6), was repeated. The patient reported relaxation effects immediately after the treatment.

### Patient education

During the second treatment session, a daily exercise routine was demonstrated to the patient and recommended. The exercises included one designed to improve and prevent abdominal somatic dysfunction, especially in the stomach area (Fig. 7.13). A routine of fascial fitness exercises was also recommended (Figs. 7.10–7.12). A telephone consultation in 2 weeks was scheduled.

### Follow up

After 2 weeks, during the phone consultation, the patient reported an improvement in sleep and in digestion, and the absence of painful cranial and cervicothoracic symptoms. Another phone consultation was done 4 weeks later, in which the patient reported a continued absence of symptoms, some weight loss and a negative response to the *Helicobacter pylori* test. The specialist recommended that she continue taking the probiotics. The next follow-up with the osteopath is scheduled in 2 months.

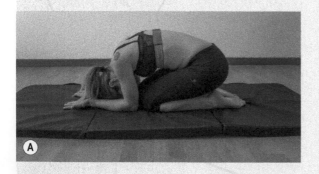 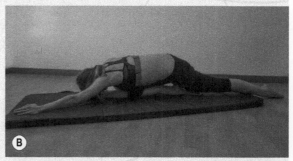

**Fig. 7.13**

Exercise for abdominal visceral mobilization.

(A) *Position 1*

Kneel, sitting on your heels, with the trunk bent on the knees, the head resting on the floor and your upper arms contacting the floor. Stretching your arms as much as possible, crawl on the floor without lifting your buttocks from your heels. Keep this stretching position while breathing deeply five times, using your diaphragm. Repeat 3 times with a break of 1–2 minutes between sets. If you cannot bring your torso to your knees, keep your knees apart, but your toes together.

## Case study continued

**Fig. 7.13 continued**

*Common mistakes:*

- Lifting your head from the floor and arching the neck.
- Raising your buttocks from the heels.
- Breathing with the chest.

**(B)** *Position 2*

Kneel, sitting on the left heel, with the right leg stretched out behind; the torso is bent forward with your arms stretched wide apart, in a laid back position, with your head on the floor. Breathe regularly with the diaphragm 5 times, and then repeat on the other side (with the left leg in the back). The alternate stretching of limbs favors the gliding of fascial planes and stimulates the area of the stomach alternately, along with the kidney and the descending colon and vice versa, the liver area, the kidney, and ascending colon.

*Common mistakes*

- Keeping your head raised, arching your neck.
- Off balance because you keep your hands in.

Photos courtesy of: Brazzo M. Inside gymnastics. Novara: Ed. Red.; 2011.

## Conclusions

The treatment proposed in the metabolic-energetic model is based on approaches with visceral, neuroendocrine, and immune system targets and is supported by nutritional and exercise programs. The connective tissue anatomical space allows for reflex manual contact with the glands and organs, as well as the modulation of their functions. Each model cannot be integrated with all the other models; however, the metabolic-energetic model, by virtue of its focus on the fascial component, appears to be an interdependent model *par excellence*, so much so that some authors have proposed an energetic metamodel over and above the classical description.[8,9] Since the dawn of osteopathic medicine, there have been different approaches directed to musculoskeletal and metabolic-systemic disorders, particularly chronic ones. This success led Still and his first students to believe that something new and revolutionary was born. They tried to explain this phenomenon by integrating the principles of "bonesetters" with those of the "magnetic healers" in a unique approach that still carries with it the elements of the original principles in the techniques used by osteopaths.[196]

Some of these need to be investigated with respect to the basic mechanisms that underlie them; however, this probably requires the use of a biophysical paradigm.[84] In fact, even biomedicine[197] is addressing some issues with the help of physicists in research labs alongside biologists and doctors, so much so that we are able to identify specific electromagnetic signals coming from plasma of patients suffering from various infections and chronic diseases.[198] Emilio Del Giudice and his team showed and proposed that water can be organized into networks of "coherence domains" involving millions of water molecules, which are the size of nanostructures.[197] We hypothesize that these nanostructures can self-renew with electromagnetic waves, which emit, and can retain faithfully, the genetic information of DNA. Of course the discoveries mentioned have raised many unanswered questions that need further work and interaction between different sciences. The DNA signal is stimulated by electromagnetic waves that propagate in biological fluids. Could it be that osteopathic attention to the fluidic-electromagnetic domains is not just a mere coincidence or a thing of the past?

## References

1. Trowbridge C. Andrew Taylor Still 1828–1917. Kirksville, MO: Truman State University Press; 1991. p. 125.

2. Bischof M, Del Giudice E. Communication and the emergence of collective behavior in living organisms: a quantum approach. Mol Biol Int. 2013;2013:987549.

3. Educational Council on Osteopathic Principles (ECOP). Glossary of osteopathic terminology usage guide. Chevy Chase, MD: American Association of Colleges of Osteopathic Medicine (AACOM); 2011. p. 25.

4. World Health Organization (WHO). Benchmarks for training in traditional/complementary and alternative medicine: benchmarks for training in osteopathy. WHO; 2010. p. 5.

5. Hruby RJ. Pathophysiologic models and the selection of osteopathic manipulative techniques. J Osteopath Med. 1992;6(4):25–30.

6. DiGiovanna EL. Goals classifications and models of osteopathic manipulation. In: DiGiovanna EL, Schiowitz S, Dowling DJ, editors. An osteopathic approach to diagnosis and treatment. 3rd ed. Philadelphia, PA: Lippincott Williams and Wilkins; 2005. p. 78.

7. De Stefano L. Greenman's principles of manual medicine. 4th ed. Baltimore, MD: Williams and Wilkins; 2011. p. 50.

8. Hendryx JT. The bioenergetic model in osteopathic diagnosis and treatment: an FAAO thesis. Part 1. Am Acad Osteop J. 2014;24(1):12–20.

9. Hendryx JT. The bioenergetic model in osteopathic diagnosis and treatment: an FAAO thesis. Part 2. Am Acad Osteop. J 2014; 24(2):10–8.

10. Seffinger MA, King HH, Ward RC et al. Osteopathic phylosophy. In: Chila A, editor. Foundations of osteopathic medicine. 3rd ed. Philadelphia, PA: Lippincott Williams and Wilkins; 2011. p. 4.

11. Navarro E, Funtikova AN, Fíto M et al. Can metabolically healthy obesity be explained by diet genetics and inflammation? Mol Nutr Food Res. 2014;59(1):75–93.

12. Seaman DR. Body mass index and musculoskeletal pain: is there a connection? Chiropr Man Therap. 2013;21:15.

13. Stone AA, Broderick JE. Obesity and pain are associated in the United States. Obesity. 2012;20:1491–5.

14. Leboeuf-Yde C. Body weight and low back pain. A systematic literature review of 56 journal articles reporting on 65 epidemiologic studies. Spine. 2000;25:226–37.

15. Vismara L, Menegoni F, Zaina F et al. Effect of obesity and low back pain on spinal mobility: a cross sectional study in women. J Neuroeng Rehabil. 2010;7:3.

16. Vismara L, Romei M, Galli M et al. Clinical implications of gait analysis in the rehabilitation of adult patients with "Prader-Willi" syndrome: a cross-sectional comparative study ("Prader-Willi" syndrome vs matched obese patients and healthy subjects). J Neuroeng Rehabil. 2007;4:14.

17. Chou R, Qaseem A, Snow V et al. Diagnosis and treatment of low back pain: a joint clinical practice guideline from the American College of Physicians and the American Pain Society. Ann Intern Med. 2007;147:478–91.

18. Bays HE, Gonzalez-Campoy M, Henry RR et al. Is adiposopathy (sick fat) an endocrine disease? Int J Clin Pract. 2008;62:1474–83.

19. Bays HE. Adiposopathy: is sick fat a cardiovascular disease? J Am Coll Cardiol. 2011;57:2461–73.

20. Bays HE. Adiposopathy diabetes mellitus and primary prevention of atherosclerotic coronary artery disease: treating "sick fat" through improving fat function with antidiabetes therapies. Am J Cardiol. 2012;110(Suppl):4B–12B.

21. Lee KH, Park SW, Ye SM. Relationships between dietary habits and allostatic load index in metabolic syndrome patients. Korean J Fam Med. 2013;34(5):334–46.

22. Galic S, Oakhill JS, Steinberg GR. Adipose tissue as an endocrine organ. Mol Cell Endocrinol. 2010;316:129–39.

23. Sell H, Eckel J. Adipose tissue inflammation: novel insight into the role of macrophages and lymphocytes. Curr Opin Clin Nutr Metab Care. 2010;13:366–70.

24. Saraiva M, O'Garra A. The regulation of IL-10 production by immune cells. Nat Rev Immunol. 2010;10:170–81.

25. Berenbaum F. Osteoarthritis as an inflammatory disease (osteoarthritis is not osteoarthrosis). Osteoarthr Cartil. 2013;21:16–21.

26. Mantyselka P, Miettola J, Niskanen L et al. Persistent pain at multiple sites connection to glucose derangement. Diabetes Res Clin Pract. 2009;84(2):e30–2.

27. Shiri R, Karppinen J, Leino-Arjas P et al. The association between obesity and low back pain: a meta-analysis. Am J Epidemiol. 2010;171:135–54.

28. Sommer C, Birklein F. Resolvins and inflammatory pain. F1000 Med Rep. 2011;3:19.

29. Das UN. Is multiple sclerosis a proresolution deficiency disorder? Nutrition. 2012;28:951–8.

30. Izzi V, Masuelli L, Tresoldi I et al. The effects of dietary flavonoids on the regulation of redox inflammatory networks. Front Biosci (Landmark Ed). 2012;17:2396–418.

31. Bistolfi F. Classification of possible targets of interaction of magnetic fields with living matter. Panminerva Med. 1987;29(1):71–3.

32. Bistolfi F. The bioelectronic connectional system (BCS): a therapeutic target for nonioizing radiation. Panminerva Med. 1990;32(1):10–8.

33. Janig W. Neurobiology of visceral pain. Schmerz. 2014;28(3):233–51.

34. Bonaccio M, Cerletti C, Iacoviello L et al. Mediterranean diet and subclinical chronic inflammation: the MOLI-SANI study. Endocr Metab Immune Disord Drug Targets. 2014 [Epub ahead of print].

35. Hirahatake KM, Slavin JL, Maki KC et al. Associations between dairy foods, diabetes and metabolic health: potential mechanisms and future directions. Metabolism. 2014:63(5):618–27.

36. Pischinger A. The extracellular matrix and ground regulation: basis for a holistic biological medicine. Berkeley, CA: North Atlantic Books; 2007.

37. Siasos G, Tousoulis D, Kioufis S et al. Inflammatory mechanisms in atherosclerosis: the impact of matrix metalloproteinases. Curr Top Med Chem. 2012;12(10):1132–48.

38. Traverso S. Mechanical signalling in tissues and its possible role in nociception. Theor Biol Forum. 2011;104(2):75–84.

39. Bei R, Masuelli L, Palumbo C et al. Long-lasting tissue inflammatory processes trigger autoimmune responses to extracellular matrix molecules. Int Rev Immunol. 2008; 27(3):137–75.

40. Di Girolamo N, Visvanathan K, Lloyd A et al. Expression of TNF-alpha by human plasma cells in chronic inflammation. J Leukoc Biol. 1997;61(6):667–78.

41. Gabay C. Interleukin-6 and chronic inflammation. Arthritis Res Ther. 2006;8(Suppl)2:S3.

42. Eijsbouts AM, van den Hoogen FH, Laan RF et al. Hypothalamic-pituitary-adrenal axis activity in patients with rheumatoid arthritis. Clin Exp Rheumatol. 2005;23(5):658–64.

43. Kyrou J, Chrousos GP, Tsigos C. Stress, visceral obesity and metabolic complications. Ann NY Acad Sci. 2006;1083:77–110.

44. Taylor BK, Corder G. Endogenous analgesia dependence and latent pain sensitization. Curr Top Behav Neurosci. 2014;20:283–325.

45. Sulli A, Montecucco CM, Caporali R et al. Glucocorticoid effects on adrenal steroids and cytokine responsiveness in polymyalgia rheumatica and elderly onset rheumatoid arthritis. Ann NY Acad Sci. 2006; 1069:307–14.

46. Richards HL, Ray DW, Kirby B et al. Response of the hypothalamic-pituitary-adrenal axis to psychological stress in patients with psoriasis. Br J Dermatol. 2005;153(6):1114–20.

47. Raap U, Werfel T, Jaeger B et al. Atopic dermatitis and psychological stress. Hautarzt. 2003;54(10):925–9.

48. Buske-Kirschbaum A, von Auer K, Krieger S et al. Blunted cortisol responses to psychosocial stress in asthmatic children: a general feature of atopic disease? Psychosom Med. 2003;65(5):806–10.

49. Buske-Kirschbaum A, Hellhammer DH. Endocrine and immune responses to stress in chronic inflammatory skin disorders. Ann NY Acad Sci. 2003;992:231–40.

50. Cutolo M, Foppiani L, Minuto F. Hypothalamic-pituitary-adrenal axis impairment in the pathogenesis of rheumatoid arthritis and polymyalgia rheumatica. J Endocrinol Invest. 2002;25(10 Suppl):19–23.

51. Parker AJ, Wessely S, Cleare AJ. The neuroendocrinology of chronic fatigue syndrome and fibromyalgia. Psychol Med. 2001;31(8):1331–45.

52. Morand EF, Leech M. Hypothalamic-pituitary-adrenal axis regulation of inflammation in rheumatoid arthritis. Immunol Cell Biol. 2001;79(4):395–9.

53. Mastorakos G, Ilias I. Relationship between interleukin-6 (IL-6) and hypothalamic-pituitary-adrenal axis hormones in rheumatoid arthritis. Z Rheumatol. 2000;59(Suppl 2):II/75–9.

54. Demitrack MA, Crofford LJ. Evidence for and pathophysiologic implications of hypothalamic-pituitary-adrenal axis dysregulation in fibromyalgia and chronic fatigue syndrome. Ann NY Acad Sci. 1998;840:684–97.

55. Buske-Kirschbaum A, Jobst S, Psych D et al. Attenuated free cortisol response to psychosocial stress in children with atopic dermatitis. Psychosom Med. 1997;59(4):419–26.

56. Crofford LJ, Engleberg NC, Demitrack MA. Neurohormonal perturbations in fibromyalgia. Baillieres Clin Rheumatol. 1996;10(2):365–78.

57. Liang Y, Pan HF, Ye DQ. Therapeutic potential of STAT4 in autoimmunity. Expert Opin Ther Targets. 2014;20:1–16.

58. Hamminga EA, van der Lely AJ, Neumann HA et al. Chronic inflammation in psoriasis and obesity: implications for therapy. Med Hypotheses. 2006;67(4):768–73.

59. Bos JD, de Rie MA, Teunissen MB et al. Psoriasis: dysregulation of innate immunity. Br J Dermatol. 2005;152(6):1098–107.

60. Mastorakos G, Ilias I. Relationship between interleukin-6 (IL-6) and hypothalamic-pituitary-adrenal axis hormones in rheumatoid arthritis. Z Rheumatol. 2000;59(Suppl 2): II/75–9.

61. Jongen-Lavrencic M, Peeters HR, Wognum A et al. Elevated levels of inflammatory cytokines in bone marrow of patients with rheumatoid arthritis and anemia of chronic disease. J Rheumatol. 1997;24(8):1504–9.

62. Nordenstrom BE. Biologically closed electric circuits. Stockholm: Nordic Medical Publications; 1983.

63. Ladik J. Solid state physics of biological macromolecules: the legacy of Albert Szent-Gyorgyi. J Mol Struc (Theochem). 2003; 666–67:1–9.

64. Gascoyne PRC, Pethig R, Gyorgyi AS. Water structure-dependent charge transport in proteins. Proc Natl Acad Sci. 1981; 78(1):261–5.

65. McMakin CR, Oschman JL. Visceral and somatic disorders: tissue softening with frequency-specific microcurrent. J Altern Complement Med. 2013;19(2):170–7.

66. Korr IM. Proprioceptors and somatic dysfunction. J Am Osteopath Assoc. 1975;74:638–50.

67. Korr IM. Sustained sympathicotonia as a factor in disease. In: Korr IM,editor. The neurobiologic mechanisms in manipulative therapy. New York: Plenum Press; 1978.

68. Johansson H, Sojka P. Pathophysiological mechanisms involved in genesis and spread of muscular tension in occupational muscle pain and in chronic musculoskeletal pain syndromes: a hypothesis. Med Hypoth. 1991;35:196–203.

69. Knutson GA, Owens EF. Active and passive characteristics of muscle tone and their relationship models of subluxation/joint dysfunction: Part I. J Can Chiropr Assoc. 2003;47:168–79.

70. Knutson GA, Owens EF. Active and passive characteristics of muscle tone and their relationship models of subluxation/joint dysfunction. Part II. J Can Chiopr Assoc. 2003;47:269–83.

71. Gabbiani G. The myofibroblast in wound healing and fibrocontractive diseases. J Pathol. 2003;200:500–3.

72. Desmoulière A, Badid C, Bochaton-Piallat ML et al. Apoptosis during wound healing, fibrocontractive diseases and vascular wall injury. Int J Biochem Cell Biol. 1997;29:19–30.

73. Cho JS, Moon YM, Park IH et al. Epigenetic regulation of myofibroblast differentiation and extracellular matrix production in nasal polyp-derived fibroblasts. Clin Exp Allergy. 2012;42(6):872–882.

74. Hinz B, Phan SH, Thannickal VJ et al. Recent developments in myofibroblast biology: paradigms for connective tissue remodeling. Am J Pathol. 2012;180(4):1340–1355.

75. Finando S, Finando D. Fascia and the mechanism of acupuncture. J Bodyw Mov Ther. 2011;15:168–76.

76. Wolff J. The law of bone remodeling. Translation of the 1892 German edition. Berlin: Springer; 1986.

77. Rolf IP. Rolfing. Reestablishing the natural alignment and structural integration of human body for vitality and well-being. Rochester, VT: Healing Arts Press; 1989. p. 129.

78. Simons DG, Travell JG. Travell & Simons' myofascial pain and dysfunction: the trigger point manual. 2nd ed. Baltimore, MD: Williams and Wilkins; 1999. pp. 8–9.

79. Selye H. The stress of life. New York: McGraw-Hill; 1956. Plate 3 or revised edition 1984 p. 219.

80. Oschman JL. Energy medicine: the scientific basis. New York: Churchill Livingstone; 2000. pp. 1–40.

81. Lee RP. Interface: mechanisms of spirit in osteopathy. Portland, OR: Stillness Press; 2005. pp. 175–253.

82. Oschman JL. Energy medicine in therapeutics and human performance. New York: Butterworth/Heinemann; 2003. pp. 1–27.

83. Burr HS. Blueprint for immortality: the electric patterns of life. UK: Neville Spearman Publishers; 1972. pp. 1–192.

84. National Center for Complementary and Alternative Medicine (NCCAM). What is complementary and alternative medicine? National Center for Complementary and Alternative Medicine; 2012. http://nccamnihgov/health/whatiscam.

85. Clyde H. Medical history of Wapello County. Photocopy of writings on Paul Caster's treatment and mentoring of A.T. Still in magnetic healing. Kirksville, MO: Osteopathic Archives at Kirksville College of Osteopathic Medicine; 1898.

86. Coues E. Biogen: a speculation of origin and nature of life. Boston, MA: Estes and Lauriat; 1884.

87. Still AT. The philosophy and mechanical principles of osteopathy. Kansas City, MO; Hudson-Kimberly Publication Co.; 1902. pp. 248–68.

88. Comeaux Z. The soul of osteopathy. USA: Boocklockercom; 2009.

89. Littlejohn JM. The physiologic basis of therapeutic law. J Am Osteopath Assoc. 1902;2:42–60.

90. Hulett GD. A textbook of the principles of osteopathy. Kirksville, MO: Journal Printing Co.; 1903. pp. 43–68.

91. Sutherland WG. The cranial bowl. Mankato, MN: WG Sutherland; 1939. pp. 24. (Reprinted by the Osteopathic Cranial Association, Meridian, ID, 1948).

92. Magoun HI. Osteopathy in the cranial field. 2nd ed. Kirksville, MO: Journal Publishing Co; 1966. pp. 23–42.

93. Comeaux Z. The role of vibration or oscillation in the development of osteopathic thought. AAO Journal. 2000;10(3):19–24.

94. Becker RE. Diagnostic touch: its principles and applications. Part I: To feel living function. In: Brooks RE, editor. Life in motion. Portland, OR: Rudra Press; 1997. pp. 153–65.

95. Becker RE. Diagnostic touch: its principles and applications. Part II: What a diagnostic touch can do. In: Brooks RE, editor. Life in motion. Portland, OR: Rudra Press; 1997. pp. 166–79.

96. Becker RE. Diagnostic touch: its principles and applications. Part III: Putting a diagnostic touch to work. In: Brooks RE, editor. Life in motion. Portland, OR: Rudra Press; 1997. pp. 180–202.

97. Becker RE. Diagnostic touch: its principles and applications. Part IV: Trauma and stress. In: Brooks RE, editor. Life in motion. Portland, OR: Rudra Press; 1997. pp. 203–16.

98. Becker RE. In: Brooks RE, editor. Life in motion: the osteopathic vision of Rollin E. Becker DO.

Portland, OR: Rudra Press; 1997.
pp. 181–2.

99. Brooks RE. Editor's note. In: Brooks RE, editor.
Life in motion. Portland, OR: Rudra Press; 1997.
p. 153.

100. Davidson SM. Neurofascial release: a course in
guided palpation and treatment. Phoenix, AZ:
Practical Publications; 1990. pp. 1–20.

101. MacDonald RC. "The energy cyst": its
ramifications and use in osteopathic
manipulative management. AAO Journal.
2003;13(3):16–8.

102. Upledger JE. 1987 Craniosacral therapy. II:
Beyond the dura. Seattle, WA: Eastland Press.
pp. 212–4.

103. Holland EC. Viscoelastic and viscoplastic axes
of motion in the cranium: the biophysics of
cranial osteopathy; 1992 [Video].

104. Holland EC. The biophysics of Fulford
techniques. Sebastopol, CA; 2012.

105. O'Connell JA. Bioelectric fascial activation and
release. Indianapolis, IN: American Academy
of Osteopathy; 2000. pp. 22–25, 59–78.

106. O'Connell JA. Myofascial release approach.
In: Chila A, editor. Foundations of osteopathic
medicine. 3rd ed. Philadelphia, PA:
Lippincott Williams and Wilkins; 2011.
pp. 699–700.

107. Comeaux ZJ. Facilitated oscillatory release – a
method of dynamic assessment and treatment
of somatic dysfunction. AAO J. 2003;13(3):30–5.

108. McConnell CP. [1939] Fundamental fragments.
Relatedness. In: Jordan T, Schuster R, editors.
Selected writings of Carl Phillip McConnell
DO. Columbus, OH: Squirrel's Tail Press; 1994.
pp. 129–30.

109. Brizhik LS, Del Giudice E, Popp FA et al.
On the dynamics of self-organization in
living organisms. Electromagn Biol Med.
2009;28(1):28–40.

110. Collebrusco L, Lombardini R. Osteopathic
manipulative treatment and nutrition: an
alternative approach to the irritable bowel
syndrome. Health. 2013;5(6A2):87–93.

111. Tozzi P. A unifying neurofasciagenic model of
somatic dysfunction. Underlying mechanisms
and treatment. Part I. J Bodyw Mov Ther.
2015;19(2):310–26.

112. Gamber RG, Shores JH, Russo DP et al.
Osteopathic manipulative treatment in
conjunction with medication relieves pain
associated with fibromyalgia syndrome:
results of a randomized clinical pilot
project. J Am Osteopath Assoc.
2002;102(6):321–5.

113. Johnson AW, Shubrook JH Jr. Role of
osteopathic structural diagnosis and
osteopathic manipulative treatment for
diabetes mellitus and its complications.
J Am Osteopath Assoc. 2013;113(11):
829–36.

114. Hundscheid HW, Pepels MJ, Engels LG et
al. Treatment of irritable bowel syndrome
with osteopathy: results of a randomized
controlled pilot study. J Gastroenterol Hepatol.
2007;22(9):1394–8.

115. da Silva RC, de Sá CC, Pascual-Vaca ÁO et
al. Increase of lower esophageal sphincter
pressure after osteopathic intervention
on the diaphragm in patients with
gastroesophageal reflux. Dis Esophagus.
2013;26(5):451–6.

116. Cohen-Lewe A. Osteopathic manipulative
treatment for colonic inertia. J Am Osteopath
Assoc. 2013;113(3):216–20.

117. Heineman K. Osteopathic manipulative treatment in the management of biliary dyskinesia. J Am Osteopath Assoc. 2014;114(2):129–33.

118. Cerritelli F, Carinci F, Pizzolorusso G. Osteopathic manipulation as a complementary treatment for the prevention of cardiac complications: 12-months follow-up of intima media and blood pressure on a cohort affected by hypertension. J Bodyw Mov Ther. 2011;15(1):68–74.

119. Daraï C, Deboute O, Zacharopoulou C et al. Impact of osteopathic manipulative therapy on quality of life of patients with deep infiltrating endometriosis with colorectal involvement: results of a pilot study. Eur J Obstet Gynecol Reprod Biol. 2015;188:70–3.

120. Goodman CC, Snyder TK. Diagnosi differenziale in fisioterapia. 3rd ed. Turin: Utet Scienze Mediche; 2005. pp. 20–2.

121. Goodman CC, Snyder TK. Differential diagnosis for physical therapists. Screening for referral. 4th ed. Philadelphia, PA: Elsevier Mosby Saunders; 2007. pp. 393–5.

122. APTA. Today's physical therapist: a comprehensive review of a 21st-century health care profession. American Physical Therapy Association; 2011.

123. Schiowitz S, Dowling DJ. Structural examination and documentation In: Di Giovanna EL, Schiowitz S, Dowling DJ, editors. An osteopathic approach to diagnosis and treatment. 3rd ed. Philadelphia, PA: Lippincott Williams and Wilkins; 2005. pp. 53–63.

124. Myers TW. Anatomy trains: myofascial meridians for manual and movement therapists. 3rd ed. Edinburgh: Churchill Livingstone Elsevier; 2014. p. 28.

125. Schleip R, Müller DG. Training principles for fascial connective tissues: scientific foundation and suggested practical applications. J Bodyw Mov Ther. 2013;17(1):103–15.

126. Myers TW. The 'anatomy trains'. J Bodyw Mov Ther. 1997;1:91–101.

127. Owens C. An endocrine interpretation of Chapman's reflexes. Carmel, CA: Academy of Applied Osteopathy; 1937, reprinted 1963.

128. Hebgen E. Visceral manipulation in osteopathy. Kandern: Georg Thieme Verlag; 2010. p. 3.

129. Hebgen E. Visceral manipulation in osteopathy. Kandern: Georg Thieme Verlag; 2010. p. 15.

130. Hebgen E. Visceral manipulation in osteopathy. Kandern: Georg Thieme Verlag; 2010. p. 18.

131. Hebgen E. Visceral manipulation in osteopathy. Kandern: Georg Thieme Verlag; 2010. p. 28.

132. Willard FH, Fossum C, Standley PR. The fascial system of the body. In: Chila A, editor. Foundations of osteopathic medicine. 3rd ed. Philadelphia, PA: Lippincott Williams and Wilkins; 2011. ch. 7.

133. Littlejohn JM. The fundamentals of osteopathic technique. Maidstone, UK: Institute of Classical Osteopathy; n.d.

134. Wernham J. The 1956 Yearbook. Maidstone, UK: Institute of Classical Osteopathy; 1956.

135. Parsons J, Marcer N. Osteopathy: models for diagnosis, treatment and practice. Edinburgh: Elsevier Churchill Livingstone; 2006. pp. 181–8.

136. Lederman E. Harmonic technique. Edinburgh: Churchill Livingstone; 1990.

137. Tozzi P. Selected fascial aspects of osteopathic practice. J Bodyw Mov Ther. 2012;16(4):503–19.

138. Dugailly PM, Fassin S, Maroye L et al. Effect of a general osteopathic treatment on body satisfaction, global self perception and anxiety: a randomized trial in asymptomatic female students. Int J Osteopath Med. 2014;17(2):94–101.

139. Bove GM, Chapelle SL. Visceral mobilization can lyse and prevent peritoneal adhesions in a rat model. J Bodyw Mov Ther. 2012;16(1):76–82.

140. Tozzi P, Bongiorno D, Vitturini C. Low back pain and kidney mobility: local osteopathic fascial manipulation decreases pain perception and improves renal mobility. J Bodyw Mov Ther. 2012;16(3):381–91.

141. Hendryx JT, O'Brien RL. Dynamic strain-vector release: an energetic approach to OMT. AAO J. 2003;10(3):19–29.

142. Chaitow L. Is a postural-structural-biomechanical model within manual therapies viable?: a JBMT debate. J Bodyw Mov Ther. 2011;15(2):130–52.

143. Malys MK, Campbell L, Malys N. Symbiotic and antibiotic interactions between gut commensal microbiota and host immune system. Medicina (Kaunas). 2015;51(2): 69–75.

144. Bach JF. The effect of infections on susceptibility to autoimmune and allergic diseases. N Engl J Med. 2002;347:911–20.

145. Devereux G. The increase in the prevalence of asthma and allergy: food for thought. Nat Rev Immunol. 2006;6:869–74.

146. Willett WC. Balancing life-style and genomics research for disease prevention. Science. 2002;296:695–8.

147. Tracy SW. Something new under the sun? The Mediterranean diet and cardiovascular health. N Eng J Med. 2013;368:1274–76.

148. Estruch R, Ros E, Salas-Salvadó J et al. Primary prevention of cardiovascular disease with a Mediterranean diet. N Engl J Med. 2013;368:1279–90.

149. Slavin J. Why whole grains are protective: biological mechanisms. Proc Nutr Soc. 2003;62:129–34.

150. Maslowski KM, Mackay CR. Diet gut microbiota and immune responses. Nat Immunol. 2011;12:5–9.

151. Pellegrini N, Serafini M, Colombi B et al. Total antioxidant capacity of plant foods beverages and oils consumed in Italy assessed by three different in vitro assays. J Nutr. 2003;133:2812–9.

152. Walker C, Reamy BV. Diets for cardiovascular disease prevention: what is the evidence? Am Fam Physician. 2009;79(7):571–8.

153. D'Alessandro A, De Pergola G. Mediterranean diet pyramid: a proposal for Italian people. Nutrients. 2014;6(10):4302–16.

154. Venti CA, Johnston CS. Modified food guide pyramid for lactovegetarians and vegans. J Nutr. 2002;132(5):1050–4.

155. Ruini LF, Ciati R, Pratesi CA et al. Working toward healthy and sustainable diets: the "double pyramid model" developed by the Barilla Center for Food and Nutrition to raise awareness about the environmental and nutritional impact of foods. Front Nutr. 2015;2:9.

156. Goodwin H, Haycraft E, Meyer C. The relationship between compulsive exercise and emotion regulation in adolescents. Br J Health Psychol. 2012;17(4):699–710.

157. Holland LA, Brown TA, Keel PK. Defining features of unhealthy exercise associated with disordered eating and eating disorder diagnoses. Psychol Sport Exerc. 2015;15(1):10.

158. Cook B, Hausenblas H, Crosby RD et al. Exercise dependence as a mediator of the exercise and eating disorders relationship: a pilot study. Eat Behav. 2015;16:9–12.

159. Renström P, Johnson RJ. Overuse injuries in sports: a review. Sports Med. 1985;2(5): 316–33.

160. Counsel P, Breidahl W. Muscle injuries of the lower leg. Semin Musculoskelet Radiol. 2010;14(2):162–75.

161. De Stefano L. Greenman's principles of manual medicine. 4th ed. Baltimore, MD: Williams and Wilkins; 2011. pp. 479–510.

162. Brazzo M. Ginnastica interna. Ed Red Novara; 2011.

163. Fulford RC, Stone G. Dr Fulford's touch of life: the healing power of the natural life force. New York: Pocket Books; 1997.

164. Decoster LC, Cleland J, Altieri C et al. The effects of hamstring stretching on range of motion: a systematic literature review. J Orthop Sports Phys Ther. 2005;35(6):377–87.

165. Stecco C, Porzionato A, Lancerotto L et al. Histological study of the deep fasciae of the limbs. J Bodyw Mov Ther. 2008;12(3):225–30.

166. Payne P, Crane-Godreau MA. Meditative movement for depression and anxiety. Front Psychiatry. 2013;24;4:71.

167. Vismara L, Romei M, Galli M et al. Clinical implications of gait analysis in the rehabilitation of adult patients with "Prader-Willi" syndrome: a cross-sectional comparative study ("Prader-Willi" syndrome vs matched obese patients and healthy subjects). J Neuroeng Rehabil. 2007;10;4:14.

168. Vismara L, Menegoni F, Zaina F et al. Effect of obesity and low back pain on spinal mobility: a cross sectional study in women. J Neuroeng Rehabil. 2010;18;7:3.

169. Vismara L, Cimolin V, Menegoni F et al. Osteopathic manipulative treatment in obese patients with chronic low back pain: a pilot study. Man Ther. 2012;17(5):451–5.

170. Zhao RH, Baig MK, Mack J et al. Altered serotonin immunoreactivities in the left colon of patients with colonic inertia. Colorectal Dis. 2002;4(1):56–60.

171. Baig MK, Zhao RH, Woodhouse SL et al. Variability in serotonin and enterochromaffin cells in patients with colonic inertia and idiopathic diarrhoea as compared to normal controls. Colorectal Dis. 2002;4(5): 348–54.

172. Smilowicz A. An osteopathic approach to gastrointestinal disease: somatic clues for diagnosis and clinical challenges associated with *Helicobacter pylori* antibiotic resistance. J Am Osteopath Assoc. 2013;113(5):404–16.

173. Wiegand S, Bianchi W, Quinn TA et al. Osteopathic manipulative treatment for self-reported fatigue, stress and depression in first-year osteopathic medical students. J Am Osteopath Assoc. 2015;115(2):84–93.

174. Heath DM, Makin IR, Pedapati C et al. Use of real-time physiologic parameter assessment to augment osteopathic manipulative treatment training for first-year osteopathic

medical students. J Am Osteopath Assoc. 2014;114(12):918–29.

175. Perrin RN, Edwards J, Hartley P. An evaluation of the effectiveness of osteopathic treatment on symptoms associated with myalgic encephalomyelitis. A preliminary report. J Med Eng Technol. 1998;22(1):1–13.

176. Perrin RN, Richards JD, Pentreath V et al. Muscle fatigue in chronic fatigue syndrome/ myalgic encephalomyelitis (CFS/ME) and its response to a manual therapeutic approach: a pilot study. Int J Osteopath Med. 2011;14(3):P96–105.

177. Wallace E, McPartland JM, Jones JM III et al. Lymphatic system: lymphatic manipulative techniques. In: Ward RC, editor. Foundations for osteopathic medicine. Baltimore, MD: Williams and Wilkins; 1997.

178. Mueller DM. The 2012–2013 influenza epidemic and the role of osteopathic manipulative medicine. J Am Osteopath Assoc. 2013;113(9):703–7.

179. Schander A, Downey HF, Hodge LM. Lymphatic pump manipulation mobilizes inflammatory mediators into lymphatic circulation. Exp Biol Med (Maywood). 2012;237(1):58–63.

180. Morhenn V, Beavin LE, Zak PJ. Massage increases oxytocin and reduces adrenocorticotropin hormone in humans. Altern Ther Health Med. 2012; 18(6):11–18.

181. Rapaport MH, Schettler P, Bresee C. A preliminary study of the effects of repeated massage on hypothalamic-pituitary-adrenal and immune function in healthy individuals: a study of mechanisms of action and dosage. J Altern Complement Med. 2012;18(8): 789–797.

182. Salamon E, Zhu W, Stefano GB. Nitric oxide as a possible mechanism for understanding the therapeutic effects of osteopathic manipulative medicine (Review). Int J Mol. Med. 2004;14(3):443–449.

183. Bokhari AR, Murrell GA. The role of nitric oxide in tendon healing. J Shoulder Elb Surg. 2012;21(2):238–244.

184. Ziche M, Morbidelli L. Nitric oxide and angiogenesis. Neurooncol. 2000;50(1–2): 139–148.

185. Garthwaite J. Concepts of neural nitric oxide-mediated 104 transmission. Eur J Neurosci. 2008;27(11):2783–2802.

186. Wink DA, Hines HB, Cheng RY et al. Nitric oxide and 105 redox mechanisms in the immune response. J Leukoc Biol. 2011;89/106(6):873–891.

187. Tozzi P. A unifying neuro-fasciagenic model of somatic dysfunction. Underlying mechanisms and treatment. Part II. Bodyw Mov Ther. 2015 (in press).

188. Arnsdorf EJ, Tummala P, Castillo AB et al. The epigenetic mechanism of mechanically induced osteogenic differentiation. J Biomech. 2010;43(15):2881–2886.

189. Bavan L, Midwood K, Nanchahal J. MicroRNA epigenetics: a new avenue for wound healing research. Bio-Drugs. 2011;25(1):27–41.

190. Kutty JK, Webb K. Vibration stimulates vocal mucosa-like matrix expression by hydrogel-encapsulated fibroblasts. J Tissue Eng Regen Med. 2010;4(1):62–72.

191. Craig AD. How do you feel? Interoception: the sense of the physiological condition of the body. Nat Rev Neurosci. 2002;3(8): 111, 655, 666.

192. Björnsdotter M, Morrison I, Olausson H. Feeling good: on the role of C fibre mediated touch in interoception. Exp Brain Res. 2010;207(3-4):149-55.

193. McGlone F, Wessberg J, Olausson H. Discriminative and affective touch: sensing and feeling. Neuron. 2014;82(4):737-55.

194. Olausson H, Wessberg J, Morrison I et al. The neurophysiology of unmyelinated tactile afferents. Neurosci Biobehav Rev. 2010;34(2):185-91.

195. Efrati C, Nicolini G, Cannaviello C et al. *Helicobacter pylori* eradication: sequential therapy and *Lactobacillus reuteri*

supplementation. World J Gastroenterol. 2012;18(43):6250-4.

196. Gevitz N. A degree of difference: the origins of osteopathy and first use of the "DO" designation. J Am Osteopath Assoc. 2014;114(1):30-40.

197. Del Giudice E, Tedeschi A. Water and the autocatalysis in living matter. Electromagnetic Biology and Medicine. 2009;28:46.

198. Montagnier L, Aïssa J, Ferris S et al. Electromagnetic signals are produced by aqueous nanostructures derived from bacterial DNA sequences. Interdiscip Sci Comput Life Sci. 2009;1:81-90.

# The behavioral-biopsychosocial model

*Paolo Tozzi*

## Synopsis

The behavioral-biopsychosocial model allows for treatment of the patient's entire physical, psychological, behavioral, and social spectrum, through a therapeutic relationship of inter-collaboration between patient and osteopath, and toward choosing a healthier lifestyle. It can be applied both as a model in its own right, complete and effective in the various therapeutic instruments at its disposal, and as a "model among the osteopathic models," by applying principles, focusing on the communicative aspect and the overall approach to the person and the context in which he or she lives. The flexibility and complexity of this approach, which guarantees its effectiveness for many conditions through various application methods, also requires as much operator effort, requiring the performance of a careful evaluation of the patient and of his or her pain, stress and related disabilities, perception and experience of his or her own condition, the behavioral response to it, family and social support, and the working environment and environmental influences, adapting the treatment accordingly.

The body responds to these stimuli from the physiological, psychological and behavioral point of view, determining the impact on itself and on its network of relationships. Such responsiveness may be deleterious, if poorly managed, or become a stimulus to the development of personal resources in dealing with the pain, stress and difficulties of life. The biopsychosocial model is aimed at leading the individual to discover in oneself the strength and the strategies needed to manage or compensate, in order to solve any destabilizing factors. Several tools are used for this purpose, such as communicative empathy, cognitive-behavioral approach, biofeedback, meditation techniques, group therapy and inter-disciplinary interventions. The patient is taught to prevent disease and promote health, and made aware of self-regulating mechanisms in order to be the protagonist of his or her own healing process, until he or she achieves optimal control of the state of wellness with himself or herself and with the social and environmental contexts in which the patient exists. In a certain sense, this is perhaps the osteopathic model that best reflects the principle of the unity of body, mind and spirit, and of the whole person, in every aspect of life.

## Introduction

It is a clear and intrinsic concept in osteopathic medicine since its founding that the complexity of the human being does not end in the physical, but expands into a dynamic triadic relationship between body, mind, and spirit.[1] Any form of dual-ism or separation of this functional unit can only be an artfact. Thus, the osteopathic concept of disease, such as anatomical alteration followed by physiological changes,[2] is also built on the principle that hereditary, psychological, and behavioral factors (such as nutrition and physical activity), and social and environmental factors exert substantial influence on the pathological process.[3,4] Littlejohn[5] recognized how many physical symptoms have underlying psychological factors (indices of a mental condition without whose resolution it would be impossible to heal the body). By the same token, Still did not forget the impact of the related responses to stress, or the importance of mental illness.[6]

In turn, osteopathic treatment was proposed to correct any form of structural, functional and environmental influence that could afflict the human body.[7] This includes emotional support and strategic advice to address and manage the condition of the patient,[6] i.e., the education of the latter toward a healthy lifestyle, enhanced by a healthy diet and appropriate physical activity, as well as abstinence from toxic substances of any type. At the Still-Hildreth Sanatorium, the first osteopathic sanatorium, active from 1914 to 1968 in Missouri, the majority of patients suffered from psychiatric disorders, and received treatments focused on the totality of each case, through specific physical activity programs (baseball, football, ice skating, tennis, swimming), recreation (music, reading, dancing, fishing, cooking, sewing), relaxation (gardening, walks, exhibitions, etc.), as well as nutritional treatments, hydrotherapy and pharmacological and osteopathic treatments.[8]

The holistic approach to the patient often expanded to the care of family members, who were often affected by physical and emotional stress because of the need for constant assistance to the needy relative; this aspect has been confirmed by recent studies in which families responsible for Alzheimer's patients care showed signs of chronic stress, impaired immune function, and delay in tissue repair.[9] Korr stressed[10] how the osteopath, in the care of the whole person, must look beyond the symptom and the identification of the disease, beyond the treatment of the single compromised organ, beyond the dysfunction, and rather explore the factors in the patient's life that might have helped develop the disease and that, if identified, modified, compensated, or deleted, could

stimulate the recovery, prevent re-occurrence of the disease and improve overall health. These factors include biological (genetic, nutritional), psychological, behavioral, sociocultural, occupational, and environmental conditions, including beliefs, ideals, prejudices, and expectations, all of which need to be approached via a collaborative relationship between patient and osteopath, and in some cases, with the concerted action of social community, national institutions or international organizations.[10]

The collaborative relationship between patient and osteopath is a partnership founded on the education process to maintain and enhance the patient's management of his or her own health, as the best form of prevention, including referral (theoretically) to the therapist as an ideal lifestyle model.[10]

In osteopathy these concepts are now articulated in a broad conceptual and application environment defined as the "behavioral-biopsychosocial" model, which considers the individual throughout all his or her physical, mental, emotional, and spiritual spectrum, including lifestyle (diet, exercise, substance abuse, etc.), but, in particular, the psychosocial context in which the patient exists, with all possible interactions with the family, work, and social environment, in order to identify any hereditary, sex, food, cultural, religious, psychological, environmental, socioeconomic, and geographic factors that might influence the person's state of health, compromise their adaptability capacities, facilitate pathological processes[11] and thus influence their perception and experience of pain, illness, or disability.[12,13] This model also fits with the concept of "total osteopathic lesion,"[14] defined as the summation of all the mechanical, physiological, and psychological stressors that interact in the life of an individual, determining a state of general "facilitation."

Consequently, every somatic dysfunction affects the musculoskeletal reaction to biopsychosocial stressors,[11] which in turn are able, also via subliminal stimuli of any origin and nature, to generate and maintain pain and other symptoms, emotional reactions, and maladaptive behaviors, which requires a multidimensional therapeutic intervention. During the evaluation, the behavioral model is also applied to "read" emotions and feelings expressed through the musculoskeletal system, or stressors that may be due to increased neuromuscular tension. Fulford,[15] for example, described how emotional shocks can appear in the diaphragm and the solar plexus, and even more commonly in the masseter, the upper trapezius, and pelvic floor, and potentially in any muscle tissue, depending on the type of the causative trauma and the specific individual reaction.

One can use several constitutional and biotypological models to evaluate the patient and the underlying pathophysiological mechanisms, as well as to select and administer the best therapeutic intervention for each case[16] to improve the operational, compensatory, or adaptive response of the person to the stressors mentioned above. This includes the conscious and appropriate use of the relationship (verbal and nonverbal) between therapist and patient, i.e., the process of empowerment of the latter in his or her own healing process.[17] This behavioral-biopsychosocial model is now one of the basic foundations of medical care,[18] as well as one of the characteristic and distinctive features of osteopathy, for the way in which it is applied to the uniqueness of the person, as well as its individual and contextual globality, with an attitude of listening and empathy[19] that transcends the exclusive focus on the symptom or pain. It is also true that understanding the impact that the pain or illness has on the person is required to understand their multidimensional effects on the individual.[20]

For example, in the presence of a painful condition, the fear of pain or of its potential recurrence seems to influence more than the pain itself,[21] being related to perceived disability levels[22] and facilitating the circumvention of physical and/or working daily activities, with risk of chronicity.[23] Conversely, various emotional influences, including memories of past experiences[24] as well as various psychological factors[25] or psychological conditions such as depression,[26] can cause physical changes and produce pain, or alter the perception of pain stimuli and the experience of pain itself, resulting in the development of chronic illness and disability. It is enough to say that even the nature of an individual's personality seems to affect the perception of pain and disability,[27] along with his belief, faith, and religion,[28] or job dissatisfaction.[29] As such, therefore, all these factors should be incorporated into the biopsychosocial model, throughout the patient's clinical and management process,[30] especially if suffering from chronic disease[31] in which the perception of persistent pain is part of a multidimensional context (genetic, chemical, biomechanical, neurophysiological, psychological, social, etc.) in which each component can play a significant role in the patient's dysfunction.[32]

Thus, there is a need to use a multidisciplinary approach,[33] above all from the active and shared participation of the patient in his or her own healing process,[34] through the proper use of information regarding posture, ergonomics, sports, employment, nutrition, education, and so on. In other words, the approach to the individual's health requires a multidimensional intervention, which should not be limited to the resolution of the stressors or somatic dysfunction, but should be extended to have a wider scope. If we intend to engage not the pain but the person, in all his or her physical, mental, spiritual, and social spectrum, it is necessary to expand the horizon to include: biopsychosocial models,[24] considered congruent even with osteopathic principles;[35] interdisciplinary paradigms,[36] recognized as consistent with osteopathic philosophy;[37] salutogenic processes,[38] which extend from treatment to health care, from protection to prevention, from education to health promotion, to improve the perception of health and quality of life;[39] coping strategies (coping),[40] self-efficacy,[41] and empowerment mechanisms.[42]

Patient information and education are essential to this process in which the therapist acts as a catalyst for change,[43] to guide the patient's expectations, beliefs, and opinions about their own condition, i.e., to encourage personal control of his or her resources and thus solve the problem[44] by acting indirectly in a positive way also on the patient's family, social and environmental context.[45] In fact, education about healthy lifestyle choices and the processes of health and disease is crucial to correct any unhealthy behaviors, strengthening the management of health and optimizing the overall response capacity, thus acting as a key element for prevention.[10]

## Historical background

In 1977, George Engel[46] proposed to the medical and scientific world a new model of care, based on the concept that disease cannot exist without a physical, psychological, and social component, in an intimate and complex dynamic interaction of high impact on the onset, course, and resolution of the disease itself. The individual's experience of his own pathological condition exercises a decisive influence on the outcome of the healing process, along with factors such as personality type, lifestyle, and social support.[47]

This was the birth of the biopsychosocial model, which offered to medicine a new way of thinking and approaching the patient, by interpreting the patient's relationship with the disease, the interaction among pathological processes in the body, the psychological component and the patient's social context.[48] The very perception of pain is a complex process influenced by different psychosocial factors that can affect the interpretation of any nociceptive stimulation.[49] Specifically, cultural or ethnic groups that gravitate toward a particular interpretation of pain may reflect individual differences in pain tolerance, from a stoic to a more emotional and expressive attitude. In addition, the quality and intensity of pain are determined by other factors such as previous experience of the individual, his or her level of anxiety, and attention to the symptom. Basically, from a biomedical model that interpreted the disease as being an infectious, traumatic or hereditary process,[50] and pain as synonymous with tissue damage, we now propose a multidimensional model of pain, made up of sensory, affective, and cognitive elements[51] (the gate control theory of Melzack and Wall).

We propose that this model involves interactions in a neural pain matrix,[52] formed by somatosensory, limbic, thalamic, and cortical units, thus determining the unique and individual experience of pain, which is then influenced by social, environmental,[53] psychological, and biological factors.[54] For example, the Whitehall studies showed significant correlations between increasing mortality/illness rates and lower socioeconomic and psychosocial outcomes, depending on the social and occupational class, and the economic and cultural life to which the tested samples belonged.[55,56] Today, sociodemographic factors such as age, gender, cultural background, and ethnic and economic aspects are recognized as factors that impact chronic disability.[57] Engel's proposed model, based on concepts and evidence from previous decades, revealed the influence of stress and emotional disturbances on the physiological processes of the body. In fact, the idea that the suppression and the unconscious repression of painful or emotionally disturbing memories might spill into the soma, through a "conversion" process, was already present at the dawn of psychoanalysis.[58]

Similarly, Wilhelm Reich associated traumatic psychological events or suppressed emotions/impulses to body response patterns, such as muscle tension, intended to repress movements or emotions.[59] If repeated or persistent, such tensions can lead to muscle stiffness and chronic unconscious patterning – defined as "armor" – with effects on the personality and its development, as well as on the free movement of fluids and physical energy. Reich proposed to address this dysfunctional process through manual intervention on the physical, while also incorporating psychoanalysis to improve the structural and emotional harmony of the individual. The autonomic nervous system was considered to be the interface between physical and emotional processes conveying cognitive and affective information processed by the central nervous system through the bloodstream to the internal organs.[60] Later, Philip Latey proposed muscles as sensory organs in the true sense of the term, able to change physical trauma into emotional reaction.[61]

This opened the door to psychosomatic medicine, i.e., the study of disorders of physiological processes based on alleged emotional origin.[62]

In 1970, the physiatrist John Sarno noticed, in patients with chronic low back pain and neck pain, the absence of correlation between pain intensity/ neurological symptoms reported and the severity of radiological findings, as well as between them and the course of the disease.[63] This was later confirmed by subsequent magnetic resonance imaging (MRI) studies, which revealed both the absence of correlation between development or persistence of low back pain and imaging findings,[64,65] and the presence of disc disease in 64% of patients without low back pain.[66] Sarno therefore advanced the hypothesis that stressful situations, as well as the patient's response to them, including the emotional component, could be the cause of physical symptoms reported in the absence of instrumental artifacts. Hence, the development of a psychoeducational approach, which aimed to identify and address the underlying psychological issues related to physical symptoms, and with which he successfully oversaw many chronic musculoskeletal disorders, frequently associated with mental disorders such as anxiety and depression. The therapeutic approach proposed was not based so much on the traditional form of psychological treatment as on a path of recognition – specifically, psychoeducative – that real physical symptoms come from mental processes, rather than as a pathological event in the body.[67]

The clinical emphasis was gradually slipping from an operator-centric approach to a biopsychosocial one, oriented to the control of the internal and external environments, and based on the patient's full involvement and participation in his or her own healing process.

In 1932, the physiologist Walter Cannon coined the term "homeostasis" to indicate the adjustment process and balance of body systems.[68] He also introduced the concept of alarm reaction,[69] meaning that the body, in situations perceived as threatening, triggers a fight-or-flight mechanism mediated by the sympathetic nervous system. On the other hand, a phase of "rest and digest" takes place, mediated by the parasympathetic system, to permit the recovery of energy resources in the absence of danger conditions.[70] In 1936, however, the physiologist Hans Selye[71] coined the term "stress," indicating the body's nonspecific response to each request made toward it, or an adaptive response to internal or external stimuli (in this case defined as "eustress"). However, stress can become pathological, regardless of its nature or origin, when environmental demands, including biochemical, physical, or psychological factors, exceed the individual's adaptive capabilities, which respond by developing a "general adaptation syndrome."[71] This syndrome consists of three distinct stages: alarm reaction, resistance, and exhaustion, of which at least the first two are reversible. Selye had observed the effects in laboratory rats subjected to stress, as a result of which they developed signs of immune dysfunction (involution of the thymus) and autonomic hyperactivity (peptic ulcer and hypertrophy of the adrenals).[72]

The three stages correspond to physiological, pathophysiological, and pathological responses (mediated by the interaction of the nervous and endocrine system) to short-term, long-term and unsustainable stress respectively (Fig. 8.1), including physical and emotional stimuli. Subsequently, Sterling and Eyer[73] advanced the concept of "allostasis," the process through which the body, facing a stress factor, can maintain homeostasis due to a response to physiological change. When the stress subsides, the body may return to a state of original balance or remain anchored in a state of hyper- or hypoactivity. Each allostatic cycle is a protective response of short duration to the stress to which the individual is exposed. However, if stress is persistent, it can cause long-term changes, with consequent deleterious effects on the entire body. This phenomenon, defined as "allostatic load," mainly consists of an imbalance of the systems that promote adaptation. It can be caused by the combined effect of multiple stress factors, but also by insufficient capacity of adaptation of the organism, or even more from its prolonged or inadequate

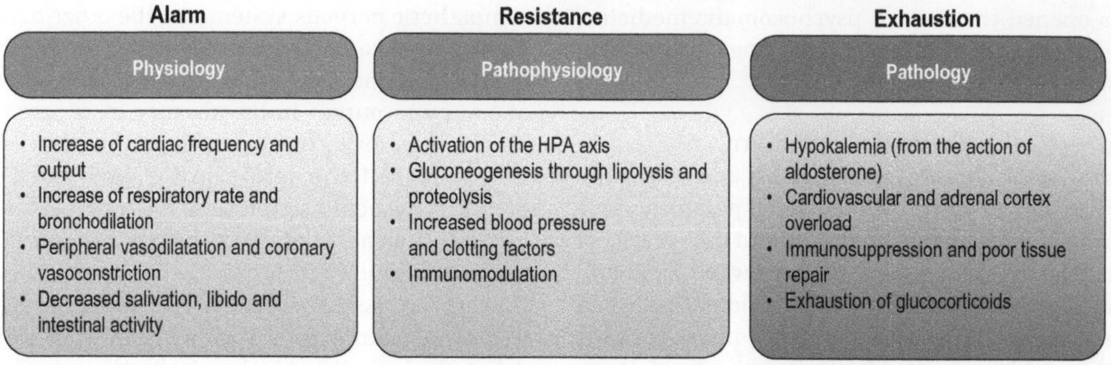

**Fig. 8.1**

The three stages of reaction to stress (alarm, resistance, exhaustion), with the corresponding organism responses (physiological, pathophysiological, pathological). Modified from: Selye H. The stress of life. New York, NY: McGraw-Hill; 1976.

response to stress – the first due to a delayed response of suppression, the second followed by compensatory hyperactivity of other physiological mechanisms.[74] In any case, the body is exposed to excessive secretion of hormones, cytokines, neurotransmitters, and other endogenous factors, with potential deleterious effects and pathological outcomes.[75]

In 1964, George Solomon[76] coined the term "psycho-neuro-immunology," indicating how emotional states may alter immune competence to the development of physical illness. The correlation between psychosis and impaired immune function has been demonstrated since the 1940s[77] and then confirmed by Levy's studies,[78] in which immune activity in women with breast cancer not only appeared to be a predictor of the course of the disease, but also a factor influenced by the level of stress of the patients, their emotional level, state of depression or fatigue, and insufficient social support. Therefore, the evaluation of the initial stress level could be a predictive factor of immune efficiency and thus the outcome of the disease itself. It is clear that there is a dynamic interaction and integration between the nervous, endocrine, and immune systems, which were considered as a single network,[79] as they operate as both sensory and effector organs, able to share physiological signals to preserve homeostasis through a "regulatory redundancy."[80] Immune

cells have receptors for hormones, neuropeptides, and neurotransmitters, thus establishing communication with the neuroendocrine system; in turn, cytokines may act directly on the activity of the nervous system via specific receptors on the neuronal walls at both central and peripheral levels.[79]

For example, the presence in the lymphocytes of receptors for ACTH and endorphins, identical to those present in the pituitary gland, proved the ability of the immune system not only to communicate with the brain via immunopeptides, but also to receive information from the brain through neuropeptides.[81] Likewise, the immune cells can produce neurohormones, such as oxytocin and gonadotropin, with impact on neural activity.[82] In addition, the presence of receptors for these peptides in unicellular organisms and plants, like those present in mammals, indicated that this molecular mechanism used for intercellular communication has probably appeared in evolution before the same endocrine, nervous, and immune systems were developed in vertebrates.[83] Nodal points of the distribution of the receptors for these peptides were identified, such as the limbic brain, posterior horn of the spinal cord, periaqueductal gray, gastrointestinal tract, kidneys, testes, and pancreas. This system operates outside of the linear neurotransmission channels, taking advantage of the extracellular matrix as a parallel-parasynaptic diffuser of neurotransmitters, to affect the target cell even at a distance, because of their receptor specificity.[79,84]

Then it became necessary to identify the interaction of molecules such as morphine, benzodiazepine, cholecystokinin, substance P, and insulin. Pert believed that the 70–80 neuropeptides identified were the biochemical substrate of emotion, with substantial impact on immune function,[85] and therefore the emotional state could affect the course and outcome of biological diseases. Therefore, he advanced the concept of a broad and unified network of endogenous peptides psychosomatic communication, not neural tissues and their corresponding receptors in the immune, endocrine, and nervous systems. In other words, the close link between the psyche, endocrinology, immunology, and neuroscience has allowed the development of a single coherent model, able to offer a more organic and unitary vision of health.

## Objectives and indications

The behavioral model has gained more and more consideration among academics and institutional environments[86] and is now recognized as the main scientific model for understanding pain, especially musculoskeletal pain.[87] Osteopathy has been frequently described as a patient-centric profession[88] oriented toward a biopsychosocial approach,[89] and thus different from other health professions,[90] although these concepts have been recently revisited[91] and considered as characteristic of osteopathy, although difficult to evaluate in osteopathic practice and in possible effects on clinical outcomes.[92] In any event, in today's osteopathy, the biopsychosocial model is proposed as a first approach to improve the biological, psychological and social components of the individual's health spectrum.[93] This includes emotional balance and reproductive processes, as well as compensation mechanisms and behavioral adaptation.

Understanding the complex interaction between psychological, physiological, environmental, and behavioral factors that influence health both directly and indirectly (such as illness and associated musculoskeletal, nervous, endocrine, and immune responses), is the basis of this model.[94] The osteopathic approach therefore needs to transcend the biological level of the sensory and neural transmission modes, of sensation and perception of pain, including the interaction of body, mind, spirit, and environment to understand the unique presentation of each patient.[95]

Recently it has been proposed that there is a need to overcome biomedical reductionism, tending to interpret all mental and emotional process as only a biochemical phenomenon, with a biocognitive model that better reflects the philosophy and holistic practice of osteopathic medicine, because it is based on natural interaction and mutual influence between mind and body.[96] In particular, the consideration of psychosocial factors is indicated for the chronic pain management for which various techniques of osteopathic manipulation have been proposed[97] and for which the integration of five osteopathic models becomes crucial to restore the optimal relationship between structure and function.[35] Patients with physical and emotional distress:[9]

- seek medical care and are hospitalized more frequently, bringing mostly physical symptoms and rarely psychological ones at the time of consultation

- have a higher morbidity and decreased response to previous therapeutic interventions

- follow medical treatments with more difficulty or less constancy, and more frequently abandon treatment

- undergo medical evaluations that do not come to a biological diagnosis about two-thirds of the time.

In these cases, osteopathic manipulative treatment employs the biopsychosocial model with specific objectives (Box 8.1), to improve the body's ability to manage, compensate, or adapt effectively to stress factors, as well as to optimize lifestyle and behavioral choices. This process starts with the education of the patient about their constitutional or hereditary predisposition to a given condition, the effects of trauma and past or current illnesses, and behaviors and trends learned that contribute to pain and suffering, along with the appropriate use of traditional and complementary medical care, or any form of care that is supported by adequate scientific evidence,[98] often provided within a transdisciplinary approach.

---

**Box 8.1**

Key elements for the clinical application of the biopsychosocial model

- Recognizing the central importance of the social relations and relationships in health assistance

- Using self-conscience as a diagnostic and therapeutic method

- Eliciting the patient's history in any contextual aspect of his or her life

- Determining which biological, psychological and social factors are dominant for framing and promoting health

- Ensuring a multidimensional treatment.

---

Certainly, osteopathic intervention aims to reduce nociception in an effort to reduce stress and improve function,[99] but the ultimate goal remains the restoration, maintenance, and enhancement of health, and thus the prevention of disease until the achievement of a state of well-being, based on the individual's ability to balance and recover,[98] promoted by the self-regulating and self-healing processes.

## Assessment

The osteopathic assessment for this model includes a comprehensive biopsychosocial case history, physical examination, the osteopathic examination and follow-up visits for the re-evaluation of pain and functional ability or of the overall management plan.[32] This leads to a limitation in terms of biopsychosocial, i.e., a biological integrated detection, psychological and social assistance.[100] This medical-clinical model has been described as patient-centric[101] or relationship-centric,[102] in that the patient is encouraged to express their preferences for diagnostic and therapeutic intervention, after discussing the relative risks and benefits.[103] The information and involvement become essential, founded on the free sharing of knowledge with the patient as an active player, in full control of the clinical decision-making, which also determines the level of involvement in the therapeutic process.[104] Through communication skills, the operator identifies and responds to the ideas and feelings of the patient about his or her own condition and then the operator establishes a basic common ground for the classification of the disease and its treatment, as well as the roles that both the therapist and the patient play.[105]

This process is based on an empathic relationship between operator and patient, which helps the patient to feel understood, and the operator to understand the uniqueness of the clinical condition and the patient.[106] Therefore, a different approach is needed, one that is the opposite to the approach defined as "paternalistic," in which the operator decides what is best for the patient, keeping dialogue and interaction to a minimum.[107] Instead, a patient-centric approach is not just a passive acceptance of the choices or the patient's opinions, but a clever approach, based on respect and empathy for the therapeutic relationship, and on the sharing of power to optimize health.

The sharing of all available information with the patient is not equally applicable in every case; for example, if the patient does not intend to take responsibility for his or her own healing process the patient-centric model should slip to a less patient-centric form.[108] The flexibility and adaptability of the model are its strength. This is the essential foundation for assessment (Box 8.2) and treatment of the whole person – body, mind, and spirit – of his or her allostatic load and responses related to it, via a personal management plan.

## Box 8.2

### Elements of assessment for the biopsychosocial model

- Pain perception and individual experience of pain and disability associated with emotional and affective reactions, mental and cognitive states, impacts on daily, work, and social life

- Range of confronting and adaptation responses to pain and stress, including the individual's willingness to constructively interact with health workers to restore a state of functional equilibrium[109]

- Constitutional factors, as well as acquired conditions such disease, trauma, abuse.

- Behavioral aspects such as nutrition, physical activity, sleep habits

- Family support, social and health systems, environmental impacts.

## Box 8.3

### Possible strategies to promote empathy with the patient during interviews

- Formulate open questions to start the discussion (which are very patient-centered and difficult to influence).

- Allow enough time for an exhaustive explanation of the reason of consultation. Some evidence has shown that on average a doctor stops listening to a patient after about 18 seconds![113]

- Ask the patient to describe the emotions related to his or her condition.[114]

- Recognize and reassure the patient's concerns (noting also elements such as breathing, tone of voice, speed of speach, signs of pain or anxiety, eye contact avoidance).

- Use empathic comments and refrain from judging.

## The interview with the patient

Empathic listening becomes even more critical in the medical history because clinical decision-making is founded upon it. The operator can establish or strengthen the relationship through empathy to create an ideal situation for the collection of not only clinical information, but also information about life, experiences, suffering, and the patient's hopes. This requires an attitude directed to listening and assertiveness, recognized as consistent with the practice and application of evidence-based medicine,[110] which is expressed in a series of specific strategies (Box 8.3). These strategies are particularly useful in the management of patients affected by pain that cannot be clinically diagnosed.[111,112]

Listening and communication skills are essential in this process: eye contact, a sitting position, being composed and attentive during the history are all examples of nonverbal language that integrate with oral communication to cultivate an environment of trust and personal care. This situation will facilitate the presentation of the history and demonstrate understanding and emotional support for the patient.[115] A patient who experiences any form of neglect by the operator is likely to limit the information about himself or herself, and may alter answers to the questions asked, based on what is perceived as acceptable or expected by the operator.[116]

The osteopath should never forget that pain is a complex phenomenon of subjective perception, with intensity, quality, course, impact, and significance that varies from person to person. And it is precisely the suffering (that is, the experience of pain), more than pain itself (defined as pain stimulus), that motivates the patient to seek medical advice in the hope of finding relief.[117] It is good practice therefore to note any possible behavioral signs of pain (Table 8.1): for example, if the patient is agitated, anxious, tense, worried, depressed, or angry; if he or she tends to dramatize his or her pain,[118] or if the experience of it is so ingrained as to refuse any logical or rational argument; if he or she fears pain[119] or movement that can generate pain,[120] thus promoting inactivity. Of course,

**Table 8.1**
Behavioral indications of pain

| | |
|---|---|
| Vocalizations | Tears, sighs, moans |
| Facial expressions | Holding the corners of the mouth in a tense horizontal position, or superiorly and posteriorly; sagging and wrinkling of the eyebrows |
| Motor activity | Slow movements and avoidance of activities for fear of pain |
| Mood | Aggressive, sad, irritable, self-effacing |
| Gestures and postures | Claudicating or antalgic, rigid and protective positions; rubs or supports the painful area; frequent changes of position |
| Behavior | Inactivity and rest to avoid pain; excessive use of drugs and medical care; poor social life |

Modified from: Turk DC. A cognitive-behavioral perspective on treatment of chronic pain patients. In: Turk DC, Gatchel RJ, editors. Psychological approaches to pain management. 2nd ed. New York NY Guilford Press; 2002. pp. 138–58.

the interview includes both current and past medical history, pharmacological, social, and family medical history, to acquire appropriate information for the formulation of a clinical and bio-psycho-social diagnosis.

### The motivational conversation

The motivational interview is a style of collaborative and oriented communication, which pays special attention to the language of change, designed to enhance personal motivation and commitment to a specific goal, through the facilitation of the exploration of the individual's reasons for change, all in an atmosphere of acceptance and support.[121] So, to make the change it is necessary to recognize the motivation oriented both toward it and to maintain the current situation, and respond to them appropriately. To evoke statements oriented to change it is necessary to formulate evocative questions, which may fall into four categories[122] (Box 8.4). The appropriate usage of the motivational interview helps to guide the patient through the stages of change (Box 8.5).

### The assessment of stress and social factors

Individual response to stress depends on a multitude of factors, such as the type of stress, chronic stress,

behavioral and emotional response of the person involved,[123] his or her genetic predispositions, health status, psychological factors, coping strategies, and

---

**Box 8.4**

### The four categories of evocative questions or change-oriented statements

1. *Capacity*: "What do you think you could change?", "If you really decide to ..., how would you do it?", "How confident are you to ...?"

2. *Desire for change*: "How would you want things to change?", "What do you hope to achieve altogether?", "Tell me what you do not like about your current condition", "How would you like your life to change in 1 year?".

3. *Need for the change*: "How important is it for you ...?", "What do you feel you should change?", "Do you see this change as serious/urgent?".

4. *Reasons for change*: "Why do you want to increase physical exercise?", "What is negative in the current situation?", "What would be a positive aspect of stop drinking?", "What would be the advantages of ...?".

## Box 8.5

### Key elements of the motivational interview and the C.A.M.B.I.A.* model

*Check*

- The current stage of change in which the patient is (also in follow-up).

- Openness to change:

  – If not available, make an informed estimate

  – If available:

    – importance (numerical scale 0–10)

    – self-efficacy (numerical scale 0–10).

*Adopt non-confrontational attitudes*

- Repeating, summarizing, stating, using other words and open questions

- Avoid direct confrontation

- Give advice only when requested and/or request permission, do health education, do not discuss your health care role, do not rush.

*Maximize resources (for each risk)*

- Give personalized advice, analyzing the resources that the patient has, his or her life priorities, and protective factors (friends, social networks)

- Build capacity, helping to build individual motivations to change.

*Barriers and needs*

- Identify social, financial, environmental barriers

- Analyze concerns and needs

- Check the pros and cons of a change, as defined by the patient.

*Intervene*

- With the feedback or with advice only if asked, without saying what to do and eventually agreeing on the objectives.

*Affirm and summarize what has been said*

- Finish any interview by setting priorities, a future plan summary and scheduling a follow-up appointment.

* Originally proposed by Miller and Rollnich.121 Amended by: Canciani L, Ostrich PL. Health promotion. In: Gasbarrini G, Cricelli C, Gasbarrini A et al., editors. Internal medicine treaty. Rome: Verducci; 2011. ch. 11.

the interactions among these and other variables. The deleterious effect that a sustained stress or the combined action of various stressors exerts on the individual can be illustrated with the Social Readjustment Rating Scale, developed by Holmes and Rahe.[124] This is a numerical scale correlating potential diseases that a person can develop within 2 years to the amount of stress endured in 1 year, with the severity of the disease that increases in a manner correlated to the amount of accumulated stress. The latter can be caused by events such as the loss of a spouse, divorce, retirement, sexual disorders, a change of residence, and so on. In addition, if the patient experiences the stressor event as a negative experience, the impact is greater.[125] The scale, however, does not consider the variable reaction of the person to stress, or the mechanisms or resources available to deal with the stressor. It is nevertheless an excellent example of a measuring tool of the allostatic load of an individual.[126] Today a biopsychosocial framework protocol also includes the assessment of social factors such as interruption of a romantic relationship, experiences in childhood, the family environment and dysfunctions in it, which can easily impact the development of symptoms, the course of the clinical condition, and the use of health care.[127]

## Pain assessment

When a patient with pain is evaluated, it is necessary to remember that this is a perception, part of a greater sensory and emotional experience – suffering – including physiological and psychological components.[128] This phenomenon is in constant dynamism because of the plasticity of the nervous system, with a significant impact on the physiology of the body[129] and a profound influence on the activity of the central nervous, musculoskeletal, and endocrine systems. Significant changes, from the molecular level to the coarse structural level, are caused by processes of gene expression and protein synthesis,[130] sometimes temporary and sometimes permanent, depending on the intensity, frequency, and duration of the nociceptive stimulus.

It is therefore essential to keep in mind this evolving nature of the pain when evaluating a person. The behavioral signs of acute patients are generally agitation, "fight-flight" type of reactions, apprehension about the intensity of pain, a hypervigilance to each stimulus, with impact on lifestyle and on themselves.[131] The musculoskeletal system is the active agent of the "attack and escape" type of response by putting in tension as well as relaxing once the cause has ceased. This acute phase is usually followed by a phase of the body's resistance, attempting to reach a compromise with the homeostatic stressors and pain. However, the latter can persist in some cases, even following adequate treatment of various kinds. Research has highlighted the psychosocial factors that can increase the risk of a sharp pain in persistent developments, with associated disability, and loss of quality of life and work.[132] These risk factors have been defined as yellow flags to distinguish them from clinical emergencies, which are the red flags (see Chapter 9) and articulated in behaviors, attitudes, emotions, family factors, work, and so on.

The clinical signs usually associated with chronic conditions are irritability, depression, concern for health and physical function, sleep and libido disorders, reduced activity, and deterioration of interpersonal relationships.[133] The general behavior regresses, requiring at all costs the control of pain by the practitioner. The family and social environments usually reinforce these behaviors,[134] which are integrated in the patient's lifestyle, until the pain becomes the central focus of existence, inevitably leading to demoralization and suffering. The patient expresses structural changes and functional disorders associated with thoughts, emotions, and typical pain response behaviors, through the musculoskeletal and visceral systems, and related immunological, neural, and endocrine responses, with profound consequences on the physical, mental, and spiritual levels.[98]

Individual behaviors in response to pain develop and change through learning and are formed based on past experiences and painful memories.[45] Since cognitive elements can promote the modulation of nociceptive stimuli, and therefore the conscious experience of them, what the individual thinks or feels about his or her own painful condition can affect the way in which he or she processes the pain and faces it. Because of this, much of the disabling effect of chronic pain resides in cognitive and affective factors and cannot be explained by objective physical measurements.[135] It is good practice to gain specific information about pain, for example asking the patient to quantify it on a scale from 0 (no pain) to 10 (unbearable pain). Among other things, the properties and the psychometric quality of this simple numerical scale of pain intensity have been shown to be valid and reliable,[136] although they always need to be verified by observation of the person's behavior (e.g., a patient reports a pain of 9/10 and then has no problems executing every movement during the visit).

Further information can be the type or nature of pain, localization, distribution, irradiation, onset, progression, daily pattern, and the alleviating and worsening factors. But the assessment also needs to include multidimensional measurements of the symptomatic picture, such as the affective response, coping skills, performance of daily activities, level of overall satisfaction,[136] which can, for example, be measured using the McGill Pain Questionnaire.[137] So, the patient's reporting of the pain, and not just the pain, must be assessed[136] (Box 8.6).

## The evaluation of environmental factors

If the operator suspects that the symptomatology is related to an environmental factor, the next step should be the assessment of the presence of:[138]

- a repetitive worsening of symptoms in the workplace or at home

Box 8.6

## Elements of the multidimensional assessment of pain[98]

It is good practice to investigate the impact that pain is causing on:

- affective and mood state, generating perhaps depression, worry, anger or fear, as well as on the cognitive state and self-esteem

- the behavior of positions and basic movements such as sitting, standing, bending forward

- daily activities such as bathing, eating, walking, cooking

- working out and the limitations caused, or disability

- physical activity and how much this has changed in consequence

- nutrition and appetite

- abuse of cigarettes, alcohol, caffeine, or other unhealthy substances

- sleep patterns, causing difficulty falling asleep or staying awake, or inability to rest sufficiently

- the family sphere, influencing the dynamics and interpersonal relationships

- the community and the patient's role in it

- the economic sphere, such as job performance, job loss

- the health care system, resulting in constant search for a medical and legal support

- the environment, including exposure to radiation and to chemicals.

- third parties in the workplace or at home who have developed the same symptoms

- industries, landfills, power plants near the home

- chemicals (solvents, glues, pesticides, etc.) routinely used indoors, outdoors or in the workplace, and if the necessary precautions and protections are taken

- risks of exposure to radiation or other forms of pollution while on the job, and if the necessary precautions and protections are taken

- pets at home or at work who have exhibited pathological signs

- recent trips abroad and contacts with third parties from other countries.

## Physical examination

The biopsychosocial assessment of pain needs to be integrated with physical examination and dysregulation of the system and the adaptive response pattern.[98] Although the interview with the patient provides meaningful information about his or her condition, physical contact through palpation in the physical examination provides an additional and unique opportunity to expand the perspective and develop a healthy and constructive relationship between the operator and the patient.[139] The patient feels better understood when examined and touched where he or she feels pain, being certain that he or she conveyed to the operator the information needed to understand the problem. Confirming this hypothesis with the pain worsening tests (e.g., by compression or drive maneuvers) reinforces the communicative relationship between the operator and the patient. Therefore, the palpation evaluation provides information not only about the tissue causing pain (as is confirmed by a positive therapeutic response to the manipulative intervention) but also on the level of response and adaptation to stress from the musculoskeletal system, as suggested by Dummer[140] (Fig. 8.2).

However, the evaluation of posture and biotypological constitution can help the osteopath formulate a hypothesis about the structure and function of the patient's body, the patient's methods of thought and communication, predispositions to develop certain conditions, as well as responses to certain modes of therapeutic intervention.

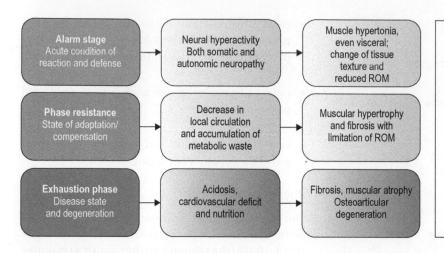

**Fig. 8.2**
The illustration shows the most common behavioral signs related to pain that may be evaluated by the operator during the interview with the patient. Modified from: Turk DC. A cognitive-behavioral perspective on treatment of chronic pain patients. In: Turk DC, Gatchel RJ, editors. Psychological approaches to pain management. 2nd ed. New York: Guilford Press; 2002. pp. 138–58.

## The biotypological evaluation/assessment

Biotypology is the study and classification of humans according to physical appearance and morphology, from which it is possible to infer generalizations about anatomical structure, physiological processes and associated psychological attitudes, as well as potential pathological processes that the patient is likely to develop (diathesis). The classical concept of diathesis, or genetic susceptibility to certain diseases, found its basis in individual histocompatibility, which includes polypeptides on the cell surface capable of identifying "not self" structures and organizing a prompt reaction against them.[141]

Compared to the concept of constitutional weakness, Pende[142] considers that weakness in a specific organ may depend on:

- excessive development of the mesenchymal tissue, affecting vegetative anabolic functions, resulting in the accumulation of waste materials and a deficit of natural immunity

- deficit in the development of the interstitial connective tissue, resulting in insufficient trophic and necessary anabolic support for morphological functional changes.

What is certain is that a given temperament and the corresponding constitution represent a biotype. Not surprisingly, the psychologist Sheldon, one of the leaders of this science, believed that the temperament and physical appearance of a person were two aspects of the same entity.[143] However, although it may seem to be a recent application, this science is very ancient in human history: from Pythagoras to Empedocles, from Hippocrates to Galen and Kant, somatotype/biotypology and constitutional psychology has fascinated and influenced the thinking of many authors and their work.

Other experts in the field, such as Goldthwait, Kretschmer, and Vannier and Martiny, despite having different backgrounds and perspectives, have come to propose biotypological classifications for many situations. In osteopathy, Dummer has integrated several models proposing an application of osteopathic significance.[144] However, these have often been criticized, since the biotypes never appear as such in reality, and are limited only to hypothetical archetypes, and sometimes prejudicial stereotypes.

In fact, an individual usually presents a mixture of characteristics belonging to more than one biotype, although in different proportions, and it is only the dominant component that defines the major biotype. These models are only estimates, because each biotype is the endpoint of a range of psychological and associated physical properties, while most of the time people embody a transition point between one biotype and another. Obviously, physical examination confirms or rejects the constitutional interpretation, which needs to be integrated with other factors, such as the environmental influences to which the individual's temperament is subjected and which could overlap with natural constitutional trends.

The osteopath Philip Latey[145] has for years explored the relationship between emotions, postural patterns and bodily tensions observed at several levels. He has proposed the distinction between postures of image, slump, residual, and of the inner tube.

The *image posture* is the social posture that is expressed when we know we are being watched. The body is kept in a "correct" posture by the action of large superficial muscles, providing an indication of how the patient is socially expressed. As soon as one relaxes, the individual reveals the posture of collapse. The *slump posture* is the most habitual posture, one that responds to gravity and is maintained by the action of postural muscles (paraspinal, suboccipital, etc.). *Residual posture* is revealed when the individual is lying down and relaxed, and is determined by the tone and the muscle activity at rest, maintained by unconscious control of the higher centers reducing the effects of gravity and social interaction. Some postural muscles may remain unintentionally hypertonic (especially the erector spinae), revealing the physical and psychological state of the individual. The muscle tissue in this posture manifests rhythmic contractions, though influenced by the emotional state. For example, in the stage of exhaustion or disease, the movements are more feeble, while, if physical or emotional trauma is present, there may be areas of rigidity and tension, which strongly evokes Reich's concept of "armor" and the psychodynamic interpretation of suppression or repression of emotions.[59] The *inner tube* consists of the involuntary smooth muscle, both visceral and vascular. The gastrointestinal system, in combination with the respiratory system, is centrally positioned in the body, strongly connected with generation and the perception of body and brain emotional processes.[146] According to this model, there are three areas in which psychophysical tensions can accumulate (Box 8.7), generating postures altered by those areas which become closed like a

"fist", along with contractions responding to specific emotions, and causing musculoskeletal or systemic dysfunctions.

---

**Box 8.7**

**The three areas of accumulation of physical and psychological stress and related dysfunctions according to Latey**

- *The pelvic girdle*: can generate lumbar, pelvic and lower limb dysfunctions, such as mechanical imbalances and musculoskeletal dysfunction, with impaired motor control and sensitivity. In the chronic phase we find stasis, inflammation, intestinal, bladder, or genital congestion, which can result in a range of clinical consequences.

- *The lower chest and the upper abdomen*: may cause effects on the respiratory muscles, as variably linked to the expression of emotions (laughing, crying, etc.), leading to respiratory problems, such as asthma and recurrent respiratory infections, and to gastrointestinal disorders such as reflux, hiatal hernia, and finally to mechanical problems such as thoracolumbar dysfunction.

- *Head, neck, and shoulders*: here emotional repression can lead to muscle tension and the development of headaches, sinusitis, temporomandibular dysfunction, or damage to the ENT (ear, nose and throat) system.

---

Similarly, Kelman's psychoemotional approach[147] divides the body into three compartments (head, thorax, abdomen), but also into three layers (outer: skin and nervous system; middle: muscles, bones, and connective tissue; inner: internal organs used for breathing, digestion, assimilation, and distribution). In a healthy individual, the three layers and the three compartments are balanced, ensuring the proper exchange of body fluids. Stress, however, can change the posture until the rigidity collapses, disrupting the balance of the compartments and therefore the exchange of fluids.

The result is four types (rigid and controlled; dense and shameful; swollen and manipulative; collapsed and compliant), each of which presents possible physical, psychological and social sequelae for the reciprocity between physical and emotional state. For the same reason, it is possible to normalize dysfunctional processes acting on the physical, for example through breathing techniques and proper nutrition.

Among the biotypological models, the most popular in osteopathy is the anterior and posterior type proposed by Littlejohn, and then developed by Wernham and Hall.[148] Both types are related to the slippage, respectively forward and backward, of the center of gravity line from its ideal position. The latter is determined by the interactions of the anteroposterior line (AP) and postero-anterior (PA), i.e., anterior-central (AC) and posterior-central (PC). When altered, it causes postural, structural, and functional changes.

- *Anterior type* (Fig. 8.3): the head is held forward; the chest and diaphragm in inhalation; the dorsal spine in extension, with a reduction of the upper

lumbar lordosis and anteversion of the pelvis; hypertonia of suboccipital muscles, spinal extensors, and external rotators of the hips; shoulder blades retracted with external rotation of the upper limbs; tension of the abdominal muscles with compression of the posterior viscera in the abdominal and pelvic cavities (also because of the descent of the diaphragm that is held in the inhalation position); increase in abdominal and pelvic pressure and decrease in thoracic pressure that alters the pressure gradient and thus the physiological gas exchange and global fluid body; slowdown in the cranial venous drainage, impaired respiratory function, congestion of the lower limbs and the pelvic organs predisposing to disorders such as migraine headaches, cystitis, and dysmenorrhea.

- *Posterior type* (Fig. 8.4): the chest is maintained in exhalation with an ascended diaphragm, with increased intrathoracic pressure, resulting

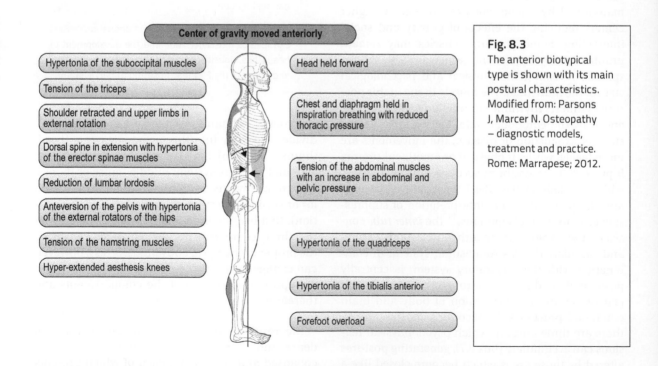

Center of gravity moved anteriorly

Hypertonia of the suboccipital muscles

Tension of the triceps

Shoulder retracted and upper limbs in external rotation

Dorsal spine in extension with hypertonia of the erector spinae muscles

Reduction of lumbar lordosis

Anteversion of the pelvis with hypertonia of the external rotators of the hips

Tension of the hamstring muscles

Hyper-extended aesthesis knees

Head held forward

Chest and diaphragm held in inspiration breathing with reduced thoracic pressure

Tension of the abdominal muscles with an increase in abdominal and pelvic pressure

Hypertonia of the quadriceps

Hypertonia of the tibialis anterior

Forefoot overload

Fig. 8.3
The anterior biotypical type is shown with its main postural characteristics. Modified from: Parsons J, Marcer N. Osteopathy – diagnostic models, treatment and practice. Rome: Marrapese; 2012.

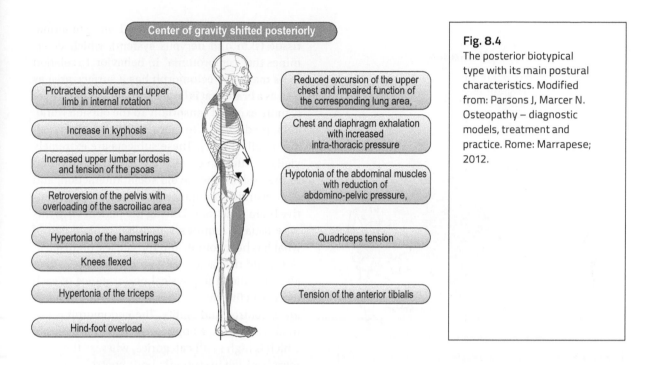

Center of gravity shifted posteriorly

Protracted shoulders and upper limb in internal rotation

Increase in kyphosis

Increased upper lumbar lordosis and tension of the psoas

Retroversion of the pelvis with overloading of the sacroiliac area

Hypertonia of the hamstrings

Knees flexed

Hypertonia of the triceps

Hind-foot overload

Reduced excursion of the upper chest and impaired function of the corresponding lung area,

Chest and diaphragm exhalation with increased intra-thoracic pressure

Hypotonia of the abdominal muscles with reduction of abdomino-pelvic pressure,

Quadriceps tension

Tension of the anterior tibialis

**Fig. 8.4**
The posterior biotypical type with its main postural characteristics. Modified from: Parsons J, Marcer N. Osteopathy – diagnostic models, treatment and practice. Rome: Marrapese; 2012.

in alteration of general respiratory function and the function of the heart and great vessels (and therefore tissue perfusion), and of the general venous return. In the abdominopelvic cavity the opposite occurs, namely a reduction of pressure, with a tendency toward congestion and the development of conditions such as hemorrhoids and constipation.

However, the biotypological model perhaps best known and applied in osteopathy is the triadic model of Sheldon,[149] for which he studied 4,000 students and estimated their embryogenetic predominance. This approach is based on embryological tissue (endoderm, mesoderm, ectoderm) predominant in the individual, influencing the physical (somatotype) and psychological, or "temperament." Unlike the physical characteristics, which are immutable, temperament is influenced by the environment. The dominance of one tissue with respect to another is rated on a scale from 1 to 7. Each subject was assigned a three-digit number, with each of the digits corresponding respectively to the intensity of the first (endomor-

phic), second (mesomorphic) or third (ectomorphic) component, so as to differentiate the definition of somatotype. Indeed, it is rare to encounter a person who belongs to a single somatotype, as the majority of the time there is the coexistence of all three types (Fig. 8.5). In this system, for example, the number 247 indicates reduced endomorphic (number 2), medium mesomorphic (number 4), and high ectomorphic (7) characteristics:

- *Endomorphic*: characterized by a relative predominance of rounded geometry from different tissues. The body's economy is dominated by the digestive viscera (of endodermic derivation), and in particular from the gastrointestinal tract, liver, pancreas, thymus, thyroid, and parathyroid. The physical dominance of these structures determines a "viscerotonic" temperament, with the tendency to enjoy food and food's presence, flavors, and aromas, especially when in the company of good friends; to put on weight; to be friendly and sociable; to enjoy elegant, sumptuous comforting and

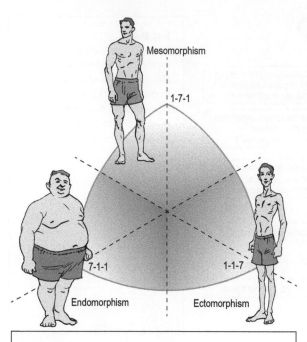

Mesomorphism

1-7-1

7-1-1

1-1-7

Endomorphism

Ectomorphism

**Fig. 8.5**
The three Sheldonian somatotypes: ectomorphic, mesomorphic, and endomorphic.

- *Ectomorphic*: this type is based on ectodermal tissue (skin and nervous system), which determines the "cerebrotonia" in behavior. In relation to its mass, the ectomorph has a surface area as well as a brain that is larger and therefore relatively more exposed sensorially to the outside world. This predisposes to sensitivity, introspection, and intellectuality. These subjects are extremely vigilant, but also careful not to attract attention to themselves; they avoid social interaction, and demonstrate dominance of inhibitory and attentive brain functions. During the patient visit, this type usually requires a detailed explanation of what has been found, and the causes, predispositions, and risk factors of their condition. Sheldon also classified the physical performance of each biotype in five categories: strength, power, endurance, control, and agility. The endomorph is low in all categories, as opposed to the mesomorph, which is high in all categories, whereas the ectomorph is high in strength, body control, and agility but low in power and strength. This system allowed for the selection of therapeutic intervention guidelines for each biotype, according to the resilience and the response of the person to treatment, especially if supported by palpatory observations and by the use of cardiovascular indices.

For example, the endomorph, with a tendency to low metabolism, may necessitate strong and deep treatments of long duration; the ectomorph, on the other hand, may need short and light approaches; the robust and athletic person, with predominant mesomorphic constitution, tends to tolerate strong treatments.[150] In addition, Chaouachi[151] investigated the correlation between aerobics and pulmonary ventilatory capacity of different somatotype groups, who underwent 12 weeks of exercise, performed twice a week. He found a significant difference between the groups: for example between ectomorph and mesomorph, increased aerobic capacity in the mesomorphic type. Other authors conducted an analysis of anthropometric somatotypes in relation to cardiovascular vegetative regulatory capacity, noting an association between somatotypes and blood

relaxing surroundings. During the patient visit, this biotype shows no particular expectations or claims but seeks to engage the operator's attention to talk about general topics of life and especially the pleasures that could arise from it.

- *Mesomorphic*: characterized by a relative predominance of connective tissue, muscles, and bones (mesoderm-derived), with rectangular geometry, firm, solid, and heavy tissues. Temperament is expressed as "somatotonia," an active somatic-muscular system, leaning toward physical activity (especially team activities), good athletic ability, with a tendency to competitiveness, hard work, and sometimes aggression. During the patient visit, usually this type is not interested in the findings or diagnosis, provided their pain can be alleviated and they can return to their work or sporting activities as soon as possible.

pressure/autonomic tone.[152–154] The cardiovascular index, i.e., the sum of systolic and diastolic pressure multiplied by the arterial rhythm detected at the wrist, has normal amplitude between 12,000 and 24,000 units. Clinical observations[155] made it possible to detect a common cardiovascular index for each somatotype (the endomorph tends to be >18,000; the ectomorph <12,000; the mesomorph demonstrates values between the two previous ones).[150]

Similarly, Martiny[156] defined the corresponding types of endoblast, mesoblast, and ectoblast, adding the cordoblast as the perfect constitution, determined by the combination of the previous three. The School of Viola, a professor at the medical clinic that created the anthropometric method, produced a brilliant student, Nicola Pende, who along with Martiny precisely described the four basic human biotypes. These authors present a biotypological pyramid, at the base of which there is genetics and whose levels represent, respectively, the morphological, physiological, ethical, and intellectual aspects of a person. They describe, depending on the stage of life and neuroendocrine status, a stenic and asthenic constitution variant, a change that would occur around an age that is called the "age of life deformation," coinciding with the fifth decade. In this phase, the tissues would have a decrease in elasticity and tone, with progressive replacement of the elastic tissue with fibrous connective tissue, manifesting a morphological portrait of what is now called "metabolic syndrome".[157]

We must also consider the description of the psychological types of Jung,[158] extroversion or introversion, in terms of inward (the subject) or outward (the object) libido orientation, as well as the four functions of consciousness, or thought, feeling, intuition, and sensation. In every individual, there would be a driving force that guides the person's approach to reality. Kretschmer[159] ranked four constitutions like those of Martini's: the pyknic type (physically equivalent to the endomorph), who can easily develop manic-depressive disorders; the asthenic (the equivalent to the ectomorph), prone to schizophrenia; the athletic (physically equivalent to the mesomorph), less prone to any psychological disorder; and the dysplastic (equivalent to cordoblast). Another type of classification is that of Leon Vannier,[160] who identified three biotypologies – carbonic, phosphoric, and fluoric – based upon human response to three homeopathic remedies, respectively, Carbonic Calcareous, Phosphoric, and Fluoric Calcareous, each with its own tendencies to develop certain pathophysiological processes.[161]

Finally, Dummer[162] proposed an empirical model of bipolar types, based on the synthesis of different sources, to support the osteopath in the clinical context. Based on Still's principles, he defined a structural and functional biotype and a third one that is a "mix" of the two, depending on the individual predisposition to respond therapeutically to structural or functional methods, or both. However, Dummer specified several times that the biotype is only one of the factors on which to establish osteopathic intervention, along with the intention of the operator or the application of a method that uses a structural or functional approach. This classification, therefore, is a dynamic process and needs a re-evaluation at every consultation.

In conclusion, the framing of a subject in a biotype is not an end in itself, but part of an open semiotic, aimed at expanding the operator's point of observation of the person. Through global indicators, the operator tries to understand where to start with a patient and how far to go, to finalize a complete treatment. Thus, the operator does not proceed by framing a biotype described in summary tables by a particular author, but rather uses the knowledge of the major typological systems to implement a multifaceted observation of the individual's reactive mode. For each biotype (Box 8.8) we observe the:

- prevalence of structures and functions derived from a germinal layer

- neuroendocrine structure

- dominance of autonomic polarity

- metabolism

- characteristic responsiveness to the environment

- biological reactivity (psycho-neuro-endocrine-metabolic) with its pathophysiological trends.

## Box 8.8

Biotypological rating

### Endoblastic

Hyper-endoblastism present with normal or deficient mesoblast and with deficit of the ectoblast:

- *Neuroendocrine signs*: vagotonic, total hypopituitarian, hypothyroid with hypertyrosinemia and hypotyroxinemia, secondary hyperthymism, hyperparathyroid with normal serum calcium, but functional hypoparathyroid with a slow basal metabolism (calcium accumulation in bone cells), hyperthermic, corticomedullar adrenal insufficiency, hypogonadic, hyperpancreatic

- *Metabolism:* anabolic-anaerobic

- *Characteristics:* calm, sleepy, lethargic, sedentary, defeatist, methodical; has a dominant instinct for preservation, oriented to nutrition and reproduction; learning is slow and methodical, intelligence is analytical, assimilative and repetitive, and imagination is linked to sensory stimuli (sensation function)

- *Pathophysiological characteristics:* resistance to physical stress and low tendency to manifest:

  – hydrophilic cell; shortage of the mesoblast element, therefore of the muscle tone, determines hypotonia in the arterial system, with small wrist and tendency to constitutional arterial hypotension; hypotonia of the venous system contributes to a tendency to peripheral cyanosis; in the lymphatic system it manifests as an excess of protein molecules due to excessive visceral assimilation. Pseudohypothyroidism results in hydrophilic tissue

  – overweight or obesity because of hypolipolysis; overdevelopment of the digestive organs; hydro-

philic tendency contributes to the tendency to be overweight and also affects endocrine factors such as the lack of somatotropic hormone (SH) (with diminution of protein anabolism) and adrenocorticotropic hormone (ACTH) (with deficiency of androgenic steroids, essential for protein anabolism), in contrast with the tendency to hyperinsulinism and consequent increase in the glucose load which is converted further into fat in adipose tissue. Allergic predisposition, lymphatic-exudative, with slowing of hepatic and reticuloendothelial functions, and tendency to circulatory and intestinal disorders of dysbiotic or parasitic type.

### Mesoblast

Excessive function of the mesodermal-derived organs, accompanied by normal endodermal and ectodermal function:

- *Neuroendocrine signs:* neurovegetative antiphony, anterior hyperpituitarism, hypercortical-adrenal hypergonadism

- *Metabolism:* anabolic-aerobic

- *Characteristics:* eager to act and to impose himself or herself, combative impulses; high intelligence with a tendency for social survival and desire for affirmation, capable and strives to finalize projects

- *Pathophysiological characteristics:* very good resistance to physical exertion, with fast reactions characterized by discrete dexterity; tendency for increased urea with a high rate of androgen hormones, both adrenal and gonadic, that results in an intense anabolism; the increase of renal tubular secretion of uric acid cannot counter the positive nitrogen balance determined by steroids and by the adrenal-gonadic androgen. The mineralocorticoids of the adrenal contribute to an osmotic mechanism of water reabsorption at the level of the distal and proximal tubules of the kidney, with expansion of the extracellular fluid and tendency to increase blood pressure.

### Ectoblast

The hyperfunctioning of the ectodermal organs is often accompanied by a functional deficiency of organs derived from the endoblast and mesoblast tissues:

- *Neuroendocrine signs:* hypersympathicotonia dominance, which can lead to dystonia and orthosympathetic dominance followed by a phase of vagotonic exhaustion; hyperpinealism, posterior hyperpituitarism, anterior hypopituitarism, hypoparathyroidism, dysthyroidism with a tendency to secondary hyperthyroidism, medullary hypoadrenalism (increased production of adrenaline and noradrenaline), cortical hypoadrenalism, hypogonadism

- *Metabolism:* anaerobic-catabolic

- *Characteristics:* emotional, imaginative and emotionally hypersensitive, unwillingness, fearful, pessimistic, with a tendency toward an "inferiority complex" in the terms in which I sense that the patient does not feel ready to face questions about his or her environment from the physical point of view; emotional, has fervid imaginative activities that reverberate with mental hyperactivity and a tendency to have hypochondriacal thoughts; has abstract intelligence, is an idealist, dreamer, not a concrete thinker

- *Pathophysiological characteristics:* during resistance to physical stress there occurs a contradiction between the sedentary physical aspect and psychic hyperactivity. The individual has rapid psychomotor reactions, but he or she tires easily. A usually slow hematopoiesis tends to develop anemia; the dominance of the adrenal medulla and sympathetic tone, as well as the plasma levels of catecholamines and thyroid hormones, contribute to a state of nervous hypertension with stimulation of the reticular activating system. This causes effects on the peripheral nervous system, such as the shortening of the reaction time of reflexes from stretching. The ectoblast manifests, alongside hypoenergetic endocrine activity, a deficiency of vitamins accentuated by a lack of endoblastic assimilation and by catabolism not compensated by a proper diet. The most frequent vitamin deficiencies are a deficiency of group B vitamins (neuritis, neuralgia, weight loss, constipation, bloating, eczema), and PP (nicotinic acid) (skin discoloration, depressive or anxious state).

This leads to the following question: is the biological reactivity of the individual consistent with his or her constitution? In fact, a characteristic reactive mode of a disorder may be consistent with the stenic phase of a constitution, for example, be coherent with the autonomic hypersympathetic-tonic nature characteristic of the ectoblastic subject showing a cervical pain, albeit in a vigilant mode, accompanied by sleep disturbances, digestive problems (swelling), and high blood pressure. The life stages defined as stenic and asthenic are to be understood as variations in a "hypo" or "hyper" sense, absolutely paraphysiological. In fact, the structures and functions of a dominant somatotype can be hyperactive in a juvenile stage (stenic), and then express hyperoactivity in old age (asthenic phase).

### Formulating a diagnosis

After relying on interpersonal communication skills, acquiring information about the biopsychosocial factors in which the patient's medical condition is engaged, including perception of pain and stress, and even more so their thoughts, emotions and behaviors that underpin the related symptoms and on the lifestyle choices made,[100] the osteopath interprets and integrates this information with that from any imaging studies, laboratory tests and the physical examination. The process leads to the formulation of a biodescription, a diagnosis and the treatment of the patient[163] (Box 8.9).

---

**Box 8.9**

Biopsychosocial diagnosis

The diagnosis must include:

- medical diagnosis, together with affective, cognitive, behavioral comorbidities

- current tissue damage and the understanding of the underlying nociceptive mechanisms, either central or peripheral

- presence and degree of suffering, musculoskeletal reactions and consequent adaptive responses

- the understanding of the biopsychosocial impact on the function and quality of the individual's life.

Decision-making requires flexibility and attention to avoid getting caught up in only the goal of recognizing something abnormal, which can lead to a misdiagnosis.[164] The diagnosis must not place the patient in a position with few or no options, and at risk for deleterious consequences. Instead, through communicative language[165] and the appropriate information, the patient is kept informed of the processes that underlie the condition from which he or she suffers, so that the operator can then assess and promote optimal adaptive responses to resolve the situation and prevent recurrence. The application of cognitive strategies[166] and regarding the patient as the primary source of resources[116] can guide clinical decision-making in an appropriate manner.

## Principles and methods of treatment

The therapeutic application of the biopsychosocial model includes all the elements of osteopathic philosophy (Table 8.2) and involves the education of the patient with coping strategies, a healthy lifestyle (exercise, diet, meditation) and abstinence from toxic substances (smoking, alcohol, drugs). However, the model is also and above all connected to the direct or indirect management of the experiential (cognitive and emotional), pain and disability aspects, as well as the behavioral (inactivity, catastrophism, sexuality), general medical (drug treatments in place, comorbidities, trauma or previous surgery), social (family, work), religious and spiritual, and environmental (pollution of any origin and nature) aspects, using a multidisciplinary intervention, focused on the patient and on the environment in which the patient exists. The aim is to forge a multidimensional therapeutic intervention to identify and address possible causes of biopsychosocial and maladaptive responses to the allostatic load of the individual. Once a diagnosis is

**Table 8.2**
Therapeutic aspects of the biopsychosocial model

| | |
|---|---|
| **Biopsychosocial perspective** | Broadening the extent of intervention, including biological, psychological, and social aspects of pain/dysfunction/disability |
| **The patient as a person** | Recognize the patient's individuality as a person, emphasizing the meanings and personal interpretations attributed to their condition (emotions, fears, and expectations) |
| **Sharing of power and responsibilities** | Building a fair and equal relationship between operator and patient, involving mutual participation, collaboration, and negotiation during the planning and implementation of the entire therapeutic process |
| **The therapeutic alliance** | Establishing a collaborative link between patient and operator to maximize therapeutic potential; this is expressed by establishing an agreement on the intervention through a negotiation of the objectives of the treatment |
| **The operator as a person** | The awareness of the influence of the operator's personal qualities and the way they are implemented (including the influence of the emotional state and technical capabilities of the osteopath) |

Modified by: Thomson OP, Petty NJ, Moore AP. Reconsidering the patient-centeredness of osteopathy. Int J Osteopath Med. 2013;16(1): 25–32.

made, we inform the patient, guiding the identification and resolution of the causative factors to better relieve or cope with the stress. In doing so, we aim to change the individual's response to stressful factors; we educate the patient about coping skills, by correcting the neuroendocrine reactions associated with somatic dysfunction, with a general impact on health.[167]

In case of acute pain caused by tissue damage and inflammation, the first objective is to reduce the acute pain and inflammation, making use of OMT, rest, topical or systemic medications, physical therapy (Tecar therapy, TENS, etc.), acupuncture, biofeedback, recommendations on the best posture and ergonomics at work and at home, at rest and during activity. This may include advice on nutrition and sleep, or other supplementary care or mind–body therapies,[168] such as tai chi, yoga, Feldenkrais and Alexander technique.[169] Finally, we may recommend surgery, if necessary. However, each management plan should be individualized and carefully re-evaluated, relative to the benefits and side effects of the treatment and the impact on daily activities.

The osteopath should support the patient in avoiding dramatization of pain,[170] as well as the fear of it;[171] have strong supportive conversations about pain,[172] advise how to handle it[173] and any psychiatric co-morbidity;[135] identify events in the environment that strengthen the pain and behaviors associated with musculoskeletal related reactions; evaluate the possible use, or inappropriate dosage of, drug treatment;[174] discourage alleged miraculous cures or potentially dangerous actions; and promote self-management and self-healing of symptoms.[175] The patient is then guided to recognize the physicality of his or her pain and reactions related to it, and to then control it without succumbing to despair and surrender, becoming aware of his or her choices, as well as of his or her own mistakes, and the willingness to forgive. The patient is finally encouraged to take note and to manage his or her resources in

pain relief, look toward a cure, or at least understand that there is more in life, and higher goals to seek.

However, such possibility of change is not always available or accessible to the patient.[176] Therefore, the operator should cultivate a caring relationship with the individual based on the current condition of the patient, rather than giving the patient an ideal target that does not exist except in the mind of the therapist.[105] In addition, not all patients being treated by the osteopath are ready to be sent to other professionals, for example to the psychotherapist. There is no doubt that, by its empathetic nature, osteopathic medical history allows psychic contents to emerge. This fact, far from negligible, has two consequences: on the one hand it helps to strengthen the relationship between the operator and the patient, with obvious positive implications in terms of the treatment profile and compliance of the patient; on the other hand it includes materials and issues that, in the case of patients with psychological disorders, require an explicitly psychotherapeutic intervention.

For this reason, the operator must be able to motivate the patient to see a specialist. Cognitive-behavioral psychotherapy is one approach that requires a qualified specialist; however, knowledge of the basic principles allows the osteopath to:

- understand behavioral traits that represent worsening factors or maintenance of the patient's condition

- "approximate" the patient to the appropriate psychotherapeutic approach through consistent communication

- manage non-pathological behavioral traits, which, although minor, add to the allostatic load of the patient.

## Cognitive-behavioral intervention

The cognitive approach is a well-structured intervention oriented to specific objectives and focused on identifying and solving the problem. It presupposes that the beliefs and attitudes that patients have influence symptoms such as anxiety and depression. Thus, we identify ways that information becomes distorted, and teach the patient to recognize, assess and respond to thoughts and dysfunctional beliefs, using a variety of techniques aimed at thinking, mood, and behavior. It is practical and realistic, and can be a general as well as a specific approach. It is also active, as it implies learning principles that lead the patient to develop new adaptive modes of behavior to normalize dysfunctional thoughts and emotions. This implies the recognition of how difficult it is to change, and the need for a schedule to minimize discouragement of both patient and operator, while constantly encouraging a positive attitude toward a lasting or permanent change. To act on the behavior, this approach also involves the systematic change of the environment, which in turn produces and/or maintains the dysfunctional behavior (even when the cause has been removed).

All this is a dynamic process that has been divided into five phases in the trans-theoretical model[177] (Box 8.10). The operator's responsibility is to assist the patient in recognition of his or her current phase and progression into the next one. Treatment should be individualized, flexible, and based on both the physical examination and the biopsychosocial findings that emerge during construction.

---

### Box 8.10

Five stages of behavior change according to the trans-theoretical model

1. Pre-contemplation: in this first stage, patients are often unaware of, or deny the negative consequences of, their behavior. This information is critical, in order to inform the individual of their current condition and then create the best basis for the therapeutic choice.

2. Contemplation: the patient reflects on his or her own behavior and assesses both negative consequences if they persevered, and the likely benefits if changed positively.

3. Preparation: the patient attempts to change and the operator's job is to negotiate a plan with a high probability of success.

4. Action: the patient and the operator implement the plan for behavioral change with clear outcome assessments to monitor progress.

5. Maintenance: the patient experiences the effects of reinforcing the plan of action, to the point that the change becomes a regular part of their lives.

Modified by: Prochaska JO, DiClemente CC. Stages of change in the modification of problem behaviors. Prog Behav. 1992; 28:183–218.

---

### The operator–patient relationship at the basis of the therapeutic process

The goal of this process is the birth and growth of a collaborative relationship between operator and patient, which aims to offer a concrete explanation of stressors and related risks by sharing experience and knowledge.[178] This gives the patient an ability to be in control, reducing the effects of stress by enhancing appropriate responses to it, promoting appropriate coping strategies, and educating the patient about reinforcing prevention and anticipation of stress.[163] By learning adaptive behaviors the individual faces the problem better during subsequent experiences. Operator and patient cooperation must be maximized and the therapeutic relationship strengthened to better promote the active participation of the individual in his or her healing journey.

The alliance and cooperation between osteopath and patient are crucial in facilitating the patient's ability to restore health and maintain a healthy relationship between body, mind, and spirit. Stoffelmayr and colleagues[179] propose four specific sequential strategies in the therapeutic relationship to ensure cooperation and motivation, and thus establish the individual's responsibility toward his or her own health:

1. *Information*: the operator should never take anything for granted regarding the knowledge and understanding of the patient, regardless of social origin or level of education. Therefore, one should first assess the current level of understanding that the patient has about his or her condition, listening to the patient's explanation, and then identifying any misinterpretations.

2. *Education*: this must be in plain language, and may also make use of images or educational material, if necessary. The operator can then verify that the patient has learned, for example by asking the patient to repeat the instructions in his or her own words. Information is the key at this stage, as patients who are unclear about what is asked of them may find it difficult to follow the given recommendations, and any resulting dissatisfaction may increase the chance that the patient will not return on subsequent visits.

3. *Gaining commitment*: this step requires the appropriate use by the operator of an authoritative attitude, making the patient feel accepted and approved. Such an attitude requires clear statements about the negative effects of the patient's current behavior, as well as a clear description of the appropriate and expected changes, so as to encourage a commitment to work together.

4. *Negotiate and individualize the path to wellness*: all recommendations require a change in lifestyle (physical activity, sexual, occupational, social, etc.). The more complex the required changes, the harder it is for the patient to cooperate. The purpose of the negotiation is to find a compromise, an agreement, after having individualized the way to changing the individual's life circumstances. One must also recognize and acknowledge the patient's emotional responses. The patient often complains, that he or she has been has not been heard or given the opportunity to adequately describe his or her condition

to cold and distant (although competent) operators. Often this view is based on the operator's ability to recognize and respond to concerns or emotions expressed. This makes the operator–patient relationship an essential requirement to promote a positive change: when the report is based on empathic listening, shared attention and compassionate understanding, cooperation with the therapeutic process becomes easily achievable. Participation and emotional support also imply a consequent reprogramming and individualization of the therapeutic process from time to time, within the context of patient responses.

---

**Box 8.11**

Example of problem solving strategy in circular sequence

1. Perceive the stress

2. Identify the reactions to stress

3. Be aware of how the stress influences the organism

4. Compare this with similar past events (including decisive actions)

5. Compare this with simultaneous perceptions

6. Define the origins of the stress

7. State a hypothesis of resolutive behavior based on the probability of efficacy and effectiveness

8. Choose the most appropriate resolutive behavior

9. Apply the chosen behavior

10. Verify its success or failure (return to point 1).

At the end of each circular sequence the individual has acquired an existential condition which is more evolved than the previous one. In this sense the stress can be used as an ally, which reveals the aspects of life that can be improved in the progress toward a healthy condition.

Modified from: Nardone G, Watzlawick P. Brief strategic therapy. New York: Jason Aronson; 2005.

Assertiveness, as well as problem-solving techniques (Box 8.11) are unparalleled tools to achieve this aim. Assertiveness is defined as the capacity of the subject to use, in each relational context, communication methods that make positive reactions with the environment highly possible and negate or reduce the possibility of negative reactions.[180] These techniques are particularly useful for those who live under stress because of difficulties of expression or poor interpersonal skills, who risk aggravating related physical symptoms. For example, a very demanding spouse or superior at work can be a common cause of stress and associated symptoms. In this case, we may, for example, teach the patient verbal response strategies, to properly manage excessive or improper requests, thus learning effective behaviors in addressing the problem.

## The development of adaptation resources and coping techniques

It is critical to recognize and activate the patient's coping strategies and resources to resist stress. These strategies consist of material (money and everything that can be purchased), physical (strength, health, etc.), intrapersonal (self-esteem, inner strength), cultural (sense of coherence and belonging to a community), and information and education resources.[126] Most of these resources are interconnected and all are needed in the planning of a management-specific and individual plan, which aims to better manage the largest number of stressors, including referral to other specialists if needed. For example, we can use specific techniques to manage conditions such as insomnia. After 3 weeks, this disorder becomes rooted and requires behavioral strategies to correct the dysfunctional habit, such as relaxation techniques, distraction, stimulus control, and education regarding sleep, as well as appropriate pharmacological support.

Usually, these behavioral strategies are applied during visits distributed over 6–8 weeks, possibly in group sessions,[181] leading to improved sleep patterns, better concentration, the ability to cope with the problems and manage stress as well as the intensity of related physical symptoms. A widely used method to develop listening and control of the patient's own body and its adaptive mechanisms is biofeedback, which teaches the patient to use physiological monitoring instrumentation to perceive their physiological processes, then to learn to manage and control them. The individual learns to perceive the close interconnection between mind and body by converting instrumentally monitored physiological responses received as auditory and visual signals and to consciously control these signals and the corresponding bodily activities.

From the osteopathic point of view, this method could be extended to the possibility of voluntarily controlling certain elements of somatic dysfunction, through the reduction of the response of somatic and visceral reflex activity, so as to develop a sense of trust and security of his or her own healing capacities.[167] Techniques are often incorporated in this process, such as Jacobson's progressive muscle relaxation,[182] which is based on the contraction and relaxation of specific muscles to make the individual aware of the state of tension in the body as a possible indicator of stress. Associated with a controlled diaphragmatic breathing and biofeedback, this method is often used in controlling the physical symptoms of anxiety.[183] Yoga, transcendental meditation, and other mind–body approaches to relaxation, including massage and acupuncture, are widely used in this model,[184] along with the integration of herbal and essential oils[185] or use of specific electromagnetic fields,[186] in order to reduce anxiety, fear of surroundings (kinesiophobia), and chronic muscle tension associated with pain.[187]

## The multidisciplinary intervention

A multidisciplinary approach is often adopted based on the best evidence-based knowledge about the biopsychosocial treatment, especially in patients suffering from chronic pain,[188] in order to assist them in the homeostatic response to recovery. Each therapeutic prescription needs to be individualized. In the interdisciplinary model, the patient, a leader and in partnership with the operator, creates his or her own team for assistance in the care and management of pain/disability.

## The development of psychosocial support

A strong resource for helping to alleviate stress is psychosocial support, understood as a social network of concentric relationships that expand from the patient in the center, offering appreciation, support, trust, and sharing.[167] Most of the time this is expressed as respect and listening offered by a spouse or friend, opening the door to sharing concerns and problems; other times it expands to include social or religious groups. But family is certainly the first social group into which the individual is born, grows, and interacts. The operator should clearly understand, while collecting medical history, the role and responsibility of each member of the family, and then promote therapeutic and effective communication between family members and the person being treated, as well as support, encouragement, and sharing of values.[189] Among other things, this approach also supports the management of the patient by the osteopath, who can, in turn, continue his or her advice and keep the treatment plan active.

Faith and religion are included in this framework, both as a spiritual support to stress management and as a source of confidence in a supernatural meaning of life and of events, resulting in the enhancement of health and healing processes.[190,191] Similarly, patient involvement in support groups who share the problem of stress can sustain the process of healing and especially the learning of new and more functional behaviors, for example by involving the patient with a group of patients who may be older and/or suffering from a more serious condition, but displaying better responsiveness, stimulates the individual to manage his or her own stress/anxiety with less pain. In this group model, patients reorganize the meaning given to pain, and the cognitive and emotional evaluation and problem-solving strategies,[192] by reconsidering how pain impacts themselves and their lives.

## The work environment

Work plays a vital role in life and in stress management. A job that is perceived as oppressive, or useless, or too challenging, or otherwise not satisfactory from any point of view should be dealt with through a plan for change. If such change is not possible, then alternatives, such as changes within the work environment could be contemplated, or the pursuit of training for a different career.

Patients should be encouraged to form friendships in the workplace. If the workplace does not offer social gatherings or other similar activities, the patient may become a promoter of recreational, sporting or social activities among colleagues.

## The behavioral component

The behavioral components of the body and mind interaction are manifested in cognitive processes, emotional or physical hazards that need to be translated into motor actions and produce physiological responses before generating a given behavior. For this reason current bio-behavioral thinking considers the mental aspect of a particular form of physical phenomenon is thus inseparable from physiological processes.[193] Bio-behavioral factors exert their influence in three main ways: first, cognitive and emotional reactions generate physiological alterations that contribute to the pathophysiology of the disease (such as response to stress, that if chronic, may predispose to systemic dysregulation, including mental and/or physical illness); second, there can be involvement of behaviors associated with increased or decreased risk of developing disease. For example, smoking is a behavior at high risk of developing various diseases, and healthy physical activity is a health support. Other behaviors include diet, sleeping, and sun exposure and so on, which can directly or indirectly influence the pattern of pain, medical intervention, and the natural course of disease. The third way includes behaviors that occur in response to the present or suspected disease or to the possibility of verifying the presence of disease. This includes screening attitudes regarding the prevention, symptom recognition, and the decision to actively participate in care and medical follow-up respecting the prescription and intervention arrangements, or risky behaviors such as discontinuities in following the care plan, or neglecting to carry out routine checks. Beliefs about health, risk perception and anxiety related to his or her disease may contribute to avoidance behavior by the patient,[194] and influence compliance with the planned medical care regime. However, nonadherence to treatment may also result from other causes such as inadequate understanding,[195] forgetfulness, confusion, beliefs or personal theories about his or her health or the best care for his or her condition.[196] In any case, good communication, patient supervision, social support, and the management of associated disability help to improve the patient's adherence to treatment.[196] Therefore, many behavioral responses to chronic pain may impact the treatment and recovery of health, as well as help to understand the mechanisms underlying the chronicity of pain[197,198] and any associated disabilities.[199]

The majority of such disorders – such as obesity, cancer, and hypertension – are generated and/or maintained by erroneous behavioral choices, as well as dysfunctional mind-body interactions.[193] The behaviors most commonly associated with disease, disability, and reduced health level are the use of tobacco, alcohol abuse, high fat diet, sedentary lifestyle, unprotected sexual activity, and various accidents.[200] Even directly related behaviors that result in seeking or avoidance of medical care may have important consequences on prevention, early diagnosis, and adherence to medical care.

## Physical activity

Physical activity is a fundamental tool to promote health (if there are no medical or pharmacological treatment conditions that contraindicate the practice or which may pose a health risk). Exercise has an impact on posture, balance, flexibility, strength, endurance, and coordination, promoting an optimal relationship between structure and function.[98] Physical activity is also useful in managing stress, by reducing episodes of anxiety and depression, normalizing blood pressure, improving the immune profile and the quality of life of healthy individuals or those with various types of pathologies.[201]

In general, regardless of the physical fitness level of the patient, the osteopath should motivate him or her to increase physical activity in daily life, or at least take the first steps in this direction, encouraging exercises that are practiced with pleasure by the patient, in companies and social contexts perceived as favorable, for easy inclusion in the patient's lifestyle in a consistent way. However, we should not underestimate that the stress to which many individuals are subjected tends to reduce the physical activity undertaken.[202] In any case, these physical activities should be proposed by an osteopath who also acts as a model of life and physical fitness. Patients, in fact, are much more prone to listen and to follow health advice by an operator whose lifestyle reflects the specified behavior.[203] Generally, the operator recommends balanced and gradual programs of aerobic daily exercise and resistance to develop strength and power, as well as stretching to increase flexibility and prevent injuries.

Clearly it is necessary to evaluate the current level of fitness, age-based, to encourage a program based on well-defined objectives and implemented with the right progression.[204] It has been shown that, if the regime of activity is individualized, supervised, and structured on stretching and strength training, it has a much better chance of success in reducing pain and improving overall function.[205] A 30-minute program performed twice a day, starting with less demanding activities, such as walking, water activities and exercise bike, and that encourages self-management, has been found to be excellent in the long term.[98] In this phase it is essential to avoid excessive fatigue, to speed recovery, and avoid dehydration, with the possibility of including beverages with mineral supplements, where the physical activity should extend to more than 1 hour.

## Nutrition

Nutrition is a key aspect for the restoration, maintenance, and enhancement of health. Usually the recommendation is for an abundant intake of fresh fruit and vegetables, as well as frequent meals with high protein content derived from fish, especially those with high levels of omega 3. Conversely, we tend to discourage the intake of red meat and limit dairy products, salt, refined grains, sweetened drinks, and alcohol.[206]

### Sexual activity

Sexual activity is a central component of the human sphere in health, as well as a healthy source of pleasure and intimacy. However, the improper practice of this activity can lead to disease. It is the responsibility of the operator to inform their patients, when appropriate, on how to practice safe sex, including the appropriate use of contraceptives. Women suffer from diseases transmitted by sexual intercourse, as well as unwanted pregnancies. A mutually monogamous relationship (besides abstinence) is certainly the safest practice to avoid contracting related diseases. When this is accepted or not possible, the operator should educate the patient about safe or low-risk sexual behaviors.

### Pollution and risks

Particular attention should be paid to educating the patient to avoid various types of common health risks and pollution (Box 8.12), considering that the research suggests that environmental factors, such as pollution, gas, chemicals, and radiation, can contribute to the development of pathology.[207]

---

**Box 8.12**

**Appropriate patient education on common risks/pollution**

- *In general*: educate the patient to wash his or her hands well after using the bathroom or changing a baby, so as to reduce the risk of contagion or infection, and the avoidance of common illnesses such as colds, respiratory or intestinal flu; to use appropriate protection when exposed for long periods to sunlight, since prolonged exposure without protection to solar ultraviolet radiation is related to the development of skin tumors;[208] to avoid practicing physical outdoor activities when air pollution levels are classified as high, especially if the patient suffers from asthma or other respiratory disorders.[209]

- *At home*: educating the patient regarding the appropriate use of chemicals that can easily contaminate areas or objects and thus facilitate poisoning; recommend the use of gloves, masks and eye or face protection where necessary, and to use extreme caution when using pesticides or when applying children's insect repellent, which should not be used on open wounds or directly on the face and hands; advise the patient to keep chemicals and pharmaceuticals away from children, and to use of biodegradable and non-toxic products. In addition, inform the patient to localize and remove as soon as possible any moisture and mold in the home, mostly in bathrooms,[210] and, finally, to take the right precautions if one suffers from allergies, such as the use of bed covers and pillows that protect against allergy to dust mites.[211]

- *At work*: encourage the patient to inform himself or herself about the risks associated with the performance of his or her job duties. For example, if the job involves the use of high noise equipment, this can cause permanent hearing damage.[212]

---

## Rationale and mechanisms

### Evidence on the bio-psycho-behavioral responses to stress and pain

Research has shown in several instances that chronic stress and emotional reactions to stress are able to generate psycho-physiological disorders such as hypertension, coronary artery disease, and peptic ulcers,[213] or even stimulate carcinogenesis through the alteration of immune function,[214] repair processes of DNA and/or apoptosis, in both healthy patients and patients suffering from cancer.[215] In addition, chronic stress can cause an increase of interleukin-6, C-reactive protein, and tissue necrosis factor,[47] which in turn stimulate the release of ACTH and cortisol, and decrease the levels of serotonin,[216] causing symptoms such as fatigue, loss of appetite, and sleep disorders, and difficulties with memory and concentration, thus predisposing to heart,[217] vascular,[218] and rheumatic[219] diseases, and viral reactivations.[220,221] It has been shown that psychological stress delays the processes of tissue repair,[219] and affects the duration and/or severity of diseases, for example oral and genital herpes, which are controlled by the immune system mediated by T lymphocytes.[222]

Decreased activity of natural killer cells has been reported in individuals during severe stressful situations,[223] with diminished immune response after the loss of loved ones,[224] in grieving widows,[225] in students before exams, in cases of depression,[226] and in hospitalized patients with major depressive disorder,[227] resulting in an increased susceptibility to infections. Depression in particular is also associated with cardiovascular disease, influencing vascular inflammation, decreasing heart rate variability and increasing platelet activation, blood coagulability and plasma cortisol levels.[228]

Levels of perceived stress appear to be strongly linked to changes in the efficiency of the immune system, as demonstrated by research evidence over the last 30 years.[229,230] Presumably this occurs through a feedforward mechanism, in which each further consequence of stress becomes an aggravating factor of a dysfunctional general level. For example, the activation of inflammatory mediators such as interleukin-6 in response to chronic stress can sensitize peripheral nociceptors, leading to hyperalgesia,[231] as well as exacerbate the adaptive response of the central nervous system,[232] resulting in neurodegeneration,[233] so much so that hypersecretion of interleukins, such as IL-2 and IL-6, has been demonstrated to be capable of generating schizophrenia and depression[234] through the stimulation of astrocytes and microglia, producing additional cytokines.[235]

Recent biological studies on the etiology of psychiatric disorders have shown a correlation between depression and decrease of platelet and neuronal membrane viscosity,[236] which would reduce the accessibility of serotonin at the central level.[237]

Such a change in the viscosity of the membrane, caused by an increase of arachidonic acid, would seem to be able to modify neural transmission, via alteration of the receptor-mediated mechanisms of serotonin reuptake,[238,239] through cytoskeletal changes (especially tubulin and the Gsα protein) and activation of phosphorylation mediated by G proteins and second messengers.[240] In fact, platelet elements involved in this process, such as adenylyl cyclase, have been proposed as the predictive peripheral biological markers of depression.[241]

Not only stress, but also the perception and interpretation of pain produce important answers: dramatizing pain, for example the tendency to misinterpret (exaggerate) situations perceived as threatening, can greatly alter the experience of pain.[242] Patients with chronic pain, often associated with depression, tend to experience and to quantify their pain as more severe,[26] to withdraw into an attitude of protection and avoidance, which, paradoxically, only adds to the pain and the related disability.[171]

Among other things, the association between depression, somatic dysfunction, and chronic low back pain has been widely observed in several studies.[243] In 202 adult patients with chronic low back pain researchers observed a rate of recurrent depressive symptoms in 22% of cases, and a significant correlation between depression and the somatic dysfunction score (p <0.01).[244] The evidence suggests that dysfunctional emotional processing, especially the deletion of the emotions, is associated with chronic low back pain, especially in males, and can be a predictive factor for the development of this condition.[245] In these cases, the result is often an avoidance of daily activities, predisposing to the development of tissue fibrosis, which in turn increases the risk of injury and inflammation, resulting in a reinforcement of the chronic pain pattern and trend toward inactivity.[246]

The bio-behavioral approach, therefore, has long highlighted the correlation between cognitive, emotional, and behavioral factors with the onset and progression of many diseases.[247] For example, stressful experiences early in life are related to decreased cognitive abilities;[248] the risk of cervical hyperplasia due to human papilloma virus increases significantly in women who have negative affective states;[249] in cancer patients, the affective component of their disease and disability, often associated with depression, may increase the risk of mortality;[250] behavioral and neuropsychiatric disorders have been associated with autoimmune and viral conditions such as lupus erythematosus and multiple sclerosis.[251]

Stress, including pain, is therefore a psychophysical-biological phenomenon to be reckoned with in the decision-making and management process of patients, as well as the individual's behavioral response to similar experiences. Inappropriate behavior, such as altered coping with stress mechanisms, or personality type A, or smoking, can cause adverse metabolic effects on serum lipid levels, or silent ischemic oxidative damage.[252] Dysfunctional daily habits, such as sleep pattern disturbance, can significantly influence the state of health (such as the use of sleeping pills, insufficient or poor quality sleep time), can foster the development of diseases, and influence the rate and risk of mortality.[253,254] The correlation between physiological and behavioral aspects can trigger acute pathologic events and/or alter the pathophysiology of pre-existing disorders.[255] For example, acute cardiovascular events, ischemic attacks, and arrhythmias have been demonstrated to be correlated with anxiety, suffering and anger.[256]

Aggressiveness, impatience, hostility, competitiveness, and poor adaptability, characteristics that characterize individuals with type A personality,[257] have often been associated with coronary heart disease. Several mechanisms have been proposed to explain these responses, including neurovegetative dystonia, altered hemodynamics and platelet function, and endothelial alteration.[258,259] These maladaptive behaviors may be the result of response patterns acquired in the past. In 1975, Robert Ader[260] administered cyclophosphamide (an alkylating chemical with powerful immunosup-

pressive agents) in saccharin containers, an unmistakable unpleasant taste to laboratory rats. The animals developed immune suppression, reproduced when simply exposed to saccharin, and therefore to a simple neurological stimulation by taste. These results, reported later in humans,[261] confirmed the theory that the mind can cause physical disorders through behavioral conditioning.

Several laboratory studies have demonstrated that subjects (animals and humans), faced with unavoidable stress, activate cognitive processes such as abandoning avoidance behaviors and receiving punishment passively, developing limited self-esteem and stress management expectations, contingent depression, helplessness, retarded learning, loss of appetite and inability to correct problems.[262,263] Therefore, it is possible for an individual to learn maladaptive processes to stress based on past experiences, like negative patterns regarding themselves and their abilities,[264] sinking into a sense of inadequacy and failure, which may lead to depression. These dysfunctional patterns can reside in the individual's unconscious sphere, only to re-emerge as defense mechanisms in difficult situations.

Approximately 95% of our thinking and affective activity is subconscious,[265] and this unconscious potential can perpetuate physical symptoms resulting from some other cause, such as trauma, for the sole purpose of circumventing situations that are difficult to deal with, such as in the workplace. In fact, stressful working environments with poor flexibility and lack of support from superiors can help generate and maintain chronic musculoskeletal pain.[29] Individuals under stress or emotional distress have been shown to be more likely to develop this unconscious (or conscious) defensive reaction and develop physical symptoms after simulation of a car accident.[266]

Conversely, a well-disposed therapy, for example manual therapy, can positively modulate the impact and the outcome, unlike a placebo intervention.[267] Patients with chronic fatigue associated with malignant disease and with positive attitude to manual therapy showed a significant increase in immune response (IgA), not observed in the control group, as a result of treatment with myofascial release (even if the evoked pain threshold to pressure showed no change).[268] Among the behavioral responses to stress, smoking, addiction to drugs, and sleep deprivation, studies have shown reduced immune efficiency, an inability to interact with others, and depression, causing further immune impairment.[269]

Stress appears to be one of the factors that contributes significantly to increasing the frequency and amount of tobacco use in smokers, as well as encouraging the resumption of the habit after stopping.[202] It is clear that the combination of stress and smoking is a behavioral self-perpetuating pattern, complicated by nicotine addiction and escape from abstinence,[270] as well as by the development of many diseases, such as cancer, autoimmune and cardiovascular diseases, cataracts, and periodontitis, not only for those who actively make use of this substance, but also for those who breath it passively,[271] especially infants and children. These individuals are in fact likely to develop cardiovascular and respiratory diseases, and cancer,[272] through well-defined physiological mechanisms.[273]

Alcoholism is considered a chronic disease with genetic, psychological, and environmental components that influence its onset and progression.[274] It interacts with different neural systems including endogenous opioid, serotonergic, and dopaminergic systems.[275,276] Alcoholism is often associated with psychiatric disorders, such as anxiety and mood disorders. Here too, there is a correlation between stress and alcohol abuse, probably through the action of CRH released in response to stress, which favors an increase in the GABA neurotransmission produced by alcohol.[277] Cerebral atrophy is seen in the frontal lobes, limbic system, and cerebellum, responsible for memory loss, and diminished cognitive and decision-making skills, depending on the severity and duration of substance abuse.[277,278]

Patients who suffer from insomnia, however, have an increased stimulation of the sympathetic nervous system and the HPA axis,[279] experiencing more physical problems, anxiety, depression, and greater propensity to abuse toxic substances.[280]

## Mechanisms of bio-psycho-behavioral responses to stress and pain

Allostasis is the set of adaptive reactions that help the individual to maintain homeostasis in the face of a given level of stress (pain, trauma, disease, etc.). Allostasis is maintained through the coordinated action of the cardiovascular, endocrine, immune, and nervous systems, which all show a different degree of activity, as a function of circadian rhythms and in response to the external and internal demands of the organism. These systems are involved in dealing with the process of adaptation and are much more effective when they are able to take action, but also to be deactivated quickly if their reaction is no longer necessary.

Usually the body responds to environmental stress by activating the HPA axis and changing some physiological parameters. Through the release of CRH, the hypothalamus stimulates the pituitary gland to produce ACTH, which in turn acts on the adrenal cortex by increasing the production of cortisol. The hippocampus records the physiological variation of cortisol and, by means of a mechanism of sending retroactive information to the hypothalamus, regulates the production. Stress and its alarm reaction also triggers an autonomic response (autonomic component), amygdala (affective component), and periaqueductal gray (pain modulation), coordinating sensory input with emotional content and cognitive attributes, in order to activate a behavior response and survival.[281]

The system is expected to slow to avoid overactivity, allowing the resumption of anabolic and recovery processes. The defense system is thus auto-activated and auto-deactivated, while the interaction of cortical, subcortical, and brainstem centers enables learning and memory, for complete management of the situation. But if stress prevails, then one reaches exhaustion, causing effects on pain, memory, sleep, and habits about the stimulus. Acute stress is capable of causing chronic increased cortisol, which can in turn cause hyperglycemia, hyperlipidemia, arterial hypertension, modulation of the immune system,[282] and the suppression of the neural mechanisms which underlie short-term memory, by acting on the hippocampus and on the temporal lobe. These effects are reversible and of relatively short duration.[283] However, acute and repeated stressful events can cause atrophy of dendrites of pyramidal neurons in some regions of the hippocampus, causing an increased secretion of glucocorticoids and excitatory amino acids. This atrophy is potentially reversible, but, in the course of chronic stress, can degenerate to the loss of any ability to regulate cortisol production.[284] This has been reported in cases of depression, post-traumatic stress disorder, and Cushing's syndrome.[285]

The hippocampus plays an important role in episodic and declarative memory and is particularly involved in the context of memory, relative to the time and place of occurrence of an event with a strong emotional impact. A decrease in hippocampus function involves a decrease in the reliability and accuracy of this type of memory mechanism that contributes to consider a stressful being perceived in circumstances that are non-threatening.[286] Even the autonomic axis is activated with devastating systemic consequences, including bone and immune system tissue. Osteoblasts[287] and lymphoid cells[269] have β-adrenergic specific receptors through which the sympathetic nervous system can modulate the activity through the release of neuropeptides such as neuropeptide Y. Orthosympathetic activation has been shown to reduce bone mass[288] and accelerate the replication of HIV,[289] as well as idiopathic arthritis.[290]

Finally, the subjective perception of the stressor event is able to activate cognitive mechanisms, which lead to the inability to directly express the "fight-or-flight" reaction at the somatic or behavioral level (action inhibition), the memory of which can lead to the onset of diseases by chronic

stress.[291] This is also observed in the brain–viscera–immunity relationship: anxiety worsens in the case of intestinal problems[292,293] and triggers inflammatory digestive problems,[294,295] maintaining a cycle of mutual aggravation of the immune-visceral response and the psychological-emotional state.[296] Neurophysiology highlights the involvement of limbic and paralimbic systems, including the insula, in the two-dimensional relationship between the brain and the gut,[297,298] showing a correlation between the intensity of general hypersensitivity and emotional instability.[299]

According to Elkiss,[98] the allostatic reaction is primarily handled by the integrated musculoskeletal, immune, neurological and endocrine system (MINE). The four components of the system are interdependent and autopoietic, forming a feedback (and in some cases feedforward) mechanism which can be interpreted as closed because of the sharing of common ligands and associated receptors. Neurotransmitters, peptides, hormones, cytokines, and endocannabinoids are the biochemical messengers responsible for the cross-talk between the systems, whose interaction is much more complex than the sum of their individual activities.

The MINE system interacts dynamically with internal and external environmental factors, to maintain health: it responds to overcome the pain and stress, ensuring defense, cohabitation with, or adaptation to both. Stress, comorbidity, the social component, as well as the inherent vulnerability of the system, could deregulate the MINE network and its response capabilities, providing the development of a nociceptive stimulation in chronic pain. This dysregulation can occur as a result of the alteration of the system response threshold, as demonstrated in chronic pain experiences and post-traumatic stress.[300]

This happens when stress is too high or repetitive, but can also occur from an imbalance of the systems themselves or their inability to be activated or deactivated in an appropriate manner. When systems are not disabled at the appropriate time, they can cause organ damage or promote a disease, whereas when not responding adequately, they can cause an increase in other system activities normally counter-regulated by them.[301] Such multisystemic dysregulation of the stress response interacts with psychosocial factors, painting a potentially responsible biological picture of a large family of vague symptoms, nonspecific, and of different nature, which only rarely results in an accurate diagnosis, but rather remains within the limits of the clinically altered situation, albeit never frankly pathological. Similar presentations are known in the international literature as MUS (medically unexplained symptoms) (Box 8.13).[302-305]

---

**Box 8.13**

Some examples of disorders related to medically unexplained symptoms (MUS)

- Frequent feeling of general tiredness
- Difficulty concentrating
- Panic attacks, crying
- Irritability
- Sleep disorders
- Change in body mass not associated with nutritional changes (metabolic alterations)
- Functional disorders of the genitourinary, cardiovascular, and gastrointestinal systems.

---

The MINE model, which is based on the biopsychosocial model, emphasizes the critical role of the muscular-neuro-immune-endocrine system and of the dysregulation system,[306] of which neurogenic inflammation is a good example. From the osteopathic point of view, one of the main mechanisms underlying the genesis and maintenance of somatic dysfunction due to irritation consists of primary afferent fibers (C fibers), following a nociceptive stimulation (thermal, chemical, physical), being able to release pro-inflammatory neuropeptides (such as substance P and somatostatin), until the eventual generation of neurogenic inflammation. If persistent, as in the case of tissue damage, the stimulation of these nerve fibers alters their own activation threshold, producing an area of hyperalgesia or peripheral sensitization,[307] with relative changes of tissue texture from vascular and immune activation.[308]

The hyperactivity of these fibers determines the release of excitatory amino acids and of substance P in the dorsal horn of the spinal cord, which induces a series of events: activation of N-methyl-D-aspartate (NMDA) channels, phosphorylation, alterations in membrane properties, resulting in induction of genes and the release of facilitatory substances such as dynorphin – which reduces the activation threshold causing hyperexitability[309] – resulting in pathological changes in the tissues, such as terminal sprouting, increase in receptor fields,[310] apoptosis of sensitization of the inhibitory neurons[311] and hyperalgesia.[312] This also causes an alteration of the anterior roots and visceral efferent fibers, causing, respectively, changes in muscle and organ tone, and sudo/vasomotor changes in the corresponding spinal segments.

These phenomena determine changes in the spinal gray matter that result in spinal facilitation (central sensitization). This is a process that can trigger a cascade of local and global responses: chronic pain and connective tissue remodeling,[246] impaired mechanoception and muscle control,[313] followed by further neural and tissue response, cortical reorganization,[314] influences on the endocrine and autonomic routes,[315] and a permanent allostatic change, called "general adaptation syndrome."[311]

The pain may alter the activity of the higher centers, reducing their ability to process sensory, cognitive, and affective information,[316] with reorganization of the motor cortex associated with change of motor control[317] and postural control deficits,[318] and alteration of the function and structure of the central nervous system.[319] There may be dysfunctional reactions of many bodily systems and abnormalities in metabolism and cerebral perfusion,[320] with neural processes completely different from those that characterize acute pain.[321]

While the lateral system is projected to the somatosensory primary and secondary cortex, passing through the lateral thalamus, allowing discrimination of duration, intensity and origin of the nociceptive stimulus, the medial system is projected toward the brainstem and then to the medial thalamus, anterior cingulate cortex, amygdala, and back to the brainstem, from which depart ascending and descending pathways for nociception modulation.[322,323] The medial nociceptive system is associated with autonomic, emotional, and motor responses, because of which sensory afferents are correlated with autonomic efferents and motor actions of defense and avoidance. Researchers have demonstrated a cortical reorganization and cell loss in the anterior insula and cingulate in patients with chronic pain, such as low back pain,[324] tension headache,[325] and irritable bowel syndrome.[326] Some changes have also been seen in the density of the thalamic gray matter in the prefrontal cortex and the ascending and descending pathways of pain modulation.[319,327,328] Perhaps due to similar processes, in migraine patients researchers observed a thickening of the somatosensory cortex,[329] as well as hyperalgesia with central sensitization in patients with fibromyalgia.[330]

Neurophysiological and neuroimaging studies[331] have shown that nociceptive stimuli induce responses in a large neural network, called the pain matrix, including the somatosensory cortex, insula, and cingulate gyrus, as well as frontal and parietal areas. This network is considered a representation of the intensity of the perception induced by a nociceptive stimulus and related physiological responses, which would make pain an entirely personal sensory, cognitive, and affective experience,[332] capable of altering the behavior, emotions, and even the perception/self-image of one's body.[333–336] Osborn and Smith[337] have shown that in cases of chronic aching the affected body regions are rejected as "self," or even perceived as foreign to the rest of the body. These responses also involve the central autonomic network, which is an integral part of an internal control system, through which the brain controls the visceral-motor, neuroendocrine, pain, posture, and behavioral responses necessary for survival.[338]

This network includes the insular cortex, amygdala, hypothalamus, periaqueductal gray, parabrachial complex, nucleus of the solitary tract, and ventral-lateral medulla and may be critically involved in panic disorder, essential hypertension, obesity, and other medical conditions or circumstances,[339] with consequent bio-behavioral responses.[340] On the other hand researchers also demonstrated the possibility of a genetic predisposition to sensitivity to pain and to amplify the sensory stimulus, thereby increasing the risk of mood disorders.[341] Zubieta and colleagues[342] found that the genes that code for the enzyme catechol-$O$-methyltransferase (COMT) modulate individual sensitivity to pain; the combination of allelic variants of COMT would play a modulation role in pain perception, and in mood and cognitive function, altering the structure of the mRNA that modulates protein expression.[343]

Therefore, the polymorphism of COMT would be able to influence the human experience of pain, by providing a biological explanation to the individual diversity of pain response to stimulus, as well as to the predisposition to develop chronicity.[344] Taken together, these findings may explain a number of local, global, and segmental effects of a given somatic dysfunction, with all its physical, emotional, cognitive, and behavioral parameters, as understood in the concept of the "total osteopathic lesion,"[345] which requires a multidimensional approach to pain and the individual.

## Evidence on the effectiveness of the biopsychosocial model

Systematic reviews have shown significant efficacy of cognitive-behavioral intervention in reducing both pain[346,347] and chronic stress, in addition to depression and the related anxiety.[348–351] However, there is little evidence that psychosocial interventions can improve the course of cancer and cardiovascular diseases,[352,353] so it has been suggested that they can only offer support to cope with the effects of such primarily biological diseases.[354] In other cases, however, such as asthma and rheumatoid arthritis, a psychosocial approach has been shown to improve the symptoms of the condition[335] by reducing the number and activity of IL-2, NK cells and receptors for IgE, as well as the frequency of asthmatic attacks, and the use of bronchodilators after 6 months of therapy.[356]

Finally, as proposed by Schubiner,[354] this is also seen with a third type of presentation, such as headaches, back pain, neck pain, fibromyalgia, chronic pelvic pain, temporomandibular joint syndrome, functional dyspepsia, irritable bowel syndrome, insomnia, and tinnitus, although it is not considered psychosomatic. These were interpreted more as a physiological and pathological disorders (Fig. 8.6), and treatable successfully with psychodynamic approaches.[357,358]

The latter appear to increase tolerance to pain by activating endogenous opioids when the patient is subjected to a painful stimulus.[359] Such approaches make use of coping strategies,[40] self-efficacy mechanisms,[41] and patient empowerment processes[42] to promote the recognition and use of available resources to overcome the experience of pain and related disability. They are also often used for stress reduction techniques, such as:

- mindfulness meditation and mind–body techniques (breathing therapy, Alexander technique, Feldenkrais, tai chi, etc.),[360] which have been shown to reduce symptoms in patients with fibromyalgia,[361] irritable bowel syndrome,[362] cardiac insufficiency,[363] kidney insufficiency,[364] and chronic pain, including musculoskeletal,[365,366] and to improve the quality of life in individuals with a precarious state of health.[367] This probably occurs via the awareness and acceptance of emotionally charged experiences,[368] the activation of specific brain areas used for this function,[369] the reduction in cortisol levels, pro-inflammatory cytokines and blood pressure,[370] and the normalization of body awareness and self-image[371]

- biofeedback techniques such as electromyographic and thermal techniques, which are effective in

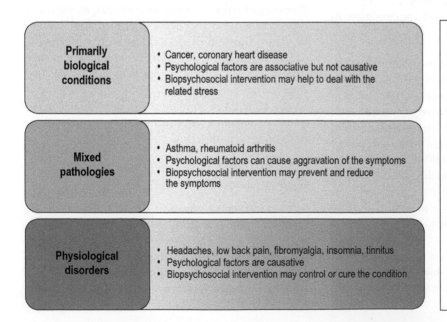

**Primarily biological conditions**
- Cancer, coronary heart disease
- Psychological factors are associative but not causative
- Biopsychosocial intervention may help to deal with the related stress

**Mixed pathologies**
- Asthma, rheumatoid arthritis
- Psychological factors can cause aggravation of the symptoms
- Biopsychosocial intervention may prevent and reduce the symptoms

**Physiological disorders**
- Headaches, low back pain, fibromyalgia, insomnia, tinnitus
- Psychological factors are causative
- Biopsychosocial intervention may control or cure the condition

**Fig. 8.6**
Examples of three types of conditions (organic, mixed, physiological) with the corresponding effects both provoked by psychological factors and achievable by biopsychosocial intervention. Modified from: Schubiner H. Mind-body medicine. In: Chila AG, editor. Foundations of osteopathic medicine. 3rd ed. Philadelphia, PA: Lippincott, Williams and Wilkins; 2011. ch. 27.)

controlling migraines,[372] Raynaud's syndrome,[373] and pain in patients with fibromyalgia[374]

- therapeutic writing techniques[375] are able to produce benefits in patients with fibromyalgia,[376] asthma, and rheumatoid arthritis[377] or in various stress or traumatic situations, even though supported by little evidence[378]

- yoga, which, when applied to patients with chronic disorders, has been shown to influence the level of cortisol, as well as pain, tendency to dramatize, and the level of acceptance of one's condition,[379] and finally to improve functional disability in patients with chronic low back pain[380] in both the short and the long term.[381]

Another integrative approach is neurolinguistic programming, which has been shown to cause neuroimmune interactions, including changing the immune response and immunological reactivity.[382] The principles of neurolinguistic programming are used to develop positive self-identity and bring order to chronologically chaotic and fragmented memories, thus helping to provide continuity and to establish goals.[383] The addition of cognitive therapy to neurolinguistic programming has been shown to alter long-standing and distorted thinking patterns, among other factors that can cause and perpetuate depression.[384]

Social media is exercising an influence that should not be underestimated in this therapeutic process, given that interdisciplinary and intersectional action, at the social level, can support quality of life,[385] as well as the process of health during the course of life.[386] To confirm this, individuals married or involved in social and religious groups demonstrated a lower mortality by 50% over the course of 9 years,[387] when compared to people with depression.[388] Spirituality and prayer assume a supporting role in dealing with disease, promoting acceptance, forgiveness, tolerance to pain, and improve physical, psychological, and social function,[389–391] and also creating a sense of optimism, as shown in patients undergoing cardiac surgery.[392]

In these cases, when spiritual support is associated with social support, regardless of the type or level of spirituality practiced, there was a 10-fold increase in survival as compared to those who did not have these support systems.[393] However, a related spirituality, church attendance and prayer, have shown a lack of correlation with cardiac morbidity or mortality in patients with acute myocardial infarction, associated with depression or poor social support.[394] Spirituality could have an impact on the health and welfare of the individual, and is considered in patient care as a placebo mechanism, relaxation, expression of positive emotions, direct or indirect influence of pain perception,[395] or even as a channel for supernatural intervention,[396] effectively supporting the coping capacity of the individual.[397] The fact is that the combination of different noetic methods (such as prayer, music, imagery, and healing touch) has been shown to reduce anxiety and emotional distress, but especially mortality compared to a single administration of such prayer, as well as the standard of care, in patients undergoing percutaneous coronary intervention[398] (although there was no indication of difference in outcome between the groups).

In the care process, communication is essential. Research has shown the value of effective communication between patient and operator in improving the outcomes of common medical conditions such as hypertension, headache, anxiety, and diabetes.[399] The choice of language is critical, since it can affect motor patterns of the listener[400] as well as the relational similarity between the interlocutors.[401] In turn, communication must be based on empathy, understood primarily as a cognitive process[402] through which the operator can act on the psychobiology of the patient. However, research with positron emission tomography has also shown this to be a neurobiological answer, via the activation of a specific neural network,[403] capable of generating synchronicity of autonomic and emotional activity, if the two parties come into full empathetic interaction.[404,405] The osteopath can therefore seek empathy as a clinical procedure that uses an "emotional resonance"[406] to reach communicative resonance able to produce a neurobiological intervention.[106] The system of mirror neurons may help to explain this response of empathic resonance.[407,408]

Recent reviews have shown a small but significant effect on the operator and patient health outcomes,[409] while others suggest that interventions prone to change the communicative relationship toward a more patient-centric approach do not show significant evidence of improved measurable health outcomes or satisfaction.[410] It is also true, however, that patients who have received more communication and patient-centric care, during a medical examination, have shown less concern about their complaints and symptoms, an increase in mental well-being 2 months after the visit, i.e., a 50% reduction in the need for referral to other specialists and a 40% reduction in the need for further diagnostic tests.[411] Interestingly, a non-correlation was observed in the study mentioned above, between the patient's subjective perception of how the visit was focused on his or her person and objective assessment of how this had actually happened, by analysis of audio recordings of the visit, which once again highlights the dominance of the perception of the experience over the experience itself, on human psycho-physiological responses.

The patient-centered communicative approach is congruent with osteopathic principles, as osteopaths seem to show a greater ability to listen and interact with the patient, discussing preventive measures, social activities, family relations, and emotional states more than the allopathic doctors.[412] However, osteopaths seem lacking in properly communicating the nature of the treatment and the related expected level of pain, as well as the potential adverse after-effects of treatment, and finally the strategies on how to prevent the pain.[413]

The multidisciplinary approach has proven essential for the achievement of the best clinical outcomes, especially in chronic patients[414,415] suffering from musculoskeletal pain,[416] and in the primary medical care sector.[417] Multidisciplinary rehabilitation is a more effective standard of care for patients with chronic low back pain, especially if organized in collaboration with various local health care authorities.[418] Behavioral outcomes such as return to work are best achieved with multidisciplinary therapeutic approaches rather than unimodal ones, both short and long term.[419]

This approach can be extended to include relaxation techniques, biofeedback, hypnosis, cognitive behavioral therapy,[420] social reinforcement, and controlled drug treatment, but may also require the integration of rehabilitation, occupational, surgical, orthotic, psychological, and nutritional care. Psychological support for patients with relationship difficulties and suffering from chronic musculoskeletal pain seems to have a significant impact on the rehabilitation process for the patients' physical condition,[421] and can enhance immune and cardiovascular function.[422,423] In addition, group therapy programs appear effective, even for patients with chronic musculoskeletal pain, and have been shown to improve the awareness and use of active coping strategies, as well as decreasing the pain experience.[424]

Finally, it has been shown that group and psycho-educational support can increase immune activity and survival rates in patients suffering from cancer.[425,426] This group model would help to increase activity levels and to effectively apply pain management skills, and allow for the treatment of a significant number of patients at relatively low cost.[427]

Physical activity is closely related to health, given that the risk of mortality decreases in both sexes with the improvement of physical fitness.[428] Regular exercise increases physical and psychological health,[429,430] enhances proprioception,[431,432] immune response,[433] and the sleep pattern,[429] reduces stress,[434] and the risk of developing cancer[435,436] and cardiovascular diseases,[437] probably by acting on mood and reducing the perception of and physiological reactivity to stress.[438] For example, research has shown that physical exercise is associated with an increase in KAT (kynurenine aminotransferase) enzyme's ability to convert kynurenine, produced during stress conditions, into kynurenic acid, a substance that cannot pass from the blood to the brain.[439] In addition, exercise also promoted the increase of irisine, which induces proliferation of peroxisomes, active γ receptors and the levels of PGC-1α1 protein, with effects on circulation, differentiation of osteoblasts, nerve cells, and the regeneration of B cells.[440] At the same time, specific stretching protocols can produce long-term benefits in patients suffering from chronic pain, such as improved function and satisfaction levels.[441] However, excessive exercise without adequate recovery may cause changes in the number and function of immune cells.[434]

A triptophanic or atherogenic diet may increase tissue oxidative damage with infiltration of inflammatory immune cells.[442] Conversely, a diet with a balanced ratio of omega 6/omega 3 seems to be crucial in maintaining health[443] or in the prevention and management of inflammatory conditions,[444] or even as a supplementary treatment of chronic arthritis.[445] The diet may be viewed as a natural approach with a specific anti-inflammatory effect.[446] It includes a reduced contribution of saturated fat and is rich in plant-based foods and dairy products,[447] beverages with a high rate of polyphenolic catechins (such as green tea), cold-water fish,[448] and herbal culinary spices with anti-inflammatory effects, such as ginger and turmeric.[449]

A group of aromatic ketones, called chalcones, present in many plants such as liquorice and mulberry, have been associated with immune-modulator, anti-inflammatory, and antioxidant effects.[450] Among the many choices, avocado and soybean oils contain biologically active substances that can produce long-term beneficial effects in cases of osteoarthritis;[451] the devil's claw is used for degenerative disorders for pain relief, and as an anti-inflammatory and antioxidant;[452] crude bilberry extract, rich in phenolic acids and flavonoids, has antinociceptive and anti-inflammatory action;[453] extracts of plants such as phyllantus or myrobalan have powerful antinociceptive properties.[454]

Avoidance of incorrect habits or vices, such as smoking, is part of the strengthening of the health process. It has been estimated that by 2020 tobacco alone will cause more death and disability than any other disease.[455] Thus prevention is the best strategy for limiting cigarette smoking and its adverse effects.[456] Behavioral strategies,[457] multimodal approaches,[458] educational programs, motivational encouragement, face to face with a therapist, group therapy to stimulate mutual support, traditional and complementary treatments, and long-term follow-up[459] have been shown to produce good results, breaking the vicious cycle of tobacco and stress.

Regarding the abuse of alcohol, however, denial and minimization are usually used as mechanisms to view the addiction as less severe than it is, especially when confronted by a health care professional. Other manipulative attitudes usually emerge to avoid admitting the problem. However, research suggests that, if abstinence is maintained for more than 6 months, partial brain function can be recovered and that 5–15 minutes of motivational counseling can reduce abuse by 25%,[460] as can family, medical, and group therapies.[461]

With regard to weight gain, obesity and excessive intake of salt and fat, interventions directed to weight loss and maintenance of ideal body weight have shown better results when they are pursued with discipline and consistency over time,[462] as well as when supported by adequate family support.[463] Finally, for the treatment of sleep disorders, cognitive-behavioral strategies directed at re-establishing normal sleep patterns have been shown to be at least as effective as sedative hypnotics in acute phases, as well as more effective in the long term,[464] including patients affected by psychiatric disorders.[465]

In conclusion, the more the evaluation is multifactorial and biopsychosocial, the more global the plan of action focused on the patient, the better the quality of life and the long-term reported pain levels.[348,466] The intensity of chronic pain, and the impact this has on the individual's life, is reduced significantly with cognitive-behavioral treatment.[467] From the point of view of health care costs, group sessions for patients in distress, patient education, social support and coping strategies, and the ability to interact individually with the doctor all increase customer satisfaction and quality of care of the patient, and reduce hospitalization costs, visits to the emergency department, and specialist referrals.[468]

## Mechanisms of effectiveness of the biopsychosocial model

It is well established that the nervous, endocrine, and immune systems interact as a "super-system," through mutual adjustment effects, which could be the basis of the interaction between mind, body, and behavior and their impact both in health and in disease. Communication takes place via molecules produced by nerve, immune, or endocrine cells equipped with receptors capable of decoding messages from the network as a whole.[469]

Neuropeptides can modulate the activity of other non-peptide neurotransmitters, with completion of their action in a way similar to that of hormones directed both to the central nervous system and to the peripheral organs. For example, the neuropeptide TRF can stimulate the secretion of thyroid hormones and simultaneously induce an increase of alertness, mood, and motor activity of the individual. The neuropeptides are also produced by immune cells: the cytokines released and transported through the bloodstream and along the major cranial nerves – particularly the vagus nerve[470] – stimulate the activity of the locus coeruleus and the hypothalamic secretion of CRF, mediating biological phenomena such as body temperature, feeding behavior, sleep-wake cycle, mood, psychomotor activity, and psychological states such as anxiety or depression.[201] Consequently, the neuroendocrine input from the pituitary and hypothalamus can affect the immune cell function and cytokine release.

Finally, emotional and behavioral states affect the nervous system, the immune response and its reactivity, such as the proliferation of lymphocytes and the levels of IL-1, IL-2, IL-4, IL-6, and interferon.[471,472] It has been shown that negative affective states lower the levels of antibodies to, for example, herpes simplex virus type 1 and 2, and Epstein-Barr virus, while the positive affective states have the opposite effect.[222]

A similar relationship also exists between the heart and brain; the cardiac atria secrete a hormone known as atrial natriuretic factor, which influences certain brain structures such as the amygdala – used for the regulation of emotional states with consequent effects on memory and the ability to learn[473] – as well as the hypothalamus and the pituitary gland, regulating the production of melatonin and thus the chronobiological rhythms and changes in mood. This process facilitates the correlation between thought and emotional states, so the expression of emotion becomes a critical instrument to preserve the individual and the company's state of health.[474] The expression of emotions, designed also as a biological phenomenon, strengthens the immune system that creates a state of relaxation, trust or joy, increasing the secretion of interferons and interleukins at the cellular level and in the brain dopamine production.

Interferons and interleukins increase the polarization of the cell membrane, making the cells more resistant to pathogenic organisms.[475] In addition, neurological signals from the heart directly influence the activity of the amygdala and basal nuclei, generating a rapid behavioral response to perceived dangers in the environment and influencing the storage process of behavioral patterns.[476] Inconsistent signals from the heart affect the amygdala activity that assesses the dangerous state according to sensory information; if the state of danger is high, it directly sends signals to the thalamus and the autonomic nervous system, activating emergency response behaviors.[477] Negative emotions cause a disorder of the heart rhythm and the autonomic nervous system, thus adversely affecting the whole body; conversely, positive emotions bring greater harmony and consistency in heart rhythms and improve balance in the nervous system.[478]

It is therefore reasonable to expect that OMT, which affects neural transmission, may have an impact on behavioral states. One of the ways in which OMT could affect the neuro-immune cross-talk consists in modulating the release of neuropeptides. Neuropeptide receptors may be found in the brain as in leukocytes, which in turn produce response cytokines (IL-1, IL-2, IL-4 and IL-6).[229,230] These cytokines can bind specifically to the hypothalamus and the pituitary gland, acting as a neurotransmitter in the central nervous system through modulation of synaptic transmission.[479] Their psycho-neural activities, considered altogether, include the stimulation and inhibition of corticotropic hormone release, β-endorphins, growth hormone, luteinizing hormone, follicle stimulating hormone, prolactin, and other pituitary hormones.[229,480] The result of these interactions is a measurable alteration in behavior and immune function.[230] For example, OMT has proven to be an effective adjunctive therapy in women with depression, with 100% of patients achieving normal psychometric values after 8 weeks of intervention (compared to 33% of the control group).[481] Researchers did not observe significant differences or trends between the groups in the levels of production of cytokines (IL-1, IL-10, IL-2, IL-4 and IL-6) and antibodies (anti-HSV-1, anti-HSV-2, anti-EBV), nor did they identify any specific pattern of structural dysfunctions.

Another way that would allow OMT to produce multisystemic effects, including behavioral and psychological effects, could be that of nitric oxide (NO), a neurotransmitter and hormone on the cardiovascular, immune, and nervous systems,[482] which showed a significant increase after OMT,[483] as much as after moderate physical activity,[484] through the activation of nitric oxide synthase. NO may play an important role in modulating and reducing inflammation,[483] in tissue repair, promoting cell proliferation and migration[485,486] and the synthesis of collagen, thus improving clinical symptoms and functional recovery after injury[487] as well as the relaxation of smooth muscles and angiogenesis. It has been shown that NO plays an important role in neurotransmission[488] and in response to immunogens,[489] but especially in decreasing heart rate, creating a sense of well-being a lessening of antibacterial and antiviral effect through the modulation of neurotransmitters and behavioral aspects,[490] perhaps also due to cross-talk between NO receptors and atrial natriuretic peptides.[491]

Another way by which OMT can affect mood, immune, and neural system activity might be by stimulating the endocannabinoid system,[492] resulting in an increase of up to 68% in serum anandamide levels after treatment. Activation of this system can reduce afferent nociception and tissue inflammation[493] by modulating the immune system (IL-2, T helper 1, etc.) and reducing blood levels of several biomarkers in patients with chronic musculoskeletal pain.[494] There is also an increase in N-palmitoylethanolamide, a powerful endogenous fatty acid amide with analgesic and anti-inflammatory properties, 30 minutes after OMT on patients with chronic low back pain, which was double the concentration observed in the control group. The endocannabinoid system has been shown to produce mood changes through interaction with the central nervous system and the HPA axis, to modulate peripheral and central sensitization processes and the activity of the autonomic system,[495] by producing cardiovascular effects and smooth muscle relaxation,[496] also by release of nitrogen monoxide by vascular,[497] neuronal, and immune endothelial cells.[498]

Through a similar process, the placebo effect may intervene as a biological process during and after administration of OMT.[499] Placebo analgesia is considered a biological phenomenon that activates opioid and non-opioid mechanisms,[500] measurable through brain imaging technologies, which may be pharmacologically blocked and exaggerated by behavior.[501] It seems to be related to the area that generates and maintains frontal cortical cognitive processes, which in turn can be reinforced by dopaminergic reward pathways (gratification).[502] Dopamine is linked through the associated stimulus-response system to free reward, essential to control behaviors learned from previous experiences. If a person experiences constant failures and believes he or she is not able to perform a given action, then the dopamine levels are markedly lower, decreasing the motivation once one achieves one's goals and making one susceptible to depression and feelings of rejection.[503] It is considered plausible today that the placebo effect modulates responsiveness of the peripheral immune system,[504] although other placebo responses originate from a less conscious process, such as classical conditioning in the case of immune, hormonal, and respiratory function.[505] The current research on placebo response, and on placebo and nocebo analgesia, showed that the psychosocial aspect of any treatment is crucial in determining the nature and degree of a placebo effect, impacting on both research and clinical practice.[506,507] In addition, complementary medicine approaches may have an increased placebo effect compared to allopathic medicine, through efficacy based on ritual,[508] in addition to the activation of areas such as the anterior cingulate cortex through manual contact.[509]

Hormonal mediation could explain the multisystemic and behavioral effects of OMT. OMT has been shown to reduce the perception of pain and the level of stress hormones.[510] Evidence suggests that manual therapy has an effect mediated by hormones that persist for days, modulating the HPA axis and immune function.[511-513] However, the hormonal response has been demonstrated to not happen in the case of isolated articulatory osteopathic techniques such as rib raising.[514] Therapy sessions twice a week have been shown to increase levels of oxytocin and reduce those of arginine-vasopressin and cortisol.[512] These changes persisted for 4 days with changes in cytokines up to 8 days after the treatment. In another study,[513] an increase of oxytocin was correlated with a decrease in adrenocorticotropic hormone after manual intervention. Oxytocin could play a role as an endogenous pain control system. After manual therapy, high levels of this hormone have been found in plasma and in the periaqueductal gray matter, showing antinociceptive effects probably through interaction with the opioid system.[515] But even more important is the strong relationship that oxytocin would have with the formation of social or interpersonal ties based on trust,[516] thus affecting the psychosocial dimension of the individual.

OMT has also been shown to indirectly produce a reduction in stress levels correlated with modulation of hyper-sympathicotonia,[517] normalization of the effects on heart rate variability,[518] endothelial function,[519] and on the levels of anxiety and depression as demonstrated in other manual therapeutic areas,[520] although in some cases reduction of psychological stress, the state of anger and stress levels, and perceived pain revealed an association with increasing orthosympathetic activities as a result of manual intervention.[521,522] Finally, an increase in parasympathetic response was observed after specific fascial treatments, with effects on blood flow turbulence and blood shear rate,[523] while an increase in cardiac vagal modulation and a decrease in oxygenation in the prefrontal brain lobes were found after application of cranial techniques.[524]

Interestingly, studies on interception[525] have discovered a representation of the information about the body's state in the lobe of the insula, a major portion of the limbic formation, thus presenting an anatomical bridge between mental state and somatic function. "Tactile C fibers" have recently been detected in the human subcutaneous connective tissue,[526] used for the conduction of distinct tactile information in humans, even though C fibers are classically described as nociceptors, or chemoreceptors. These fibers are activated during light touch, as happens during many manual therapies (but also in sham control groups), by sending signals to the rear insular area (but not to the somatosensory area), where sensory and affective information are integrated by generating the "limbic tract," with consequent chain effects on behavior, psycho-endocrine function, immune system activity, autonomic regulation, and modulation of pain.[527] Therefore, tactile stimuli, such as those applied during the OMT, would activate multimodal receptors and consequent tissue and neural responses[528,529] through rapid myelinated ways and access the discriminative cortical and cognitive systems, allowing an analytical assessment of touch while using slower pathways to the limbic brain, resulting in affective and emotional impressions to tactile stimulation[530] and the coloring of experience and past memories, to determine bio-behavioral responses and possible changes of interception, self-image, and body awareness.[531]

## Further development of the biopsychosocial model

The crisis of the "biomedical" paradigm has opened the way for a broader consideration of the factors involved in sickness and in health, toward an approach which includes:

- the inseparability of mind and body in the influence on health and disease

- the multifactorial nature of the causes that affect health and disease and the effects generated by them

- the interaction between macro-processes (such as social support) and micro-processes (such as

imbalances in biochemical and cellular level) and intermediate processes (such as cognitive affective attributes and contents) in the establishment of the state of health or disease

- the concept that health is a goal that must be achieved positively, through attention to the needs of biological, psychological, and social order, and not as a state that should only be safeguarded.

Health is therefore seen as a resource for everyday life, and not as the goal of life; it is a positive concept emphasizing personal and social resources, as well as physical capacities. An individual or group must be able to change the surrounding environment or cope, to identify and to realize aspirations, to satisfy his or her own needs to achieve a state of complete physical, mental and social well-being (Fig. 8.7).

The Ottawa Charter, promoted by the World Health Organization in 1986,[532] defines health promotion as the process of enabling people to exercise more control over their health and to improve it by reducing the obvious differences in the current social stratification, and giving everyone equal

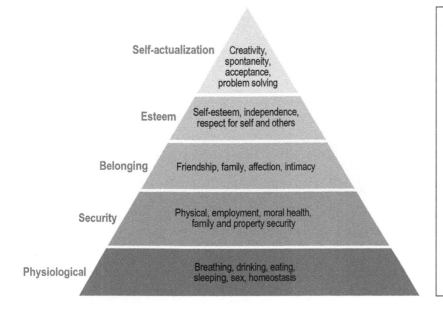

**Fig. 8.7**
The main needs of man presented in a pyramidal organization, according to the Maslow model. The needs are divided into five categories: physiological, safety, belonging, esteem, and self-actualization needs. Modified from: Maslow A. Motivation and personality. New York: Harper; 1954.

Self-actualization — Creativity, spontaneity, acceptance, problem solving

Esteem — Self-esteem, independence, respect for self and others

Belonging — Friendship, family, affection, intimacy

Security — Physical, employment, moral health, family and property security

Physiological — Breathing, drinking, eating, sleeping, sex, homeostasis opportunities and resources to achieve the maximum health potential possible. This includes:

- the skills necessary for life

- the ability to make healthy and appropriate choices about one's own health, through the development of individual skills and the appropriate information and education toward an always increasing health control

- the creation of welcoming environments and offering adequate support for the pursuit of health

- the strengthening of local communities so that citizens can make autonomous health decisions

- the reorientation of health services, making them more suitable for interaction with each other, in an approach called "cross-sector" providing, that is, the intervention, collaboration, and coordination

of different sectors of society (education, culture, transport, agriculture, tourism, etc.) to implement initiatives for improving community health.

Consequently, we must propose strategies that address in parallel disease prevention and health promotion policies, understood as the analysis and understanding of the determinants of health (Fig. 8.8). The Dahlgren and Whitehead model[533] is the main determinant of health viewed as a series of concentric arcs around the individual, ranging from genetic factors (age, sex, and genetic) which cannot be modified by more general social conditions, such as social and community networks and individual lifestyles (Fig. 8.9). The closest arcs are the ones most influenced by individual human behaviors, while those further away require the involvement of all institutions and forces of the community. Social forces can act collectively, shaping the individual's biology, risk behaviors, environmental exposures, and access to resources that promote health. Not surprisingly, people with fragile social

**Socioeconomic and macroeconomic determinants and income distribution mode**

- Wealth of the country and redistribution policies
- Level of education and type of work
- Structure of the family and social networks

**Lifestyle**

- Tobacco addiction, abuse of alcohol and/or drugs
- Diet and power quality
- Physical activity and sexual behavior

**Environment**

- Pollutants: outdoor (dioxins, fine particulates, heavy metals, ozone); indoor (cigarette smoke); water (microbial agents, metals, pesticides and nitrates)
- Food contaminants
- Environmental noise; modification of the biosphere

**Health promotion**

- Active protective measures (home security and prevention of accidents, use of seat belts and helmets, prevention of fire and heat stroke) and risk intervention
- Disease prevention (screening and vaccinations)
- Health promotion in several key settings (workplaces, schools, health institutions, etc.)

Fig. 8.8
The main determinants of health, divided into four levels (socioeconomic, lifestyle, environment, health promotion), as described by the Ministry of Health, Italy (www.salute.gov.it/imgs/C_17_pubblicazioni_1144_ulteriorialle-gati_ulterioreallegato _1_alleg.pdf)

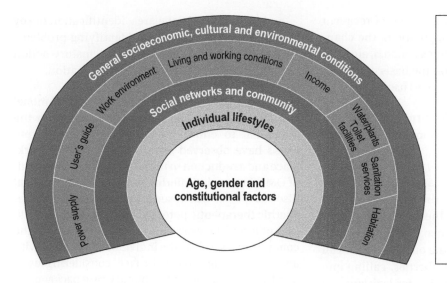

**Fig. 8.9**
The determinants of health according to the Dahlgren and Whitehead model.

networks have a higher risk of becoming ill or dying prematurely,[534] while a good psychosocial balance strengthens disease resistance.[535] Increased understanding of these determinants is therefore crucial to reduce disparities in the health of the population and to ensure maximum possible longevity. Some researchers have proposed the following ideal balance of these factors: socioeconomic factors and lifestyles (40–50%), the state and the conditions of the environment (20–33%), genetic inheritance (20–30%), and health services (10–15%).[536]

The analysis of traditional epidemiological data has shown that incongruous lifestyles are not evenly distributed in the population. It was pointed out, for example, that tobacco smoking is higher in men and women with low levels of formal education, low income, and low employment level.[537] We must therefore investigate the conditions that determine the risks. According to the World Health Organization in 2008, 86% of deaths, 77% of the loss of years of healthy life, and 75% of health care costs in Europe and Italy are caused by certain chronic diseases (cardiovascular disease, cancer, diabetes, respiratory disease, mental health problems, and musculoskeletal disorders), which have in common modifiable risk factors, such as tobacco smoking, obesity and

being overweight, alcohol abuse, low consumption of fruits and vegetables, a sedentary lifestyle, excess lipids in the blood, and high blood pressure. These risk factors alone are responsible for 60% of the loss of years of healthy life in Europe and in Italy.

To counter these trends, it is necessary to enact policies that promote health. This includes research and upgrading of health resources, i.e., every factor that increases the capacity of individuals, communities, populations, systems, and institutions to maintain wellness. It is possible to identify the resources in all the determinants of health, including genetic determinants, social circumstances, environmental conditions, choices of behavior, and health services. At the individual level, these resources include social skills, techniques for resisting negative stimuli, the presence of positive values, self-esteem and strengthening of individual resources (empowerment).

The types of intervention refer to different strategies[538] that can be categorized as follows:

- *Communication strategies*: allowing transmittal of a message regarding knowledge, attitudes, and health behaviors, reaching a large number of subjects. They differ in the type of recipient (individual, community, population), the channel (personal, media technology, media, etc.) and languages (differentiated on the basis of characteristics of the target population) used.

- *Educational strategies*: adopt traditional teaching methods (lectures, workshops, laboratories).

- *Strategies relating to health policies* include the issuance of guidelines, laws and regulations governing behavior relative to the health of individuals and the community. The use of this type of strategy is controversial, since, on the one hand it ensures public health, on the other, it borders on the territory of individual liberties, calling into question an ethical dimension for legislators to take into account.

- *Strategies of health "engineering"*: dealing with change at a structural level (the services and systems of care) in order to provide health promotion conditions. These are intended to influence the environment rather than to act directly on the individual (e.g., to equip cars with proper safety equipment).

- *Strategies relating to health services for the community*: these concern treatments (screening, childhood vaccinations, preventive examinations) that can easily reach a large number of people and put them in contact with health professionals.

- *Community activation strategies*: provide for the involvement and participation of the community in the processes of identification of problems and resources related to the health and decision-making phase of interventions for health promotion programming. The aim here is to promote social support, provide information, and motivate people to be active protagonists with a significant process of commitment and within a dedicated time level. It implies the creation of relations of trust among individuals and institutions in the area, identification of key people in the community, identifying problems in which to intervene, and participatory action planning, implementation, and evaluation.

The osteopath applying the biopsychosocial model can then calibrate the therapeutic focus from the individual to entire social environments. Recent works have observed less absence from the workplace and a reduction in the intake of drugs as a result of OMT in people suffering from painful functional disorders,[539,540] which suggests that there is an osteopathic therapeutic potential for a category of workers subjected to stress, and thus an impact on the community as well as the individual, especially with an integrated approach. In fact, considering osteopathy within a "multidisciplinary care package,"[541] several studies have shown that it is also a valuable support tool for special categories, such as military personnel, because it improves quality of life, work efficiency,[542] and acute back pain symptoms.[543]

A recent study shows that osteopaths have been able to bridge the cultural gap between the people of Haiti and evidence-based medicine, by using manipulative approaches similar to traditional ethnomedical Haitian practices. This study showed that facilitating trust in Western medicine stimulates integration between the two medical approaches, with significant impact on a disadvantaged population's health status.[544] Moreover, there are increasing voluntary organizations in the community of osteopathic practice.[545-547] They always seem to attract more professionals willing to engage directly in improving living conditions in rural communities. The osteopath, using an empathetic approach in his or her work, can therefore shift the focus from the individual to the community, using treatment based on beliefs or evidence to a practice based on his or her conscience. Research in cognitive and emotional development shows that the empathic process begins when the child acquires skills in the use of language, is able to express and reveal emotions, and develops a sense of reciprocity and social duty, including the most evolved form of empathic response, or the ability to feel the suffering of an entire group of people, or even of another species, as if it were his or her own.[548] It conquers the concept of consciousness (universal communion) – a process that never ends, but that osteopathy seems to have already marked with milestones and biopsychosocial achievements.

## Conclusions

Stress and pain can have multisystemic effects on the body, and cause profound changes in human behavior, with an impact on the physical state, the psyche, and quality of life. Numerous biological diseases can manifest with psychological symptoms, and many medical diseases may precipitate emotional distress, which complicates the treatment and increases health care costs. Maladaptive behaviors, fears, and emotional experiences of pain, catastrophism, helplessness, expectations, trust, cognitive factors, faith, beliefs and personality all need to be taken into account through an integrative conceptual model and comprehensive evaluation, intervention, and management of patients with pain, particularly if persistent.[549]

Osteopathic medicine, at its most basic level, is a way to modify the changes related to pain[550,551] by local, segmental, regional, and global effects on neuro-musculoskeletal activity, resulting in effects on the autonomic and limbic systems, attempts to change behavior, offering the patient a chance to feel better, approaching not the symptom, but the cause of it, through an intervention that incorporates evidence-based guidelines.[17] Educating the patient to achieve understanding and self-management

of pain, of its generators and management mechanisms, until one gains full control of it, is therapeutic; indeed, adequate information, in plain language, allows one to improve clinical outcomes.[552–554]

The individual must then become the protagonist of his or her own healing process, made conscious and aware of his or her individual resources for a life of well-being and quality, in keeping with the family and social environment from which he or she comes and to which he or she belongs. Osteopathic intervention has holistic properties directed to the person, not only to pain, and a multidimensional impact, i.e., in the context in which the person exists, characterized more as a process than as an act of care, especially in the application of the behavioral-biopsychosocial model. This multidimensional approach is more successful in decreasing the perception of pain and the resulting behavior,[555] although it is the combination of the five osteopathic models in a global and person-centered treatment that increases the chances of success and the quality of the outcome.[555]

In conclusion, the goal is to plan a treatment that simultaneously addresses the biological, psychological, and social factors of the individual affected by stress and/or pain, especially if chronic, and based on the interaction between body, mind, behavior, and environment. This is crucial for mental and physical health and is used in the biopsychosocial model to improve coping strategies and overall quality of life.[556] More research is needed on the incorporation of the complex interaction of the physical, psychological and social to inform and enhance the practice of osteopathy.[557,558]

## References

1. Still AT. The philosophy and mechanical principles of osteopathy. Kansas City, MO: Hudson-Kimberly; 1902. pp. 16–7.

2. Still AT. Osteopathy research and practice. Kirksville, MO: AT Still; 1910. p. 15.

3. Booth ER. Summation of causes in disease and death. J Am Osteopath Assoc. 1902;2(2):33–41.

4. Lyne ST. Osteopathic philosophy of the cause of disease. J Am Osteopath Assoc. 1904;3(12): 395–403.

5. Littlejohn JM. Psychology and osteopathy. J Osteopath. 1898;5(2):67–72.

6. Still AT. Osteopathy research and practice. Kirksville, MO: AT Still; 1910.

7. Comstock ES. The larger concept (editorial). J Am Osteopath Assoc. 1928;(2):463–4.

8. Still-Hildreth Osteopathic Sanatorium Records 1914–1967. Kirksville, MO: Museum of Osteopathic Medicine (SM).

9. Baron DA, Julius RJ, Willard FH. Psycho-neuro-immunology basic mechanisms. In: Chila A, editor. Foundations of osteopathic medicine. 3rd ed. Philadelphia, PA: Lippincott Williams and Wilkins; 2011. ch. 17.

10. Korr IM. An explication of osteopathic principles. In: Ward RC, editor. Foundations of osteopathic medicine. 2nd ed. Philadelphia: Lippincott Williams and Wilkins; 2002. pp. 12–17.

11. Seffinger MA, King HH, Ward RC et al. Osteopathic philosophy. In: Chila A, editor. Foundations of osteopathic medicine. 3rd ed. Philadelphia, PA: Lippincott Williams and Wilkins; 2011. p. 7.

12. Quintner JL Cohen ML Buchanan D et al. Pain medicine and its models: helping or hindering? Pain Med. 2008;9(7):824–34.

13. Flor H, Hermann C. Biopsychosocial models of pain. In: Dworkin RH, Breitbart WS, editors. Psychosocial aspects of pain: a handbook for health care providers, progress in pain research and management. Seattle: IASP Press; 2004. pp. 47–76.

14. Fryette HH. Principles of osteopathic technique. Reprint. Colorado Springs: American Academy of Osteopathy; 1980.

15. Comeaux Z. Robert Fulford DO and the philosopher physician. Seattle: Eastland Press; 2002.

16. Parsons J, Marcer N. Osteopathy: models for diagnosis, treatment and practice. Edinburgh: Elsevier Churchill Livingstone; 2006. ch. 5.

17. Rogers FJ, D'Alonzo GE, Glover J et al. Proposed tenets of osteopathic medicine and principles for patient care. J Am Osteopath Assoc. 2002;102(2):63–5.

18. Trilling JS. Selections from current literature. Psycho-neuro-immunology: validation of the biopsychosocial model. Fam Pract. 2000;17(1):90–3.

19. Shubrook JH Jr, Dooley J. Effects of a structured curriculum in osteopathic manipulative treatment (OMT) on osteopathic structural examinations and use of OMT for hospitalized patients. J Am Osteopath Assoc. 2000;100(9):554–8.

20. Gamsa A. The role of psychological factors in chronic pain II. A critical appraisal. Pain. 1994;57(1):17–29.

21. Waddell G, Newton M, Henderson I et al. A fear-avoidance beliefs questionnaire (FABQ) and the role of fear-avoidance beliefs in chronic low back pain and disability. Pain. 1993;52(2):157–68.

22. Asmundson GJ, Norton PJ, Norton GR. Beyond pain: the role of fear and avoidance in chronicity. Clinical Psych Rev. 1999;19(1):97–119.

23. Vlaeyen JW, Kole-Snijders AM, Boeren RG. Fear of movement/(re)injury in chronic low back pain and its relation to behavioural performance. Pain. 1995;62(3):363–72.

24. Flor H, Turk DC. Psychophysiology of chronic pain: do chronic pain patients exhibit symptom-specific psycho-physiological responses? Psychol Bull. 1989;105(2):215–59.

25. Pincus T, Burton AK, Vogel S et al. A systematic review of psychological factors as predictors of

chronicity/disability in prospective cohorts in low back pain. Spine. 2002;27(5):E109–20.

26. Parmelee PA, Katz IR, Lawton MP. The relation of pain to depression among institutionalized aged. J Gerontol. 1991;46(1):P15–21.

27. Radnitz CL, Bockian N, Moran A. Assessment of psychopathology and personality in people with physical disabilities. In: Frank RG, Elliot TR, editors. Handbook of re-habilitation psychology. Washington DC: American Psychological Association; 2000. pp. 287–309.

28. Koenig HG. Depression in chronic illness:does religion help? J Christ Nurs. 2004;31(1):40–6.

29. Kaila-Kangas L, Kivirnaki M, Riihimaki H. Psycho-social factors at work as predictors of hospitalisation for back disorders: a 28-year follow-up of industrial employees. Spine. 2004;29(16):1823–30.

30. Nicholas MK, Linton SJ, Watson PJ et al. Early identification and management of psychological risk factors ("yellow flags") in patients with low back pain: a reappraisal. Phys Ther. 2011;91(5):737–53.

31. Lima DD, Alves VL, Turato ER. The phenomenological-existential comprehension of chronic pain: going beyond the standing healthcare models. Philos Ethics Humanit Med. 2014;9:2.

32. Kuchera ML. Osteopathic manipulation medicine consideration in patient with chronic pain. J Am Osteopath Assoc. 2005;105(9 Suppl 4):S29–36.

33. Golden BA. A multidisciplinary approach to non-pharmacologic pain management. J Am Osteopath Assoc. 2002;102(Suppl 3):S1–5.

34. Ballard-Reisch DS. A model of participative decision making for physician-patient

interaction. Health Communication. 1990;2(2):91–104.

35. Penney JN. The biopsychosocial model of pain and contemporary osteopathic practice. Int J Osteopath Med. 2010;13(2):42–7.

36. Gatchel RJ. Clinical essentials of pain management. Washington DC: American Psychological Association; 2005.

37. Mackintosh SE, Adams CE, Singer-Chang G et al. An osteopathic approach to implementing and promoting inter-professional education. J Am Osteopath Assoc. 2011;111(4):206–12.

38. Antonovsky A. Health stress and coping. San Francisco: Jossey-Bass; 1979.

39. Eriksson M, Lindström B. A salutogenic interpretation of the Ottawa Charter. Health Promot Int. 2008;23(2):190–9.

40. Jensen MP, Turner JA, Romano JM et al. Coping with chronic pain: a critical review of the literature. Pain. 1991;47(3):249–83.

41. Bandura A. Self-efficacy mechanism in human agency. Am Psychol. 1982;37:122–47.

42. Ramsay Wan C, Vo L, Barnes CS. Conceptualizations of patient empowerment among individuals seeking treatment for diabetes mellitus in an urban public-sector clinic. Patient Educ Couns. 2012;87(3):402–4.

43. Gafni A, Charles C, Whelan T. The physician-patient encounter: the physician as a perfect agent for the patient versus the informed treatment decision-making model. Soc Sci Med. 1998;47(3):347–54.

44. Weisenberg J. Cognitive aspects of pain. In: Wall PD, Melzack R, editors. Textbook of pain 2. Edinburgh: Churchill Livingston; 1989. pp. 231–41.

45. Fordyce WE. Behavioral methods for chronic pain and illness. St Louis, MO: CV Mosby; 1976.

46. Engel GL. The need for a new medical model: a challenge for biomedicine. Science. 1977;196(4286):129–36.

47. Kiecolt-Glaser JK, McGuire L, Robles TF et al. Psychoneuroimmunology: psychological influences on immune function and health. J Consult Clin Psychol. 2002;70(3): 537–47.

48. Engel GL. The clinical application of the biopsychosocial model. Am J Psychiatry. 1980;137(5):535–44.

49. Melzack R, Wall P. The challenge of pain. 2nd ed. London: Penguin Books; 1988.

50. Alonso Y. The biopsychosocial model in medical research: the evolution of the health concept over the past two decades. Patient Educ Couns. 2003;53(2):239–44.

51. Melzack R, Wall PD. Pain mechanisms: a new theory. Science. 1965;150(3699):971–9.

52. Melzack R. From the gate to the neuromatrix. Pain. 1999;S121–6.

53. Smith GC, Strain JJ. George Engel's contribution to clinical psychiatry. Aust N Z J Psychiat. 2002;36(4):458–66.

54. Lutgendorf SK, Costanzo ES. Psycho-neuro-immunology and health psychology: an integrative model. Brain Behav Immun. 2003;17(4):225–32.

55. Breeze E, Fletcher AE, Leon DA et al. Do socioeconomic disadvantages persist into old age? Self reported morbidity in a 29-year follow-up of the Whitehall study. Am J Public Health. 2001;91(2):277–83.

56. Stansfeld SA, Head J, Fuhrer R et al. Social inequalities in depressive symptoms and physical functioning in the Whitehall II study: exploring a common cause explanation. J Epidemiol Community Health. 2003;57(5):361–8.

57. Truchon M. Determinants of chronic disability related to low back pain: towards an integrative biopsychosocial model. Disabil Rehabil. 2001;23(17):758–67.

58. Breuer J, Freud S. Studies on hysteria. In: Strachey J, editor. The standard edition of the complete psychological works of Sigmund Freud. London: Hogarth Press; 1955. vol. 2.

59. Reich W. Analisi del carattere. Milan: Sugarco Ed; 1933.

60. Reich W. Dalla psicoanalisi all'elettrofisiologia e all'orgonomia (1933–1942). Rome: Scritti II Andromeda Ed; 2014.

61. Latey P. The muscular manifesto. 2nd ed. London: Philip Latey; 1979.

62. Lipowski ZJ. What does the word "psychosomatic" really mean? A historical and semantic inquiry. Psychosom Med. 1984;46(2):153–71.

63. Sarno J. Mind over back pain. New York: Harper Collins; 1984.

64. Borenstein DG, O'Mara JW Jr, Boden SD et al. The value of magnetic resonance imaging of the lumbar spine to predict low-back pain in asymptomatic subjects: a seven-year follow-up study. J Bone Joint Surg Am. 2001;83-A(9):1306–11.

65. Savage RA, Whitehouse GH, Roberts N. The relationship between the magnetic resonance imaging appearance of the lumbar spine and low back pain age and occupation in males. Eur Spine J. 1997;6(2):106–14.

66. Jensen MC, Brant-Zawadzki MN, Obuchowski N et al. Magnetic resonance imaging of the lumbar spine in people without back pain. N Engl J Med. 1994;331(2):69–73.

67. Sarno JE. The mindbody prescription: healing the body, healing the pain. New York NY: Warner Books; 1998.

68. Cannon WB. The wisdom of the body. New York, NY: Norton; 1932.

69. Cannon WB. The mechanism of emotional disturbance of bodily functions. N Engl J Med. 1928;198:877–84.

70. Kandel ER, Schwartz JH, Jessell TM, editors. Principles of neural science. New York: McGraw-Hill; 2000. ch. 49.

71. Selye H. The stress of life. New York: McGraw-Hill; 1976.

72. Selye H. The physiology and pathology of exposure to stress: a treatise based on the concepts of the general adaptation syndrome and the diseases of adaptation. Montreal, AR: Acta Incorporated Medical Publishers; 1950.

73. Sterling P, Eyer J. Allostasis: a new paradigm to explain arousal pathology. In: Fisher S Reason J, editors. Handbook of life stress, cognition and health. New York: John Wiley; 1988.

74. McEwen BS. Protective and damaging effects of stress mediators. New Engl J Med. 1998;338(3):171–9.

75. Seeman TB, Singer BH, Rowe JW et al. Price of adaptation – allostatic load and its health consequences. MacArthur studies of successful ageing. Arch Intern Med. 1997;157(19):2259–68.

76. Solomon GF, Moos RH. Emotions, immunity and disease: a speculative theoretical integration. Arch Gen Psychiatry. 1964;11:657–74.

77. Freeman H, Elmadjan F. The relationship between blood sugar and lymphocyte levels in normal and psychotic subjects. Psychosom Med. 1947;9(4):226–32.

78. Levy SR, Lippman M, d'Angelo T. Correlation of stress factors with sustained depression of natural killer cell activity and predicted prognosis in patients with breast cancer. J Clin Oncol. 1987;5(3):348–53.

79. Pert CB, Ruff MR, Weber RJ et al. Neuropeptides and their receptors: a psychosomatic network. J Immunol. 1985;135(2 Suppl):820s-26s.

80. Rubinow DR. Brain behavior and immunity: an interactive system. J Natl Cancer Inst Monogr. 1990;(10):79–82.

81. Blalock JE. A molecular basis for bidirectional communication between the immune and neuroendocrine systems. Physiol Rev. 1989;69(1):1–32.

82. Blalock JE. The syntax of immune-neuroendocrine communication. Immunol Today. 1994;15(11):504–11.

83. Roth J, Leroith DL, Collier ES et al. Evolutionary origins of neuropeptides, hormones and receptors: possible applications to immunology. J Immunol. 1985;135(2 Suppl):816s-9s.

84. Schmitt FO. Molecular regulation of brain function: a new view. Neuroscience. 1984;13(4):991–1001.

85. Pert CB, Dreher HE, Ruff MR. The psychosomatic network: foundations of mind-body medicine. Altern Ther Health Med. 1998;4(4):30–41.

86. Alonso Y. The biopsychosocial model in medical research: the evolution of the health concept over the past two decades. Patient Educ Couns. 2003;53(2):239–44.

87. Australian Acute Musculoskeletal Pain Guidelines Group. Evidence-based management of acute musculoskeletal pain. Brisbane: Australian Academic Press; 2003.

88. Butler R. The patient encounter: patient-centered model. In: Chila A, editor. Foundations of osteopathic medicine. 3rd ed. Philadelphia, PA: Lippincott Williams and Wilkins; 2011. ch. 29.

89. World Health Organization (WHO). Benchmarks for training in osteopathy. Geneva: WHO; 2010.

90. Howell JD. The paradox of osteopathy. N Engl J Med. 1999;341(19):1465–8.

91. Penney NJ. The biopsychosocial model: redefining osteopathic philosophy? Int J Osteopath Med. 2013;16(1):33–7.

92. Thomson OP, Petty NJ, Moore AP. Reconsidering the patient-centeredness of osteopathy. Int J Osteopath Med. 2013;16(1):25–32.

93. Educational Council on Osteopathic Principles (ECOP). Glossary of osteopathic terminology usage guide. Chevy Chase, MD: American Association of Colleges of Osteopathic Medicine (AACOM); 2011. p. 26.

94. Baum A, Posluszny DM. Health psychology: mapping bio-behavioral contributions to health and illness. Annu Rev Psychol. 1990;50:137–63.

95. Gatchel RJ, Maddrey AM. The biopsychosocial perspective of pain. In: Raczynski J, Leviton L, editors. Healthcare psychology handbook. Vol II. Washington DC: American Psychological Association Press; 2004.

96. McLaren N. Toward an osteopathic psychiatry: the biocognitive model of mind. J Am Osteopath Assoc. 2010; 110(12):725–32.

97. Anderson GB, Lucente T, Davis AM et al. A comparison of osteopathic spinal manipulation with standard care for patients with low back pain. N Engl J Med. 1999;341(19):1426–31.

98. Elkiss ML, Jerome JA. Chronic pain management. In: Chila A, editor. Foundations of osteopathic medicine. 3rd ed. Philadelphia, PA: Lippincott Williams and Wilkins; 2011. ch. 16.

99. Nielson WR, Weir R. Biopsychosocial approaches to the treatment of chronic pain. Clin J Pain. 2001;17(4 Suppl):S114–27.

100. Smith RC. Patient-centered interviewing: an evidence-based method. Philadelphia, PA: Lippincott Williams and Wilkins; 2002.

101. Stewart M. Evidence for the patient-centered clinical method as a means of implementing the biopsychosocial approach. In: Frankel RM, Quil TE, McDaniel SH, editors. The biopsychosocial approach: past present future. Rochester, NY: University of Rochester Press; 2003. p. 123.

102. Tresolini CP. Health professions, education and relationship-centered care: report of the Pew-Fetzer Task Force on advancing psychosocial education. The Pew-Fetzer Task Force. San Francisco, CA: Pew Health Professions Commission; 1994.

103. Austoker J. Gaining informed consent for screening. Br Med J. 1999;319(7212):722–3.

104. Fraenkel L, McGraw S. Participation in medical decision making: the patient's perspective. Med Decis Making. 2007;27(5):533–8.

105. Epstein RM. The science of patient-centered care. J Fam Pract. 2000;49(9):805–7.

106. Adler H. Toward a biopsychosocial understanding of the patient-physician

relationship: an emerging dialogue. J Gen Intern Med. 2007;22(2):280–5.

107. Coulter A. Paternalism or partnership? Br Med J. 1999;319(7212):719–20.

108. Zandbelt LC, Smets EMA, Oort FJ et al. Determinants of physicians' patient-centred behaviour in the medical specialist encounter. Soc Sci Med. 2006;63(4):899–910.

109. Morris DB. The challenges of pain and suffering In: Jensen TS, Wilson PR, Rice AS, editors. Clinical pain management: chronic pain. London: Arnold; 2003. pp. 3–13.

110. Sackett DL, Straus SE, Richardson WS et al., editors. Evidence-based medicine: how to practice and teach EBM. London: Churchill Livingstone; 2000. p. 1.

111. Olde Hartman TC, Hassink-Franke LJ, Lucassen PL et al. Explanation and relations. How do general practitioners deal with patients with persistent medically unexplained symptoms: a focus group study. BMC Fam Pract. 2009;10:68.

112. Henningsen P, Zipfel S, Herzog W. Management of functional somatic syndromes. Lancet. 2007;369(9565):946–55.

113. Roter DL, Stewart M, Putnam SM et al. Communication patterns of primary care physicians. JAMA. 1997;277(4):350–6.

114. Lo B, Ruston D, Kales LW et al. For the working group on religious and spiritual issues at the end of life. Discussing religious and spiritual issues at the end of life: a practical guide for physicians. JAMA. 2002;287(6):749–54.

115. Novack D, Suchman A, Clark W et al. Calibrating the physician, personal awareness and effective patient care. J Am Med Assoc. 1992;278(6):502–9.

116. Groopman J. How doctors think. New York: Houghton Mifflin; 2007.

117. Loeser JD. Pain and suffering. Clin J Pain. 2000;16(2 Suppl):S2–6.

118. Sullivan MJ, Thorn B, Haythornthwaite JA et al. Theoretical perspectives on the relation between catastrophizing and pain. Clin J Pain. 2001;17(1):52–64.

119. Albaret MC, MunozSastre MT, Cottencin A et al. The fear of pain questionnaire: factor structure in samples of young, middle-aged and elderly European people. Eur J Pain. 2004;8(3):273–81.

120. Roelofs J, Goubert L, Peters ML et al. The Tampa Scale for kinesiophobia: further examination of psychometric properties in patients with chronic low back pain and fibromyalgia. Eur J Pain. 2004;8(5):495–592.

121. Miller WR, Rollnick S. Motivational interviewing: preparing people to change addictive behaviour. New York: Guilford Press; 1991.

122. Miller WR, Rollnick S. Il colloquio motivazionale. 3rd ed. Trento: Erickson; 2014. ch. 13.

123. Spiegel D. Healing words:emotional expression and disease outcome. JAMA. 1999;281(14):1328–9.

124. Holmes TB, Rahe RH. The social readjustment rating scale. J Psychosom Res. 1967;11(2):213–8.

125. Sarason IG, Johnson JH, Siegel JM. Assessing the impact of life changes development of the life experiences survey. J Consult Clin Psychol. 1978;46(5):932–46.

126. Sheridan CL, Radmacher SA. Health psychology challenging the biomedical model. New York: Wiley; 1992.

127. Ringel Y, Sperber AD, Drossman DA. Irritable bowel syndrome. Ann Rev Med. 2001;52: 319–38.

128. International Association for the Study of Pain (IASP). Pain terms: a list with definitions and notes on usage. Recommended by the IASP Subcommittee on Taxonomy. Pain. 1979;6(3):249.

129. Gatchel RJ, Robinson RC, Peng YB et al. Pain and the brain. Pract Pain Manage. 2008;8(5):28–40.

130. May A. Chronic pain may change the structure of the brain. Pain. 2008;137(1):7–15.

131. Jerome JA. Transmission or transformation? Information processing theory of chronic human pain. Am Pain Society J. 1993;2(3):160–71.

132. Kendall N, Linton S, Main C. Guide to assessing psychosocial yellow flags in acute low back pain: risk factors for long-term disability and work loss. Wellington, New Zealand: ACC and National Health Committee; 1997.

133. Wörz R. Pain in depression-depression in pain. Seattle: IASP Press; 2003. 11(5):2–6.

134. Turk DC, Monarch ES. Biopsychosocial perspective on pain. In: Turk DC, Gatchel RJ, editors. Psychological approaches to pain management: a practitioner's handbook. 2nd ed. New York: Guilford Press; 2002. pp. 3–39.

135. Banks SM, Kerns RD. Explaining high rates of depression in chronic pain: a diathesis-stress framework. Psychol Bull. 1996;119(1):95–110.

136. Turk DC, Melzack R. Handbook of pain assessments. 2nd ed. New York: Gilford Press; 2001.

137. Melzack R. The McGill Questionnaire: major properties and scoring methods. Pain 1975;1(3):277–99.

138. Nevins NA. Environmental issues. In: Chila A, editor. Foundations of osteopathic medicine. 3rd ed. Philadelphia, PA: Lippincott Williams and Wilkins; 2011. ch. 23.

139. Elkiss ML, Jerome JA. Touch – more than a basic science. J Am Osteopath Assoc. 2012;112(8):514–7.

140. Dummer T. A textbook of osteopathy. Hadlow Down: JoTom Publications; 1999. vol. 1, pp. 171.

141. Burgio GR. Biological individuality and disease. From Garrod's chemical individuality to HLA associated diseases. Acta Biotheor. 1993;41(3):219–30.

142. Pende N. Le debolezze di costituzione. Rome: Libreria Scienze e lettere; 1928. p. 36.

143. Sheldon WH, Stevens SS. The varieties of temperament: a psychology of constitutional differences. New York: Harper and Brothers; 1942.

144. Dummer T. Specific adjusting technique. Hove: JoTom Publications; 1995. pp. 36–43.

145. Latey P. Feelings muscles and movement. J Bodyw Mov Ther. 1996;1(1):44–52.

146. Latey P. Maturation – the evolution of psychosomatic problems: migraine and asthma. J Bodyw Mov Ther. 1997;1(2):107–16.

147. Kelman S. Emotional anatomy. Berkeley: Center Press; 1985.

148. Littlejohn JM, Wernham J, Hall TE. The mechanics of the spine and pelvis. Maidstone, UK: Maidstone College of Osteopathy; 1960.

149. Sheldon WH. The varieties of human physique: an introduction to constitutional psychology. New York: Harper and Brothers; 1940.

150. Chaitow L. Naturopathic physical medicine. Theory and practice for manual therapists and naturopaths. Edinburgh: Churchill Livingstone Elsevier; 2008. pp. 89–90.

151. Chaouachi M, Chaouachi A, Chamari K et al. Effects of dominant somatotype on aerobic capacity trainability. Br J Sports Med. 2005;39(12):954–9.

152. Kalitchman L, Livshits G, Kobyliansky E. Association between somatotypes and blood pressure in an adult Chuvasha population. Ann Hum Biol. 2004;31(4):466–76.

153. Salivon I, Polina N. Constitution and reactivity of the organism. J Physiol Anthropol Appl Human Sci. 2005;24(4):497–502.

154. Kriege T. Fundamental basis of iris diagnosis. London: Fowler; 1969.

155. Priest AW. The iridological assessment of the patient and its relationship to subsequent therapeutics. London: Proceedings of the Research Society for Natural Therapeutics; 1959.

156. Martiny M. Essai de biotypologie humaine. Paris: J Peyronnet; 1948.

157. Pende N, Martiny M. Traité de medicine bio-typologique. Paris: Doin; 1955.

158. Jung CG. Tipi psicologici. In: Opere. Torino: Boringhieri; 1969. vol. 6.

159. Kretschmer E. Körperbau und Charakter Untersuchungen zum konstitutionsproblem und zur lehre von den tempera-menten. Berlin: Springer; 1921.

160. Vannier L. Typology in homoeopathy. Beaconsfield, UK; 1992.

161. Marino F. Biotypology II: modern concepts. Br Homeopath J. 1999;88(4):178–83.

162. Dummer T. A textbook of osteopathy. Hadlow Down: JoTom Publications; 1999. vol. 1, pp. 133–54.

163. Brody H. The biopsychosocial model patient-centered care and culturally sensitive practice. J Fam Prac. 1999;48(8):585–7.

164. Cain RA. Clinical decision making. In: Chila A, editor. Foundations of osteopathic medicine. 3rd ed. Philadelphia, PA: Lippincott Williams and Wilkins; 2011. ch. 25.

165. Pettegrew LS, Logan R. The health care context. In: Berger C, Chaffee ST, editors. Handbook of communication science. Newbury Park: SAGE; 1987.

166. Croskerry P. Cognitive forcing strategies in clinical decision making. Ann Emerg Med. 2003;41(1):110–20.

167. Jerome JA, Osborn GG. Psychoneuroimmunology - stress management. In: Chila A, editor. Foundations of osteopathic medicine. 3rd ed. Philadelphia, PA: Lippincott Williams and Wilkins; 2011. ch. 18.

168. Astin JA, Shapiro SL, Eisenberg OM et al. Mind-body medicine: state of the science implications for practice. J Am Board Fam Pract. 2003;16(2):131–47.

169. Mehling WE, Wrubel J, Daubenmier JJ et al. Body awareness: a phenomenological inquiry into the common ground of mind-body therapies. Philos Ethics Humanit Med. 2011;6:6.

170. Sullivan MJ, Thorn B, Rodgers W et al. Path model of psychological antecedents to pain experience: experimental and clinical findings. Clin J Pain. 2004;20(3):164–73.

171. Vlaeyen JW, Linton SJ. Fear-avoidance and its consequences in chronic musculoskeletal pain: a state of the art. Pain. 2000;85(3):317–32.

172. Kerns RD, Haythornthwaite J, Southwick S et al. The role of marital interaction in chronic pain and depressive symptom severity. J Psychosom Res. 1990;34(4):401–8.

173. Loeser JD. Pain as a disease. Handb Clin Neurol. 2006;81:11–20.

174. Galluzzi KE. Management of neuropathic pain. J Am Osteopath Assoc. 2005;105(9 Suppl 4):S12–9.

175. Kerns RD, Habib S. A critical review of the pain readiness to change model. J Pain. 2004;5(7):357–67.

176. Rollnick S, Mason P, Butler C, editors. Health behavior change: a guide for practitioners. London: Churchill Livingstone; 1999. pp. 34–6.

177. Prochaska JO, DiClemente CC. Stages of change in the modification of problem behaviors. Prog Behav Modif. 1992;28:183–218.

178. Taal E, Rasker JJ, Wiegman O. Patient education and self-management in the rheumatic diseases: a self-efficacy approach. Arthritis Care Res. 1996;9(3):229–38.

179. Stoffelmayr B, Hoppe RB, Weber N. Facilitating patient participation: the doctor-patient encounter. Prim Care. 1989;16(1):265–78.

180. Libet JM, Lewinsohn PM. Concept of social skill with special reference to the behavior of depressed persons. J Consult Clin Psychol. 1973;40(2):304–12.

181. Verbeek IH, Konings GM, Aldenkamp AP et al. Cognitive behavioral treatment in clinically referred chronic insomniacs: group versus individual treatment. Behav Sleep Med. 2006;4(3):135–51.

182. Jacobson E. Progressive relaxation. Chicago: University of Chicago Press; 1938.

183. Kennerley H. Managing anxiety: a training manual. Oxford, UK: Oxford University Press; 1990.

184. Jacobs GD. Clinical applications of the relaxation response and mind-body interventions. J Altern Complement Med. 2001;7(Suppl l):S93-S101.

185. Price S, Price L. Aromatherapy for health professionals. 3rd ed. Philadelphia, PA: Churchil Livingstone; 2007.

186. Bassett CAL. Bioelectromagnetics in the service of medicine. In: Blank M, editor. Electromagnetic fields: biological interactions and mechanisms. Advances in Chemistry series 250. Washington DC: American Chemical Society; 1995. pp. 261–75.

187. Arena JG, Blanchard EB. Biofeedback and relaxation therapy for chronic pain disorders. In:Gatchel RJ, Turk DC, editors. Chronic pain: psychological perspectives on treatment. 2nd ed. New York: Guilford Press; 2002. pp. 159–86.

188. Gatchel R, Okifuji A. Evidence based scientific data documenting the treatment and cost effectiveness of comprehensive pain programs for chronic nonmalignant pain. J Pain. 2006;7(11):779–93.

189. Sawa RJ. Family health care. Newbury Park, CA: SAGE; 1992.

190. Thoresen CE, Harris AHS. Spirituality and health: what's the evidence and what's needed? Ann Behav Med. 2002;24(1):3–13.

191. Katerndahl DA. Impact of spiritual symptoms and their interactions on health services and life satisfaction. Ann Fam Med. 2008;6(5): 412–20.

192. Turk DC. A cognitive-behavioral perspective on treatment of chronic pain patients. In: Turk DC, Gatchel RJ, editors. Psychological approaches to pain management. 2nd ed. New York: Guilford Press; 2002. pp. 138–58.

193. Jerome JA, Foresman BA, D'Alonzo GE. Bio-behavioral research. In: Chila A, editor. Foundations of osteopathic medicine. 3rd ed. Philadelphia, PA: Lippincott Williams and Wilkins; 2011. ch. 73.

194. Aiken LS, West SG, Woodward CK et al. Health beliefs and compliance with mammography-screening recommendations in asymptomatic women. Health Psychol. 1994;13(2): 122–9.

195. Hussey LC, Gilliland K. Compliance low literacy and locus of control. Nurs Clin North Am. 1989;24(3):605–11.

196. Cameron C. Patient compliance: recognition of factors involved and suggestions for promoting compliance with therapeutic regimens. J Adv Nurs. 1996;24(2):244–50.

197. Gerber WD, Schoenen J. Biobehavioral correlates in migraine: the role of hypersensitivity and information-processing dysfunction. Cephalalgia. 1998;18(Suppl 21):5–11.

198. Naliboff BD, Munakata J, Chang L et al. Toward a biobehavioral model of visceral hypersensitivity in irritable bowel syndrome. J Psychosom Res. 1998;45(6):485–92.

199. Feuerstein M, Beattie P. Biobehavioral factors affecting pain and disability in low back pain: mechanisms and assessment. Phys Ther. 1995;75(4):267–80.

200. Murray CJL, Lopez AD. The global burden of disease: a comprehensive assessment of mortality and disability from diseases, injuries and risk factors in 1990 and projected to 2020. Cambridge, MA: Harvard University Press; 2000.

201. Bottaccioli F. Geni e comportamenti. Scienza e arte della vita. Milan: Red; 2009. pp. 11–35.

202. Steptoe A, Wardle J, Pollard TM et al. Stress social support and health related behavior: a study of smoking, alcohol consumption and physical exercise. J Psychosom Res. 1996;41(2):171–80.

203. Osborn GG, Jerome JA. Health promotion and maintenance. In: Chila A, editor. Foundations of osteopathic medicine. 3rd ed. Philadelphia, PA: Lippincott Williams and Wilkins; 2011. ch. 30.

204. Kisner C, Colby LA. Therapeutic exercise:foundations and techniques. 5th ed. Philadelphia, PA: FA Davis; 2007.

205. Hayden JA, vanTulder MW, Tomlinson G. Systematic review: strategies for using exercise therapy to improve outcomes in chronic low back pain. Ann Intern Med. 2005;142(9): 776–85.

206. McCullough ML, Feskanich D, Stampfer MJ et al. Diet quality and major chronic disease risk in men and women: moving toward improved dietary guidance. Am J Clin Nutr 2002;76(6):261–71.

207. Wright L. Looking deep deep into your genes: discoveries about the impact of the environment on our DNA could revolutionize our concept of illness. OnEarth 2007;29(2):32–5.

208. Katsambas A, Nicolaidou E. Cutaneous malignant melanoma and sun exposure. Recent developments in epidemiology. Arch Dermatol. 1996;132(4):444–50.

209. Cakmak S, Dales RE, Judek S. Respiratory health effects of air pollution gases: modification by education and income. Arch Environ Occup Health. 2006;61(1):5–10.

210. Cummings KJ, Van Sickle D, Rao CY et al. Knowledge attitudes and practices related to mold exposure among residents and remediation workers in post-hurricane New Orleans. Arch Environ Occup Health. 2006;61(3):101–8.

211. Nurmatov U, van Schayck CP, Hurwitz B et al. House dust mite avoidance measures for perennial allergic rhinitis: an updated Cochrane systematic review. Allergy. 2012;67(2):158–65.

212. Verbeek JH, Kateman E, Morata TC et al. Interventions to prevent occupational noise-induced hearing loss: a Cochrane systematic review. Int J Audiol. 2014;3 (Suppl 2): S84–96.

213. Cohen S, Tyrell DAJ, Smith AP. Psychological stress and susceptibility to the common cold. N Engl J Med. 1991;325(9):606–12.

214. Lutgendorf SK, Sood AK, Anderson B et al. Social support psychological distress and natural killer cell activity in ovarian cancer. J Clin Oncol. 2005;23(28):7105–13.

215. Keicolt-Glaser JK, Glaser R. Psycho-neuro-immunology and cancer: fact or fiction? Eur J Cancer. 1999;35(11):1603–7.

216. Müller N, Schwarz MJ. The immune-mediated alteration of serotonin and glutamate: towards an integrated view of depression. Mol Psychiatry. 2007;12(11):988–1000.

217. Ridker PM, Cushman M, Stampfer MJ et al. Inflammation, aspirin and the risk of cardiovascular disease in apparently healthy men. N Engl J Med. 1997;336(14):973–9.

218. Dinenno FA, Jones PP, Seals DR et al. Age associated arterial wall thickening is related to elevations in sympathetic activity in healthy humans. Am J Physiol Heart Circ Physiol. 2000;278(4):H1205–10.

219. Kemeny ME, Schedlowski M. Understanding the interaction between psychosocial stress and immune-related diseases: a stepwise progression. Brain Behav Immun. 2007;21(8):1009–18.

220. Benschop RJ, Geenen R, Mills PJ et al. Cardiovascular and immune responses to acute psychological stress in young and old women: a metaanalysis. Psychosom Med. 1998;60(3):290–6.

221. Pariante CM, Carpiniello B, Orru MG et al. Chronic caregiving stress alters peripheral blood immune parameters: the role of age and severity of stress. Psychother Psychosom. 1997;66(4):199–207.

222. Kemeny M, Cohen F, Zegans S et al. Psychological and immunological predictors of genital herpes recurrence. Psychosomatic Med. 1989;51(2):195–208.

223. Irwin MR, Miller AH. Depressive disorders and immunity: 20 years of progress and discovery. Brain Behav Immun. 2007;21(4): 374–83.

224. Bartrop RW, Luckhurst E, Lazarus L et al. Depressed lymphocyte function after bereavement. Lancet. 1977;1(8016):834–6.

225. Schleifer SJ, Keller SE, Camerino M et al. Suppression of lymphocyte stimulation following bereavement. JAMA. 1983;250(3):374–7.

226. Glaser R, Rice J, Sheridan J et al. Stress-related immune suppression: health implications. Brain Behav Immun. 1987;1(1):7–20.

227. Irwin M, Daniels M, Bloom ET et al. Life events, depressive symptoms and immune function. Am J Psychiatry. 1987;144(4):437–41.

228. Evans DL, Charney DS, Lewis L et al. Mood disorders in the medically ill: scientific review and recommendations. Biol Psychiatry. 2005;58(3):175–89.

229. Reichlin S. Neuroendocrine-immune interactions. N Engl J Med. 1993;329(17):1246–53.

230. Weigant A, Blalock JE. Role of neuropeptides in the bi-directional communication between the immune and neuroendocrine systems. In: Scharrer B, Smith EM, Stefano GB, editors. Neuropeptides and immunoregulation. Berlin: Springer-Verlag; 1994.

231. Cunha TM Verri WA Jr Silva JS et al. A cascade of cytokines mediates mechanical inflammatory hypernociception in mice. Proc Natl Acad Sci USA. 2005;102(5):1755–60.

232. Goujon E, Laye S, Parnet P et al. Regulation of cytokine gene expression in the central nervous system by glucocorticoids: mechanisms and functional consequences. Psycho-neuroendocrinology. 1997;22(Suppl 1):S75–80.

233. Sapolsky RM. Is impaired neurogenesis relevant to the affective symptoms of depression? Biol Psychiatry. 2004;56(3):137–9.

234. Müller N, Ackenheil M. Psycho-neuro-immunology and the cytokine action in the CNS: implications for psychiatric disorders. Prog Neuro-psycho-pharmacol Biol Psychiatry. 1998;22(1):1–33.

235. Haas HS, Schauenstein K. Neuroimmunomodulation via limbic structures–the neuroanatomy of psychoimmunology. Prog Neurobiol. 1997;51(2):195–222.

236. Tonello L, Cocchi M. The cell membrane: is it a bridge from psychiatry to quantum consciousness? Neuroquantology. 2010;8(1):54–60.

237. Cocchi M, Tonello L, Rasenick MM. Human depression: a new approach in quantitative psychiatry. Ann Gen Psychiatry. 2010; 9:25.

238. Donati RJ, Dwivedi Y, Roberts RC et al. Postmortem brain tissue of depressed suicides reveals increased Gs localization in lipid raft domains where it is less likely to activate adenylyl cyclase. J Neurosci. 2008;28(12): 3042–50.

239. Heron DS, Shinitzky M, Hershkowitz M et al. Lipid fluidity markedly modulates the binding of serotonin to mouse brain membranes. Proc Natl Acad Sci USA. 1980;77(12):7463–7.

240. Dowlatshahi D, MacQueen GM, Wang JF et al. G protein-coupled cyclic AMP signaling in postmortem brain of subjects with mood disorders: effects of diagnosis suicide and treatment at the time of death. J Neurochem 1999;73(3):1121–6.

241. Hines LM, Tabakoff B. Platelet adenylyl cyclase activity: a biological marker for major depression and recent drug use. Biol Psychiatry 2005;58(12):955–62.

242. Turner JA, Jensen MP, Romano JM. Do beliefs coping catastrophizing independently predict functioning in patients with chronic pain? Pain 2000;85(1–2):115–25.

243. Licciardone JC, Gatchel RJ, Kearns CM et al. Depression, somatization and somatic dysfunction in patients with nonspecific chronic low back pain: results from the osteopathic trial. J Am Osteopath Assoc. 2012;112(12):783–91.

244. Angstman KB, Bansal S, Chappell DH et al. Effects of concurrent low back conditions on depression outcomes. J Am Osteopath Assoc. 2013;113(7):530-7.

245. Esteves J, Wheatley L, Mayall C et al. Emotional processing and its relationship to chronic low back pain: results from a case-control study. Man Ther. 2013;18(6):541-6.

246. Langevin HM, Sherman KJ. Pathophysiological model for chronic low back pain integrating connective tissue and nervous system mechanisms. Med Hypotheses. 2007;68(1):74-80.

247. Krantz DS, Grunberg NE, Baum A. Health psychology. Annu Rev Psychol. 1985;36:349-83.

248. McEwen BS, Sapolsky RM. Stress and cognitive function. Curr Opin Neurobiol. 1995;5(2):205-16.

249. Goodkin K, Antoni MH, Helder L et al. Psycho-neuro-immunological aspects of disease progression among women with human papilloma-virus-associated cervical dysplasia and human immunodeficiency virus type 1 co-infection. Int J Psychiatry Med. 1993;23(2):119-48.

250. Stommel M, Given BA, Given CW. Depression and functional status as predictors of death among cancer patients. Cancer. 2002;94(10):2719-27.

251. Stein M. Future directions for brain behavior and the immune system. Bull N Y Acad Med. 1992;68(3):390-410.

252. Knox SS. Bio-behavioral mechanisms in lipid metabolism and atherosclerosis: an overview. Metabolism. 1993;42(9 Suppl 1):1-2.

253. Kojima M, Wakai K, Kawamura T et al. Sleep patterns and total mortality: a 12-year follow-up study in Japan. J Epidemiol. 2000;10(2): 87-93.

254. Kripke DF, Garfinkel L, Wingard DL et al. Mortality associated with sleep duration and insomnia. Arch Gen Psychiatry. 2002;59(2):131-6.

255. Kop WJ, Verdino RJ, Gottdiener JS et al. Changes in heart rate and heart rate variability before ambulatory ischemic events. J Am Coll Cardiol. 2001;38(3):742-9.

256. Wielgosz AT, Nolan RP. Biobehavioral factors in the context of ischemic cardiovascular diseases. J Psychosom Res. 2000;48(4-5):339-45.

257. Friedman M, Ulmer D. Treating type-A behavior and your heart. New York: Knopf; 1984.

258. Hasser EM, Moffitt JA. Regulation of sympathetic nervous system function after cardiovascular deconditioning. Ann N Y Acad Sci. 2001;940:454-68.

259. Sitruk-Ware R. Progestins and cardiovascular risk markers. Steroids. 2000;65(10-11):651-8.

260. Ader R, Cohen N. Behaviorally conditioned immuno-suppression. Psychosom Med. 1975;37(4):333-40.

261. Goebel MU, Trebst AE, Steiner J et al. Behavioral conditioning of immunosuppression is possible in humans. FASEB J. 2002;16(14):1869-73.

262. Overmier JB, Seligman ME. Effects of inescapable shock upon subsequent escape and avoidance responding. J Comp Physiol Psychol. 1967;63(1):28-33.

263. Musty RE, Jordan MP, Lenox RH. Criterion for learned helplessness in the rat: a redefinition. Pharmacol Biochem Behav. 1990;36(4):739-44.

264. Beck AT. Cognitive theory and the emotional disorders. New York: International Universities Press; 1976.

265. Wilson TD. Strangers to ourselves: discovering the adaptive unconscious. Cambridge, MA: Belknap Press of Harvard University; 2002.

266. Castro WHM, Meyer SJ, Becke ME et al. No stress–no whiplash? Prevalence of "whiplash" symptoms following exposure to a placebo rear-end collision. Int J Legal Med. 2001;114(6):316–22.

267. Fernández-Lao C, Cantarero-Villanueva I, Díaz-Rodríguez L. Attitudes towards massage modify effects of manual therapy in breast cancer survivors: a randomised clinical trial with crossover design. Eur J Cancer Care (Engl). 2012;21(2):233–41.

268. Fernández-Lao C, Cantarero-Villanueva I, Díaz-Rodríguez L et al. The influence of patient attitude toward massage on pressure pain sensitivity and immune system after application of myofascial release in breast cancer survivors: a randomized controlled crossover study. J Manipulative Physiol Ther. 2012;35(2):94–100.

269. Irwin MR. Human psychoneuroimmunology: 20 years of discovery. Brain Behav Immun. 2008;22(2):129–39.

270. Kassel JD. Smoking and attention: a review and reformulation of the stimulus-filter hypothesis. Clin Psychol Rev. 1997;17(5):451–78.

271. Hausberg M, Mark AL, Winniford MD et al. Sympathetic and vascular effects of short-term passive smoke exposure in healthy nonsmokers. Circulation. 1997;96(1):282–7.

272. Surgeon General. The health consequences of smoking – 50 years of progress: a report of the Surgeon General. Rockville, MD: US Department of Health and Human Services; 2014.

273. Girdler SS, Jamner LD, Jarvik M et al. Smoking status and nicotine administration differentially modify hemodynamic stress reactivity in men and women. Psychosom Med. 1997;59(3):294–306.

274. Morse RM, Flavin DK. The definition of alcoholism. The Joint Committee of the National Council of Alcoholism and Drug Dependence and the American Society of Addiction Medicine to study the definition and criteria for the diagnosis of alcoholism. JAMA. 1992;268(8):1012–4.

275. Sass H, Soyka M, Mann K et al. Relapse prevention by acamprosate. Results from a placebo-controlled study on alcohol dependence. Arch Gen Psychiatry. 1996;53(8):673–80.

276. Wise RA. Drug-activation of brain reward pathways. Drug Alcohol Depend. 1998; 51(1–2):13–22.

277. Nie Z, Schweltzcr P, Roberts AJ et al. Ethanol augments GABAergic transmission in the central amygdala via CRF1 receptors. Science. 2004;303(5663):1512–4.

278. Gordis E. The neurobiology of alcohol abuse and alcoholism: building knowledge creating hope. Drug Alcohol Depend. 1998; 51(1–2):9–11.

279. Redwine L, Haufer RL, Gillin JC et al. Effects of sleep and sleep deprivation on interleukin-6 growth hormone cortisol and melatonin levels in humans. J Clin Endocrinol Metab. 2000;85(10):3597–603.

280. Buysse DJ, Reynolds CF. Insomnia. In: Thorpy MJ, editor. Handbook of sleep disorders. New York: Marcel Dekker; 1990. pp. 375–433.

281. Sternberg EM, Gold PW. The mind-body interaction in disease. Scientific American special edition: The Hidden Mind. 2002;12(1):82–29.

282. Glaser R, Kennedy S, Lafuse WP et al. Psychological stress-induced modulation of IL-2 receptor gene expression and IL-2 production in peripheral blood leukocytes. Arch Gen Psychiatry. 1990;47(8):707–12.

283. Webster JI, Tonelli L, Sternberg EM. Neuroendocrine regulation of immunity. Annu Rev Immunol. 2002;20: 125–63.

284. Conti A. Neuroimmunomodulation. New York: Ann NY Acad Sci. 2001.

285. McEwen BS, Biron CA, Brunson KW et al. The role of adrenocorticoids as modulators of immune function in health and disease: neural endocrine and immune interactions. Brain Res Rev. 1997;23(1–2):79–133.

286. McEwen BS, Stellar E. Stress and the individual: mechanisms leading to disease. Arch Intern Med. 1993;153(18):2093–101.

287. Tam J, Trembovler V, Di Marzo V et al. The cannabinoid CB1 receptor regulates bone formation by modulating adrenergic signaling. FASEB J. 2008;22(1):285–94.

288. Yadav VK, Oury F, Suda N et al. A serotonin-dependent mechanism explains the leptin regulation of bone mass, appetite and energy expenditure. Cell. 2009;138(5):976–89.

289. Cole SW, Kemeny ME, Fahey JL et al. Psychological risk factors for HIV pathogenesis: mediation by the autonomic nervous system. Biol Psychiatry. 2003;54(12):1444–56.

290. Kuis W, de Jong-de Vos van Steenwijk C, Sinnema G et al. The autonomic nervous system and the immune system in juvenile rheumatoid arthritis. Brain Behav Immun. 1996;10(4):387–98.

291. Laborit H. La vie antérieure. Paris: Grasset; 1989.

292. Banovic I, Gilibert D, Cosnes J. Crohn's disease and fatigue: constancy and co-variations of activity of the disease depression, anxiety and subjective quality of life. Psychol Health Med. 2010;15(4):394–405.

293. Graff LA, Walker JR, Bernstein CN. It's not just about the gut: managing depression and anxiety in inflammatory bowel disease. Practical Gastroenterology. 2010;34(7):11–25.

294. Savignac HM, Hyland NP, Dinan TG et al. The effects of repeated social interaction stress on behavioural and physiological parameters in a stress-sensitive mouse strain. Behav Brain Res. 2011;216(2):576–84.

295. Hoge EA, Brandstetter K, Moshier S et al. Broad spectrum of cytokine abnormalities in panic disorder and post-traumatic stress disorder. Depress Anxiety. 2009;26(5):447–55.

296. McEwens BS, Gianaros PJ. Central role of the brain in stress and adaptation: links to socioeconomic status health and disease. Ann N Y Acad Sci. 2010;1186:190–222.

297. Bansal V, Costantini T, Kroll L et al. Traumatic brain injury and intestinal dysfunction: uncovering the neuro-enteric axis. J Neurotrauma. 2009;26(8):1353–9.

298. Hall GB, Kamath MV, Collins S et al. Heightened central affective response to visceral sensations of pain and discomfort in IBS. Neurogastroenterol Motil. 2010;22(3): 276-e80.

299. Iovino P, Tremolaterra F, Boccia G et al. Irritable bowel syndrome in childhood: visceral hypersensitivity and psychosocial aspects. Neurogastroenterol Motil. 2009;21(9):940-e74.

300. Roth RS, Geisser ME, Bates R. The relationship of post-traumatic stress symptoms to depression and pain in patients with accident related chronic pain. J Pain. 2008;9(7):588–96.

301. Silverman MN, Heim CM, Nater UM et al. Neuroendocrine and immune contributors to fatigue. Phys Med Rehab. 2010;2(5):338–46.

302. Epstein RM, Shields CG, Meldrum SC et al. Physicians' responses to patients' medically unexplained symptoms. Psychosom Med. 2006;68(2):269–76.

303. Woivalin T, Krantz G, Mantyranta T. Medically unexplained symptoms: perceptions of physicians in primary health care. Fam Pract. 2004;21(2):199–203.

304. Smith RC, Lein C, Collins C et al. Treating patients with medically unexplained symptoms in primary care. J Gen Intern Med. 2003;18(6):478–89.

305. Reid S, Whooley D, Crayford T et al. Medically unexplained symptoms – GPs' attitudes towards their cause and management. Fam Pract. 2001;18(5):519–23.

306. Chapman CR, Tuckett RP, Song CW. Pain and stress in a systems perspective: reciprocal neural endocrine and immune interactions. J Pain. 2008;9(2):122–45.

307. Deising S, Weinkauf B, Blunk J et al. NGF-evoked sensitization of muscle fascia nociceptors in humans. Pain. 2012;153(8):1673–9.

308. Mense S. [Pathophysiology of low back pain and the transition to the chronic state – experimental data and new concepts] [Article in German]. Schmerz. 2001;15(6):413–7.

309. Urban MO, Gebhart GF. Central mechanisms in pain. Med Clin North Am. 1999;83(3):585–96.

310. Pillemer SR, Bradley LA, Crofford LJ et al. The neuroscience and endocrinology of fibromyalgia. Arthritis Rheum. 1997;40(11):1928–39.

311. Willard FH. Neuro-endocrine-immune network nociceptive stress and the general adaptive response. In: Everett T, Dennis M, Ricketts E, editors. Physiotherapy in mental health. A practical approach. Oxford: Butterworth-Heinemann; 1995. pp. 102–26.

312. Bennett RM. Emerging concepts in the neurobiology of chronic pain: evidence abnormal sensory processing in fibromyalgia. Mayo Clin Proc. 1999;74(4):385–98.

313. Panjabi MM. A hypothesis of chronic back pain: ligament subfailure injuries lead to muscle control dysfunction. Eur Spine J. 2006;15(5):668–76.

314. Flor H. Cortical re-organisation and chronic pain: implications for rehabilitation. J Rehabil Med. 2003;41(Suppl):66–72.

315. Benarroch EE. Pain-autonomic interactions. Neurol Sci. 2006;27(Suppl 2):S130–3.

316. Peyron R, Laurent B, García-Larrea L. Functional imaging of brain responses to pain. A review and meta-analysis (2000). Neurophysiol Clin. 2000;30(5):263–88.

317. Schabrun SM, Jones E, Kloster J et al. Temporal association between changes in primary sensory cortex and corti-comotor output during muscle pain. Neuroscience. 2013;235:159–64.

318. Tsao H, Galea MP, Hodges PW. Reorganization of the motor cortex is associated with postural control deficits in recurrent low back pain. Brain. 2008;131(8):2161–71.

319. Apkarian AV, Sosa Y, Sonty S et al. Chronic back pain is associated with decreased prefrontal and thalamic gray matter density. J Neurosci. 2004;24(46):10410–5.

320. Raichle ME, MacLeod AM, Snyder AZ et al. A default mode of brain function. Proc Natl Acad Sci USA. 2001;98(2):676–82.

321. Apkarian AV, Bushnell MC, Treede RD et al. Human brain mechanisms of pain perception and regulation in health and disease. Eur J Pain. 2005;9(4):463–84.

322. Baliki MN, Chialvo DR, Geha PY et al. Chronic pain and the emotional brain: specific brain activity associated with spontaneous fluctuations of intensity of chronic back pain. J Neurosci. 2006;26(47):12165–73.

323. deCharms RC, Maeda F, Glover GH et al. Control over brain activation and pain learned by using real-time functional MRI. Proc Natl Acad Sci USA. 2005;102(51):18626–31.

324. May A. Chronic pain may change the structure of the brain. Pain. 2008;137(1):7–15.

325. Couch JR, Lipton RB, Stewart WF et al. Head or neck injury increases the risk of chronic daily headache: a population-based study. Neurology. 2007;69(11):1169–77.

326. Davis KD, Pope G, Chen J et al. Cortical thinning in IBS: implications for homeostatic attention and pain processing. Neurology. 2008;70(2):153–4.

327. Schmidt-Wilcke T, Leinisch E, Straube A et al. Gray matter decrease in patients with chronic tension type headache. Neurology. 2005;65(9):1483–6.

328. Grachev ID, Ramachandran TS, Thomas PS et al. Association between dorsolateral prefrontal N-acetyl aspartate and depression in chronic back pain: an in vivo proton magnetic resonance spectroscopy study. J Neural Transm. 2003;110(3):287–312.

329. Alexandre FM, Granzlera C, Snyder J et al. Thickening in the somatosensory cortex of patients with migraine. Neurology. 2007;69(21):1990–5.

330. Vierck CJ Jr. Mechanisms underlying development of spatially distributed chronic pain (fibromyalgia). Pain. 2006;124(3):242–63.

331. Legrain V, Iannetti GD, Plaghki L et al. The pain matrix reloaded: a salience detection system for the body. Prog Neurobiol. 2011;93(1):111–24.

332. Moseley GL. A pain neuromatrix approach to patients with chronic pain. Man Ther. 2003;8(3):130–40.

333. Moseley GL, Flor H. Targeting cortical representations in the treatment of chronic pain: a review. Neurorehabil Neural Repair. 2012;26(6):646–52.

334. Bushnell MC, Ceko M, Low LA. Cognitive and emotional control of pain and its disruption in chronic pain. Nat Rev Neurosci. 2013;14(7):502–11.

335. Giummarra MJ, Gibson SJ, Georgiou-Karistianis N et al. Mechanisms underlying embodiment disembodiment and loss of embodiment. Neurosci Biobehav Rev. 2008;32(1):143–60.

336. Moseley GL. I can't find it! Distorted body image and tactile dysfunction in patients with chronic back pain. Pain. 2008;140(1): 239–43.

337. Osborn M, Smith JA. Living with a body separate from the self. The experience of the

body in chronic benign low back pain: an interpretative phenomenological analysis. Scand J Caring Sci. 2006;20(2):216–22.

338. Benarroch EE. The central autonomic network: functional organization, dysfunction and perspective. Mayo Clin Proc. 1993;68(10): 988–1001.

339. Tracey I. Imaging pain. Br J Anaesth. 2008;101(1):32–9.

340. Craig A. A new view of pain as a homeostatic emotion. Trends Neurosci. 2003;26(6):303–7.

341. Mogil JS, Max MB. The genetics of pain. In: McMahon SB, Koltzenburg M, editors. Wall and Melzack's textbook of pain. 5th ed. Philadelphia, PA: Elsevier Churchill Livingstone; 2006. pp. 159–74.

342. Zubieta JK, Heitzeg MM, Smith YR et al. COMT val158met genotype affects mu-opioid neurotransmitter responses to a pain stressor. Science. 2003;299(5610):1240–3.

343. Diatchenko L, Nackley AG, Slade GD et al. Catechol-O-methyltransferase gene polymorphisms are associated with multiple pain-evoking stimuli. Pain. 2006;125(3):216–24.

344. Diatchenko L, Slade GD, Nackley AG et al. Genetic basis for individual variations in pain perception and the development of a chronic pain condition. Hum Mol Genet. 2005;14(1):135–43.

345. Fryette HH. Principles of osteopathic technique. Reprint. Colorado Springs: American Academy of Osteopathy; 1980. p. 41.

346. McCarberg B, Wolf J. Chronic pain management in a health maintenance organization. Clin J Pain. 1999;15(1):50–7.

347. Haugli L, Steen E, Laerum E et al. Learning to have less pain – is it possible? A one-year follow-up study of the effects of a personal construct group learning programme on patients with chronic musculoskeletal pain. Patient Educ Couns. 2001;45(2):111–8.

348. Hoffman BM, Papas RK, Chatkoff DK et al. Meta-analysis of psychological interventions for chronic low back pain. Health Psychol. 2007;26(1):1–9.

349. Compton SN, March JS, Brent D et al. Cognitive-behavioral psychotherapy for anxiety and depressive disorders in children and adolescents: an evidence-based medicine review. J Am Acad Child Adolesc Psychiatry. 2004;43(8):930–59.

350. Bell AC, D'Zurilla TJ. Problem-solving therapy for depression: a meta-analysis. Clin Psychol Rev. 2009;29(4):348–53.

351. Dickens C, Cherrington A, Adeyemi I et al. Characteristics of psychological interventions that improve depression in people with coronary heart disease: a systematic review and meta-regression. Psychosom Med. 2013;75(2):211–21.

352. Stephen JE, Rahn M, Verhoef M et al. What is the state of the evidence on the mind-cancer survival question and where do we go from here? Support Care Cancer. 2007;15(8): 923–30.

353. Linden W, Stossel C, Maurice J. Psychosocial interventions for patients with coronary artery disease: a meta-analysis. Arch Intern Med. 1996;156(7):745–52.

354. Schubiner H. Mind-Body medicine. In: Chila A, editor. Foundations of osteopathic medicine. 3rd ed. Philadelphia, PA: Lippincott Williams and Wilkins; 2011. ch. 27.

355. Smyth JM, Stone AA, Hurewitz A et al. Effects of writing about stressful experiences on symptom reduction in patients with asthma or rheumatoid arthritis: a randomized trial. JAMA. 1999;281(14):1304–9.

356. Castés M, Hagel I, Palenque M et al. Immunological changes associated with clinical improvement of asthmatic children subjected to psychosocial intervention. Brain Behav Immun. 1999;13(1):1–13.

357. Hsu MC, Schubiner H. Recovery from chronic musculoskeletal pain with psychodynamic consultation and brief intervention: a report of three illustrative cases. Pain Med. 2010;11(6):977–80.

358. Turner JA, Mancl L, Aaron LA. Short- and long-term efficacy of brief cognitive-behavioral therapy for patients with chronic temporomandibular disorder pain: a randomized controlled trial. Pain. 2006;121(3):181–94.

359. Bandura A, O'Leary A, Taylor CB et al. Perceived self-efficacy and pain control: opioid and nonopioid mechanisms. J Pers Soc Psychol. 1987;53(3):563–71.

360. Astin JA. Mind-body therapies for the management of pain. Clin J Pain. 2004;20(1):27–32.

361. Astin JA, Berman BM, Bausell B et al. The efficacy of mindfulness meditation plus Qigong movement therapy in the treatment of fibromyalgia: a randomized controlled trial. J Rheumatol. 2003;30(10):2257–62.

362. Eriksson EM, Möller IE, Söderberg RH et al. Body awareness therapy: a new strategy for relief of symptoms in irritable bowel syndrome patients. World J Gastroenterol. 2007;13(23):3206–14.

363. Baas LS, Beery TA, Allen G et al. An exploratory study of body awareness in persons with heart failure treated medically or with transplantation. J Cardiovasc Nurs. 2004;19(1):32–40.

364. Christensen AJ, Wiebe JS, Edwards DL et al. Body consciousness, illness-related impairment and patient adherence in hemodialysis. J Consult Clin Psychol. 1996;64(1):147–52.

365. Burns JW. The role of attentional strategies in moderating links between acute pain induction and subsequent psychological stress: evidence for symptom-specific reactivity among patients with chronic pain versus healthy nonpatients. Emotion 2006;6(2):180–92.

366. Merkes M. Mindfulness-based stress reduction for people with chronic diseases. Aust J Prim Health. 2010;16(3):200–10.

367. Fernros L, Furhoff AK, Wändell PE. Improving quality of life using compound mind-body therapies: evaluation of a course intervention with body movement and breath therapy guided imagery chakra experiencing and mindfulness meditation. Qual Life Res. 2008;17(3):367–76.

368. Lutz A, Brefczynski-Lewis J, Johnstone T et al. Regulation of the neural circuitry of emotion by compassion meditation: effects of meditative expertise. PLoS One. 2008;3(3):e1897.

369. Xu J, Vik A, Groote IR et al. Nondirective meditation activates default mode network and areas associated with memory retrieval and emotional processing. Front Hum Neurosci. 2014;26;8:86.

370. Carlson LE, Speca M, Faris P et al. One year pre-post intervention follow-up of

psychological immune endocrine and blood pressure outcomes of mindfulness-based stress reduction (MBSR) in breast and prostate cancer outpatients. Brain Behav Immun. 2007;21(8):1038–49.

371. Mehling WE, Gopisetty V, Daubenmier J et al. Body awareness: construct and self-report measures. PLoS ONE. 2009;4(5):e5614.

372. Andrasik F. Biofeedback in headache: an overview of approaches and evidence. Cleve Clin J Med. 2010;77(Suppl 3):S72–6.

373. Karavidas MK, Tsai PS, Yucha C et al. Thermal biofeedback for primary Raynaud's phenomenon: a review of the literature. Appl Psychophysiol Biofeedback. 2006;31(3): 203–16.

374. Glombiewski JA, Bernardy K, Häuser W. Efficacy of EMG- and EEG-biofeedback in fibromyalgia syndrome: a meta-analysis and a systematic review of randomized controlled trials. Evid Based Complement Alternat Med. 2013:962741.

375. Pennebaker JW. Traumatic experience and psychosomatic disease: exploring the roles of behavioural inhibition obsession and confiding. Can Psychol. 1985;26(2):82–95.

376. Gillis ME, Lumley MA, Mosley-Williams A et al. The health effects of at-home written emotional disclosure in fibromyalgia: a randomized trial. Ann Behav Med. 2006;32(2):135–46.

377. Smyth M, Stone A, Hurewitz A et al. Effects of writing about stressful experiences on symptom reduction with asthma or rheumatoid arthritis: a randomized trial. JAMA. 1999;281(14):1304–9.

378. Mogk C, Otte S, Reinhold-Hurley B et al. Health effects of expressive writing on stressful

or traumatic experiences – a meta-analysis. Psychosoc Med. 2006;3:Doc06.

379. Curtis K, Osadchuk A, Katz J. An eight-week yoga intervention is associated with improvements in pain psychological functioning and mindfulness and changes in cortisol levels in women with fibromyalgia. J Pain Res. 2011;4:189–201.

380. Holtzman S, Beggs RT. Yoga for chronic low back pain: a meta-analysis of randomized controlled trials. Pain Res Manag. 2013;18(5):267–72.

381. Cramer H, Lauche R, Haller H et al. A systematic review and meta-analysis of yoga for low back pain. Clin J Pain. 2013;29(5):450–60.

382. Field ES. Neurolinguistic programming as an adjunct to other psychotherapeutic/ hypnotherapeutic interventions. Am J Clin Hypn. 1990;32(3):174–82.

383. MacKinnon RA, Yudofsky SC. The psychiatric evaluation in clinical practice. Philadelphia, PA: Lippincott; 1986.

384. Burns DD. Feeling good: the new mood therapy. New York: New American Library; 1980.

385. Drageset J, Eide GE, Nygaard HA et al. The impact of social support and sense of coherence on health-related quality of life among nursing home residents – a questionnaire survey in Bergen, Norway. Int J Nurs Stud. 2009;46(1):65–75.

386. Eriksson M, Lindström B. A salutogenic interpretation of the Ottawa Charter. Health Promot Int. 2008;23(2):190–9.

387. Berkman LF, Syme SL. Social networks host resistance and mortality: a nine-year follow-up study of Alameda County residents. Am J Epidemiol. 1979;109(2):186–204.

388. Carney RM, Freedland KE, Steinmeyer B et al. Depressions and five year survival following acute myocardial infarction: a prospective study. J Affect Disord. 2008;109(1–2): 133–8.

389. Carson JW, Keefe FJ, Goli V et al. Forgiveness and chronic low back pain: a preliminary study examining the relationship of forgiveness to pain anger and psychological distress. J Pain. 2005;6(2):84–91.

390. Viane I, Crombez G, Eccleston C et al. Acceptance of the unpleasant reality of chronic pain: effects upon attention to pain and engagement with daily activities. Pain. 2004;112(3):282–8.

391. McCracken LM, Vowles KE. Psychological flexibility and traditional pain management strategies in relation to patient functioning with chronic pain: an examination of a revised instrument. J Pain 2007;8(9):700–7.

392. Ai AL, Pederson C, Tice TN et al. The influence of prayer coping on mental health and cardiac surgery patients: the role of optimism and acute distress. J Health Psychol. 2007;12(4):580–96.

393. Oxman TE, Freeman DH Jr, Manheimer ED. Lack of social participation or religious strength and comfort as risk factors for death after cardiac surgery in the elderly. Psychosom Med. 1995;57(1):5–15.

394. Blumenthal JA, Babyak MA, Ironson G et al. Spirituality, religion and clinical outcomes in patients recovering from an acute myocardial infarction. Psychosom Med. 2007;69(6): 501–8.

395. Rippentrop EA. A review of the role of religion and spirituality in chronic pain populations. Rehab Psychol. 2005;50(3):278–84.

396. Jantos M, Kiat H. Prayer as medicine: how much have we learned? Med J Aust. 2007;186(10 Suppl):S51–3.

397. McCord G, Gilchrist VJ, Grossman SD et al. Discussing spirituality with patients: a rational and ethical approach. Ann Fam Med. 2004;2(4):356–61.

398. Krucoff MW. Crater SW. Gallup D et al. Music imagery touch and prayer as adjuncts to interventional cardiac care: the monitoring and actualisation of noetic training (MAN-TRA) II randomised study. Lancet. 2005;366(9481):211–7.

399. Stewart M. Effective physician-patient communication and health outcomes: a review. CMAJ. 1995;152(9):1423–33.

400. Bargh JA, Chen M, Burrows L. Automaticity of social behavior: direct effects of trait construct and stereotype activation on action. J Pers Soc Psychol. 1996;71(2):230–44.

401. Coulehan JL, Platt FW, Egener B et al. "Let me see if I have this right": words that help build empathy. Ann Intern Med. 2001;135(3):221–7.

402. Hojat M, Gonnella JS, Nasca TJ et al. Physician empathy: definition components measurement and relationship to gender and specialty. Am J Psychiatry. 2002;159(9):1563–9.

403. Shamay-Tsoory SG, Lester H, Chisin R et al. The neural correlates of understanding the other's distress: a positron emission tomography investigation of accurate empathy. Neuro-image. 2005;27(2):468–72.

404. Levenson RW, Ruef AM. Empathy: a physiological substrate. J Pers Soc Psychol. 1992;63(2):234–46.

405. Gottman JM, Levenson RW. A valid procedure for obtaining self-report of affect in marital interaction. J Consult Clin Psychol. 1985;53(2):151–60.

406. Halpern J. Empathy: using resonance emotions in the service of curiosity. In: Spiro H, Cunen

M, Peschel E et al., editors. Empathy and the practice of medicine: beyond pills and scalpel. New Haven, CT: Yale University Press; 1993. pp. 160–73.

407. Rizzolatti G, Craighero L. The mirror-neuron system. Ann Rev Neurosci. 2004;27:169–92.

408. Carr L, Iacoboni M, Dubeau MC et al. Neural mechanisms of empathy in humans: a relay from neural systems for imitation to limbic areas. Proc Natl Acad Sci USA. 2003;100(9):5497–502.

409. Kelley JM, Kraft-Todd G, Schapira L et al. The influence of the patient-clinician relationship on healthcare outcomes: a systematic review and meta-analysis of randomized controlled trials. PLoS ONE. 2014;9(4):e94207.

410. Griffin SJ, Kinmonth AL, Veltman MW et al. Effect on health-related outcomes of interventions to alter the interaction between patients and practitioners: a systematic review of trials. Ann Fam Med. 2004;2(6): 595–608.

411. Stewart M, Brown JB, Donner A et al. The impact of patient-centered care on outcomes. J Fam Pract. 2000;49(9):796–804.

412. Carey TS, Motyka TM, Garrett JM et al. Do osteopathic physicians differ in patient interaction from allopathic physicians? An empirically derived approach. J Am Osteopath Assoc. 2003;103(7):313–8.

413. Leach J, Cross V, Fawkes C et al. Investigating osteopathic patients' expectations of osteopathic care: the OPEn project. Research Report, University of Brighton, May 2011.

414. Loeser J, Turk DC. Multidisciplinary pain management. In: Loeser JD, Butler SD, Chapman CR et al., editors. Bonica's management of pain. 3rd ed. Baltimore, MD: Williams and Wilkins; 2001. pp. 2069–79.

415. Pergolizzi J, Ahlbeck K, Aldington D et al. The development of chronic pain: physiological CHANGE necessitates a multidisciplinary approach to treatment. Curr Med Res Opin. 2013;29(9):1127–35.

416. Hildebrandt J, Pfingsten M, Franz C et al. [Multi-disciplinary treatment program for chronic low back pain part 1 Overview] [Article in German]. Schmerz. 1996;26;10(4):190–203.

417. Kim MM, Barnato AE, Angus DC et al. The effect of multidisciplinary care teams on intensive care unit mortality. Arch Intern Med. 2010;170(4):369–76.

418. Lang E, Liebig K, Kastner S et al. Multidisciplinary rehabilitation versus usual care for chronic low back pain in the community: effects on quality of life. Spine J. 2003;3(4):270–6.

419. Flor H, Fydrich T, Turk D. Efficacy of multidisciplinary pain treatment center: a meta-analytic review. Pain. 1992;49(2):221–30.

420. Golden BA. A multidisciplinary approach to non-pharmacologic pain management. J Am Osteopath Assoc. 2002;102(9 Suppl 3):S1–5.

421. Hamberg K, Johansson E, Lindgren G et al. The impact of marital relationship on the rehabilitation process in a group of women with long-term musculoskeletal disorders. Scand J Soc Med. 1997;25(1):17–25.

422. Kiecolt-Glaser JK, Newton TL. Marriage and health: his and hers. Psychol Bull. 2001;127(4):472–503.

423. Kiecolt-Glaser JK, Gouin JP, Hantsoo L. Close relationships inflammation and health. Neurosci Biobehav Rev. 2010;35(1):33–8.

424. Steen E, Haugli L. From pain to self-awareness – a qualitative analysis of the significance of group participation for persons with chronic

musculoskeletal pain. Patient Educ Couns. 2001;42(1):35–46.

425. Spiegel D, Bloom JR, Kraemer HC et al. Effect of psychosocial treatment on survival of patients with metastatic breast cancer. Lancet. 1989;2(8668):888–91.

426. Fawzy FI, Fawzy NW, Hyun CS et al. Malignant melanoma: effects of early structured psychiatric intervention coping and affective state on recurrence and survival 6 years later. Arch Gen Psychiatry. 1993;50(9):681–9.

427. Leo RJ. Concise guide to pain management for psychiatrists. Arlington, VA: American Psychiatric; 2003.

428. Blair SN, Kohl WH, Paffenbarger RC Jr. Physical fitness and all-cause mortality. A prospective study of healthy men and women. JAMA. 1989;262(17):2395–401.

429. Blair SN, Horton E, Leon AS et al. Physical activity, nutrition and chronic disease. Med Sci Sports Exerc. 1996;28(3):335–49.

430. Bouchard C, Shephard RJ, Stephens T, editors. Physical activity fitness and health: international proceedings and consensus statement. Champaign, IL: Human Kinetics; 1994.

431. Ribeiro F, Oliveira J. Aging effects on joint proprioception: the role of physical activity in proprioception preservation. Eur Rev Aging Phys Act. 2007;4(2):71–6.

432. Jola C, Davis A, Haggard P. Proprioceptive integration and body representation: insights into dancers' expertise. Exp Brain Res. 2011;213(2–3):257–65.

433. Simpson RJ, Lowder TW, Spielmann G et al. Exercise and the aging immune system. Ageing Res Rev. 2012;11(3):404–20.

434. Perna FM, Schneiderman N, LaPerriere A. Psychological stress exercise and immunity. Int J Sports Med. 1997;18(Suppl 1): S78–83.

435. Drake DA. A longitudinal study of physical activity and breast cancer prediction. Cancer Nurs. 2001;24(5):371–7.

436. Shephard RJ. Exercise and cancer: linkages with obesity? Crit Rev Food Sci Nutr. 1996;36(4):321–39.

437. Rosenwinkel ET, Bloomfield DM, Arwady MA et al. Exercise and autonomic function in health and cardiovascular disease. Cardiol Clin. 2001;19(3):369–87.

438. Anshel M. Coping styles among adolescent competitive athletes. J Soc Psychol. 1996;136(3):311–23.

439. Agudelo LZ, Femenía T, Orhan F et al. Skeletal muscle PGC-1α1 modulates kynurenine metabolism and mediates resilience to stress-induced depression. Cell. 2014;159(1):33–45.

440. Liu J. Irisin as an exercise-stimulated hormone binding crosstalk between organs. Eur Rev Med Pharmacol Sci. 2015;19(2):316–21.

441. Digiovanni BF, Nawoczenski DA, Malay DP et al. Plantar fascia-specific stretching exercise improves outcomes in patients with chronic plantar fasciitis. A prospective clinical trial with two-year follow-up. J Bone Joint Surg Am. 2006;88(8):1775–81.

442. Ronen N, Livne E, Gross B. Oxidative damage in rat tissue following excessive L-tryptophan and atherogenic diets. Adv Exp Med Biol. 1999;467:497–505.

443. Gómez Candela C, Bermejo López LM, Loria Kohen V. Importance of a balanced omega 6/ omega 3 ratio for the maintenance of health:

nutritional recommendations. Nutr Hosp. 2011;26(2):323–9.

444. Simopoulos AP. Omega-6/omega-3 essential fatty acids: biological effects. World Rev Nutr Diet. 2009;99:1–16.

445. James MJ, Cleland LG. Dietary n-3 fatty acids and therapy for rheumatoid arthritis. Semin Arthritis Rheum. 1997;27(2):85–97.

446. Marcason W. What is the anti-inflammatory diet? J Am Diet Assoc. 2010;110(11):1780.

447. Pomari E, Stefanon B, Colitti M. Effect of plant extracts on H2O2-induced inflammatory gene expression in macrophages. J Inflamm Res. 2014;7:103–12.

448. Kris-Etherton PM, Harris WS, Appel LJ. Fish consumption fish oil omega-3 fatty acids and cardiovascular disease. Circulation. 2002;106(21):2747–57.

449. Tapsell LC, Hemphill I, Cobiac L et al. Health benefits of herbs and spices: the past the present, the future. Med J Aust. 2006;21;185(4 Suppl):S4–24.

450. Yadav VR, Prasad S, Sung B et al. The role of chalcones in suppression of NF-κB-mediated inflammation and cancer. Int Immunopharmacol. 2011;11(3):295–309.

451. Ragle RL, Sawitzke AD. Nutraceuticals in the management of osteoarthritis: a critical review. Drugs Aging. 2012;29(9):717–31.

452. Akhtar N, Haqqi TM. Current nutraceuticals in the management of osteoarthritis: a review. Ther Adv Musculoskelet Dis. 2012;4(3):181–207.

453. Torri E, Lemos M, Caliari V et al. Anti-inflammatory and antinociceptive properties of blueberry extract (Vaccinium corymbosum). J Pharm Pharmacol. 2007;59(4):591–6.

454. Gorski F, Corrêa CR, Filho VC et al. Potent anti-nociceptive activity of a hydroalcoholic extract of Phyllanthus corcovadensis. J Pharm Pharmacol. 1993;45(12):1046–9.

455. World Health Organization (WHO). Smoking statistics fact sheet. Geneva: WHO; 2002.

456. Eckhardt L, Woodruff SI, Elder JP. Related effectiveness of continued lapsed and delayed smoking prevention intervention in senior high school students. Am J Health Promot. 1997;11(6):418–21.

457. Brandon TH. Behavioral tobacco cessation treatments: yesterday's news or tomorrow's headlines? J Clin Oncol. 2001;19(18 Suppl):64S–68S.

458. Coleman T. Smoking cessation: integrating recent advances into clinical practice. Thorax 56(7):579–82.

459. Kottke TE, Battista RN, DeFriese et al. Attributes of successful smoking cessation interventions in medical practice. A meta-analysis of 39 controlled trials. JAMA. 1988;259(19):2883–9.

460. Fleming MF, Mundt MP, French MT et al. Brief physician advice for problem drinkers: long-term efficacy and benefit-cost analysis. Alcohol Clin Exp Res. 2002;26(1):36–43.

461. Whitclock EP, Green CA, Polen MR et al. Behavioral counseling interventions in primary care to reduce risky/harmful alcohol use systematic evidence review. Rockville, MD: Agency for Healthcare Research and Quality; 2004.

462. Metz JA, Kris-Etherton PM, Morris CD et al. Dietary compliance and cardiovascular risk reduction with a prepared meal plan compared with a self-selected diet. Am J Clin Nutr. 1997;66(2):373–85.

463. Fitzgibbon ML, Stolley MR, Avellone ME et al. Involving parents in cancer risk reduction: a program for Hispanic American families. Health Psychol. 1996;15(6):413–22.

464. Sivertsen B, Omvik S, Pallesen S et al. Cognitive behavioral therapy vs zopiclone for treatment of chronic primary insomnia in older adults: a randomized controlled trial. JAMA. 2006;295(24):2851–8.

465. Morgenthaler T, Kramer M, Alessi C et al. Practice parameters for the psychological and behavioral treatment of insomnia: an update. An American Academy of Sleep Medicine report. Sleep. 2006;29(11):1415–9.

466. vanTulder MW, Ostelo R, Vlaeyen JW et al. Behavioral treatment for chronic low back pain: a systematic review within the framework of the Cochrane Back Review Group. Spine. 2001;26(3):270–81.

467. Morley S, Eccleston C, Williams A. Systematic review and meta-analysis of randomized controlled trials of cognitive behavior therapy for chronic pain in adults excluding headache. Pain. 1999;80(1–2):1–13.

468. Scott J, Gade G, McKenzie M et al. Cooperative health care clinics: a group approach to individual care. Geriatrics. 1998;53(5):68–70.

469. Chrousos G. Neuroendocrine and immune crosstalk. Ann NY Acad Sci New York; 2006.

470. Pert CB. Molecules of emotion: why you feel the way you feel. London: Simon and Schuster; 1997. p. 143.

471. Futterman AD, Kemeny ME, Shapiro D et al. Immunological variability associated with experimentally induced positive and negative affective states. Psychol Med. 1992;22(1): 231–8.

472. Calabrese JR, Kling M, Gold PW. Alterations in immunocompetence during stress bereavement and depression: focus on neuroendocrine regulation. Am J Psychiatry. 1987;144(9):1123–34.

473. LeDoux JE. Emotion circuits in the brain. Annu Rev Neurosci. 2000;23:155–84.

474. Damasio AR. Descartes' error emotion, reason and the human brain. New York: Quill; 1994.

475. Marques-Deak A, Cizza G, Sternberg E. Brain-immune interactions and disease susceptibility. Mol Psychiatry. 2005;10(10): 972.

476. Hamel E. Perivascular nerves and the regulation of cerebro-vascular tone. J Appl Physiol. 2006;100(3):1059–64.

477. Golanov EV, Yamamoto S, Reis DJ. Spontaneous waves of cerebral blood flow associated with a pattern of electro-cortical activity. Am J Physiol. 1994;266(1/2): R204–14.

478. Tscharnuter I. Clinical application of dynamic theory concepts according to Tscharnuter Akademie for Movement Organization (TAMO) therapy. Pediatr Phys Ther. 2002;14(1):29–37.

479. Adler MW, Geller EB, Chen X et al. Viewing chemokines as a third major system of communication in the brain. AAPS J. 2006;7(4):E865–70.

480. Felten DL, Felten SY, Bellinger DL et al. Noradrenergic sympathetic neural interactions with the immune system: structure and function. Immunol Rev. 1987;100:225–60.

481. Plotkin BJ, Rodos JJ, Kappler R et al. Adjunctive osteopathic manipulative treatment in women with depression: a pilot study. J Am Osteopath Assoc. 2001;101(9):517–23.

482. Stefano GB, Goumon Y, Bilfinger TV et al. Basal nitric oxide limits immune nervous and cardiovascular excitation: human endothelia express a mu opiate receptor. Prog Neurobiol. 2000;60(6):513–30.

483. Salamon E, Zhu W, Stefano GB. Nitric oxide as a possible mechanism for understanding the therapeutic effects of osteopathic manipulative medicine (Review). Int J Mol Med. 2004;14(3):443–9.

484. Overberger R, Hoyt JA, Daghigh F et al. Comparing changes in serum nitric oxide levels and heart rate after osteopathic manipulative treatment (OMT) using the Dalrymple pedal pump to changes measured after active exercise. J Am Osteopath Assoc. 2009;109(1):41–2.

485. Dodd JG, Good MM, Nguyen TL et al. In vitro biophysical strain model for understanding mechanisms of osteopathic manipulative treatment. J Am Osteopath Assoc. 2006;106(3):157–66.

486. Cao TV, Hicks MR, Standley PR. In vitro biomechanical strain regulation of fibroblast wound healing. J Am Osteopath Assoc. 2013;113(11):806–18.

487. Bokhari AR, Murrell GA. The role of nitric oxide in tendon healing. J Shoulder Elbow Surg. 2012;21(2):238–44.

488. Garthwaite J. Concepts of neural nitric oxide-mediated transmission. Eur J Neurosci. 2008;27(11):2783–802.

489. Wink DA, Hines HB, Cheng RY et al. Nitric oxide and redox mechanisms in the immune response. J Leukoc Biol. 2011;89(6): 873–91.

490. Stefano GB, Ottaviani E. The biochemical substrate of nitric oxide signaling is present in primitive non-cognitive organisms. Brain Res. 2002;924(1):82–9.

491. Kotlo KU, Rasenick MM, Danziger RS. Evidence for cross-talk between atrial natriuretic peptide and nitric oxide receptors. Mol Cell Biochem. 2010; 338(1–2):183–9.

492. McPartland JM, Giuffrida A, King J et al. Cannabimimetic effects of osteopathic manipulative treatment. J Am Osteopath Assoc. 2005;105(6):283–91.

493. McPartland JM. Expression of the endocannabinoid system in fibroblasts and myofascial tissues. J Bodyw Mov Ther. 2008;12(2):169–82.

494. Degenhardt BF, Darmani NA, Johnson JC et al. Role of osteopathic manipulative treatment in altering pain bio-markers: a pilot study. J Am Osteopath Assoc. 2007;107(9):387–400.

495. McPartland JM. The endocannabinoid system: an osteopathic perspective. J Am Osteopath Assoc. 2008;108(10):586–600.

496. Ralevic V, Kendall DA, Randall MD et al. Cannabinoid modulation of sensory neurotransmission via cannabinoid and vanilloid receptors: roles in regulation of cardiovascular function. Life Sci. 2002;71(22):2577–94.

497. Deutsch DG, Goligorsky MS, Schmid PC et al. Production and physiological actions of anandamide in the vasculature of the rat kidney. J Clin Invest. 1997;100(6):1538–46.

498. Stefano GB, Esch T, Cadet P et al. Endocannabinoids as autoregulatory signaling molecules: coupling to nitric oxide and a possible association with the relaxation response. Med Sci Monit. 2003;9(4): RA63–75.

499. Lucas N. To what should we attribute the effects of OMT? Int J Osteopath Med 2005;8(4):121–3.

500. Carlino E, Pollo A, Benedetti F. Placebo analgesia and beyond: a melting pot of concepts and ideas for neuroscience. Curr Opin Anaesthesiol. 2011;24(5):540–4.

501. Greene CS, Goddard G, Macaluso GM et al. Topical review: placebo responses and therapeutic responses. How are they related? J Orofac Pain. 2009;23(2):93–107.

502. Faria V, Fredrikson M, Furmark T. Imaging the placebo response: a neurofunctional review. Eur Neuropsychopharmacol. 2008;18(7):473–85.

503. Damasio AR. Looking for Spinoza. Joy sorrow and the feeling brain. Orlando: Harcourt; 2003.

504. Pacheco-López G, Engler H, Niemi MB et al. Expectations and associations that heal: immunomodulatory placebo effects and its neurobiology. Brain Behav Immun. 2006;20(5):430–46.

505. Price DD, Finniss DG, Benedetti F. A comprehensive review of the placebo effect: recent advances and current thought. Annu Rev Psychol. 2008;59:565–90.

506. Koshi EB, Short CA. Placebo theory and its implications for research and clinical practice: a review of the recent literature. Pain Pract. 2007;7(1):4–20.

507. Marchand S, Gaumond I. Placebo and nocebo: how to enhance therapies and avoid unintended sabotage to pain treatment. Pain Manag. 2013;3(4):285–94.

508. Kaptchuk TJ. The placebo effect in alternative medicine: can the performance of a healing ritual have clinical significance? Ann Intern Med. 2002;4;136(11):817–25.

509. Lindgren L, Westling G, Brulin C et al. Pleasant human touch is represented in pregenual anterior cingulate cortex. Neuroimage. 2012;59(4):3427–32.

510. Nadler SF. Nonpharmacologic management of pain. J Am Osteopath Assoc. 2004;104(11 Suppl 8):S6–12.

511. Rapaport MH, Schettler P, Bresee C. A preliminary study of the effects of a single session of Swedish massage on hypothalamic-pituitary-adrenal and immune function in normal individuals. J Altern Complement Med. 2010;16(10):1079–88.

512. Rapaport MH, Schettler P, Bresee C. A preliminary study of the effects of repeated massage on hypothalamic-pituitary-adrenal and immune function in healthy individuals: a study of mechanisms of action and dosage. J Altern Complement Med. 2012;18(8):789–97.

513. Morhenn V, Beavin LE, Zak PJ. Massage increases oxytocin and reduces adrenocorticotropin hormone in humans. Altern Ther Health Med. 2012;18(6):11–8.

514. Henderson AT, Fisher JF, Blair J. Effects of rib raising on the autonomic nervous system: a pilot study using non-invasive biomarkers. J Am Osteopath Assoc. 2010;110(6): 324–30.

515. Lund I, Ge Y, Yu LC et al. Repeated massage-like stimulation induces long-term effects on nociception: contribution of oxytocinergic mechanisms. Eur J Neurosci 2002;16(2):330–8.

516. Lieberwirth C, Wang Z. Social bonding: regulation by neuropeptides. Front Neurosci. 2014;8:171.

517. Fernández-Pérez AM, Peralta-Ramírez MI, Pilat A et al. Effects of myofascial induction techniques on physiologic and psychologic

parameters: a randomized controlled trial. J Altern Complement Med. 2008;14(7):807–11.

518. Henley CE, Ivins D, Mills M et al. Osteopathic manipulative treatment and its relationship to autonomic nervous system activity as demonstrated by heart rate variability: a repeated measures study. Osteopathic Med Prim Care. 2008;5;2:7.

519. Lombardini R, Marchesi S, Collebrusco L et al. The use of osteopathic manipulative treatment as adjuvant therapy in patients with peripheral arterial disease. Man Ther. 2009;14(4): 439–43.

520. Lindgren L, Rundgren S, Winso O et al. Physiological responses to touch massage in healthy volunteers. Auton Neurosci. 2010;158(1–2):105–10.

521. Hatayama T, Kitamura S, Tamura C et al. The facial massage reduced anxiety and negative mood status and increased sympathetic nervous activity. Biomed Res. 2008;29(6):317–20.

522. Toro-Velasco C, Arroyo-Morales M, Fernández-de-Las-Peñas C et al. Short-term effects of manual therapy on heart rate variability mood state and pressure pain sensitivity in patients with chronic tension-type headache: a pilot study. J Manipulative Physiol Ther. 2009;32(7):527–35.

523. Queré N, Noël E, Lieutaud A et al. Fasciatherapy combined with pulsology touch induces changes in blood turbulence potentially beneficial for vascular endothelium. J Bodyw Mov Ther. 2009;13(3):239–45.

524. Shi X, Rehrer S, Prajapati P et al. Effect of cranial osteopathic manipulative medicine on cerebral tissue oxygenation. J Am Osteopath Assoc. 2011;111(12):660–6.

525. Craig AD. How do you feel? Interoception: the sense of the physiological condition of the body. Nat Rev Neurosci. 2002;3(8): 655–66.

526. Björnsdotter M, Morrison I, Olausson H. Feeling good: on the role of C fiber mediated touch in interoception. Exp Brain Res. 2010;207(3–4):149–55.

527. Olausson H, Wessberg J, Morrison I et al. The neurophysiology of unmyelinated tactile afferents. Neurosci Biobehav Rev. 2010;34(2):185–91.

528. Bialosky JE, Bishop MD, Price DD et al. The mechanisms of manual therapy in the treatment of musculo-skeletal pain: a comprehensive model. Man Ther. 2009;14(5):531–8.

529. Simmonds N, Miller P, Gemmell H. A theoretical framework for the role of fascia in manual therapy. J Bodyw Mov Ther. 2012;16(1):83–93.

530. Rolls ET. The functions of the orbitofrontal cortex. Brain Cogn. 2004;55(1):11–29.

531. Ribera d'Alcalà C, Webster DG, Esteves JE. Interoception body awareness and chronic pain: results from a case-control study. Int J Osteopath Med. 2014 (in press).

532. World Health Organization (WHO). The Ottawa charter for health promotion. Ottawa, Ontario: WHO; 1986.

533. Dahlgren G, Whitehead M. Policies and strategies to promote social equity in health. Stockholm: Institute for Futures Studies; 1991.

534. Orth-Gomer K. International epidemiological evidence for a relationship between social supper and cardiovascular diseases. In: Shumaker SA, Czajkowski SM, editors. Social

support and cardiovascular diseases. New York: Plenum Press; 1994. pp. 97–117.

535. Sternberg EM, Gold PW. The mind-body interaction in disease. Sci Am. 1997;7(1):8–15.

536. Badura B. What is and what determines health? In: Laaser U, de Leeuw E, Stock Chr, editors. Scientific foundations for a public health policy in Europe. München: Juventa Weinheim; 1995. pp. 80–8.

537. Faggiano F, Versino E, Lemma P. Decennial trends of social differentials in smoking habits in Italy. Cancer Causes Control. 2001;12(7):665–71.

538. McKenzie JF, Neiger B, Smeltzer JL. Planning implementing and evaluating health promotion programs: a primer. 4th ed. San Francisco, CA: Pearson Benjamin Cummings; 2005.

539. Prinsen JK, Hensel KL, Snow RJ. Response: observational study demonstrates that OMT is associated with reduced analgesic prescribing and fewer missed work days. J Am Osteopath Assoc. 2014;114(7):530–1.

540. Prinsen JK, Hensel KL, Snow RJ. OMT associated with reduced analgesic prescribing and fewer missed work days in patients with low back pain: an observational study. J Am Osteopath Assoc. 2014;114(2):90–8.

541. Goff MB, Nelson MA, Deighton MM et al. Pain management and osteopathic manipulative medicine in the Army: new opportunities for the osteopathic medical profession. J Am Osteopath Assoc. 2011;111(5):331–4.

542. Ross EM, Darracq MA. Complementary and alternative medicine practices in military personnel and families presenting to a military emergency department. Mil Med. 2015;180(3):350–4.

543. Cruser dA, Maurer D, Hensel K et al. A randomized controlled trial of osteopathic manipulative treatment for acute low back pain in active duty military personnel. J Man Manip Ther. 2012;20(1):5–15.

544. Coupet S, Howell JD, Ross-Lee B. An international health elective in Haiti: a case for osteopathic medicine. J Am Osteopath Assoc. 2013;113(6):484–9.

545. http://divinityfoundationcom/.

546. http://wwwfurahait/.

547. http://osteopathywithoutborderscom/.

548. Rifkin J. La civiltà dell'empatia. La corsa verso la coscienza globale nel mondo in crisi. Milano: Mondadori; 2010.

549. Keefe FJ, Rumble ME, Scipio CD et al. Psychological aspects of persistent pain: current state of the science. J Pain. 2004;5(4):195–211.

550. Licciardone JC, Brimhall AK, King LN. Osteopathic manipulative treatment for low back pain: a systematic review and meta-analysis of randomized controlled trials. BMC Musculoskelet Disord 2005;6:43.

551. Stanton DF, Dutes JC. Chronic pain and the chronic pain syndrome: the usefulness of manipulation and behavioral interventions. Phys Med Rehabil Clin North Am. 1996;7:863–75.

552. Petrie KJ, Müller JT, Schirmbeck F et al. Effect of providing information about normal test results on patients' reassurance: randomised controlled trial. BMJ. 2007; 334(7589):352.

553. Burton AK, Waddell G, Tillotson KM et al. Information and advice to patients with back pain can have a positive effect: a randomized

controlled trial of a novel educational booklet in primary care. Spine 1999;24(23):2484–91.

554. Roberts L, Little P, Chapman J et al. The back home trial: general practitioner supported leaflets may change back pain behavior. 2002;27(17):1821–8.

555. Friedrich M, Gittler G, Arendasy M et al. Long term effect of a combined exercise and motivational program on the level of disability of patients with chronic low back pain. Spine. 2005;30(9):995–1000.

556. Gimpel C, von Scheidt C, Jose G et al. Changes and interactions of flourishing mindfulness sense of coherence and quality of life in patients of a mind-body medicine outpatient clinic. Forsch Komplementmed. 2014;21(3):154–62.

557. Thomson OP, Petty NJ, Ramage CM et al. Qualitative research: exploring the multiple perspectives of osteopathy. Int J Osteopath Med. 2011;14(3):116–24.

558. Foster N, Pincus T, Underwood M et al. Understanding the process of care for musculoskeletal conditions and why a biomedical approach is inadequate. Rheumatology. 2003;42(3):401–4.

# Selection and integration of the models in osteopathic treatment and management

*Paolo Tozzi*

## Synopsis

The intention of this chapter is to provide guidelines for the planning and management of osteopathic treatment, based on the information gained from the assessment, through the integrated application of the models, and with a specific focus on the totality of the person. The aim is therefore to outline the principal stages of a complex, multidimensional, dynamic and flexible decision-making process in every phase, adaptable to the needs and potential of each individual case. The reorganization of this path is always possible and necessary whenever newly acquired elements require a different and more appropriate strategy. This allows the osteopath to show flexibility and program management based on an accurate and personalized assessment of the relationship between the potential risks and benefits to be obtained. The five osteopathic models now become just one of many components involved in the actual therapy, although essential in the added value they can provide.

However, one must integrate the models in a complex way on several fronts, which inevitably change methods, timing, and application dosages. There are many factors that can influence the course of treatment, inherent both to the individual osteopath and to the patient being treated, and specific to the context in which the therapeutic relationship is shaped. This path obviously requires scientific knowledge, technical skills, clinical expertise, and professional competence on the part of the operator, who must support the patient from the beginning, and take care of the individual until discharge and the long-term management of his or her welfare. Patients should also be active participants in this process, through proper motivation and the adoption of all the necessary strategies to restore, maintain and promote their own health.

Information, education, care, and physical family and societal support are fundamental requirements for achieving the goals of treatment. The multidimensional approach to the person requires in most cases an interdisciplinary approach and cooperation of experienced professionals who consider every aspect of the individual, promoting homeostatic capability and protecting the patient from potential risks of recurrence. The ultimate goal remains the strengthening of resources, and the autonomy and independence of the individual from any support necessary for the attainment and maintenance of his or her physical, mental, and social well-being.

## Introduction

Osteopathic concepts state that osteopathic intervention is centered on the person, understood in the full range of his or her physical, mental, and spiritual expressiveness, and that this will promote the inherent ability for self-regulation, using mostly the musculoskeletal system as a key tool.[1] This is a concept that has been recognized by international organizations[2] as an essential foundation in the training of our profession.[3] How this can be implemented in everyday clinical practice through decision-making and management decisions on a personal basis remains an open debate, as well as being a field not yet fully explored.

The ability to formulate a coherent treatment and rely on a precise rationale for technique choice through a critical and reflective process is now considered an essential requirement in European osteopathic practice.[4] The fact is that the choice of when and how to act is largely left to the operator's discretion, with the "excuse" that each treatment is unique and unrepeatable for each patient and therefore cannot be limited to recipes and protocols, which undoubtedly reflects part of the reality and the fundamental principles of osteopathy, but in fact does not help the osteopath to navigate the complexity of the decision-making that involves "taking care" of the person. Fortunately, our traditional literature provides general guidance on how to unravel the puzzle of osteopathic treatment planning,[5] the selection of the techniques and forces to apply,[6] possible variations in technique, factors that may influence the choice,[7] and finally the critical thinking that should support this decision-making process.[8]

Several contemporary authors have also delineated the concepts useful in the planning of osteopathic treatment in general,[9,10] the selection of models based on the specific clinical presentation,[11] the most suitable choice of intervention for the most frequent systemic diseases,[12] or for different age groups[13] or single pathologies,[14] including indications and contraindications for the most common osteopathic techniques.[15] However, the information currently available remains fragmented and sometimes conflicting, often leaving final decisions to the clinical experience of the operator.

## The osteopath–patient relationship

The way in which an osteopath understands and conceives osteopathy will inevitably influence clinical decision-making. The perception that a health professional has of his or her profession and the subjective manner in which he or she interprets the principles and their application seem to be crucial in the clinical choice of action and type of intervention applied.[16] The same clinical information can be read and interpreted differently by operators who hold different views of the same profession[17] or have different ways of interpreting the body.[18] This determines a different selection of what is relevant, possibly resulting in a different therapeutic approach and a different interaction with the patient.

A recent qualitative study has proposed, for the first time, an evidence-based model, outlining some factors that influence the clinical decision-making process of the osteopath and the resulting therapeutic intervention.[19] This study, by 12 expert osteopaths, revealed three different qualitative types of osteopathic clinical strategy, which correspond to different ways of understanding the practice itself: the treater, the communicator, and the educator. In the first case, that of the treater, the approach was therapist-centric, with the treater assuming total control over and responsibility for the healing process. Here the osteopath is the only true protagonist. He or she understands osteopathy as a science of cause and effect, and perceives himself or herself as the expert in anatomy and biomechanics, whose purpose is to interpret the patient as a body, to discover what is wrong, and so identify the cause of pain. Then, through a mostly rational-technical process, he or she determines how best to remove the cause of the problem.

With the communicative type there is a mutual and equal partnership between therapist and patient based on sharing. Osteopathy is conceived as a professional art, based on the relationship with the person who is guided toward healing, in a mutually collaborative process negotiated around shared responsibilities. The osteopath's knowledge, as well as the information acquired, along with the expectations and the active participation of the patient interact in a partnership relationship to establish and to pursue together the best course of treatment. This path is focused on the person and based on listening to and understanding the individual's personal experience in perceiving illness or disability.

Finally, in the case of the educator, the relation is patient-centric, with the latter as the main pursuer of healing and with the operator as a facilitator. Here osteopathy is conceived as knowledge to be communicated to the patient to inform and educate them to develop their ability to manage pain, illness, disability, and then choose the most appropriate course of treatment, within the knowledge and the full control of their resources. The osteopath is a facilitator of the healing process, entrusting to the patient the leadership of the decision-making process, after receiving adequate information, consent and education.

Although this is a pilot study and therefore requires further exploration with larger samples, it is evident that a substantial variability emerged among participating osteopaths. Their ways of conceiving osteopa-

thy and osteopathic practice was strongly influenced by clinical decision-making, therapeutic objectives, and the technical approach, thus influencing the amount of interaction with the patient and the level of involvement of the patient in the healing process (Fig. 9.1). This phenomenon, also widely discussed by other authors,[17,20] seems to be characteristic of osteopathy as well as other professions.[21]

There seem to be different ways of understanding and implementing osteopathy, with many resulting therapeutic and management processes, despite the various national and international attempts to share principles and render teaching and practice. However,

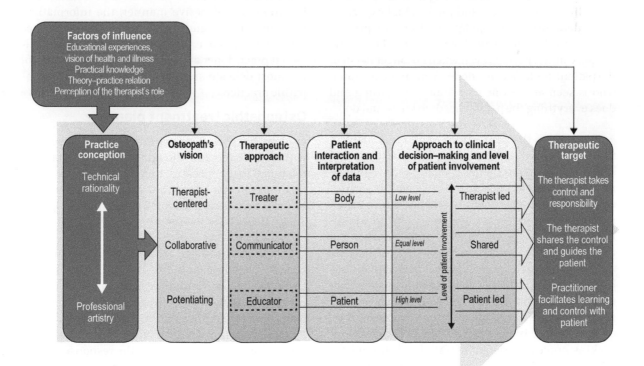

**Fig. 9.1**
Summary of the elements that characterize the theory of clinical decision-making in osteopathy formulated by Thomson et al.[19] First is a list of various factors that influence the different ways of thinking about osteopathic practice, from which are derived as many different perspectives on osteopathy. Next, three different therapeutic approaches, with three different foci with their relative levels of patient involvement and therapeutic target. Modified from: Thomson OP, Petty NJ, Moore AP. Clinical decision-making and therapeutic approaches in osteopathy – a qualitative grounded theory study. Man Ther. 2014;19(1):44–51.

it is the author's opinion that the three types described above could (and perhaps should) coexist in an osteopath, representing three different archetypes of therapeutic and managerial focus. These can be applied in different contexts to achieve optimal results. Imagine, for example osteopathically treating a hospitalized patient, perhaps postoperatively, a person with severe cognitive deficits, or someone with a pharmacologically altered state of consciousness.

It is clear that in these cases the manipulative intervention cannot rely heavily on the active participation of the patient or on his or her leadership in the therapeutic process. Therefore the temporary "leadership" of the operator is needed, for applying technical skills to the body, removing somatic dysfunction, and promoting resilience in the light of the operator's own clinical experience and professional expertise, using decision-making judgment. Here the priority is recovery. It is also true, however, that if this type of intervention persists even when no longer needed, the patient could become dependent on the operator, who is seen as the one who knows everything and does everything the patient needs to know and do.[22]

This ignores the perceptions and expectations of the patient, making him or her unable to control specific risks and the general health state. Using the previous example, once we have reached good clinical stability and a satisfactory functional recovery, it is possible, and perhaps only right, to slip into a jointly held share of the therapeutic process, aiming at the restoration of health, or at least the best possible condition. Here the priority is health. When this has happened, it will be appropriate to fully empower the patient in maintaining his or her well-being, facilitating the use of health-promoting resources, and giving the patient full control of the decision-making process, through informed and appropriate education choices. Here the priority is well-being.

In conclusion, it is the author's opinion that the coexistence of different ways of conceiving and applying osteopathy is not necessarily contrary to the principles and standards of its practice. Rather, these therapist–patient relationship models should be thoroughly known by every professional, so they can be consciously chosen and appropriately applied within the context of fulfilling the therapeutic act. The focus may move from the operator to the patient, or both, in a decision-making process, guided by the skilled and competent osteopath, who evaluates and determines the most appropriate strategy for the individual case.

We now intend to present a model of the decision-making process for osteopathic treatment and management. It represents an attempt to gather and integrate, in a cohesive manner, the information, elements, factors, and variables that should be considered at this stage. The goal is to offer to the individual practitioner a grid to which to refer in one of the most delicate and decisive processes of osteopathic practice.

## Osteopathic treatment planning

Osteopathic treatment planning can be structured with a dynamic and thoughtful choice of targets, relational foci, processes, and methods of intervention and re-evaluation. They represent the goals to be pursued during the course of treatment (Fig. 9.2). They can be the following:

*Resolutive*: to provide, for the treatment of disease, complete healing and the restoration of health, as might be the resolution process for infection, trauma, or any other event that results in mostly transient sequelae. The priority is to relieve symptoms, restore impaired function, reduce the duration of the condition, optimize the response to drug treatment, where present, or surgery, if necessary, to

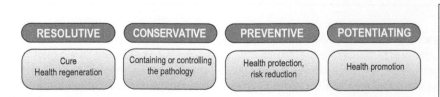

| RESOLUTIVE | CONSERVATIVE | PREVENTIVE | POTENTIATING |
|---|---|---|---|
| Cure Health regeneration | Containing or controlling the pathology | Health protection, risk reduction | Health promotion |

**Fig. 9.2**
The four objectives of osteopathic treatment – from the resolutive to the potentiating – with their respective purposes.

restore normal physical and mental health and the proper social context.

*Conservative*: use if the condition afflicting the patient is not curable, but is controllable (diabetes, hypertension) or containable in terms of systemic effects (cancer, HIV infection). Many hereditary, congenital, metabolic, autoimmune, and neoplastic diseases fit into this picture. Osteopathic treatment strives to decrease the intensity and frequency of acute episodes, to slow the progression of the disease, to optimize the response to pharmacologic agents, and to potentiate self-regulation capacity in order to improve the quality of life. An interdisciplinary approach is often essential to achieve satisfactory results, with the help of psychological and other support where necessary, but always with the active participation of the patient and his or her responsibility in the maintenance of his or her health process (see Chapter 8). It is also an essential requirement for all the objectives listed here.

*Preventive*: in this case, the patient does not complain of particular ailments but that does not mean the patient is necessarily healthy, if we understand health as a state of physical, mental and social well-being.[23] The focus will therefore be on identifying recurring patterns in the clinical history or physical examination, understood as predispositions or tendencies to develop certain conditions. The purpose of the preventive objective will therefore be protective, that is, focused on avoiding trends that precipitate overt diseases by reducing risks, possibilities, and chances of this happening, and aimed at using any means available to optimize the homeostatic and adaptive capacities of the individual, supporting and maintaining the overall health status. Much here focuses on information, patient education, and patient habits in social contexts.

*Potentiating*: these are usually luxury "objectives" in the sense that they are "applicable only to a few," although they are available to all. Even when viable, they are rarely perceived and pursued by patients. However, they represent the ultimate osteopathic approach, as they aim to bring the patient to the strongest and most independent state of health, possibly not even needing osteopathy any longer!

As an example, this can be a sportsman who wishes to improve his physical performance, but also the ordinary man who wants to feel better about how he is. This is the sphere of health promotion, where each therapeutic act is aimed at enhancing physical, mental, and social well-being in all its aspects. This approach includes diet, physical activity, occupational ergonomics, postural habits, mental health, sexual activity, social interaction and family, emotional balance, job satisfaction, play activities, environmental health, and spirituality; these are some of the aspects on which to focus listed objectives, but particularly in the potentiating objective in order to promote a healthy, stable and durable lifestyle. It is obvious that once the objective has been established it can and should be changed if the context and the conditions that led to the previous choice are altered. If, for example, during a preventive program, the patient suffers a trauma, it is clear that the target will become healing; or if a condition can only be controlled, it might be necessary to activate a conservative plan.

*Relational focus*: this represents osteopathic modes of the therapist–patient relationship[19] for the achievement of goals. They can be (Fig. 9.3): osteopath-centric, osteopath patient-centered, and patient-centered. With an *osteopath-centric* mode the operator has the responsibility for, and control of, the therapeutic process, applying strategies and measures deemed necessary for the case, through a technical rationale. It is the author's opinion that this focus is particularly indicated in cases where healing is a priority but the patient's participation is not contextually possible. With an *osteopath patient-centric* mode, the healing process is mutually shared between the two protagonists, together establishing clinical decision-making in its entire spectrum, through a relational rationale. The author suggests that this focus be adopted when health is compromised, but when there exists at least an adequate homeostatic potential to entrust that the patient has his or her own share of responsibility. It is especially indicated for conservative goals. With a *patient-centered* approach, the patient is given full decision-making control, both in the intervention and in the management, with adequate information, and an educational rationale. It is the opinion

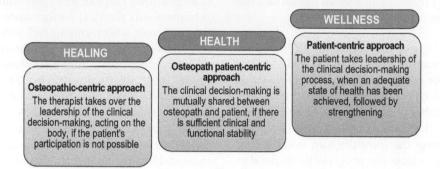

**Fig. 9.3**
The three modes of clinical decision-making exhibited by Thomson et al.[19] are adapted and presented by the author as three possible methods of osteopathic intervention that every osteopath may apply and modulate to achieve three progressive therapeutic targets (from healing to wellness), depending on the severity of the clinical context and the relative participation of the patient.

of the author that this focus may be particularly appropriate after reaching a discrete state of health, then leading the patient toward the full control of his or her salutogenic resources and the enhancement of his or her general well-being. It is especially indicated for preventive and potentiating objectives. As specified in the objectives, here it will be important to dynamically adapt the most appropriate focus according to ongoing changes.

*Processes*: once goals (and focus) have been established, the operator should define the processes through which to achieve them, as recognized (among others) by Korr:[24]

*Corrective*: these aim to bring a dysfunctional or pathological condition into normal relations. In osteopathy this could be accomplished by the correction of one or more somatic dysfunctions; in the medical field an example might be the reduction of a fracture or a dislocation.

*Reparative*: aimed at ensuring optimal conditions for the natural processes of regeneration and tissue repair because of any organic lesion, such as after a trauma or surgery. In osteopathy, this could be implemented to ensure good circulation and oxygenation of the fluids, in support of reparative tissue processes, and to balance connective tissue tensions and normalize neural reflexes correspond-

ing to the compromised area. A medical example might be the use of traction or immobilization for a fracture.

*Rehabilitative*: consists of the restoration of the impaired function toward the optimal performance allowed under current conditions. In both osteopathy and medicine, this would mean, for example, to work for the functional rehabilitation of a fractured limb and then immobilize it. At this stage one must interact with the physiatrist and the physiotherapist, with whom one can cooperate in order to restore joint mobility, normalize tensions and/or connective adhesions, and integrate the impaired function with other related regions.

*Re-educative*: focuses on the development of new alternative strategies to complete an impaired and unrestorable function, if its physical and physiological requirements have been damaged permanently. This is what happens, for example, in an individual suffering from hemiplegia or amputation of a limb or part of it. Here also, integration with the physical therapist and the occupational therapist is fundamental and necessary. The aim is to promote physical and physiological reorganization through reorganization of the overall energy economy, autonomic balance, and adequate circulation and oxygenation of fluids. Fundamental to this phase is the behavioral approach to support the patient toward the integration into his or her social context, although with different and better strategies.

*Restorative*: are intended to improve function that was only reduced in its intensity. It could be, for example, the case of a functional recovery process of a sportsman, after a respiratory infection. In this case, an integrated approach using biomechanical, circulatory-respiratory, and metabolic-energetic models becomes a priority.

*Palliative*: these are processes used to reduce symptoms, if one cannot remove the cause. They may include the placebo effect – as for any of the processes described above – but they are used mostly in terminally ill patients, or in cases where treatment of the root cause of the condition is not possible. This is essentially a symptomatic approach which indirectly aims to improve the quality of life, focusing on spiritual, social, and psychological aspects of the case. The behavioral approach is crucial in this process, as well as any osteopathic treatment to reduce pain or other symptoms, and to support the patient in as active a life as possible.

As explained above, one can, and should, change the selected process if there are no longer the original requirements that motivated the choice, or if new data suggest other processes as the most appropriate and beneficial to the individual case. Finally, it should be noted that curative objectives are often combined with corrective and rehabilitation processes; conservative objectives with rehabilitative and palliative processes; preventative and potentiating goals with corrective and recuperative processes.

**General modalities**: these refer to the definition of the general mode of osteopathic intervention, through an individualized and accurate choice. They include: the number, frequency and duration of treatments:

*Number*: the approximate number of osteopathic sessions to be carried out according to the objectives and the selected processes. For a curative aim the number of sessions may be relatively reduced, while for a conservative approach the number may vary, taking into consideration factors such as how long the patient has had the condition, financial considerations, and so on.

*Frequency*: refers to the time interval between treatments, usually based on the severity of symptoms. For example, for prevention, the frequency may be limited to one visit per year, while with an acute condition, with the objective being to cure, treatment might occur several times a week; in chronic conditions, one might apply a regular frequency that continues for months. However, most of the time, frequency also depends on the age of the patient: infants typically require a higher frequency, as compared to adults or elderly patients, because generally the homeostatic processing capacity in infants and children is more rapid and efficient than in adults. However, as always, each case requires an individual program. The general rule is that each treatment should build upon the previous treatments, and should lead to increased chance for further success with the next treatment.[5]

*Length*: indicates the length of the entire therapeutic cycle, determined by the combination of the number and frequency of sessions.

**Specific modalities** include choosing treatment methods for each working session. This includes (Fig. 9.4) dosage, pattern, level, method, technique, and design variants:

*Dosage*: the quantity and quality of therapeutic input to be administered, including how many dysfunctions are to be treated and the approaches used, and also giving consideration to the impact that their resolution will have on the entire body–mind–spirit system. The dosage should always be appropriate to the individual's physiological responsiveness. Otherwise, the therapeutic overload can result in adverse reactions or destabilization. Generally, the more ill the patient, or the more his or her adaptation potential is compromised, the more the dosage should be reduced. In infants and the elderly, low doses are preferred. It should be noted that it is not so much the number or

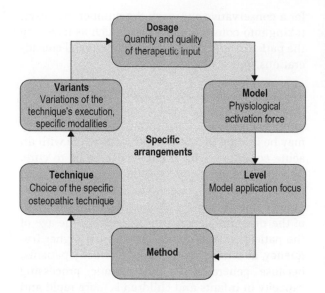

Fig. 9.4
The main stages of the decision-making process for the specific modalities of osteopathic treatment are illustrated: from the choice of dose to the models (from biomechanical to the biopsychosocial) most suitable to apply, followed by the application level of the chosen model (from local to global); the choice of method (from structural to biodynamic); finally, the technique and the variants with which to perform it.

duration of the techniques that determines the dosage of a session, but rather the administered therapeutic input, i.e., the quality and the amount of dysfunction released and the resulting tissue response. Thus, 5 minutes of articulatory technique may correspond to 1 second of recoil in terms of dosage, if both result in the same homeostatic response and equal impact on the dysfunctional system.

*Model*: refers to which of the five osteopathic models is chosen and applied; it also refers to the strength of the most appropriate physiological activation force applied with respect to the patient's condition. This often includes the integration of multiple models that best approach the complexity of the case and promote the healing process in its entire spectrum. The reader is referred to specific chapters on each model for more details on the indications and applications of each of them. It is to be noted that each model focuses on specific targets in the session in which it is applied – objectives which fall within the therapeutic cycle described above. An example is the restoration of joint mobility in the biomechanical model, or the normalization of fluid circulation in the respiratory-circulatory model.

*Level*: indicates the application focus of the model, in line with the choice of the selected dose. It can

extend to the following: (1) *local level*: in the dysfunctional area that may or may not coincide with the symptomatic area (e.g., a biomechanical model focused on normalizing a T4 in ERS left; (2) *segmental level*: for governing physiological dysfunction for example (in the case of liver dysfunction, a neurological model that operates with reflex techniques at T7–T9 and the vagus nerve); (3) *global level*: acting on the effects of the dysfunction on the patient and his or her psychophysical equilibrium systems (for example, the respiratory-circulatory model applied to reactivate the diaphragmatic lymphatic system in the case of pneumonia). Generally, if the patient's physiological response capabilities are low, with alteration of the general function that results in failure of the structure (GAS), there is a preference for action at global level to increase homeostatic capacity. This could coincide with a minimum therapeutic administration locally, but extend to the whole body, as is the case for maximalist approaches, such as the GOT,[25] in which "the part is treated by the whole."

In contrast, in cases with good energy capacity adaptive responses, where there is a dysfunctional dominance of a single structure on the general function (LAS), it is also possible to act only locally, in specific regions with dysfunctional impact. This could coincide with minimum therapeutic administration, as is the case with minimalist approaches, such as the SAT[26] or the mechanical link,[27] in which "the whole is treated through the part." It should be noted that maximalist approaches usually require time to be performed by the operator, but also short intervals between sessions; on the contrary, minimalist approaches may require less time for a treatment session, but longer periods of time between sessions to allow adequate reorganization of the body after being treated.

*Method*: refers to the specific osteopathic approach, choosing from a wide variety of available manual approaches. (See Chapter 1 for more details.) The choice of method depends primarily on the type of structure or tissue to be treated and the effects that the operator wishes to achieve, which should be consistent with the choice of the model and the application level.

*Technique*: this step involves the specification of the technique choice, consistent with the model, level, and selected method. For example, in a metabolic-energetic model, with a craniosacral approach to a global level, one can choose a homeostatic technique such as the CV4 to normalize and optimize the body's overall energy distribution; or a neurological model, with a vibratory method to a segmental level; or, one can choose an indirect technique to work on the celiac plexus and treat a stomach dysfunction.

*Execution variants*: once a technique is chosen, one must establish its implementation rules. The variants may include, but not be limited to:

- *use of tools* such as plows, wedges, or any other support that can be recruited to facilitate the accomplishment of the maneuver. In a broad sense, this may also include the possible contribution of a second therapist, using four-handed osteopathic techniques

- *position of the patient and the operator*: the same technique can be performed in different patient positions (supine, prone, sitting, or standing, with flexed legs, arms folded, etc.); there are also variations for operator positioning

- *contact*: can be of various types, mono-digital, bi-digital, single- or two-handed, palmar or volar surface, elbow, knee, chest, etc., although it is generally a good idea to choose the least contact possible but still accomplish the maneuver in an optimal, safe and effective fashion

- *lever and fulcrum*: often the same technique can be performed by choosing short or long levers, using physical fulcrums on the table or on the body of the patient or the operator, or no physical fulcrums, as in the biodynamic approach. Generally, the greater the force or the distance to be applied the more one needs to use long levers, but when more control and accuracy are needed the lever must be short.[8] Sometimes the two can be combined, so that even a long lever can be applied with precision

- *direction*: describes the use of anatomical and biomechanical knowledge to spatially orient the technique along the permitted movement axes, thus ensuring specificity and efficacy of the maneuver

- *speed and rhythm*: are two other key variables that can determine properties and completely different effects in the same technique, by varying the given speed and/or the applied rhythm (as for many oscillatory, vibrational, fluid, or articulatory techniques). Generally, high speed or rapid rhythms have a stimulatory effect and increase physiological processes, while low speed and slow rhythms are used to inhibit or slow down certain bodily activities. This variant can determine the choice of a thrust at high velocity and low amplitude (HVLA), or high amplitude and low velocity (HALV), or intermediate amplitude and low velocity (springing)[5]

- *strength/intensity*: the same technique can be performed with variable strength or variable intensity, depending on what is required, producing different tissue responses. The strength should be such as to obtain the desired tissue response while minimizing the risk of adverse reactions

- *intention*: this is perhaps the most profound essence and characteristic of a technique. Intention focused on one tissue or structure rather than another, and with the same technique, might produce completely different physiologic reactions, resulting in the application of a completely different osteopathic model. An occipitofrontal technique, for example, with the patient in the supine position, could become a myofascial release technique (in the biomechanical model) with a connective tissue focus; or a balanced membranous tension technique, with a focus on effects directed to the hypothalamus, pituitary, and brainstem (metabolic-energetic and/or neurological model); or balancing fluid circulation, with a focus on venous sinus drainage or release of the tentorial diaphragm (circulatory-respiratory pattern)

- *approach to the tissue barrier*: sometimes a technique itself (e.g., myofascial or visceral) can be applied in different ways, such as: (1) direct, moving against the barrier; (2) indirect, moving away from the barrier; (3) combined, alternating from indirect to direct in the same maneuver; (4) homeostatic, ignoring the tissue barrier but aiming to stimulate specific physiological responses (e.g., the CV4, lymphatic techniques). Direct techniques are usually recommended for chronic somatic dysfunction, as they have a strong impact on the fibrotic component of tissues; indirect techniques are commonly recommended for acute somatic dysfunction, which tends to be reactive, swollen and painful; combined techniques are recommended for intermediate conditions

- *patient contribution*: required when performing a maneuver which may include: (1) *volun-*

*tary forces*: respiratory involvement (inspiratory or expiratory breath-holding), muscle cooperation (isometric contraction of a muscle group), eye movements, tongue, jaw or any other voluntary act, aimed to facilitate the issue at fault; (2) *involuntary forces*, including the recruitment of potential homeostatic involuntary cranial, fascial, fluidic, or bioelectrical rhythms.

It must be stressed that when we speak of "intention," it is not so much the technique itself that determines the model, but rather the intention of the operator and the corresponding depth of tissue on which the operator is focused. An articulatory or oscillatory technique, for example, can be applied with the intention of improving the range and quality of joint mobility, using direction, pace, speed, and intensity for this purpose (biomechanical model); or playing on the same variants, it can focus on the remodeling of neural activity, both local and segmental (neurological model); it can also focus on fluid dynamics, creating pressure gradients that promote blood _circulation and venous and lymphatic drainage (circulatory model). It is also true, however, that some techniques have particular usefulness for some structures, such as balanced ligamentous tension techniques, which are specific for joint capsules and ligaments. Finally, one should always apply the general principle of using only the amount of activating force necessary to achieve a given purpose, and not wasting available homeostatic resources.

## Verification

Verification is the process of re-evaluating the results achieved, and is carried out at several levels: contextual, local, global, intermediate, and final:

- *Contextual*: during the performance of an osteopathic manipulation, the constant feedback of the tissue is evaluated and integrated, with the objective of calibrating the technique and optimizing the performance.

- *Local*: immediately after each corrective technique the operator evaluates its effectiveness. If the technique is not successful, it should either be repeated or the operator can use different techniques to achieve the same end.

- *Global*: from the beginning to the end of each therapeutic session the operator checks that the manipulative intervention has achieved the expected results. If not, the operator may finalize the treatment with additional techniques, or may need to re-evaluate the patient and/or consider different strategies for the next session.

- *Intermediate*: during therapy one must ensure that the pattern of results obtained is compatible with what is expected. This re-evaluation can be performed at varying intervals throughout the duration of treatment. This is a critical step in understanding the direction and timing of the therapeutic response, as well as the appropriateness of the treatments used and how they are applied. At this stage one can still "make the necessary adjustments," modify the path taken, and optimize evaluation and intervention strategies in the best fashion for the individual case.

- *Final*: at the end of the course of therapy, this is a final verification of the results achieved, which should correspond with those expected and shared with the patient. If not, more treatment sessions can be considered, if there is a real possibility of achieving the intended goal. Otherwise, one must search for the possible causes of failure, and plan further therapeutic strategies, including collaboration with other specialists. It should be stipulated that this phase may require specific imaging techniques (resonance, ultrasound, X-ray, etc.). The osteopath may require the patient's assistance to identify the changes made or the reasons for failure. Functional imaging techniques, such as postural tests, electro-acupuncture, gait analysis, etc., may also be used for this purpose.

In the broadest sense, the verification phase can be understood as a continuous monitoring process, throughout the course of treatment. Every moment of decision-making requires reflective listening skills, and acquisition, processing, and integration of new data, and any consequent implementation of the most appropriate actions, the effects of which will be also subject to re-evaluation. An example would be when the patient returns for second visit, having had an adverse reaction to the first treatment which may require a change in dose, pattern, and method used. In other words, for the entire procedure so far described, the aim of verification (Fig. 9.5), should not be construed as a rigid and unchangeable scheme, but rather it is to be applied as a dynamic, flexible and adaptable approach to individual needs.

For this to happen in a suitable and effective manner, it is necessary to develop and always maintain self-reflection,[28] recognized as an essential element in the teaching of osteopathic practice.[29] This is the operator's ability to modify his or her clinical decisions if the circumstances that have supported the choice were to require new measures of action. This can only happen in the mature and open osteopath, who is responsible and competent and does not limit himself or herself to decisions once made, or perpetuate the initial parameters when they have changed, as this would mean losing the overview and clinical context. It is not easy, but it is achievable.

Every single decision-making step thus far described, from objectives to verification, is based solely on a fundamental relationship: the risk and the costs that a given choice would entail on the one hand, and, on the other, the benefits that would follow. This concept extends from a broad perspective, such as the optimal route choice, to the final choice of technique to apply and how to apply it. Whatever the level considered, the rule of thumb is to pursue the greatest possible benefit with the least risk/cost possible. If such a relationship poses more risk it is right to utilize alternative approaches which, albeit in different ways, pursue the desired result.

Even with this approach, osteopathy could be inappropriate or ineffective, or even contraindicated,

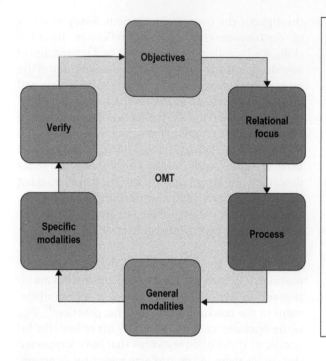

**Fig. 9.5**
The decision-making process for osteopathic treatment planning, including the choice of target (from resolutive to potentiating), the relational focus with the patient (as therapist-patient-centric), the process to apply for the achievement of the objective (from corrective to palliative), the general modalities of manipulative intervention (the number of treatments and the duration of the entire course of therapy), the specific modalities (dosage and performance of the technique variants), and the verification (contextual to final). The entire decision-making process is consistently thoughtful and based on the risk:benefit ratio, influenced by both the osteopath and the patient, and the therapeutic environment.

requiring the choice of alternative therapeutic avenues, and discussion and exploration with the patient. Generally speaking, the patient should be made an active participant of this decision-making process, being informed from the beginning about the course of treatment to be undertaken and its implementation.[4] The proposal becomes the implementation only when it is shared with the patient: otherwise it misses the therapeutic purpose.

The osteopath should also be aware that there may be many factors that affect, directly or indirectly, each phase of the clinical decision-making process so far described. They can be, but are not limited to, the following:[30]

1. *Factors inherent to the operator*, such as physical condition and constitution, level of technical skills, clinical experience, professional expertise, scientific knowledge, communication skills, age, sex, and his or her psycho-emotional state at the time of the consultation. Just think, for example, how it could affect the entire range of decision-making if a female osteopath is pregnant, or if an osteopath is taller than 1.9 meters (6 feet 3 in)

or less than 1.4 meters (4 feet 7 in), or has suffered a sprained ankle, a recent surgery, or has just lost a loved one, or is under the influence of immunosuppressive agents or antidepressants, or has just recently graduated vs. having practiced for 30 years. Each of these factors may influence, consciously or unconsciously, the choice of models, methods, techniques, locations, contacts, levers, fulcrums, and so on. Note also that every technique, direct or indirect, has no value to the osteopath who does not possess the skills needed to use them appropriately.

2. *Factors relating to the patient*, including age, sex, ethnicity and mother tongue, constitution, clinical condition, symptomatic presentation (acute, chronic), inability to assume or maintain certain positions, taking medication, previous trauma, surgeries and therapies, psycho-emotional state, general allostatic load, nutrition, social origin, property, trust in the osteopath or osteopathy in general, response to treatment, perception of their condition, expectations, motivation, and participation in the therapeutic process are some of the factors that gravitate to the patient–therapist

relationship, and may affect interpersonal dynamics, technical decisions, and clinical results.

3. *Factors inherent to the therapeutic context*: these are certainly among the most underrated, but equally influential in the decision-making process. They include contingent elements, such as the type of treatment table available (electrical, fixed, folding, reclining, etc.) or some other arrangement (e.g., a chair or a bed or a couch in a home treatment), the treatment environment (hospital, clinic, private practice, home). One must also consider material factors, such as the presence of other people in the treatment room (parents, spouses, relatives, patient's friends or colleagues, students, trainees, the osteopath's assistants) and finally, the possibility or not for immediate interaction with other professionals available in the study.

In conclusion, it is not intended that all of the procedural choices described in this chapter be used in all cases. Rather, they should be seen as a concept map for use in developing a treatment plan for each individual case. The point here is to avoid proceeding without knowing all possible treatment choices. This avoids the degeneration of healthy clinical decision-making into a mere repetition of habitual interventions, reiterative but ineffective. This is very dangerous and burdensome both for the therapist and for the patient, and can result in risky or embarrassing situations, or at least an unprofessional one, where, for example, the patient gets treatment once a week for years by his trusted osteopath, ignoring both the why and how, and having no clear objectives or expected outcomes. Rather, the osteopath must establish and share clear and achievable goals, and decide the best route to achieve them. This is the foundation of a healthy and professional relationship between therapist and patient, fueled by mutual accountability for the healing process, but based on objectives, timing and well-defined methods.

## Criteria for model selection

Every osteopathic treatment is a dynamic process that integrates all of the models. Inevitably the osteopath appeals to the five forces of activation/adaptive capacity in each of his or her interventions, drawing on the correlation between corresponding body elements. However, it is possible to arrange the manual work with specific emphasis on one or more of the models, by directing the therapeutic stimulation of a structural component and associated function, depending on the type of allostatic overload in the patient.

Therefore, although the selection and the application of the models are partly conceptual, the authors propose the following criteria in choosing where and how to direct the emphasis of treatment. These criteria consider both the constellation of factors affecting the patient (narration), and clinical and tissue evidence obtained during the osteopathic visit (observation and evaluation). The operator will integrate the information acquired and reach a conclusion supported by the majority of the available findings.

### History

Analysis of the following information obtained from the narrative will determine the anatomical region and the dominant dysfunctional physiological activity, leading the osteopath to choose the most suitable model for the patient (Box 9.1):

- Reason for consultation: a qualitative description, quantitative and chronological framework of the current symptomatic presentation

- Past medical, surgical, and social history: including disease, trauma, previous surgery and its after-effects, work activities, sports and recreation

- Systems review: signs and/or symptoms which indicate overload of a specific organ or system and/or its function, resulting in the reason for consultation.

### Observation

It is the opinion of the authors that the bio-behavioral model plays a crucial role at this stage, as a reference guide in establishing the relationship with the patient, not only in cases where it is used as a primary model, but also if one or more of the remaining four models are applied (see Chapter 8). The communicative aspect and the overall approach to the patient becomes an essential component within each biomechanical, neurological, circulatory, or metabolic approach, guiding the evaluation and clinical application processes in an empathetic relationship for health promotion. It is a kind of pattern among the patterns that drive the osteopath toward the most appropriate selection approach to the patient under treatment, as well as the education of the patient to become a protagonist of his or her own healing process. The following are examples in which the behavioral pattern might suggest the selection of the other models:

- *Evaluation of the bio-constitutional component* (see Chapter 8): the bio-typological classification of Sheldon, for example, might suggest the application of a neurological model for an ecto-morphic biotype, of a biomechanical and/or circulatory pattern for a mesomorphic type, and a metabolic-energetic model for an endomorphic type. Similarly, it may be applied to Kelman's classification with the involvement of the head compartment and the outer layer as indicative for the neurological model, the chest compartment, and the intermediate layer as indicative for the biomechanical and/or circulatory model, and the abdominal compartment and inner layer as an indicator for the metabolic-energetic model

- *Postural evaluation* (see Chapter 8): for example, by applying the Latey model, one might prefer a biomechanical model for a collapsed posture that is primarily compromised, a neurological model for a residual posture, or a metabolic-energetic model for an altered posture of the inner tube.

## Manual evaluation

The osteopathic manual evaluation captures three levels of clinical and tissue information, all of which would suggest three levels of choice and application of models:

1. The *dominant tissue dysfunction*: tissue characteristics such as stiffness, density, restriction of mobility and/or motility, low vitality, etc., are some parameters that can emerge from the osteopathic assessment of a given tissue (see Chapter 2). The latter is generally recognized as the most dominant in the dysfunctional pattern as these parameters are high in terms of severity and persistent in each position taken by the patient during the assessment (seated, supine, etc.). In addition, temporary inhibition on the tissue, using a slight manual pressure at the site, will help the operator confirm the dysfunctional dominance, leading to the improvement of semeiological test response, such as the Lasègue or Soto Hall test. This would determine the dominance of the tissue not only based on qualitative parameters, but also on the response of clinical tests. The dominant type of tissue would then suggest WHICH model to apply, or at least the most appropriate therapeutic emphasis (see Box 9.1).

2. The *fascial compartment involved*: the authors suggest the application of specific tests of fascial compartments (see Chapter 1), such as axial/appendiceal, visceral, or meningeal, for guidance as to which of them present an allostatic overload and WHERE to apply greater emphasis on the model selected.

3. The *allostatic load*: the Zink test provides useful information at this stage on the general adaptation capacity of the patient in response to the allostatic load supported (see Chapter 6), which also suggests HOW to administer the selected model. For example, a test response showing a highly decompensated Zink pattern (such as four transitional areas that rotate in the same side) indicates the need for a maximalist treatment, and then activation of the peculiar physiological strength of the model (biomechanical, neurological, respiratory-circulatory, metabolic-energetic). A compensated response may be associated with a minimalist type of treatment, i.e., related to the dominant dysfunctional structure and clinical relevance for the patient.

## Box 9.1

### Elements of selection of the osteopathic models

**Biomechanical model (see Chapter 4) (Fig. 9.6)**

- Disorders: myalgia, tendonitis, capsulitis, arthralgia, chondropathies, etc.

- Overloaded structure: musculoskeletal, the axial end of the appendix, ectoskeleton, muscles with antigravity function.

- Overloaded function: mobility and postural control, i.e., the correlation between muscle coordination, motor control and HRMT.

**Neurological model (see Chapter 5) (Fig. 9.7)**

- Disorders: changes in sensation (paresthesia, dysesthesia, allodynia, etc.), neuralgia, radiculopathies, autonomic disorders (hyperthermia, perspiration, etc.), disorders of the sense organs.

- Overloaded structure: meningeal fascia, brain, bone marrow, peripheral nerves, ganglia and plexuses, the integumentary system.

- Overloaded function: exteroceptive, proprioceptive, interoceptive, coordination, levels of nociception and awareness.

**Respiratory-circulatory model (see Chapter 6) (Fig. 9.8)**

- Disorders: mucosal congestion, lymphatic, venous, inflammation or infection of the respiratory tract, heart disease, circulatory failure.

- Overloaded structure: cervical-thoracic portion of the visceral fascia, diaphragm, lymph nodes, cardiovascular system, respiratory and urogenital.

- Overloaded function: ventilatory, circulatory (arterial-venous-lymphatic-CSF-interstitial), immune.

**Metabolic-energetic model (see Chapter 8) (Fig. 9.9)**

- Disorders: fatigue, infections, toxicity, poor ability to repair tissue, sleep disorders, thyroid disorders.

- Overloaded structure: abdominal-pelvic portion of the visceral fascia, neuroendocrine axis, the extracellular matrix of the surrounding regions internal organs.

- Overloaded function: energy balance, metabolic processes of immune regulation, levels of inflammation, digestion, absorption of nutrients, elimination of metabolic wastes, reproductive capacity.

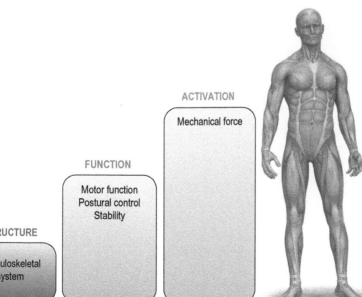

ACTIVATION

Mechanical force

FUNCTION

Motor function
Postural control
Stability

STRUCTURE

Musculoskeletal system

**Fig. 9.6**
Biomechanical-postural model, with related structure, function and activation force of reference.

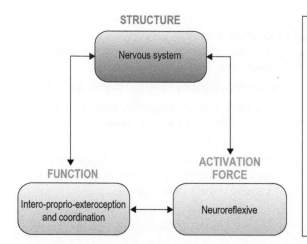

STRUCTURE

Nervous system

FUNCTION

Intero-proprio-exteroception and coordination

ACTIVATION FORCE

Neuroreflexive

**Fig. 9.7**

Neurological model, with related structure, function, and activation force of reference.

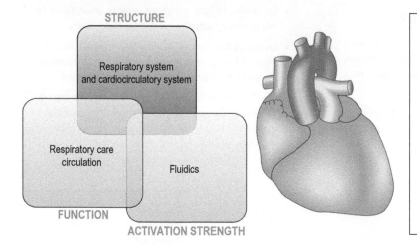

STRUCTURE

Respiratory system and cardiocirculatory system

Respiratory care circulation

Fluidics

FUNCTION

ACTIVATION STRENGTH

**Fig. 9.8**

The respiratory-circulatory model, with related structure, function, and activation force of reference. The respiratory-circulatory model, with related structure, function, and activation force of reference.

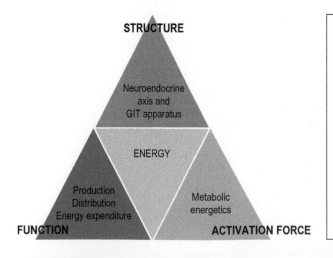

STRUCTURE

Neuroendocrine axis and GIT apparatus

ENERGY

Production Distribution Energy expenditure

Metabolic energetics

FUNCTION

ACTIVATION FORCE

**Fig. 9.9**

The metabolic-energetic model, with related structure, function, and activation force of reference.

## Osteopathic management

The planning and management of the osteopathic intervention must be based on the following:[1]

- Optimize the self-healing capacity of the body.

- Approach the primary cause of the disease.

- Incorporate evidence-based guidelines.

- Emphasize the maintenance of health and prevention of disease.

However, the topic is much more complex and requires more exploration to support the osteopath who intends to pursue the above points. In fact, osteopathic treatment is on one hand aimed at facilitating the natural self-healing mechanisms of the body, approaching areas with somatic dysfunction, and on the other hand it is based on a perspective oriented toward health and globality, so it is essential to refrain from exclusive focus on the dysfunction. It is never a good idea to focus exclusively on the symptomatic area for the manipulative treatment, because of the first principle of osteopathy, focused on the unity of the body, and also considering the multidimensional complexity that often characterizes pain, especially if chronic.[31] For this, the holistic osteopathic principles were described by the five models of structure–function relationship, addressed to the whole person, although also applicable to the location and the specificity of a single dysfunction.

However, if one intends to approach the person in the totality of his or her physical, mental, spiritual, and social being, it is necessary to expand the horizon to include both biopsychosocial models,[32] considered congruent with osteopathic principles,[33] both interdisciplinary paradigms,[34] recognized as consistent with osteopathic philosophy[35] and salutogenic processes,[36] whose different phases have been described[37] (Fig. 9.10) as follows:

1. *From treatment to treatment*: it is important to focus on healing whilst also being aware of the expense in terms of time, energy, individual and social costs. We must not fail at this stage, as it may inhibit healing and lead to chronic disease or even death.

2. *From protection of health to prevention*: protection occurs by limiting or containing the risk that a given population can develop in certain conditions, usually through specific social measures. Prevention occurs when working individually, by sensitizing the individual to be actively involved in avoiding the risk of the disease, through enhancement of health attitudes.

3. *From education to health promotion*: education takes place through the transmission of information and communication with competent and experienced professionals, but must also include the active participation of the individual. With health promotion, health is seen as a human right, with an emphasis on social and individual resources, coordinated by professionals and aimed at achieving the highest quality of life. The process of health promotion aims to increase the individual's ability to control his or her physical, mental, spiritual, and social status.

4. *Improved perceptions of health and quality of life*: this is the last stage of health promotion. It focuses on the individual's perception of his or her own health, and helps achieve the optimal quality of life, through the recognition and strengthening by the individual of his or her own resources and the development of the ability to use them as well as possible.

In conclusion, osteopathic treatment should be based on a multimodal humanistic approach that places man and his salutogenic rights in the spotlight; restores, protects, and promotes health and well-being; and is addressed to the triadic unity of body, mind, and spirit through different models that address the relationship between structure and function and aim to improve as many physiological response forces of the patient as possible. The individual must become the main protagonist of his or her own healing process, and be made conscious

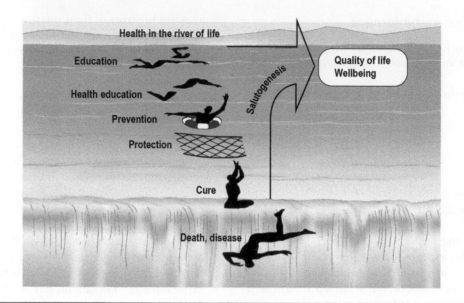

**Fig. 9.10**

The paradigm of health is schematically represented in this image, defined by the authors as 'the river of life.'[37] From the bottom up, they illustrate the different stages: (1) cure of the disease (that may progress to death); (2) protection of health; (3) prevention of the disease; (4) health education; 5) health promotion. Modified from: Eriksson M, Lindström B. A salutogenic interpretation of the Ottawa Charter. Health Promot Int. 2008;23(2):190–9.

and aware of his or her individual resources for a life of comfort and quality, in keeping with the family and social situation from which he or she comes and to which he or she belongs.

Translating these concepts into clinical practice, the management of a patient first requires a time schedule for reaching achievable goals, one that permits optimal investment of available resources without overestimating (or underestimating) the goals of treatment. This requires a careful assessment of any risk factors and the adoption of preventive measures. Osteopathic management should therefore consider the following deadlines:

1. *Short-term*: these aim to restore health through cure or control of the disease. Included in this management program are objectives such as reducing pain, restoration of function, and control/treatment of any condition affecting the patient.

2. *Medium-term*: these aim for health protection and the prevention of any recurrence or relapse. This may be achieved by a careful evaluation of personal risk factors, resulting in the adoption of appropriate preventive measures or containment.

3. *Long-term*: these aim to promote and enhance health and focus resources toward improving the quality of life in all its expressions.

## The "flags" and their osteopathic influences

The patient management approach is also profoundly influenced by what have been called "flags", shown with different colors[38], i.e., a range of factors that interact with each other and impact on clinical decision-making, as well as the way in which it is handled. The flags, are described below and shown in Fig. 9.11.

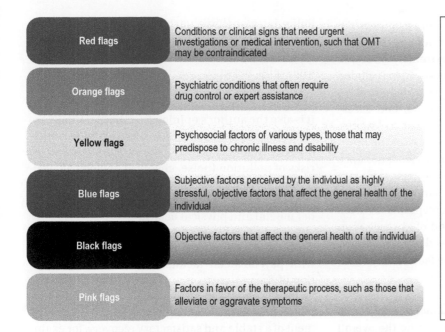

| Red flags | Conditions or clinical signs that need urgent investigations or medical intervention, such that OMT may be contraindicated |
| Orange flags | Psychiatric conditions that often require drug control or expert assistance |
| Yellow flags | Psychosocial factors of various types, those that may predispose to chronic illness and disability |
| Blue flags | Subjective factors perceived by the individual as highly stressful, objective factors that affect the general health of the individual |
| Black flags | Objective factors that affect the general health of the individual |
| Pink flags | Factors in favor of the therapeutic process, such as those that alleviate or aggravate symptoms |

**Fig. 9.11**
The various factors that may affect clinical decision-making and achievement of the appropriate therapeutic goals. They are described as different flag colors depending on the severity of the conditions affecting the patient (from red to yellow); the context in which these conditions are set (blue and black); and finally, factors that are of relative advantage for the healing process (pink flags).

- *Red*:[39] identifies conditions or undiagnosed clinical signs which may underlie states of emergency that could compromise the individual's clinical stability. There may be a need for urgent investigations or medical interventions to restore a stable clinical level. Therefore, red flags can demand the immediate suspension of osteopathic evaluation or intervention. The conditions to which this applies include: acute abdominal pathology (peritonitis, pancreatitis, etc.), cardiovascular events (myocardial infarction, stroke, hemorrhage, etc.), or other conditions such as aortic aneurysms, status epilepticus, cauda equina syndrome, tumors, and undiagnosed infections. However, the color of the flag can also refer to different clinical signs, the combination of which may suggest the presence of one of the severe conditions described above. These include progressive, constant, unremitting pain and night pain that gets worse when lying down; absence of a clear onset; systemic signs such as fever, vomiting, fatigue, anorexia, and lymphadenopathy; few or no alleviation or aggravation factors; symptoms present for more than 1 month with little or no response to treatment.

- *Orange*[40] represents psychological or psychiatric conditions, such as personality disorders, depression, post-traumatic stress, and addictions to drugs or alcohol that interfere with achieving therapeutic goals. These conditions often require psychological or psychiatric care, as well as pharmacological intervention, which can also be substituted for, or included with, osteopathic treatment.

- *Yellow*:[41] includes psychosocial factors that work against the achievement of therapeutic goals and that predispose to the development of chronic illness and disability. Catastrophism, anxiety, reluctance to return to activities for fear that the pain may recur, improper or inappropriate expectations or beliefs for recovery, concerns about the therapeutic intervention to be taken, excessive dependence or reliance on passive external treatment (injections, medicines), or shy and reluctant behavior in society. Recognition of these factors is critical to understanding the perception and the meaning that the patient attaches to his or her pain.

- *Blue*:[42] includes all relevant factors relating to the patient's occupation and which may be perceived as hostile, threatening, or extremely stressful, even if they were not actually so. Also included here are dissatisfaction with work, a perception of poor management by superiors, and excessive pressure or poor support from colleagues. Finally, the perception that the work environment is dangerous or that it increases the chance of relapse. Given that expectations to regain health and return to work seem decisive prognostic indicators,[43] these perceptions of work stress may lengthen the period of absence from work and the psychological and physical recovery after an illness. Also, these factors may result in frequent job changes.

- Black:[44] these are objective factors relating to the single professional activity, affecting the overall health of the individual. They include such things as collective bargaining, wages, minimum or maximum length of work shifts, professional ergonomics, benefit systems and reimbursement of expenses, allotted number of sick days or annual leave, company financial problems and staff salary levels. These often require the intervention of specialized personnel for support and assistance.

- Pink[45] are the only flags that relate to factors in favor of the therapeutic process and should therefore be properly exploited, by both therapist and patient, to achieve their goals. These are factors that alleviate the symptoms (such as rest and joint elevation for post-traumatic edema), as well as factors aggravating the symptoms that should be avoided (such as avoiding lifting in cases with acute disc disease). Education is essential, including discouraging inappropriate expectations or beliefs.

It should be noted that these flags are to be recognized properly and applied with a critical sense, considering not only their validity and reproducibility, but also the value they can offer to the patient and therapist in the clinical decision-making process.[46] However, these are not easy to distinguish, especially between the blue and black flags, as they often coexist independently or influence each other, or interact in combination with other factors. It is also the author's opinion that the black flags are primarily associated, with inadequate work environment elements, such as the numerous forms or risks of pollution (noise, chemical, biological, electromagnetic, etc.) to which the individual may be exposed, and that may pose a real threat to his or her mental and physical health.

Similarly, yellow flags are traditionally associated with psychosocial factors related to the perception of the patient's pain. However, one should not neglect other social factors in the patient's life that may represent an ongoing obstacle to the achievement of a stable and satisfactory recovery, for example, a sport, hobby, or family status issues that can interfere in the decision-making process. Examples can be the intense practice of a sport such as swimming in a patient with shoulder pain, an ongoing divorce for a patient who complains of headache and insomnia, any psychological dynamics, such as transference, which could interfere with a healthy patient–therapist relationship; finally, there is the possibility that a patient involved in a lawsuit about an accident or injury may cause him or her to voluntarily feign persistence or aggravation of his or her symptoms, for whatever advantage.[47]

## The multidimensional and multidisciplinary approach to the individual

Relative to the five osteopathic models, the therapeutic process considers: the removal of somatic disorders that compromise tissue mobility and free circulation and oxygenation of fluids, resulting in an alteration of the normal energy economy system; normalization of aberrant neural reflexes and spinal facilitation, as well as the impact of the biopsychosocial intervention that is followed, providing the necessary context to the natural restoration of health. The osteopath should intervene with processes, methods, frequencies, dosages, and individualized methods, to optimize self-regulating mechanisms, but with the least possible risk of adverse reactions, damage, failure, or destabilization, all based on the latest evidence.

Assessment and risk prediction become crucial, especially when considering psychological influence in the development of chronic pain and disability.[48] Understanding the impact that the pain or illness has on people is also needed to understand the multidimensional effects[49] on the individual. The fear of pain or its potential recurrence seems to increase the debilitating pain,[50] and is highly correlated with the patient's perceived disability levels.[51] This can lead to avoidance of daily activities, with risk of chronicity. Fear of returning to physical or work activities may pose the same risk,[52,53] so they should not be neglected.

Even dissatisfaction with work has been shown to be a significant factor in studies on disability or persistent pain, especially if there is poor support from colleagues, or a generally harsh and inflexible environment, which can lead to stress and even disease if it persists.[54] Typically, different psychic influences, such as emotions and memories, can cause physical changes and produce pain, as demonstrated by psychophysiological studies.[55] Also, the patient's thought processes can alter the perception of painful stimuli and the experience of pain, as in the case of catastrophic attitudes.[56] Even the type of personality of an individual appears to influence the perception of a disability,[57] as well as the person's belief, faith, and religion,[58] which relates to the concept of osteopathic triadic unity of body–mind–spirit. In addition, expectations, beliefs, and attributions about one's status are crucial to the personal control of one's own resources and for the resolution of the problem, as suggested by the cognitive model.[59]

All these factors should be incorporated throughout the patient's decision-making and management process,[60] and oriented toward self-efficacy mechanisms[61] and reinforcement,[62] rather than neglected or mismanaged in favor of persistence of pain.[63] Information gathering and patient education are essential in this therapeutic process,[64] and also act indirectly on the family and social environment of the patient, which can reinforce pain and its generative or maintenance mechanisms, as suggested by the classic behavioral model.[65]

The osteopath should always be conscious of his or her own limitations, as well as of the fact that not all conditions are treatable; sometimes they can only be contained, or they may be progressive, worsening, or terminal. Finally, we must remember that not all patients respond favorably to osteopathic manipulation, requiring the operator to reassess his or her goals at each session, making sure they are still valid, appropriate, and achievable. If they are not, new goals should be formulated and shared with the patient. If this is not possible, the therapeutic relationship should be discontinued, referring the patient to a more appropriate specialist.

At any stage of the therapeutic process the osteopath should always consider the utility of integrating osteopathic assistance with that of any other specialist, which would enhance the healing process and benefit the overall health of the patient, in light of recent evidence that such an inter-collaborative approach can improve care.[66,67] The osteopath should always interact with various experts in the field whenever appropriate.

The need to implement this interdisciplinary model not only in a clinical setting,[68] but also during osteopathic[69,70] and medical training,[71] has become increasingly important and is promoted by the World Health Organization.[72] This interaction must take place using appropriate communication methods, shared among different health professions, and based on clinical findings, objectives, and the latest scientific evidence. Dialogue, comparison, sharing, and integration of different medical models are the basic requirement of a multi- and interdisciplinary approach, resulting in a competent and experienced treatment approach, along with support and protection for the multidimensional sphere of the patient.

We now provide brief guidelines on the strategic priorities for osteopathic treatment in different clinical settings and clinical phases, based on available evidence. However, these sections are intended only as guidelines and practical tips, not as a recipe for the treatment of conditions, which would contravene the fully multi-dimensional approach to the person to which this book is dedicated.

## Obstetrics and gynecology

Many pregnant patients complain about pelvic pain and low back pain associated with mechanical disorders of the musculoskeletal system, especially pain in the thoracic and lumbar regions and functional asymmetry of the lower limbs.[73] The load sustained during pregnancy makes back pain one of the main problems for the patient.[74] In the third trimester of pregnancy, OMT aims to prevent and alleviate pain by eliminating somatic dysfunction and related aberrant reflexes, and especially autonomic effects on hemodynamics.[75] However, in general, it aims to improve overall homeostasis, comfort, and quality of life of the patient while the body adapts to the physiological and structural changes of pregnancy.[76]

In addition, in preparation for childbirth, it is essential to ensure maximum freedom of movement of each joint of the pelvis spine and lower limbs, as well as normal tension of the pelvic diaphragm, and the psoas and piriformis muscles. Indirectly the objectives are the reduction of complications during pregnancy, labor, or delivery, reducing the need for surgery or other invasive interventions.[77] Muscle energy techniques, inhibitory pressure, cranial, myofascial, articulatory, and soft tissue techniques are usually applied in this situation.[78]

## Pediatrics

The goal of pediatric OMT mainly concerns the correction of somatic dysfunction as potential causes of functional disorders which may be at the root of conditions such as infantile colic and compression of the cranial structures, such as the demonstrated correlation between lateral strain of the sphenobasilar synchondrosis and sleep disorders.[79] Recommended treatments are generally functional, myofascial, and cranial, applied to the sacrum, chest, diaphragm and skull.[80] Usually the patient responds quickly to small therapeutic doses, although constant monitoring of the treatment response is crucial. There are frequent cases of infections, such as recurrent otitis media, for which it will be important to reduce the symptoms, frequency, and intensity of acute episodes and restore a more functional fluid circulation.[81] It is important to note that the OMT should also be directed to the mechanics of infants, especially idiopathic postural asymmetries.[82] Finally, in the pre-term infant OMT can reduce the length of hospital stay and gastrointestinal symptoms.[83]

## Geriatrics

Since the individual capacity to adapt gradually decreases in this age group, while the physiological causes of stress increase, OMT is generally applied to support the patient in dealing with any failure caused by aging, especially when considering the frequent presence of combinations of different disorders in the geriatric patient (hypertension, diabetes, etc.). The goals of treatment focus on improving pain and musculoskeletal function,[84] balance and postural stability,[85] as well as the quality of life, for example in patients with osteoporosis.[86] Other goals include improvement in fluid flow, cardiorespiratory function, and the diaphragm system, especially in cases of infection[87] or hospitalization.[88] Usually we opt for at least a few days to 2 weeks between treatments.

The therapeutic movements (including thrust) should be applied slowly, administered accurately, and adapted to various patient positions depending on the patient's condition, avoiding techniques with excessive pressure on the sternum and ribs, with a preference for indirect techniques in cases of osteoporosis.[89] Counterstrain techniques, positional release, articulatory, soft tissue, and muscle energy are often used in this age group, aimed at maximizing respiratory efficiency in particular.

Possible adverse reactions, such as fatigue and increased pain for 12–48 hours, especially after the first or second treatment, may occur, especially if soft tissue techniques are used.[90] Moderate exercise, breathing exercises, Pilates, or even just walking can be effective tools for prevention or control of various disorders often suffered in this age group.[91]

## Hospital and surgical care

The preoperative phase focuses on the overall metabolic efficiency and optimization of homeostatic resources,[92] including ensuring adequate nutrition and hydration. To reduce the effects of anesthesia and of bed confinement, the goal is to increase efficiency of the circulation and diaphragms, and the expansion of the ribcage, using lymphatic, cranial, or soft tissue techniques, or treating the middle cervical region, which seems to reduce postoperative pulmonary complications.[93] The primary goal in the postoperative phase, however, is recovery of function, oxygen saturation, cardiac[94] and respiratory[95] efficiency, the reduction of symptoms and use of postoperative analgesics,[96] the reduction of hospital length of stay[97,98] and the risk of complications.[99] OMT can also be applied as soon as 1 day after surgery to reduce pain that in turn influences respiratory and diaphragmatic efficiency. The OMT should be of a low dose, even daily or several times a day, although in cases of postoperative infections it may be appropriate to avoid manipulative treatment.[100] Atelectasis is the most common cause of postoperative fever.[101] The most commonly used approaches are indirect techniques, cranial (such as CV4) techniques, soft tissue techniques, fascial techniques for the scar, lymphatic techniques, and autonomic balancing techniques.

## Psychiatry

The goal is to improve mental function, acting on somatic dysfunction and its somatic-psychological reflections.[102] Usually the aim is to reduce musculoskeletal tension, as well as orthosympathetic hyperactivity found in many psychiatric conditions, such as schizophrenia,[103] depression,[104] anxiety,[105] and also present in children[106] and the elderly.[107] Thrust techniques are generally to be avoided,[105] and less invasive techniques are preferred. It is advisable to start at the least painful regions, perhaps with the soft tissues and, where spinal manipulation is necessary, apply oscillatory and springing techniques.[108] OMT is contraindicated if the patient does not want to be touched, or if surgery is not tolerated in any way.[105] It should be noted that osteopathic treatment can be addictive, given the desperate need for care and attention that a given patient may require,[107] and this may trigger the transfer mechanism.[109] The biopsychosocial approach is fundamental, and can be integrated with psychotherapy.

## Sports medicine

This field emphasizes biomechanics and sports specific movements. It is common to schedule a first visit in preparation for competition, to determine any existing somatic dysfunction that may predispose to biomechanical stress, incorrect posture, or painful symptoms. In general, the aim is to allow the athlete to deal with these problems to improve competitive performance in terms of endurance, strength, speed, control, and precision.[110] It should be remembered that in professional sports one strives for healthy tissue, fully functional structure, good coordination of the neuromuscular network, and a clear and focused mind. Therefore, proper recovery during training and proper rest between training sessions are essential.

Osteopathic sessions are set according to the type of sport and the schedule for competition. Usually the biomechanical and metabolic-energetic model, including muscle energy techniques (isotonic type) and stretching,[111] go perfectly with the treatment objectives, which usually aim to increase sports performance and metabolic and musculoskeletal efficiency but prevent trauma and injuries.[112] Among the most frequent injuries are those affecting the musculoskeletal system, because of the strong or prolonged physical stress to which the patient is subjected. In this case, it is essential to ensure the proper rest to allow for adequate tissue repair.

Compensation for trauma can often be abnormal and painful, requiring osteopathic treatment.[113] Even when surgery is necessary, it is often possible to continue alternative physical activity during recovery to maintain the efficiency of the cardiorespiratory system. Any recovery activity should be gradual. Supervision of athletes requires excellent collaboration between medical and paramedical professionals, including the osteopath,[114] in cases of traumatic or overload pathologies as well as functional disorders.[115] It is crucial to the biopsychosocial approach based on the relationship with the team and the coach that treatment is integrated with relaxation and concentration techniques and with appropriate nutritional education.

## Performing arts

The incidence of musicians' performance injuries has been estimated at 70% in the course of their career.[116] Such injuries can result in devastating physical, emotional, and financial consequences for an artist and require a comprehensive treatment plan to allow for the best opportunity for restoration of health or its maintenance, as well as being able to return to performance. The osteopathic approach then considers all possible causes of the injury and requires a treatment rationale that often leads to a multidisciplinary approach, with attention to the performer's lifestyle, practice habits, exercise routine, diet, level of stress, and concomitant medical conditions. The performing artist needs proper functioning musculoskeletal and respiratory systems to meet the high demands that require their activities. Somatic dysfunctions at the expense of these systems thus have priority, considering the energy expenditure required of the artist. It follows that a normalization of dysfunction can be a valuable aid in recovery after an injury, in maintaining the performer's health, as well as optimization of posture and overall performance.[117,118]

## Acute phase

Here the primary objectives are to reduce the symptoms and physical stress on the involved area, with attention to the restoration of circulatory dynamics. Edema and muscle spasm are often associated with this phase, which makes it ideal to integrate the respiratory-circulatory model with the biomechanical approach to the soft tissue.[119] In the early stages, more frequent treatments (even daily) can be performed, gradually reducing the frequency to one session every 2–3 weeks.

Acute conditions usually have a rapid response to treatment, sometimes requiring only one treatment, although usually between four and six.[120] However, it is always necessary to ensure sufficient time to process the therapeutic input that has been administered, to avoid adverse reactions. Nelson and Glonek[121] recommend evaluating how much treatment the patient is able to tolerate and, in the acute phase, administering only half of it. Indirect techniques are usually preferred in this phase, where the movement is severely limited or painful. Kuchera[122] suggests that osteopathic treatment planning should also be set according to the dysfunctional stage of the patient: first degree, as in the case of a single acute dysfunction (L5 in ERS left); second degree, when it involves compensations which themselves become symptomatic, altering the corresponding functions (a group in NSR as compensation to L5 dysfunction); third degree, which includes the above dysfunctions along with the more global effects that could arise (dysfunctional adaptations of the skull, sacrum, and lower limbs).

## Chronic phase

The objectives here are to achieve symptom reduction, restoration of function, the reduction of acute episodes, a better response to drug treatment, and a reduction of co-morbidity and complications. Treatment varies depending on the condition. In the early treatment of chronic conditions one can opt for a frequency of one session per week, gradually reducing to one session per month, or one every 2 months, or in some cases every 3 or 6 months, but always re-evaluating the response to treatment to calibrate the most appropriate frequency.[120] The operator usually provides maintenance strategies to be followed between sessions. Direct techniques and isolytic muscle energy are recommended for treatment of fibrotic areas and to increase fluid movement,[111] while indirect techniques are preferred for acute exacerbations in chronic conditions.[119] An interdisciplinary approach is often necessary to cure or control these phases.

## Terminal phase

The objectives for this phase are the reduction of symptoms and the risk of complications, and improvement of quality of remaining life during the natural course of the patient's condition. The operator also strives to provide comfort for the "total pain" in these patients, meaning directing osteopathic treatment to reduce noxious stimuli, emotional reactions, interpersonal conflicts, and non-acceptance of the condition.[123] Homeostatic potential is severely compromised usually at this stage, associated with high co-morbidity, pharmacological interventions and hospitalization, there may be consequent musculoskeletal disorders, gastrointestinal and cardiorespiratory disorders. If so, then keep the dosage of osteopathic treatment low, possibly using very short treatments several times a day, but monitoring the patient closely over the next 24–48 hours, as this is the time period when any treatment reactions may occur.

The presence of muscle spasms, autonomic reactions (vasomotor, thermal), or increased heart and respiratory rate are indicators of the maximum tolerance of the patient to treatment, which should then be stopped.[124] Indirect techniques, such as counterstrain, diaphragmatic release, inhibition, soft tissue, and Chapman reflexes are usually indicated, avoiding pain as much as possible. Heart or lung impairment may be approached with lymphatic, diaphragmatic, and cervical techniques.[125] The biopsychosocial approach is crucial during the different stages that can characterize this phase: denial, anger, bargaining, depression, and acceptance.[126]

It is clear that, when applied by qualified and competent personnel, principles and osteopathic models can be applied in specific clinical conditions and in all age groups. However, the osteopaths are also required to refer patients for medical, surgical, or other therapeutic consultation and treatment when necessary, or in relevant non-osteopathic cases.[127]

## Contraindications and side effects of osteopathic treatment

The osteopath should be able to recognize when approaches and specific techniques are contraindicated. It is appropriate to note that a contraindication to OMT in one area of the body does not preclude its application to other regions. Similarly, a contraindication for any specific technique does not preclude the use of an alternative approach with the same patient. In the World Health Organization's guidance on safety issues, contraindications to direct and indirect techniques are divided into absolute and relative, both in cases of systemic diseases and when applied locally.[127]

However, the evidence regarding conditions in which certain techniques should be avoided or not is still lacking. In general, contraindications to manipulative treatment are based on the technique employed, and the osteopath is responsible for making the safest and most appropriate choice. Most frequently, understanding of the pathophysiological condition of the patient and the mechanism of action of the osteopathic technique being considered is used to establish the absolute and relative contraindications.[127] According to Greenman's *Principles of Manual Medicine*,[128] there are no contraindications to OMT if the diagnosis is accurate and adequate and the treatment is congruent and appropriate.

The patient should be informed of the potential risks and side effects (as well as benefits) of a particular approach or technique. In addition, the operator should not proceed without proper patient consent to perform a maneuver,[129] especially if the patient clearly expresses refusal of the proposed technique. The operator may encounter a patient who explicitly asks not to have thrust technique during the treatment session. Not infrequently, however, the author has encountered patients traumatized by past experiences with other colleagues or professionals, who, after reassuring the patient that thrust technique would not be used, have performed it anyway. The author believes that such behavior is an assault against the patient, who should be respected. Such an operator should be prosecuted according to current regulations in the country where this happens.

Osteopathic manipulative treatment is generally considered safe and effective as primary in some cases, or as adjuvant treatment in others. However, an adequate risk assessment, including precautions, side effects, complications, and contraindications, is crucial in formulating the treatment plan. Few medical or surgical interventions have a level of safety equal to that of osteopathy, where it is estimated that the incidence of post-treatment adverse events is between 1:400,000 and 1:3,000,000 of cases.[120] Note that the side effects of treatment can vary from minor to serious. The overwhelming majority of side effects are minor, and usually resolve within 24–48 hours. They may include fatigue after a cranial treatment or soreness after fascial work. Other complications, however, are more serious, such as dizziness or vascular accidents after cervical manipulation. Insufficient technical skills and excessive force are often the most frequent cause of these reactions, as are unrecognized or misdiagnosed diseases or abnormalities that may predispose to serious complications.[120]

However, the definition of what constitutes an adverse reaction is not as clear as might be desirable. A recent study has tried to achieve a consensus and define what an adverse event is in manual treatment.[130] Although the classification is not easy without defining the context in which an adverse reaction may occur, the following definitions are proposed:

- *Severe adverse reactions*: medium to long term, moderate to severe in intensity and usually require additional treatments

- *Moderate adverse reactions*: as above, but only of moderate severity

- *Mild adverse reactions:* transient and reversible, short-lived and mild in severity, which do not require alterations in treatment.

The General Osteopathic Council (GOsC), which in the author's judgment has developed an excellent model for osteopathic record keeping, recently commissioned the Clinical Risk Management and Osteopathy (CROaM) Study.[131] This research project investigated the type and incidence of adverse events associated with OMT and the risks related to osteopathic treatment and management. The researchers surveyed 1082 osteopaths enrolled in GOsC and 2,057 patients.

Among the many results obtained, the survey showed that the most commonly used techniques are articulatory and soft tissue techniques. Most osteopaths were unable to predict the risk of adverse reactions, but could predict certain benefits of manipulation. There was no difference in outcome between patients who had, and those who had not, received thrust techniques. The majority still reported an improvement in symptoms, which were reduced by at least 30% in half of the cases after the second day of treatment. The best responses were reported by patients describing their first visit and in patients with a new symptomatic episode. The most frequent reaction was increased pain after OMT for 20% of patients, although the pain was described as acceptable and manageable.

Four percent of patients reported temporary incapacity or disability, perceived to be caused by the treatment. There were no documented cases of life-threatening events, referral to the hospital, or permanent disability. About 12% of osteopaths reported that they had treated patients who had experienced severe adverse reactions after manipulative treatment. The study found that the estimated incidence of serious adverse reactions was 1 in 36,000, showing that they are rare but possible. Finally, the study suggests that similar research is needed to assess the actual effectiveness of OMT, its benefits and mechanisms of action, and to determine the minimum therapeutic effect that is beneficial relative to outcome, cost, and patient risk.

To properly assess clinical risk, osteopaths should be aware of the nature and frequency of mild, moderate, or severe adverse reactions to treatment, as well as the statistical data available on the subject. The risks and benefits should be communicated to the patient in an appropriate and comprehensive manner.[132]

A recent systematic review[133] showed that adverse events after treatment (not only osteopathic, but also chiropractic, medical, and physiotherapeutic) occurred in approximately 40–50% of patients, but incidents of death, vascular accidents, and neurological injuries are very rare. The incidence of cerebrovascular accidents after cervical manipulation range between 1:120,000 and 1:1,666,666 (median 1:1,000,000); that of lumbar disc herniations after manipulation is 1:38,013; and that of cauda equina syndrome between 1:3,700,000 and 1:100,000,000 lumbar manipulations. Most adverse events (an average of 79%) occur within 24 hours after treatment.

Most side effects (on average 67%), such as muscle soreness and headaches, resolve spontaneously within 24 hours. The risk of developing adverse events after manual intervention include being a woman, and the first visit, while those related to serious adverse reactions are unusual pain and stiff neck, high neck manipulation, and consultation with another physician or therapist in the weeks prior to the event (indicating the concern the patient has about his or her condition, rather than being the cause of the problem). More-

over, cervical manipulation should be avoided in the presence of pain and neck stiffness, cardiovascular failure, and in cases of recent trauma and headache. However, the risk of adverse events is very low, less than that related to the use of drugs, inherent in all health interventions, and must always be evaluated against the benefit obtained.

The study concludes that adverse reactions are not always documented and described in the scientific literature and that the majority of the available data comes from the chiropractic literature. Side effects can consist of stiffness or muscle soreness after

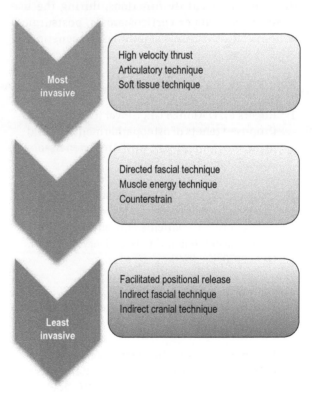

**Fig. 9.12**
From top to bottom, the osteopathic approaches are listed from the most to the least invasive respectively.[136] Based on this, it is possible to select the most appropriate intervention with respect to the clinical presentation and the therapeutic goals.

muscle energy techniques, and more acute pain if the technique has made use of excessive force of contraction; fatigue after cranial techniques; myalgia after myofascial or balanced ligamentous tension techniques; soreness after positional techniques; and bruising after inhibition or compression techniques.[134] However, these effects should resolve within 24–48 hours and can be minimized with the application of ice to the involved area for about 20 minutes after treatment.[135]

Precautions should be taken in cases of pregnancy, discopathy with radicular signs, posttraumatic cervical dysfunctions, during the use of anticoagulants or corticosteroids, postsurgical patients,[134] osteoporosis, joint laxity, genetic diseases such as Down syndrome (especially for cervical manipulation), primary or secondary bone tumors, rheumatoid arthritis and vertebral artery insufficiency,[128] hemophilia, congenital abnormalities, cerebral or spinal trauma, and connective tissue disorders.[135]

We recommend avoiding techniques that cause worsening of symptoms, and reduced dosage, method, and duration of treatment in cases where adverse reactions persist for more than 24–48 hours. Usually the sicker the patient, the lower should be the dose of treatment, especially with infants and healthy elderly patients. The choice of technique is also influenced by its level of invasiveness, and should be carefully and judiciously applied to the individual case[136] (Fig. 9.12).

## References

1. Rogers FJ, D'Alonzo GE, Glover JC et al. Proposed tenets of osteopathic medicine and principles for patient care. J Am Osteo Assoc. 2002;102(2):63–5.

2. Osteopathic International Alliance (OIA). Osteopathy and osteopathic medicine – a global view of practice patients education and the contribution to healthcare delivery. Chicago: OIA; 2013. pp. 9–10.

3. World Health Organization (WHO). Benchmarks for training in osteopathy. Geneva: WHO; 2010. pp. 3–5.

4. Forum for Osteopathic Regulation in Europe (FORE). European framework for standards of osteopathic practice. London: FORE; 2007. pp. 13–14.

5. Kimberly PE. Formulating a prescription for osteopathic manipulative treatment. J Am Osteopath Assoc. 1980;79(8):506–13.

6. Peckham RR. Method of determining the most applicable technic. J Am Osteopath Assoc. 1933;32:431–4.

7. Beal MC. Teaching of basic principles of osteopathic manipulative techniques. J Am Osteopath Assoc. 1982;81(9):607–9.

8. Allen PVB, Stinson JA. The subjective factors of skillful technic. J Am Osteopath Assoc. 1941;40:297–301 (pt 1); 40:348–56 (pt 2).

9. DeStefano LA. Greenman's principles of manual medicine. 4th ed. Baltimore, MD: Williams and Wilkins; 2011. ch. 4.

10. DiGiovanna EL. The manipulative prescription. In: DiGiovanna EL, Schiowitz S, Dowling DJ, editors. An osteopathic approach to diagnosis and treatment. 3rd ed. Philadelphia, PA: Lippincott Williams and Wilkins; 2005. ch. 118.

11. Hruby RJ. Pathophysiologic models and the selection of osteopathic manipulative techniques. J Osteopath Med. 1992;6(4): 25–30.

12. Kuchera M, Kuchera W. Osteopathic consideration in systemic dysfunction. Columbus, OH: Greyden Press; 1994.

13. Nelson KE, Glonek T. Somatic dysfunction in osteopathic family medicine. Philadelphia, PA: Lippincott Williams and Wilkins; 2006. ch. 8–13.

14. Chila A, editor. Foundations of osteopathic medicine. 3rd ed. Philadelphia, PA: Lippincott Williams and Wilkins; 2005. chs 53–69.

15. Kuchera ML, Kuchera WA. Osteopathic principles in practice. Greyden Press Columbus, OH: 1994. pp. 281–96.

16. Trede F, Higgs J. Clinical reasoning and models of practice. In: Higgs J, Jones MA, Loftus S et al., editors. Clinical reasoning in the health professions. 3rd ed. Oxford: Elsevier Butterworth-Heinemann; 2008. pp. 31–41.

17. Fish D, Coles C. Developing professional judgment in health care: learning through the critical appreciation of practice. Oxford: Butterworth-Heinemann; 1998.

18. Thornquist E. Face-to-face and hands-on: assumptions and assessments in the physiotherapy clinic. Med Anthropol. 2006;25(1):65–97.

19. Thomson OP, Petty NJ, Moore AP. Clinical decision-making and therapeutic approaches in osteopathy – a qualitative grounded theory study. Man Ther. 2014;19(1):44–51.

20. Schön DA. Educating the reflective practitioner. San Francisco, CA: Jossey-Bass; 1987.

21. Öhman A, Hägg K. Attitudes of novice physiotherapists to their professional role:a gender perspective. Physiother Theory Pract. 1998;14(1):23–32.

22. Beisecker AE, Beisecker TD. Using metaphors to characterize doctor-patient relationships: paternalism versus consumerism. Health Communication. 1993;5(1):41–58.

23. World Health Organization (WHO). Health promotion glossary. Geneva: WHO; 1998. p. 1.

24. Korr IM. An explication of osteopathic principles. In: Ward RC, editor. Foundations for osteopathic medicine. Baltimore, MD: Williams and Wilkins; 1997. pp. 7–12.

25. Parsons J, Marcer N. Osteopathy: models for diagnosis, treatment and practice. Edinburgh: Elsevier Churchill Livingstone; 2006. ch. 10.

26. Dummer TG. Specific adjusting technique. Hove: JoTom Publications; 1995.

27. Chauffour P, Prat E. Mechanical link: fundamental principles, theory and practice following an osteopathic approach. Berkeley, CA: North Atlantic Books; 2002.

28. Forum for Osteopathic Regulation in Europe (FORE). European framework for standards of osteopathic practice. London: FORE; 2007. pp. 9–15.

29. World Health Organization (WHO). Benchmarks for training in osteopathy. Geneva: WHO; 2010. p. 12.

30. Kuchera ML, Kuchera WA. Osteopathic principles in practice. Columbus, OH: Greyden Press; 1994. p. 297.

31. Pergolizzi J, Ahlbeck K, Aldington D et al. The development of chronic pain: physiological CHANGE necessitates a multidisciplinary approach to treatment. Curr Med Res Opin. 2013;29(9):1127–35.

32. Flor H, Hermann C. Biopsychosocial models of pain. In: Dworkin RH, Breitbart WS, editors. Psychosocial aspects of pain: a handbook for health care providers: progress in pain research and management. Seattle: IASP Press; 2004. pp. 47–76.

33. Penney JN. The biopsychosocial model of pain and contemporary osteopathic practice. Int J Osteopath Med. 2010;13(2):42–7.

34. Gatchel RJ. Clinical essentials of pain management. Washington DC: American

Psychological Association; 2005.

35. Mackintosh SE, Adams CE, Singer-Chang G et al. An osteopathic approach to implementing and promoting inter-professional education. J Am Osteopath Assoc. 2011;111(4):206–12.

36. Antonovsky A. Health stress and coping. San Francisco: Jossey-Bass; 1979.

37. Eriksson M, Lindström B. A salutogenic interpretation of the Ottawa Charter. Health Promot Int. 2008;23(2):190–9.

38. Fawkes C, Carnes D. What is the relevance of colored flags to osteopathic practice? The Osteopath Magazine. 2012;15(5):20–2. London: General Osteopathic Council (GOsC).

39. Stephenson C. The complementary therapist's guide to red flags and referrals. Edinburgh: Elsevier Churchill Livingstone; 2011.

40. Main CJ, Sullivan MJL, Watson PJ. Pain management:practical applications of the biopsychosocial perspective in clinical and occupational settings. Edinburgh: Elsevier Churchill Livingstone; 2008. ch. 3.

41. Kendall NA. Psychosocial approaches to the prevention of chronic pain: the low back paradigm. Baillieres Best Pract Res Clin Rheumatol. 1999;13(3):545–54.

42. Main CJ, Sullivan MJL, Watson PJ. Pain management: practical applications of the biopsychosocial perspective in clinical and occupational settings. Edinburgh: Elsevier Churchill Livingstone; 2008. ch. 2.

43. Turner JA, Franklin G, Fulton-Kehoe D et al. Worker recovery expectations and fear-avoidance predict work disability in a population-based workers' compensation back pain sample. Spine. 2006;31(6):682–9.

44. Ford J. Rehabilitation for work matters. Oxon UK: Radcliffe Publishing; 2008. ch. 3.

45. Gifford L. Now for pink flags. Physiother Pain Assoc J. 2005;20:1.

46. Stewart J, Kempenaar L, Lauchlan D. Rethinking yellow flags. Man Ther. 2011;16(2):196–8.

47. Kuchera ML, Kuchera WA. Osteopathic principles in practice. Columbus, OH: Greyden Press; 1994. p. 296.

48. Pincus T, Burton AK, Vogel S et al. A systematic review of psychological factors as predictors of chronicity/disability in prospective cohorts in low back pain. Spine. 2002;27(5):E109–20.

49. Gamsa A. The role of psychological factors in chronic pain II. A critical appraisal. Pain. 1994;57(1):17–29.

50. Waddell G, Newton M, Henderson I et al. A fear-avoidance beliefs questionnaire (FABQ) and the role of fear-avoidance beliefs in chronic low back pain and disability. Pain. 1993;52(2):157–68.

51. Asmundson GJ, Norton PJ, Norton GR. Beyond pain the role of fear and avoidance in chronicity. Clinical Psych Rev. 1999;19(1):97–119.

52. McCracken LM, Sorg PJ, Edmands TA et al. Prediction of pain in persistent pain sufferers with CLBP: effects of inaccurate predictions and pain related anxiety. Behav Res Ther. 1993;31(7):647–52.

53. Vlaeyen JW, Kole-Snijders AM, Boeren RG. Fear of movement/(re)injury in chronic low back pain and its relation to behavioral performance. Pain. 1995;62(3):363–72.

54. Kaila-Kangas L, Kivirnaki M, Riihimaki H. Psycho-social factors at work as predictors of

hospitalisation for back disorders: a 28-year follow-up of industrial employees. Spine. 2004;29(16):1823–30.

55. Flor H, Turk DC. Psychophysiology of chronic pain: do chronic pain patients exhibit symptom-specific psycho-physiological responses? Psychol Bull. 1989;105(2):215–59.

56. Turner JA, Jensen MP, Romano JM. Do beliefs coping catastrophizing independently predict functioning in patients with chronic pain? Pain. 2000;85(1–2):115–25.

57. Radnitz CL, Bockian N, Moran A. Assessment of psychopathology and personality in people with physical disabilities. In: Frank RG, Elliot TR, editors. Handbook of rehabilitation psychology. Washington: American Psychological Association; 2000. pp. 287–309.

58. Koenig HG. Is religion good for your health? Binghampton, NY: Haworth Pastoral Press; 1997.

59. Weisenberg J. Cognitive aspects of pain. In: Wall PD, Melzack R, editors. Textbook of pain 2. Edinburgh: Churchill Livingston; 1989. pp. 231–41.

60. Nicholas MK, Linton SJ, Watson PJ et al. Early identification and management of psychological risk factors ("yellow flags") in patients with low back pain: a reappraisal. Phys Ther. 2011;91(5):737–53.

61. Bandura A. Self-efficacy mechanism in human agency. Am Psychol. 1982;37:122–47.

62. Ramsay Wan C, Vo L, Barnes CS. Conceptualizations of patient empowerment among individuals seeking treatment for diabetes mellitus in an urban public-sector clinic. Patient Educ Couns. 2012;87(3):402–4.

63. Keefe FJ, Rumble ME, Scipio CD. Psychological aspects of persistent pain: current state of the science. J Pain. 2004;5(4):195–211.

64. Gafni A, Charles C, Whelan T. The physician-patient encounter: the physician as a perfect agent for the patient versus the informed treatment decision-making model. Soc Sci Med. 1998;47(3):347–54.

65. Skinner BF. Science and human behaviour. New York: MacMillan; 1953.

66. Grubmbach K, Bodenheimer T. Can health care teams improve primary care practice? JAMA. 2004;291(10):1246–51.

67. Kim MM, Barnato AE, Angus DC et al. The effect of multidisciplinary care teams on intensive care unit mortality. Arch Intern Med. 2010;170(4):369–76.

68. Golden BA. A multidisciplinary approach to non-pharmacologic pain management. J Am Osteopath Assoc. 2002;102(Suppl 3):S1–5.

69. Shannon SC. Osteopathic medical education in 2011: adapting to changes in the healthcare system. J Am Osteopath Assoc. 2011; 111(4):203–4.

70. Mészáros K, Lopes IC, Goldsmith PC. Interprofessional education:cooperation among osteopathic medicine pharmacy and physician assistant students to recognize medical errors. J Am Osteopath Assoc. 2011;111(4):213–8.

71. Frenk J, Chen L, Bhutta ZA et al. Health professionals for a new century: transforming education to strengthen health systems in an interdependent world. Lancet. 2010;376(9756):1923–58.

72. World Health Organization (WHO). Department of Human Resources for Health. Framework for action on interprofessional education and collaborative practice. Geneva: WHO; 2010.

73. Tettambel M. Obstetrics. In: Ward RC editor. Foundations of osteopathic medicine. 2nd ed.

Philadelphia: Lippincott Williams and Wilkins; 2002. pp. 450–61.

74. Nelson KE. The managment of low back pain. Am Acad Osteopath J. 1999;9(1):33–9.

75. Hensel KL, Pacchia CF, Smith ML. Acute improvement in hemodynamic control after osteopathic manipulative treatment in the third trimester of pregnancy. Complement Ther Med. 2013;21(6):618–26.

76. Lavelle JM. Osteopathic manipulative treatment in pregnant women. J Am Osteopath Assoc. 2012;112(6):343–6.

77. King HH, Tettambel MA, Lockwood MD et al. Osteopathic manipulative treatment in prenatal care: a retrospective case control design study. J Am Osteopath Assoc. 2003;103(12):577–82.

78. Nelson KE, Glonek T. Somatic dysfunction in osteopathic family medicine. Philadelphia, PA: Lippincott Williams and Wilkins; 2006. ch. 9.

79. Sergueef N, Nelson KE, Glonek T. Palpatory diagnosis of plagiocephaly. Complement Ther Clin Pract. 2006;12(2):101–10.

80. Nelson KE, Glonek T. Somatic dysfunction in osteopathic family medicine. Philadelphia, PA: Lippincott Williams and Wilkins; 2006. pp. 90–1.

81. Mills MV, Henley CE, Barnes LL et al. The use of osteopathic manipulative treatment as adjuvant therapy in children with recurrent acute otitis media. Arch Pediatr Adolesc Med. 2003;157(9):861–6.

82. PhiLippi H, Faldum A, Schleupen A et al. Infantile postural asymmetry and osteopathic treatment: a randomized therapeutic trial. Dev Med Child Neurol. 2006;48(1):5–9; discussion 4.

83. Pizzolorusso G, Turi P, Barlafante G et al. Effect of osteopathic manipulative treatment on gastrointestinal function and length of stay of preterm infants: an exploratory study. Chiropr Man Ther. 2011;28;19(1):15.

84. Knebl JA, Shores JH, Gamber RG et al. Improving functional ability in the elderly via the Spencer technique, an osteopathic manipulative treatment: a randomized controlled trial. J Am Osteopath Assoc. 2002;102(7):387–96.

85. Lopez D, King HH, Knebl JA et al. Effects of comprehensive osteopathic manipulative treatment on balance in elderly patients: a pilot study. J Am Osteopath Assoc. 111(6): 382–8.

86. Papa L, Mandara A, Bottali M et al. A randomized control trial on the effectiveness of osteopathic manipulative treatment in reducing pain and improving the quality of life in elderly patients affected by osteoporosis. Clin Cases Miner Bone Metab. 2012;9(3):179–83.

87. Hodge LM. Osteopathic lymphatic pump techniques to enhance immunity and treat pneumonia. Int J Osteopath Med. 2012;15(1): 13–21.

88. Noll DR, Degenhardt BF, Morley TF et al. Efficacy of osteopathic manipulation as an adjunctive treatment for hospitalized patients with pneumonia: a randomized controlled trial. Osteopath Med Prim Care. 2010;19;4:2.

89. Kuchera ML, Kuchera WA. Osteopathic principles in practice. Columbus, OH: Greyden Press; 1994. p. 289.

90. Nelson KE, Glonek T. Somatic dysfunction in osteopathic family medicine. Philadelphia, PA: Lippincott Williams and Wilkins; 2006. p. 164.

91. Hardman AE, Stensel DJ. Physical activity and health: the evidence explained. London: Taylor and Francis; 2009.

92. Larson NJ. Manipulative care before and after surgery. Osteopath Med. 1977;2(1):41–9.

93. Henshaw RE. Manipulation and postoperative pulmonary complications. The DO. 1963;4(1):132–3.

94. YurvatiAH, Carnes MS, Clearfield MB et al. Hemodynamic effects of osteopathic manipulative treatment immediately after coronary artery bypass graft surgery. J Am Osteopath Assoc. 2005;105(10):475–81.

95. Sleszynski SL, Kelso AF. Comparison of thoracic manipulation with incentive spirometry in preventing postoperative atelectasis. J Am Osteopath Assoc. 1993;93(8):834–8, 843–5.

96. Goldstein FJ, Jeck S, Nicholas AS et al. Preoperative intravenous morphine sulfate with postoperative osteopathic manipulative treatment reduces patient analgesic use after total abdominal hysterectomy. J Am Osteopath Assoc. 2005;105(6):273–9.

97. Radjieski JM, Lumley MA, Cantieri MS. Effect of osteopathic manipulative treatment of length of stay for pancreatitis: a randomized pilot study. J Am Osteopath Assoc. 1998;98(5):264–72.

98. Crow WT, Gorodinsky L. Does osteopathic manipulative treatment (OMT) improves outcomes in patients who develop postoperative ileus: a retrospective chart review. Int J Osteopath Med. 2009;12(1):32–7.

99. Stiles EG. Osteopathic treatment of surgical patients. Osteopath Med. 1976;1(3):21–3.

100. Nelson KE, Glonek T. Somatic dysfunction in osteopathic family medicine. Philadelphia, PA: Lippincott Williams and Wilkins; 2006. p. 131.

101. Nelson KE, Glonek T. Somatic dysfunction in osteopathic family medicine. Philadelphia, PA: Lippincott Williams and Wilkins; 2006. p. 129.

102. Korr M. Clinical significance of the facilitated state. J Am Osteopath Assoc. 1955;54(5):277–82.

103. Dunn FE. Osteopathic concepts in psychiatry. J Am Osteopath Assoc. 1950;49:354–57.

104. Plotkin BJ, Rodos JJ, Kappler R et al. Adjunctive osteopathic manipulative treatment in women with depression: a pilot study. J Am Osteopath Assoc. 2001;101(9):517–23.

105. Osborn GG. Manual medicine and its role in psychiatry. Am Acad Osteopath J. 1994;4(1): 16–21.

106. Hildreth AG, Still FM. Schizophrenia. J Am Osteopath Assoc. 1939,38:422–26. Reprint: Hildreth AG, Still FM. J Am Osteopath Assoc. 2000 ;100(8):506–10.

107. Bradford SG. Osteopathic considerations in psychiatric disorders of the elderly. Osteopath Ann. 1974;2:26–7, 29–31.

108. Dunn FE. The osteopathic management of psychosomatic problems. J Am Osteopath Ass. 1948;48:196–99.

109. Nelson KE, Glonek T. Somatic dysfunction in osteopathic family medicine. Philadelphia, PA: Lippincott Williams and Wilkins; 2006. pp. 83–4.

110. Brolinson GP, McGinley SMG, Kerger S. Osteopathic manipulative medicine and the athlete. Curr Sports Med Rep. 2008;7(1):49–56.

111. Kuchera ML, Kuchera WA. Osteopathic principles in practice. Columbus, OH: Greyden Press; 1994. pp. 290–2.

112. Brumm LF, Janiski C, Balawender JL et al. Preventive osteopathic manipulative treatment and stress fracture incidence among collegiate cross-country athletes. J Am Osteopath Assoc. 2013;113(12):882–90.

113. Brolinson PG, Heinkirrg KP, Kozar AJ. An osteopathic approach to sports medicine. In: Ward RC, editor. Foundations of osteopathic medicine. 2nd ed. Philadelphia: Lippincott Williams and Wilkins; 2002. pp. 534–50.

114. Maffetone P. Complementary sports medicine. Human Kinetics; 1999.

115. Larequi Y. Physiotherapy and osteopathy: a real holistic supervision of athletes. Rev Med Suisse. 2010;6(258):1504–7.

116. Fishbein M, Middlestadt SE, Ottati V. Medical problems among ICSOM musicians: overview of a national survey. Med Probl Perform Art. 1998;3(3):1–8.

117. Shoup D. Survey of performance related problems among high school and junior high school musicians. Med Probl Perform Art. 1995;10(3):100–5.

118. Shoup D. An osteopathic approach to performing arts medicine. Phys Med Rehabil Clin N Am. 2006;17(4):853–64 viii.

119. DeStefano LA. Greenman's principles of manual medicine. 4th ed. Baltimore, MD: Williams and Wilkins; 2011. p. 52.

120. DiGiovanna EL. The manipulative prescription. In: DiGiovanna EL, Schiowitz S, Dowling DJ, editors. An osteopathic approach to diagnosis and treatment. 3rd ed. Philadelphia, PA: Lippincott Williams and Wilkins; 2005. p. 671.

121. Nelson KE, Glonek T. Somatic dysfunction in osteopathic family medicine. Philadelphia, PA: Lippincott Williams and Wilkins; 2006. p. 31.

122. Kuchera ML, Kuchera WA. Osteopathic principles in practice. Columbus, OH: Greyden Press; 1994. pp. 298–300.

123. Leleszi JP, Lewandowski JG. Pain management in end-of-life care. J Am Osteopath Assoc. 2005;105(3 Suppl 1):S6–11.

124 Sergueef N, Nelson K. Osteopathy for the over 50s. Maintaining function and treating dysfunction. East Lothian, UK: Handspring Publishing; 2014. p. 83.

125. Stretanski MF, Kaiser G. Osteopathic philosophy and emergent treatment in acute respiratory failure. J Am Osteopath Assoc. 2001;101(8):447–9.

126. Kubler-Ross EO. On death and dying. New York: Scribner; 1969. p. 7.

127. World Health Organization (WHO). Safety issues. In: Benchmarks for training in osteopathy. Geneva: WHO; 2010. pp. 15–7.

128. DeStefano LA. Greenman's principles of manual medicine. 4th ed. Baltimore, MD: Williams and Wilkins; 2011. p. 53.

129. Forum for Osteopathic Regulation in Europe (FORE). European framework for codes of osteopathic practice. London: FORE; 2007. pp. 9–10.

130. Carnes D, Mullinger B, Underwood M. Defining adverse events in manual therapies: a modified Delphi consensus study. Man Ther. 2010;15(1):2–6.

131. Vogel S, Mars T, Keeping S et al. Clinical risk osteopathy and management (CROaM). Scientific report. London: National Council for Osteopathic Research (NCOR); 2013. wwwncororguk/wp-content/uploads/2013/05/croam_full_re-port_0313pdf.

132. Leach J, Mandy A, Hankins M et al. Communicating risks of treatment and informed consent in osteopathic practice. A literature review and pilot focus groups.

London: National Council for Osteopathic Research (NCOR); 2011. www ncororguk/wp-content/uploads/2012/10/communicating-riskpdf.

133. Carnes D, Mars T, Mullinger B et al. Adverse events in manual therapy: a systematic review. London: National Council for Osteopathic Research (NCOR); 2009. wwwncororg uk/wp-content/uploads/2012/10/adverse-events_in_manual_ therapy_a_systematic_review_full_reportpdf.

134. DiGiovanna EL. The manipulative prescription. In: DiGiovanna EL, Schiowitz S, Dowling DJ, editors. An osteopathic approach to diagnosis and treatment. 3rd ed. Philadelphia, PA: Lippincott Williams and Wilkins; 2005. pp. 672–3.

135. Seffinger MA, Hruby RJ. Evidence-based manual medicine: a problem-oriented approach. Philadelphia, PA: Saunders Elsevier; 2007. p. 61.

136. Nelson KE, Glonek T. Somatic dysfunction in osteopathic family medicine. Philadelphia, PA: Lippincott Williams and Wilkins; 2006. p. 29.

Note: Page number followed by f and t indicates figure and table respectively.